Palliative care nursing

Palliative care nursing

Principles and evidence for practice

Edited by Sheila Payne, Jane Seymour and Christine Ingleton

Open University Press

Open University Press
McGraw-Hill Education
McGraw-Hill House
Shoppenhangers Road
Maidenhead
Berkshire
England
SL6 2QL

email: enquiries@openup.co.uk
world wide web: www.openup.co.uk

and Two Penn Plaza, New York, NY 10121–2289, USA

First published 2004

A catalogue record of this book is available from the British Library

ISBN 0 335 21243 3 (pb)   0 335 21492 4 (hb)

Library of Congress Cataloging-in-Publication Data
CIP data has been applied for

Typeset by RefineCatch Limited, Bungay, Suffolk
Printed in the UK by Bell & Bain Ltd, Glasgow

Contents

Contributors

Julia Addington-Hall, Professor, Department of Palliative Care and Policy, King's College London, London, UK

Hilde Ahmedzai, Research Associate, Trent Palliative Care Centre, The University of Sheffield, Sheffield, UK

Sam H. Ahmedzai, Professor of Palliative Medicine, Academic Palliative Medicine Unit, The University of Sheffield, Sheffield, UK

Sanchia Aranda, Professor, Director of Cancer, Peter MacCallum Cancer Institute, Melbourne, Victoria, Australia

Liz Barker, Director of Quality by Peer Review in Specialist Palliative Care, York, UK

Jon Birtwistle, Clinical Trials Monitor, Radcliffe Infirmary, Oxford, UK

Katie Booth, Macmillan Practice Development Unit, The University of Manchester, Manchester, UK

Bert Broeckaert, Professor, Centre for Religious Studies, University of Leuven, Leuven, Belgium

Margaret Camps, Clinical Nurse Specialist, Campden and Islington Community NHS Trust, London, UK

David Clark, Professor of Medical Sociology, Lancaster University, Lancaster, UK

Reverend Mark Cobb, Professional Services Directorate, Sheffield Teaching Hospitals NHS Trust, Sheffield, UK

Jessica Corner, Professor, Chair in Cancer and Palliative Care, University of Southampton, Southampton, UK

Karen Cox, Professor in Cancer and Palliative Care, University of Nottingham, Nottingham, UK

Sue Davies, Senior Lecturer, School of Nursing and Midwifery, The University of Sheffield, Sheffield, UK

Deborah Fitzsimmons, Research Fellow/Lecturer, School of Nursing and Midwifery, University of Southampton, Southampton, UK

Katherine Froggatt, Senior Lecturer, School of Nursing and Midwifery, The University of Sheffield, Sheffield, UK

Merryn Gott, Lecturer, Sheffield Institute for Studies on Ageing, The University of Sheffield, Sheffield, UK

Elizabeth Hanson, Research Fellow, University College of Borås, Borås, Sweden

Sue Hawkett, Nursing Advisor, Department of Health, London, UK

Matthew Hopkins, Assistant General Manager, Diagnostic and Therapeutic Services Directorate, Guy's and St Thomas' Hospital Trust, London, UK

Christine Ingleton, Senior Lecturer, School of Nursing and Midwifery, The University of Sheffield, Sheffield, UK

Veronica James, Professor, School of Nursing, University of Nottingham, Nottingham, UK

Nikki Jarrett, Lecturer, School of Nursing and Midwifery, University of Southampton, Southampton, UK

Gail Johnston, Department of General Practice, Queen's University of Belfast, Belfast, Northern Ireland

Jeanne Samson Katz, Senior Lecturer, School of Health and Social Welfare, The Open University, Milton Keynes, UK

David Kissane, Professor, Sloan Kettering Institute, New York, USA

Jonathan Koffman, Lecturer in Palliative Care, King's College London, London, UK

Carol Komaromy, Lecturer in Health Studies, The Open University, Milton Keynes, UK

Mari Lloyd-Williams, Director of Community Studies/Professor and Consultant in Palliative Medicine, University of Liverpool, Liverpool, UK

Sian Maslin-Prothero, Senior Lecturer, School of Nursing and Midwifery, University of Southampton, Southampton, UK

Kay Mitchell, Department of Psychology, University of Auckland, Auckland, New Zealand

Margaret O'Connor, Chair in Palliative Care Nursing, Monash University, Melbourne, Australia

Sheila Payne, Professor, Chair in Palliative Care, The University of Sheffield, Sheffield, UK

Silvia Paz, Specialist Registrar, Trent Palliative Care Centre, The University of Sheffield, Sheffield, UK

Marilyn Relf, Head of Education, Sir Michael Sobell House, Oxford, UK

Liz Rolls, School of Health and Social Care, University of Gloucestershire, Gloucester, UK

Jane Seymour, Senior Lecturer, School of Nursing and Midwifery, The University of Sheffield, Sheffield, UK

Paula Smith, Lecturer, School of Nursing and Midwifery, University of Southampton, Southampton, UK

Margaret Sneddon, Macmillan Lecturer in Palliative Care, School of Nursing and Midwifery, University of Glasgow, Glasgow, UK

Magi Sque, Senior Lecturer, School of Nursing and Midwifery, University of Southampton, Southampton, UK

Vanessa Taylor, Lecturer in Nursing, School of Nursing, University of Bradford, Bradford, UK

Joanne Wells, Research Fellow, European Institute of Health and Medical Sciences, University of Surrey, Guildford, UK

Reverend Dr Michael Wright, Research Fellow, Lancaster University, Lancaster, UK

Acknowledgements

The Editors would like to thank Jacinta Evans for proposing the book and encouraging us to write it. We appreciate the help of Rachel Gear and the rest of the production team at McGraw-Hill. We would also like to thank the reviewers for their helpful comments.

Introduction

Sheila Payne, Jane Seymour and Christine Ingleton

Fifty-six million people die in the world each year (World Health Organization 2002). Some infants may die after just a few hours or days of life, while other people die many decades after birth in late old age (Nuland 1994). Death may come in many different ways, such as after an acute illness, as a result of a sudden violent road accident, on the battlefield, following a chronic illness or after a prolonged decline in physical fitness in late old age. While all of us will die, most of us cannot determine the manner of our dying. According to the World Health Organization (2002), approximately 40 per cent of deaths worldwide are related to 11 risks: being underweight (especially for women and children), unsafe sexual behaviour, hypertension, tobacco use, alcohol consumption, unsafe water, lack of sanitation, high cholesterol, indoor smoke from cooking and heating fires, iron deficiency anaemia and obesity. There are stark contrasts between causes of death in different parts of the world, and in overall life expectancy and in healthy life expectancy. In the developed world, death is no longer common in infants and young people, but it is most frequently associated with chronic illness and occurs in later life. It has been estimated that approximately 60 per cent of all deaths worldwide could be amenable to palliative care interventions. However, health care agendas, the organization and funding of health care services, and resources for health and social care are remarkably variable throughout the world (Sepulveda *et al.* 2002). So the majority of dying people do not benefit from supportive and palliative care or even have sufficient access to medication to relieve suffering.

This book is about the care of people facing death, both those who will die and those who accompany them – families, friends, community supporters, volunteer workers, health and social care workers. In particular, the book focuses on the role of nurses in providing care during the trajectory of advanced illness, through the process of dying and in the respectful care of the dead person. Nurses generally work closely with family members, supporting them through the process of illness and bereavement. We have focused attention on those who die as adults rather than those who die as babies and young children. Paediatric palliative nursing care is an important topic but requires the attention of a different book. However, dying adults are often in relationships with children as parents, grandparents or guardians, so to ensure the needs of children are not overlooked a chapter about services for bereaved children has been included.

The palliation of distressing symptoms, the care of patients approaching death, the laying out of the body and the care of newly bereaved relatives have long formed an important part of nursing work. In the latter part of the twentieth century, the emergence of the modern hospice movement has provided an impetus to reconceptualizing the delivery of some aspects of this care (Clark and Seymour 1999). Nursing has been central to a new style of end-of-life care, both in specialist contexts such as in hospices, hospital teams and community teams, and more broadly in delivering care to terminally ill people in a range of settings. Specialist education for nurses in 'care of the dying' has been available in post-qualifying courses in the UK since the 1980s. Nursing roles have been extended to develop specialist expertise and practice, such as Macmillan nurses, clinical nurse specialists and nurse consultants. Current debates in health care recognize a number of tensions that are likely to impact upon specialist palliative care services. They include: concerns about the medicalization of dying; issues around lack of access for certain groups, such as those with non-cancer diagnoses, minority ethnic groups, older people, poor people, socially excluded groups; and problems with funding sources. The relationship of specialist palliative care services and central health care planning and policy remains controversial in some countries because hospices have arisen independently of central control (Clark and Wright 2003). This means these services do not form part of the main health care agenda and therefore do not secure necessary resources. However, they have offered opportunities for innovation in care and pioneering new ways of working.

What is palliative care?

The use and evaluation of specialist palliative care services is based on an assumption that people share a common understanding of the terminology and purpose of palliative care. But most of the evidence indicates that definitions and terminology are poorly understood and not agreed (Praill 2000; Payne *et al.* 2002). Terminology is influenced by the historical development and the nature of end-of-life health care services in different countries and changes over time (see Box 1). In the UK, terminology relating to end-of-life care has undergone several transitions from hospice care and terminal care in the early period of the hospice movement (1960s and 1970s) to palliative care towards the turn of the last century (1980–2000). Clark and Seymour (1999) provide an account of these transitions in terminology in relation to

---

Box 1   Terms associated with caring for dying people

- Hospice care
- Terminal care
- Continuing care
- Care of the dying
- Palliative care
- End-of-life care
- Supportive care

the UK context. They have noted how terminology has changed as tensions in the boundaries between generalist and specialist skills, activities and services have become more contentious.

Recently, supportive care has emerged as an accepted term within the context of services that are provided in addition to curative treatments for cancer patients (Department of Health 2000). Although the term end-of-life care was first applied to care of dying patients in Canada, this term is now widely used in North America.

There are several reasons for the increasing number of terms used to describe health and social care services provided for those near the end of life. While the early hospice movement in the UK was unambiguously concerned with terminal care, predominantly for those with cancer, subsequent developments have sought to extend the range of services in terms of both client groups (non-cancer) and types and timing of interventions during the illness trajectory. Current policies in the UK have sought to introduce palliative or supportive care much earlier in the illness trajectory (Department of Health 2000; National Institute for Clinical Excellence 2003). Most discussion of supportive care and the definition offered by the National Council for Hospices and Specialist Palliative Care Services (NCHSPCS 2002) are located in the context of cancer care, but there is no good reason why supportive care could not be applicable to those with other chronic illnesses (Addington-Hall and Higginson 2001; NCHSPCS 2003). Praill (2000) has argued that the transition in terminology from 'terminal care' to 'palliative care' reflects a 'death-denying' tendency. These changes in terminology have paralleled the growth in medical involvement in end-of-life care services more generally. Writing from an Australian perspective, McNamara (2001) has observed how the medical component has gradually come to frame and dominate definitions of palliative care. It is therefore hardly surprising that most major medical and nursing textbooks in palliative care prioritize symptom control as a key function (e.g. Doyle *et al.* 1998; Ferrell and Coyle 2001).

In an attempt to establish greater clarity, predominantly directed at an audience within specialist palliative care, the National Council for Hospices and Specialist Palliative Care Services (2002) published a briefing paper that offers a series of definitions of common terms. Many other organizations and countries have sought to establish working definitions and standards to guide service provision, for example in Australia and New Zealand. There has yet to be a consensus view. For the purposes of this book, we will draw upon the working definitions proposed by the National Council for Hospices and Specialist Palliative Care Services (2002) and the World Health Organization's recently revised definitions (Sepulveda *et al.* 2002). However, we do not agree with the abrupt demarcation between supportive/palliative care and bereavement depicted in the National Council for Hospices and Specialist Palliative Care Services (2002) model; instead, we regard it as a transition, in that preparation for bereavement care for families may start before the death of the patient, as will be explained in greater detail in Part Three of this book.

Sepulreda *et al.* define palliative care as follows:

Palliative care is an approach that improves the quality of life of patients and their families facing the problems associated with life-threatening illness, through the prevention and relief of suffering by means of early identification and impeccable assessment and treatment of pain and other problems, physical, psychosocial and spiritual.

(Sepulveda *et al.* 2002: 94)

Palliative care:

- provides relief from pain and other distressing symptoms;
- affirms life and regards dying as a normal process;
- intends neither to hasten nor postpone death;
- integrates the psychological and spiritual aspects of patient care;
- offers a support system to help patients live as actively as possible until death;
- offers a support system to help the family cope during the patient's illness and in their own bereavement;
- uses a team approach to address the needs of patients and their families, including bereavement counselling, if indicated;
- will enhance quality of life and may also have a positive influence on the course of illness;
- is applicable early in the course of illness, in conjunction with other therapies that are intended to prolong life, such as chemotherapy or radiation therapy, and include those investigations needed to better understand and manage distressing clinical complications.

The National Council for Hospices and Specialist Palliative Care Services (2002: 2) differentiate between *general palliative care*, which 'is provided by the usual professional carers of the patient and family with low to moderate complexity of palliative care need', and *specialist palliative care services*, which 'are provided for patients and their families with moderate to high complexity of palliative care need. They are defined in terms of their core service components, their functions and the composition of the multi-professional teams that are required to deliver them.'

In the following sections, several key debates and questions in contemporary palliative care will be highlighted. Many of these topics will be discussed in greater depth in the ensuing chapters.

Is palliative care about dying or symptom control?

The twentieth century was remarkable in the successful development of a large range of new health technologies (e.g. blood transfusion, radiotherapy), pharmaceutical agents (e.g. antibiotics, insulin, antiretroviral agents) and preventive health care procedures (e.g. immunization). Combined with improved nutrition, better housing, sanitation and clean water, many of the citizens of the developed world have opportunities for healthy living, unrivalled in history. The profession of medicine was seen to contribute to these developments and a culture of 'cure' was seen to marginalize the dying. However, the rise in medical power did not go unchallenged (Illich 1976) and from the 1950s there was a growing interest in improving the welfare of dying people (Clark's chapter provides a fuller account of the history of hospice development).

Contemporary debates focus on whether palliative care services should concentrate attention on terminal care or extend its remit to those at earlier stages of the illness. Arguably, the success of the early 'hospice' period was because it had a clear goal in improving the quality of dying, especially for those dying of cancer. The advantage of this approach is that it makes good use of limited resources and practitioners develop specific skills in controlling difficult symptoms associated with the dying phase. Moreover, professionals can also concentrate their efforts on addressing the psychosocial and spiritual concerns of patients and supporting family members. The disadvantage of offering services just to those who are imminently dying is the difficulty in accurate prognostication. Therefore, people who have precipitous deaths may miss out and those whose final illness is very protracted may exhaust the resources of some charitable services. In the UK, palliative care services generally have a great deal of expertise in caring for people with cancer but rather less expertise in caring for patients dying of other conditions. There have been concerns raised about the arbitrary definitions of 'dying' applied to different groups of people. In the USA, access to insurance-funded hospice care programmes has been dependent upon people agreeing to no longer seek curative treatment. This has created great dilemmas and conflict within families, as different members may or may not wish to continue to seek active interventions. The consequence is that many people are admitted to palliative care programmes when it is almost too late for them or their families to benefit from care.

An emerging model of palliative care emphasizes the supportive role of health and social care practitioners throughout the trajectory of illness. This model, which is arguably driven by a medical agenda, suggests that symptom control is the main priority. There are now many more well-established medical interventions than were available in the early days of hospice care. For example, the syringe driver has revolutionized the way medication may be delivered in those with advanced illness. Its use has become pervasive in many palliative care contexts because it offers many benefits for people who are unable to take oral medication. The advantage of a supportive care model is that skilled medical and nursing symptom control interventions are not limited to one period of a patient's life (the final stage), so that suffering can be relieved at all stages of their illness. In the UK, the most frequent reason for admission to in-patient palliative care is for treatment of complex symptoms. Once there is resolution of symptoms or acceptable management, patients are discharged home or to other types of care. The use of skilled specialist palliative care resources can be targeted at those with severe and/or complex symptoms, rather than people being admitted to palliative care programmes 'just' because they have cancer. The disadvantage of this model of palliative care is the lack of clarity in its implementation. In particular, there are concerns about territorial disputes between generalists (such as general practitioners and community nurses, or hospital-based practitioners) and specialist palliative care providers. This model has the potential to deskill other health and social care providers because they come to believe that only specialist palliative care professionals are competent to work with dying people. Caring for patients with advanced disease and those who are dying is an important aspect of many health care professionals' workload. It is therefore important not to disempower them but instead to work in collaboration while acknowledging the skills that each practitioner may bring. This model of care also raises concerns about boundaries between the areas of expertise in specialist workers. Since many older patients have a number of co-morbidities that may be treated by different specialists, such as a cardiologist, a neurologist and an oncologist, there are real dangers of over-treatment. By extending the remit of specialist palliative care to patients who are at earlier stages of their disease, this raises issues about availability of funding and resources, and their optimal use.

Who gets palliative care? Who should get palliative care?

In the UK, approximately 95 per cent of patients referred to specialist palliative care services have cancer. But not everyone with cancer receives specialist palliative care. The preponderance of patients with cancer accessing palliative care in the UK is probably related to the historical development of early hospices and funding from key cancer charities. The only other medical condition with a history of specialist hospices is HIV/AIDS. In the UK during the 1990s, several reports and other documents explored what came to be known as the cancer–non-cancer debate (Field and Addington-Hall 1991). These publications rehearsed arguments for and against extending specialist palliative care to non-cancer patients. One of the chief concerns was that if access was widened to those with other conditions, there would be insufficient resources (the 'flood gates' argument) and current services would be overwhelmed. This prediction has proven not to be convincing since, despite repeated calls to widen access, little has changed in the last 5 years, indicating that either patients without cancer may be reluctant to be admitted to institutions so closely associated with cancer or that practitioners remain unwilling to refer them. In our view, these debates have largely been superseded by a public health agenda that calls for a recognition that access to specialist palliative care should be based on levels of distress and disease burden rather than diagnostic category (Foley 2003). In this book, we make no assumption that palliative care is restricted to people with cancer.

Where is palliative care delivered?

As we have reiterated before, most patients receive palliative care from their usual health care providers. In the UK, this means that most patients with advanced illness are in the care of the primary health care team, consisting of general practitioners, community nurses and allied health and social care professionals. Care is therefore delivered in patients' homes where they spend the majority of their time, even during the final year of life. Moreover, home is overwhelmingly the preferred place of care for most people. General practitioners and community nurses may make referrals to specialist palliative care providers. Specialist palliative care services themselves offer a range of provision, from a single specialist nurse to a comprehensive multidisciplinary team. Specialist palliative care services have developed an array of different types of provision including in-patient units (hospices), hospital teams, community teams, out-patient clinics, day care, respite services, bereavement support services, complementary therapies, counselling and psychological support, and spiritual and religious support.

What constitutes specialist palliative care and hospice care varies both within and across countries. In the UK, the early development was marked by the construction of dedicated separate buildings as in-patient hospices. In the USA, a hospice programme tends to refer to community-based support. There is a need to understand more clearly how the provision of palliative care is linked to the availability of resources in each country, to the political prioritization of different aspects of health care and attitudes to the use of opioid medication (Clark and Wright 2003).

Who provides palliative care?

There is a danger when providing a list of who provides palliative care that some people may be overlooked. With this proviso in mind, Box 2 offers a broad overview of the types of individuals who may be engaged in providing both paid and unpaid palliative care.

Corner (2003) discriminates between two types of nurses working in specialist palliative care – those who have additional post basic qualifications in palliative care and provide direct patient care in various contexts, including in-patient hospices and in the patient's home, and the clinical nurse specialist. The latter nursing role has been developed in the UK largely through the funding made available from a cancer charity now called Macmillan Cancer Relief. These specialist nurses tend to use the title 'Macmillan' nurse. Research evidence demonstrates that a large part of their role involves direct face-to-face contact with patients (89 per cent) and that the most common reason for referral is for emotional support (Corner *et al.* 2002; Skilbeck *et al.* 2002). Most of these nurses do not provide 'hands-on' physical care but instead offer support and information to patients. They also

---

Box 2   Palliative care work force

Patient's carers:	families; friends; neighbours
Nursing care:	general nurses; specialist nurses
Medical care:	general practitioners; specialists in palliative medicine; specialists in other areas of medicine
Social care:	social worker
Spiritual care:	chaplaincy; faith advisors
Therapists:	occupational therapists; physiotherapists (physical therapists), speech and language therapists; art, drama and music therapists
Psychological care:	counsellors; clinical and health psychologists; psychotherapists; liaison psychiatrists;
Specialist staff:	nutritionists; dieticians; pharmacists
Support staff:	care assistants; administrative and domestic staff; gardeners; transport and other workers
Volunteer workers	

---

work behind the scenes in coordinating care and offering specialist advice to generalists, including general practitioners and community nurses. Their work serves to promote better standards of palliative care by disseminating good practice and current evidence. They are, therefore, an important resource in trying to improve palliative care provision. An earlier study from the USA described the practice of a single palliative care nurse and emphasized the emotional and supportive elements of the role (Davis and Oberle 1990), rather than the networking and liaison functions. Much remains unknown about how clinical nurse specialists develop and sustain their role, what attributes are required and how they may be supported. Skilbeck and Payne (2003) have drawn attention to the ambivalence in these nurses about taking on emotional labour and emotional support functions when they are often poorly prepared and inadequately supported in this aspect of their role. Many of the subsequent chapters in this book will explore how nurses work to provide palliative care and the challenges this may create for them.

Overview of the book

In the final part of this Introduction, we will introduce ourselves as editors and explain how we selected the authors of the chapters.

The editors

This book has been a pleasure and a challenge to produce. We are all academics, nurses and researchers in palliative care. We share attributes as well as contributing our unique perspectives. We have drawn upon our academic

disciplines of health psychology and medical sociology. We have also practised as nurses. In addition, we have expertise in education for health and
social care professionals at basic level and in higher and continuing education. The experience of designing, coordinating and teaching on Masters
level courses in palliative care has been very influential in developing this
book. The many students on these courses have taught us much, and we are
grateful to them. We are indebted to Elaine Craigie, who has helped us
manage the clerical work involved in this book.

Sheila Payne has worked as an academic health psychologist for the last
20 years. Her background is in nursing. Her main research interests are in
palliative care and bereavement. She has conducted numerous research studies in palliative care and worked with colleagues in developing palliative care
and bereavement services. Sheila has offered doctoral degree supervision to
over 20 students. She has published widely in academic and professional
journals.

Jane Seymour is a nurse and sociologist. Jane has worked in palliative
care research and education since 1994, before which she pursued a career
in clinical nursing. Her PhD was an ethnographic study of the management
of death, dying and end-of-life decision making in intensive care units. Her
current research interests are advance care planning and the palliative care
needs of older people and their families.

Christine Ingleton qualified as a nurse in 1978 and has worked as a
clinician, manager, educationalist and researcher. Her doctoral thesis was
concerned with the development of a model for palliative care service evaluation and she has published widely in this area. She has been involved in a
variety of funded research projects in the area of end-of-life care, including
service evaluation, needs assessment, satisfaction with bereavement care,
the provision and quality of respite services, and the role of non-specialist
providers of palliative care.

The authors

We have been most fortunate in obtaining chapters from some of the leading
experts in palliative care. We have selected authors who represent a range of
expertise and are drawn from different professional and academic backgrounds. They include academics, researchers, professional practitioners,
managers, policy makers and educators. We believe that the diversity of
backgrounds and perspectives enhance the depth of coverage. However, it
does mean that the writing styles vary and while some editorial work has
been undertaken, we are keen that the chapters reflect the views and attitudes of our authors rather than conform to our perspectives. We have urged
authors to take an international perspective when possible, but each person
is likely to know their own country's health care systems and issues best. We
realize that there are some important omissions; namely, we have decided
not to include a chapter written by a patient or carer presenting the 'user'
perspective. Although this has become fashionable, we are concerned about
tokenism and we also acknowledge that people hold multiple roles – in

that some of our chapter authors may also be a patient and/or a carer. Second, we are aware that our authors do not represent all areas of the world, especially palliative care services in developing countries with limited resources. We regard this not as a failing but as an opportunity for another book.

Aims of the book

This textbook aims to draw together principles and evidence in palliative care nursing that underpin practice in order to support both nurses working in specialist palliative care settings and those whose work involves end-of-life care in other settings. The book will focus on palliative care for adults. The textbook uses a novel organizing framework – the trajectory of life-limiting illness – and will revisit key issues in association with important transitions in that trajectory (e.g. suspecting illness, diagnosis confirmation, living with dying and bereavement). Organizing the book like this enables the examination of complex issues in a longitudinal way and from a variety of perspectives. We have rejected the old four-part framework of physical, psychological, social and spiritual care because it tends to prevent an acknowledgement of the integration of patient experience, and there is a tendency to privilege physical aspects of care. The book has dedicated sections on research issues as well as integrating research findings throughout. The book draws extensively from literature in fields related to, and informing, nursing: history, psychology, sociology, social policy, anthropology and ethics. The book emphasizes the phenomenology or experience of care giving and care receiving and offers an agenda for change and future research.

Explanation of the 'trajectory of illness' framework

We have explicitly decided to move beyond an approach based on a traditional model of palliative care involving physical, psychological, social and spiritual aspects of care, as we believe this is not compatible with a holistic and person-centred approach. We are mindful that people experiencing these transitions in their lives are often connected with families and friends and a wider social network, and we will attempt to suggest how nursing interventions may encompass a socially embedded approach to care. We make no assumptions that end-of-life care is concerned merely with those who have cancer, but much of current specialist palliative care is provided for those with cancer and, therefore, the research literature reflects this reality.

Who is this book for?

This book is aimed at post qualifying level and is likely to be useful as a core text for students undertaking Master's level courses in palliative care and related courses in health and social care. The book will contribute to courses predominately aimed at developing a conceptual understanding of the theories and evidence that underpin clinical skills. In addition, the book will function as a resource for clinical nurse specialists and nurse consultants, and those working in nurse education and management. The book is aimed at those working in the UK and other English-speaking countries such as Australia, New Zealand and Canada. We also believe that it will be useful for readers in Europe, especially as specialist palliative care education for nurses becomes more widely developed. While aimed primarily at nurses, we hope that this book will be read widely by a range of health and social care practitioners, helping them to think more critically about palliative care. This book is not primarily a 'how to do' book or a practical guide to delivering care; instead, it seeks to intellectually challenge the reader and promote debate and discussion about the nature and purpose of palliative care.

Overview of Parts One to Four

This book is structured around a framework of four major parts; the first three are based on a trajectory of illness model, and the final part addresses contemporary issues in nursing and inter-professional working. Each part is introduced by an overview chapter dealing with the principles and theoretical issues underpinning practice, which is authored by one or more of the editors. This is followed by shorter and more focused chapters written by experts in the area, which deal with specific contexts, conditions and practical issues. These are meant to be illustrative of the issues raised in the overview chapter. Chapters conclude with advice on further reading.

| References

Addington-Hall, J.M. and Higginson, I.J. (2001) *Palliative Care for Non-Cancer Patients*. Oxford: Oxford University Press.

Clark, D. and Seymour, J. (1999) *Reflections on Palliative Care*. Buckingham: Open University Press.

Clark, D. and Wright, M. (2003) *Transition in End of Life Care: Hospice and Related Developments in Eastern Europe and Central Asia*. Buckingham: Open University Press.

Corner, J. (2003) Nursing management in palliative care. *European Journal of Oncology Nursing*, 7(2): 83–90.

Corner, J., Clark, D. and Normand, C. (2002) Evaluating the work of clinical nurse specialists in palliative care. *Palliative Medicine*, 16: 275–7.

Davis, B. and Oberle, K. (1990) Dimensions of the supportive role of the nurse in palliative care. *Oncology Nursing Forum*, 17(1): 87–94.

Department of Health (2000) *The NHS Cancer Plan: A Plan for Investment, A Plan for Reform*. London: HMSO.

Doyle, D., Hanks, W.C. and MacDonald, N. (1998) *Oxford Textbook of Palliative Medicine*, 2nd edn. Oxford: Oxford University Press.

Ferrell, B.R. and Coyle, N. (2001) *Textbook of Palliative Nursing*. Oxford: Oxford University Press.

Field, D. and Addington-Hall, J. (1991) Extending specialist palliative care to all? *Social Science and Medicine*, 48: 1271–80.

Foley, K. (2003) Lessons learned to improve end of life care. Invited lecture at the *European Association of Palliative Care Conference*, The Hague, The Netherlands.

Illich, I. (1976) *Limits to Medicine*. Harmondsworth: Penguin.

McNamara, B. (2001) *Fragile Lives: Death, Dying and Care*. Buckingham: Open University Press.

National Council for Hospice and Specialist Palliative Care Services (2002) *Definitions of Supportive and Palliative Care*. London: NCHSPCS.

National Council for Hospices and Specialist Palliative Care Services (2003) *Palliative Care for Adults with Non-malignant Diseases*. London: NCHSPCS.

National Institute for Clinical Excellence (2003) *Supportive and Palliative Care Guidance for Cancer*. London: NICE.

Nuland, S.B. (1994) *How We Die*. London: Chatto & Windus.

Payne, S., Sheldon, F., Jarrett, N. *et al.* (2002) Differences in understandings of specialist palliative care amongst service providers and commissioners in South London. *Palliative Medicine*, 16: 395–402.

Praill, D. (2000) Who are we here for? (editoral). *Palliative Medicine,* 14: 91–2.

Sepulveda, C., Marlin, A., Yoshida, T. and Ullrich, A. (2002) Palliative care: the World Health Organization's global perspective. *Journal of Pain and Symptom Management*, 24(2): 91–6.

Skilbeck, J. and Payne, S. (2003) Emotional support and the role of clinical nurse specialists in palliative care. *Journal of Advanced Nursing*, 43(5): 521–30.

Skilbeck, J., Corner, J., Bath, P. *et al.* (2002) Clinical nurse specialists in palliative care (1): a description of the Macmillan nurse caseload. *Palliative Medicine*, 16: 285–96.

World Health Organization (2002) Report on 'Preventing Risks, Promoting Healthy life' (http://www.who.int/mediacentre/releases/pr84/en/), accessed March 2003.

PART ONE

Encountering illness

1

Overview

Sheila Payne and Jane Seymour

It might strike readers as rather strange to start at the beginning of a patient's experience of illness when palliative care is usually thought of as being about services provided at the end of life to people with a serious illness like advanced cancer. We have already challenged this view in the Introduction by examining new and emerging models of palliative and supportive care. This chapter explores what it means for people who become ill to take up the social role of 'patient' and the implications this has for family members and friends who will be designated as 'carers' or 'care-givers'. We examine various perspectives on the self and introduce models of illness drawn from anthropology, sociology and psychology. In each case, we examine how they inform our understandings of palliative care nursing and how they have influenced the development of palliative care both over time and across geographical boundaries. In addition, we draw upon current conceptualizations of palliative care to consider how very ill and dying people are perceived by different societies, how the 'good death' has been constructed and reshaped over time, and what is considered to be 'normal' care for those with end-stage disease. For example, in developed societies, people with diseases such as heart failure are more likely to be treated with intensive medical and nursing interventions like artificial ventilation in intensive care units right to the end of their lives, whereas others with conditions such as dementia are less likely to receive such treatments (Seymour 2001).

In the latter part of this chapter, we discuss the impact of disease and illness upon those people who are in close relationships with the ill person. These are usually assumed to be family members or relatives, but the changes wrought by divorce, geographical mobility, increased longevity and declining birth rates may mean that friends or employed care workers provide more significant and meaningful relationships. Human beings are social animals and are embedded within social systems, kinship networks and cultural groups: the lack of such networks is potentially problematic for those reaching the end of their life, particularly the socially excluded, such as refugees and asylum seekers. We therefore introduce the reader to some concepts about social support, social networks and social relationships. Overall, this chapter aims to provide a clear framework to guide the reader through the ensuing chapters in Part One.

What does it mean to become a patient?

The sociological and anthropological literature has long emphasized the impact of illness and subsequent contact with health care services on personal identity and feelings of personhood (Kleinman 1980; Helman 2000). While early functionalist accounts of the 'patient's role' (in which patient-hood was conceptualized as a 'social role' with its own set of expectations, responsibilities and constraints) are now largely discounted, there remain a few elements that are highly salient for consideration when thinking about palliative and health care. The use of the label 'patient' continues to be dominant in the language of health care workers, health care managers and policy makers, and is widely used by the public. It serves to differentiate the 'well' from the 'ill', the 'cared for' from the 'care workers'.

Typically, life-threatening illness changes the outlook of the person it affects and alters the possibilities available to them. One's taken-for-granted life and the expectation of an almost limitless future diminish, and with increasing physical and/or mental decline imposed by illness comes creeping social isolation as treasured roles are modified and eventually relinquished. For example, employment provides many opportunities, including financial security, interactions and social relationships with work colleagues, social status, power and enhanced self-esteem. Of course, although not all work-related experiences are life-enhancing, to be forced to leave work because of illness is particularly symbolic of the way in which life-threatening illness eventually leads to a transition from activity to passivity. At this point, there may also be an incremental dismantling of essential features of personhood, such as the appearance of the physical body, as in cachexia, the destruction of cognitive and emotional capacity, as in end-stage dementia, and a withdrawal of social relationships, as in the 'social death' described by Sudnow (1967).

Concepts of the self and identity

Nurses have traditionally engaged with the physical body of the patient by providing comfort care, observing and recording physiological changes, assisting with activities of living and administering medical treatments. These complex skills are often referred to as 'basic' nursing care. However, research by Lawler (1991) has shown how nursing work also involves a detailed *social* understanding of the body. Her research has demonstrated

Box 1.1 An example of a study of people with lung cancer from the Netherlands (The 2002)

A social science researcher, Anne-Mei The (2002), conducted an ethnographic study in a cancer centre focusing on the experience of a group of patients with advanced small-cell lung cancer. Ethnography has been defined as 'that form of inquiry and writing that produces descriptions and accounts about the ways of life of the writer and those written about' (Denzin 1997: xi). Ethnographers typically develop a close relationship with people to gain access to their understandings and the social culture they inhabit. Anne-Mei The spent a great deal of time in the clinics listening to the doctors and nurses and sharing the experiences of the patients and their families as they underwent diagnosis, initial treatment, recurrence and through to their final days and deaths. We are introduced to the key players: Mr van der Ploeg, Mr Dekker, Mr Henvel, Mr Wiersema, Mr Wessels and other patients early in their illness, their spouses and families. We also learn about medical and nursing staff not as stereotypical consultant oncologists, junior doctors and ward nurses, but as complex individuals who vary both between each other and also between their handling of each patient. The research sought to address the questions about why and how patients remain so optimistic throughout their illness when the outcome is known (by medical staff) to be almost invariably fatal. This research offers an antidote to simplistic communication research in cancer care that focuses solely on 'the bad news' interview as though it were a single event. It demonstrates the complex interactions between patients, families, medical and nursing professionals in constructing what is 'known', and when and how it is 'known'. Anne-Mei The argues that both patients and their doctors collude in minimizing the significance of the disease in the early stages by concentrating their attention on short-term outcomes such as planning and starting treatment. In her view, this serves to deflect attention away from the more unpleasant long-term outcome that will be the patient's inevitable death. This analysis confirms other research such as that by Christakis (1999), which indicates that doctors are less likely to offer a prognosis than a diagnosis.

Patients and their families come to understand the implications of their disease through processes of social comparison with other patients. Once again, this is rarely acknowledged in the communication literature, where health professionals are often portrayed as virtually the only sources of information. By comparison, in this research we are shown how patients hear about the recurrences and deaths of their peers, and how they both learn from, and distance themselves from, these events. Anne-Mei The also describes how nurses are placed in the difficult position of having to 'fish' for information about the level of awareness of patients because they are not party to the communication that has occurred between medical consultants and patients. The picture of fluctuating awareness is akin to that described by Field and Copp (1999) as 'conditional awareness'. The research paints a complex picture of the tangled web of truths, half-truths and deceptions that are, in our view, the pattern of communication that most patients, families and health care workers participate in creating.

This research study is a very good example of ethnography. Ethnographic methodology has a long tradition in social research about end-of-life care, from the influential work of Glaser and Strauss (1965) in which 'awareness contexts' were described in acute care hospitals in the USA, to more recent UK examples in a cancer hospital (Costain Schou and Hewison 1999), in a hospice (Lawton 2000) and in intensive care (Seymour 2001). It is a powerful research methodology that enables rich analytical accounts to be developed. One of the markers of a good ethnographic account is an acknowledgement of the role of the researcher in the collection of the data and the construction of the analysis. In the Epilogue, Anne-Mei The demonstrates how she coped with the emotional involvement in the participants' lives and deaths. She addresses the dilemma between over-involvement and academic detachment which are faced by all researchers who see themselves as part of the process of research. It is a pity that positivist positions in research serve to marginalize this method and, therefore, findings from ethnographies are generally not included in evidence-based practice guidelines.

that nurses are skilled at managing intimate bodily care while engaging in strategies to minimize embarrassment and discomfort for the patient. Changes in nursing education, knowledge and concepts of professional role in the latter part of the twentieth century opened up new possibilities for how nurses engage with and 'know' patients. May (1992) argues that nurses now seek to 'know' patients in terms of 'foreground' and 'background' knowledge. 'Foreground' knowledge relates to the clinical definition of the body: this allows nurses to establish what nursing work needs to be undertaken. 'Background' knowledge concerns the person as an individual, and it is this engagement of nurses with a person who is a complex social being with an unique identity that is arguably new to nursing rhetoric. Although there are evident benefits for nurses and patients in moving beyond stereotypical portrayals of patients (such as 'the lung cancer in bed 6'), this rhetoric can represent a challenge to nurses because it requires sensitive communication and an openness to the full extent of each person's experience of suffering. It is also potentially more invasive for patients because they are expected to reveal to nurses not only their physical bodies, but also their thoughts, feelings and existential concerns. Demands to 'know' the whole person and to deliver 'holistic' care have been made particularly loudly in palliative care (e.g. Buckley 2002).

If 'knowing the person' is regarded as fundamental to palliative care nursing, what theories of the self and identity influence our understanding? In this section, we consider how concepts of the self and identity are described from various perspectives. Psychological approaches to questions of self and identity fall into four major groups: psychoanalytic and psychodynamic therapists have drawn upon their clinical work (e.g. Freud 1923), humanistic psychologists have drawn upon insights from psychotherapeutic work (e.g. Kelly 1955; Rogers 1961; Maslow 1970), social psychologists have used experimental methods (e.g. Bem 1972) and, more recently, social constructivist theorists have drawn upon narrative methods (e.g. Crossley 2000). Sociologists tend to emphasize the influence of socialization or 'cultural programming' (Giddens 1998) on self-identity. Critically important here are the accidents of birth that tend to give individuals differential educational and employment opportunities and thus ensure that they occupy particular positions in society. Traditional sociological approaches have emphasized: the influence of historical, cultural and economic circumstances (for example, the theories of Karl Marx about the way in which social conditions shape human existence); the influence of ethical or 'normative' standards on identity (for example, Talcott Parson's idea of 'sick role' as a set of normative expectations that shape the identity of patients); and how self-perception is fashioned through the way in which others respond to us during social interaction. This latter idea has emerged in different ways in the work of symbolic interactionists who have followed George Herbert Mead and in the work of those who follow Erving Goffman. Goffman showed how the small rituals of everyday life constrain our behaviour and shape our sense of self as we learn to 'play the game' (May 1996). Contemporary sociologists have used these traditional perspectives in new ways. Most notable among these is Giddens' theory of 'structuration', in which he draws together a range of perspectives to argue that social structures (of which culture is pre-eminent) do not merely *influence* a person's sense of self, but are manifest *through* individuals' engagement with the practices that make up social life (Giddens 1976).

Identity has been posited to be derived predominantly from one's social position at birth (e.g. being born to wealthy or poor parents), acquired through education and employment, or derived from performance of social roles like being a parent, a widower or widow, which determine to some extent what are regarded as appropriate behaviours and ways of interacting with others. More recently, identity has been presented as a more flexible and negotiated construct, and it has been suggested that people living in contemporary Western societies take a more reflexive and internalized position to identity in which traditional belief systems play little part. Thus Taylor (1989) argues that in many countries people now spend more time pondering existential questions about the meaning of life and their role in it, because there is less acceptance of broad frameworks like religion.

Lawler (1997) has emphasized that the outward presentation of the body has become very influential in defining identity and individuality, and conveys powerful messages about culture. For example, our choice of clothing and accessories can signify wealth, culture, age and gender. Similarly, body art (e.g. tattoos, ear rings and nose studs) is closely linked with the way we wish to convey both our identity as cultural group members and as individuals. Wearing make-up and styling hair in certain ways are gender markers in most cultures. Thus, difficulty in maintaining one's usual standards of personal dress and grooming may be profoundly challenging for people with advanced disease. For example, the thinness associated with cachexia or the swelling arising from ascites may be difficult to mask by clothing and may lead people and their families to feel depersonalized by the experience of illness.

Narratives, or stories, have become a powerful and popular way to reveal identity (Radley 1993). Biographies and autobiographies are popular in everyday life and, in a recent book, they have also been used to provide insights into how Canadians experience dying (see Barnard *et al.* 2000). Crossley (2000) argues that people use stories to create accounts of themselves that are flexible over time. Stories also provide an opportunity for people to make sense of experiences and find meanings (Launer 2003). For example, you may have dealt with patients and families who have been involved in a traumatic road traffic accident, and found them constantly needing to tell their story about what happened. Arguably, one of the functions of counselling is to provide the space for people to tell their story, from which they may gain insights into themselves and may even find the storytelling healing (Frank 1995). Many bereavement counsellors report that being available to listen and hear the story of the death is an important aspect of their role (Payne *et al.* 2002). Crossley (2000) suggests that the way the story is told and the language used serve to shape people's understanding of their own identity. Thus, some people with cancer object strongly to the term 'cancer victim' because it positions them as passive, helpless and deserving of pity. They prefer to use language which indicates a more active and positive stance, such as 'cancer survivor'.

Sociologists highlight how serious and chronic illness disrupts individuals' sense of identity and the taken-for-grantedness of continuity that characterizes most people's lives (see, for example, Bury 1982; Charmaz 1991). Most of us optimistically assume that we will live to a happy and healthy old age and we plan and live our lives based on these assumptions. Therefore, when illness occurs, especially if this is sudden like a stroke, there are major psychological and social adjustments to be made, as well as the challenges of managing the physical and functional changes associated with illness. 'Narrative medicine' is a new development that seeks to take account of how people understand their identity and how illness impacts on their sense of self and the meaning that illness has at each stage in their life (Greenhalgh and Hurwitz 1998). It also seeks to redefine the role of medicine by emphasizing the more fundamental and humanitarian aspects of care. It is argued that by using narrative (stories), patients can be encouraged to share their experiences, which provides an insight into their predicaments.

The distinction between *illness* and *disease*

In this book, we make the distinction between *illness*, which refers to the subjective experience of being unwell and may or may not be linked to an organic disease, and *disease*, which refers to a recognized pathological state (see Chapter 7). It is therefore possible for a person to have a life-threatening disease and to describe themselves as 'well'. Similarly, it is also possible for a person to feel ill but not have a disease. The recognition and labelling of disease states (i.e. diagnosis) has traditionally been the role of medicine, but a diagnostic label takes no account of the meaning a person places on the set of symptoms. There are worldwide agreed systems of classification of diseases that are useful in cross-cultural research trials, for example DSM-IV-R (American Psychiatric Association 1994) for psychiatric conditions. The fact that disease classification systems are revised and modified indicates that notions of disease change over time and across cultures.

Research indicates that nurses find diagnostic labels highly salient. In a study of information transfer between nurses working in wards for older people, most nurses reported that the essential information they required during handovers (reports between nursing shifts) included patient's name, age, diagnosis and resuscitation status (Payne *et al.* 2000). During observations in the same wards, it was noted that nurses always provided information about the original diagnosis at admission even if subsequent investigations had altered the diagnosis and made the old one redundant. This information was always exchanged between nurses at handovers before nursing care information was given. This indicates that nurses prioritize medical information and the authors suggested that diagnostic labels

Box 1.2 An example of a study of one person with oral cancer (Crossley 2003)

John Diamond, a British broadcaster and journalist, wrote an account of his experience of oral cancer in a series of articles in *The Times* newspaper over a period of 4 years, from diagnosis to 1 week before his death. His account provided a narrative of one man's experience of living with cancer. Through writing the articles in the form of a diary, he attempted to find meaning in his experiences and, according to his brother-in-law, the writing was his method of coping with illness. Crossley (2003), a health psychologist, undertook a narrative analysis of Diamond's articles, which she interpreted in the context of Del Vecchio Good and co-workers' (1994) notion of 'therapeutic emplotment'. Del Vecchio Good *et al.* (1994) have argued that oncologists and patients creatively manage time and the patients' experience of illness as part of 'a larger therapeutic story' (p. 855). This serves to highlight particular events and episodes that appear to maintain the possibility of hope. Crossley examined Diamond's articles for evidence of his unfolding story. She categorized them into six sequential stages.

1 *Pre-cancer: touch wood*. In the first article on 14 September 1996, he reported the possibility that his mouth swelling *might be* cancer but distanced himself.
2 *Learning to live in 'therapeutic emplotment'*. Over the next 6 months, Diamond's articles were full of accounts of various medical and surgical treatments and their associated side-effects. His language appeared to be optimistic, with an emphasis on the future expectation that after 6 weeks of daily radiotherapy and surgery, he would achieve full recovery. He was encouraged by health professionals to live in the 'immediacy of treatment' while the future held the promise of a certainty of outcome (cure).
3 *In limbo: holding one's breath*. Following treatment, he came to realize that 'the truth is . . . I still don't know whether I'm cured. Nor will I know for weeks, or months, or possibly years'. This period is sometimes described as 'watchful waiting' and can be even more stressful than undergoing active medical treatment (Jones and Payne 2000).
4 *Recurrence: 'therapeutic emplotment' continued*. Ten months after what appeared to be the 'end' of treatment, his cancer recurred. Diamond tried to be optimistic in the face of further radical head and neck surgery. He wrote, 'if the surgeons slash and burn in the right way, then I have a reasonable chance of a cure'.
5 *Through the mirror: the 'unspoken narrative'*. Following surgery, there was evidence that Diamond started to abandon his previous expectations of cure and gave up his 'almost childish belief in the power of modern medicine'. However, he consented to chemotherapy, which he described as 'stale hell' and some 4 months later another swelling in his neck was confirmed as cancer recurrence.
6 *Endings or the end?* The final period of writing was characterized by a lethargy and resignation. Further recurrence and spread to his lungs were responded to by his agreement to a further three courses of chemotherapy but with no optimistic expectations. One week later, he died in hospital.

This is a tale of one person's experience of oral cancer. As readers we know the outcome, but as Crossley points out in her analysis, Diamond did not. How he engaged with this uncertainty is powerfully revealed in his writing.

functioned to stereotype patients and were used to determine the types of care to be given. Moreover, attention appeared to be focused on the current diagnosis, with less attention being paid to the co-morbidities experienced by these older people.

Patterns of disease have traditionally been categorized as chronic or acute. Palliative care services have predominantly been concerned with providing care for people with chronic rather than acute diseases. This distinction has, arguably, become blurred by changes in diseases themselves, in medical technology and in treatment. For example, 50 years ago childhood leukaemias were regarded as acute and rapidly fatal diseases but now most children with leukaemia survive. Similarly, antiretroviral agents have transformed AIDS into a chronic disease, or at least for those who have access to appropriate medication. Many cancers are now also experienced as an intermittent chronic condition, as patients encounter repeated episodes of recurrence and further treatment. However, the public perception of cancer remains of a rapidly fatal disease.

In the UK, palliative care services have been closely identified with cancer and it is only in the last 5 years that serious attempts have been made to broaden the scope of palliative care to those with other life-threatening conditions (Addington-Hall and Higginson 2001). Arguably this change in focus has paralleled the growth in medical treatments for such conditions that prolong life and thus create space for the greater use of palliative interventions. For example, ACE inhibitors have prolonged the lives of those with heart failure and the quality of palliative care delivered to patients with heart failure has, at the same time, come under the spotlight (British Heart Foundation 2001). Out of this has come recognition that the prognosis of those with heart failure is worse than for those with breast or prostate cancer, with one in five patients dying within a year of diagnosis. Moreover, retrospective UK data gathered from carers indicate that end-of-life symptoms for those dying of heart failure are distressing and poorly controlled (McCarthy *et al.* 1996), suggesting that much remains to be done to enhance the quality of care for those dying of heart failure. While attention is beginning to be focused on the need to improve end-of-life care in a range of chronic physical diseases, those with mental health conditions and cognitive deficits remain largely neglected (Lloyd-Williams and Payne 2002).

Underpinning much of the palliative care literature is an assumption that people have a single identifiable disease. Yet evidence from Western countries suggests that the majority of older people and an increasing proportion of younger people are living with at least one chronic disease and a range of co-morbidities (Williams and Botti 2002). There is evidence that with increasing age there is a rise in the number of co-morbidities. For example, an 88-year-old person may live with pain from osteoarthritis, asthma that results in acute episodes of breathlessness and is complicated by recurrent chest infections, and osteoporosis that has resulted in hip fractures. This person has, therefore, several chronic diseases that result in chronic pain and also a number of acute problems requiring a complex range of health and social care interventions. The outcome of experiencing a number of chronic diseases may include reduced quality of life, repeated and sometimes unpredictable requirements for health and social care services, and increased health care costs. Unfortunately, the organization of medical services generally focuses on specific types of pathology (e.g. oncology or orthopaedics) with little integration between services, which necessitates visits to different physicians at different clinics and possibly in different hospitals.

There is some evidence that the end-of-life care needs of older people have been relatively neglected by palliative care services (Seymour *et al.* 2001). Seymour *et al.* argue that expertise in gerontology and elderly care medicine may provide useful insights for palliative care workers who may be unfamiliar with working with people over 85 years. For these people, patterns of deterioration and dying may be less clear-cut than in younger people. Their physical and mental decline, which will often be combined with social withdrawal, may be drawn out over many years, and it is more difficult to recognize a clearly terminal phase. It has been highlighted that there is a need to build collaboratively upon the skills and expertise of care workers located in nursing and care home environments rather than assume that specialist palliative care workers are expert in all types of dying (Froggatt 2001; Froggatt *et al.* 2002).

So far, we have differentiated between illness and disease and highlighted how important these are for understanding the experience of patients. But we have not yet mentioned or sought to define 'health' in the context of palliative care. Readers may be surprised to consider this as an outcome of palliative care. Yet Kellehear (1999) has argued for a 'health promoting palliative care', and enhanced quality of life is widely regarded as a successful outcome for palliative and supportive care. Another way to construe this is that the outcome of palliative care interventions and nursing care is to foster and enhance remaining opportunities for healthy living. This does not just mean eating more fruit and vegetables or stopping smoking, but enhancing perceived well-being and health. Of course, 'health' is a notoriously difficult concept to define. However, it is possible to identify a number of differing perspectives on health and illness to provide a foundation to thinking about health in advanced disease. Within each perspective there are numerous debates and we do not claim to do justice to the complexity of the positions introduced here. The following is merely an introduction to these and readers are encouraged to seek more information from specialist texts.

Models of health and illness

Anthropologists have emphasized that Western notions of biomedicine are just one of a number of ways to understand health, illness and the body (Kleinman 1980). Moreover, Western medicine should not be thought of as a static or uniformly agreed set of ideas, as caricatured in the 'medical model'. Biomedicine is constantly evolving; for example, recent research on genetics and the human genome project bring new ways to conceive of the body and to think about the genetic and foetal origins of disease. As well as Western biomedicine, there are other well-accepted medical systems such as that used by Chinese medical practitioners. And, of course, people also have access to their own culturally defined folk beliefs that may incorporate aspects of other health beliefs, such as those derived from biomedicine. These health and illness beliefs may be complex and influence health-seeking behaviours, especially in relation to common ailments and normal life transitions. Thus, as we will see in Part Three, folk beliefs about what are 'normal' bereavement experiences incorporate psychological models of phases and beliefs that bereavement represents a 'process' (Payne *et al.* 1999).

In the UK and in North America, a heterogeneous group of therapies, dietary practices and types of healing have been labelled as 'complementary medicine'. The use of this term to describe a diverse range of therapeutic and diagnostic interventions positions them as adjuncts to biomedicine, although this relationship is ambivalent. The critics of complementary medicine highlight the lack of scientific evidence to support the use of many of the therapies, while their supporters emphasize the popularity of these interventions with the general public and how some therapies have gained acceptance as supportive treatments in hospice and palliative care contexts. In many areas, nurses have been active in including complementary therapies – especially 'touch therapies' like aromatherapy and massage – in the repertoire of interventions available to palliative care patients.

Evidence from major surveys in the UK (e.g. Blaxter 1990) has been used by sociologists to demonstrate that health and illness are regarded in different ways by different groups of people. Field (1993) reminds us that social factors such as gender, age, social class, economic and educational abilities, all influence what people regard as normal health and how they define themselves as ill. For example, in some communities where smoking is common, older people have described a cough as 'normal'. The apparent paradox in contemporary societies is that there appears to be greater mistrust and disillusionment with medical practitioners and health care institutions than in the past but, at the same time, greater attention is devoted to risk management and seeking health care (Lupton 1994). There are a plethora of health information sources but access to them, especially via electronic computer-based media, are known to be related to socio-demographic factors such as age and economic resources, which may exacerbate health inequalities.

Psychological perspectives on health and illness have tended to focus upon trying to understand the thought processes (cognitions) and behaviours of individuals. It is recognized that people are influenced by the views and beliefs of others, especially those important to them. A number of the early models, such as the Health Belief Model (Becker and Maiman 1975) and the Theory of Planned Behaviour (Ajzen 1991), focused on behavioural intention and trying to predict how people make choices about health behaviours, such as stopping smoking or attending for breast cancer screening. These theories are popular with health psychologists but have a limited ability to predict actual behaviour because they tend to assume that people behave rationally, are not heavily influenced by their emotional state and have to make all their decisions at one time (for a more detailed critique, see Crossley 2000). Recently, Petrie and Weinman (1997) have developed Leventhal's model of illness representation to take account of both cognitive and emotional elements in how illness is understood. In contrast, Prochaska and DiClemente (1983) developed the Transtheoretical Model, which takes account of the extent to which people are prepared to change their health behaviours. This suggests that interventions such as smoking cessation should be linked to the motivational stage of the person. When people are thinking about changing (that is when providing information about *how* to change) makes the most impact. In contrast, giving information about *why* they should change their behaviour is needed at an earlier stage when they are contemplating making changes; such information becomes redundant once the decision has been made.

The impact of the illness on the family and the social context of the family

So far, we have concentrated on people facing the end of their lives and not the people who populate their lives and social worlds. This has been a criticism of palliative care (Field 2000). Field has argued that while specialist palliative care workers acknowledge the psychosocial impact of illness and the need to recognize psychosocial care needs, the emphasis has tended to be on the psychological care of patients with much less attention being directed to social aspects. Whatever your views are about this criticism, in this book we intend to consider explicitly the social relationships and social contexts in which people live. The remainder of this chapter is therefore devoted to an account of how 'social support' and 'social network' are conceptualized in the literature. We focus on the impact of illness and approaching death upon families and friends, who are often described as carers or care-givers. In many nursing textbooks, these people remain marginal in the text and therefore, by implication, in the lives and deaths of patients. But the reality of palliative care nursing both in community or institutional contexts means that we are constantly working with the families and friends of our patients.

Who are the family?

We suggest that a broad definition of 'family' is necessary to encapsulate those people who share biological, social or legal ties. It includes those related by continuing heterosexual and same-sex relationships. It also includes wider culturally recognized groups such as the New Zealand Maori *whanau* and other extended families through birth, adoption or legal contract (marriage). Nurses should be aware that notions of what constitute a 'family' may vary between cultures, from a dyad (for example, a mother and child) to a multi-generational dynasty. Perhaps a defining feature of a family is the sense of enduring emotional and social bonds experienced by members.

Whatever the definitional problems with the term 'family', it should be acknowledged that families are dynamic social structures. Families change over time as members are added through marriage, birth and adoption or lost through death and, in some cultures, following marriage. There are role expectations, responsibilities and commitments that are often related to economic provision, child-bearing and child-raising activities and in some cultures the roles may be defined by gender. Theories tend to describe family relationships in terms of complex systems of reciprocal demands and support.

Social changes in Western countries have influenced family structures and the availability of family members to fulfil caring roles. These changes include increasing divorce and separation, with some individuals experiencing a series of marital relationships. Their children thus experience a series of family relationships with step-parenting and step siblings becoming more common. Increased longevity may result in greater numbers of people enjoying being grandparents or great grandparents, but also an increased possibility of experiencing the loss of, or distancing from, family members in late old age. In many countries there is a declining birth rate, with some people remaining childless (approximately 10 per cent in the UK) and family size declining to one or two children per partnership. This reduces the potential number of people related by kinship who may be available to offer care near the end of life. Economic pressures for two incomes combined with other factors has increased female employment rates, while male employment patterns have become less stable with greater geographical mobility and more part-time working. One of the most dramatic changes of recent years relates to the disease trends in Africa that relate to AIDS: this has massively increased the numbers of children orphaned and growing up in unprotected or institutional environments.

Certain groups in society are less likely to have close family ties. Socially disadvantaged or socially excluded people such as refugees, homeless people and prisoners are less likely to have access to families or friends to support them during times of crisis. Other people may reject, or have been rejected by, their families. It is important to remember that not all families are mutually supportive or beneficial to their members. Rather, some may be constituted by abusive, exploitative or threatening relationships that undermine or threaten an individual's welfare.

Older people, especially those in later old age (more than 85 years), are an increasing proportion of the population in many developed countries, and are vulnerable to social isolation as their families disperse and their friends die. Approximately a fifth of all people over 85 years in the UK die in residential or nursing homes. For many, close emotional and social relationships with their peers and with staff members assume a special importance.

▌Who are the carers?

Lay people who take on unpaid caring roles in relation to the person facing the end of life are usually defined as 'carers' or 'care-givers'. They may be family members, friends or neighbours, although it should not be assumed that all family members are able to, or wish to, take on a caring role. Evidence suggests that more women than men take on a caring role (Payne and Ellis-Hill 2001), and that in palliative care there is more within-generational than cross-generational care-giving. Being a carer is a social relationship that can only be undertaken in the context of another person, even if that person rejects the carer or is reluctant to be cared for. Research undertaken with older people indicates that many people are fearful of becoming dependent upon family members and do not wish to 'burden' their adult children (Seymour *et al.* in press). So becoming a 'carer' and becoming a 'cared for' person are roles that many people approach with some ambivalence. It should not be assumed that family members or patients are necessarily comfortable with the term 'carer' or attribute it to themselves.

There are a number of ways to conceptualize and categorize caring. Drawing on the work of Nolan *et al.* (1995), who built upon the earlier formulations of Bowers (1987), the following offers one way of conceptualizing types of caring:

- anticipatory care

- preventative care

- supervisory care

- instrumental care

- protective care

- preservative care

- (re)constructive care

- reciprocal care

While lists may not be very helpful in a practical sense because types of care may overlap considerably, they are useful in highlighting 'hidden' elements of caring. For example, in caring for a person with a terminal condition, the carer may spend time in the early stages, when there are relatively few physical problems, anticipating and planning for deterioration in the ill person's physical abilities. It may only be during the later stages of the illness that physical caring, such as washing, become necessary. During much of the illness trajectory, care-giving involves 'being there' both physically and emotionally for the ill person but this is rarely construed as 'caring' by professionals. Evidence from The's (2002) study in the Netherlands (see Box 1.1) showed how the spouses of people with lung cancer spent many hours accompanying their relatives to cancer clinics and helped them as advocates and as mediators in acquiring information from health care staff.

Social support and social network

Here, we briefly explore the concepts of 'social support' and 'social network' to provide a wider theoretical context within which to situate the subsequent chapters about carers. We only provide brief examples from a much wider literature that readers may want to explore for themselves (see Payne and Ellis-Hill 2001). Social support has been defined as information leading individuals to believe they are cared for and loved, esteemed and valued, and belong to a network of communication and mutual obligation (Cobb 1976). Several different types of social support have been identified. They function in different ways and may involve 'doing for' the cared-for person, encouraging activity in others, taking responsibility or just 'being there' for others. The following list defines key types of social support:

- *Informational support* refers to the provision of knowledge relevant to the situation the individual is experiencing.

- *Tangible support* refers to specific activities that others provide which are perceived to be helpful.

- *Emotional support* is the perceived availability of thoughtful, caring individuals who can share thoughts and feelings.

- *Affirmatory or validatory support* is given when others acknowledge the appropriateness of a person's beliefs and feelings.

- *Social affiliation* refers to an individual's system of mutual obligations and reciprocal help with other individuals and institutions.

Social support can be differentiated from 'social network', which is a system of social ties such as those formed between family, relatives and friends. Simmons (1994) suggested that there are seven functions of a social network: intimacy, social integration, nurturing others, reassurance of worth, assistance, guidance and access to new contacts. Social networks are generally defined in terms of their structural properties, including:

- *Size*: the number of people within the network.

- *Network density*: the amount of contact between members.

- *Accessibility*: the ease with which members can be contacted.

- *Stability over time*: the duration of the relationship.

- *Reciprocity*: the amount of give and take in the relationship.

- *Content*: the nature of the involvement in the relationship.

- *Intensity*: the degree of closeness within the relationship.

The mechanism by which social support mediates the effects of stress upon health remains controversial. Two main hypotheses have been postulated: the main effects hypothesis, which suggests that social support is beneficial whether or not the individual is experiencing stress, and the stress buffering hypothesis, which suggests that social support influences individual appraisals of stressful stimuli. No one model adequately explains all the variance found in the literature. However, it is generally accepted that the extent of the social network is not sufficient to account for the health-enhancing effects; rather, it is the perception of the availability of appropriate support and the social skills needed to elicit them that are the key determinants.

Much of the literature emphasizes the positive effects of social support. For example, a literature review of social support for those with breast cancer concluded that social support is important for psychological adjustment and survival (Carlsson and Hamrin 1994). Frequently, psychological need constitutes the largest proportion of self-identified needs for both patient and carer, above physical, financial, informational and household needs (e.g. Hileman and Lackey 1990). The opportunity to confide in others appears to be an important component and function of social support, although research indicates differences between the sexes in the number of available confidantes, with more women appearing to utilize multiple confidantes and men tending to confide in fewer people, usually just their spouse (Harrison *et al.* 1995). Social support may break down when there is a mismatch between the expectations of cancer patients and their relatives, because relatives make assumptions about what the cancer patient's needs might be (Gurowka and Lightman 1995).

Three types of support have been identified as critical for patients receiving radiotherapy: 'being there' (physically, emotionally and spiritually), 'giving help' (instrumental) and 'giving information and advice' (Hinds and Moyer 1997). These authors state that 'While support was hierarchical in nature, with levels of support linked to the closeness of relationship, it was also multi-faceted' (p. 375). In other words, different people provided different types of support at different times. Nevertheless, family and friends were found to be the primary source of all types of support. Professional support was mainly perceived to be at an informational level.

Social relationships associated with care-giving may also have negative aspects. Rook and Pietromonaco (1987) highlighted four unsupportive factors:

- ineffective help;
- excessive help that increased recipient dependence;
- unwanted or unpleasant interactions;
- encouragement of unhealthy behaviours.

Conflict about care-giving may be experienced in all families, but in families where conflict is unresolved, long-standing or violent, the establishment of caring relationships for an ill person is especially problematic. Conflict may be more intense in small kinship networks where increasingly heavy demands are placed upon relatively few people, compared with larger more diverse social networks were there may be more resources for people to draw upon and the potential for overloading each individual is less. This has implications for nurses working with certain groups of people, such as those with few social contacts (e.g. people who have moved to a new area to retire), those who are alienated from others because of poor social skills, alcohol or substance abuse, and those living in socially disadvantaged communities.

In a study of carers of people with dementia in Canada by Neufeld and Harrison (2003), two main categories of non-support were identified. Unmet expectations were described as:

- unfulfilled or missing offers;
- unmet expectations for social interactions;
- mismatched aid;
- incompetence.

Negative interactions included:

- disparaging comments;
- conflict in appraisal of the care recipient's health status;
- criticism;
- spillover of conflict from other issues.

This study provides a useful reminder that social support may function in undesirable as well as desirable ways. Moreover, both aspects may be experienced during the course of care-giving relationships. Research from Israel provides evidence from carers of people with dementia that their feelings of competence and satisfaction with their role of carer can co-exist with feelings of burden (Greenberger and Litwin 2003). The last two cited studies have been drawn from the experience of care-giving to those with dementia where, typically, the illness trajectory is more prolonged than in some other types of illness such as cancer or heart failure. Less research has focused on the needs of those caring for people likely to experience a quicker dying trajectory.

Overview of chapters in Part One

In the remainder of this chapter, we introduce the other eight chapters in Part One. Our aim is to guide the reader by providing a conceptual framework to understand the content.

The experience of dying differs by race, ethnicity, social position and time in the life span of the person. Paradoxically, it is an experience which all of us will undergo, but it is arguably highly individual (Nuland 1994) and is shaped by our social position, culture and location in the world. In Chapter 2, David Clark presents an historical analysis of the care provided for dying people. He traces back the roots of modern palliative care to before the mid-twentieth-century developments led by Cicely Saunders in the UK. He highlights the important role of women, some of whom were nurses, in responding to the needs of dying people. People are shaped by the understanding of death in their culture and the resources available to them. Many of the early pioneers trying to improve the care of dying people were inspired and motivated by religion, especially Christian teaching.

Arguably, nursing as a profession was born out of a sense of Christian 'calling' or vocation but was forged in the catalyst of war. Thus nursing builds upon the 'normal' work of women, caring for the sick, child-raising and tending to dependent family members, both young and old. Religious institutions had, for a long time, attracted men and women who wished to dedicate their lives to serving their god through caring for the sick and needy. Key influences in British nursing history have been war and military medical services. As most readers will know, Florence Nightingale came to prominence following the Crimean War (1854), but it was the mobilization of large numbers of young women from all social classes during the First World War (1914–18) that established the importance of nursing. It also exposed large numbers of women, the majority working as untrained nurses, to the realities of dying.

Chapter 2 concludes with an account of global developments, indicating how services for dying people have responded to socio-political context and culture.

In Chapter 3, Jane Seymour explores the differences in terminology used by nurses and others to describe their contribution to palliative care. Readers may wonder why we have devoted a whole chapter to deconstructing key terms. We would argue that words are not neutral and do not serve merely to reflect experience and understandings. Rather, language fundamentally determines the way in which the world is understood and shaped. Seymour's analysis shows how nurses' definitions of what constitutes nursing care have made available a number of discourses which open up and also limit possible interactional styles with patients. Drawing upon May's (1995) account of 'knowing the patient', Seymour argues that in the last 10 years nurses have reframed their engagement with patients from an attention on care of the body to an attempt to work with the 'whole' person. This account privileges the psychological status of the person, especially their need for 'support'.

There is evidence from a large-scale evaluation of Macmillan nurses (clinical nurse specialists) working in 12 areas of the UK (Corner *et al.* 2003) that the majority of referrals were for 'psychosocial support', which is a poorly defined intervention. Corner and co-workers reported that the majority of nursing input could be loosely regarded as psychosocial support. They indicate that there were considerable methodological problems in conducting the research because standardized measures of quality of life were insensitive to detect the subtle changes resulting from nurses' contributions to complex and dynamic palliative and cancer care environments.

Seymour's critique of key concepts in palliative care nursing highlights the assumptions that are made by nurses; for example, new approaches to 'knowing' patients are predicated upon open disclosure of their concerns but patients may not want to lay bare their soul or reveal their long-held secrets. The resistance of patients to this style of nursing has not been explored; nor has there been an adequate investigation of the expectations and wishes of patients. For some people in some cultures, stoicism and emotional containment are highly valued. Do nurses have the right to challenge these ways of coping?

Merryn Gott focuses in Chapter 4 on the debates surrounding how patients and others are engaged in shaping palliative care services and research. The policy of involving people other than professionals in influencing health and social care services has been growing in popularity since the early 1990s in the UK. It has arisen from social changes that have challenged medical hegemony and paternalism, and involves a broader recognition of consumer rights.

Gott differentiates between the terms 'user' and 'consumer'. Neither word is entirely appropriate, as not all people may be current service users and in some health care systems, such as the British NHS, patients are not active purchasers of health care. They may not, therefore, perceive themselves to be 'consumers'. Moreover, Gott points out there is little evidence that the preferences for terms of those most involved, patients and carers, have been sought.

Most of the literature advocates the benefits of user involvement by enhancing self-esteem and empowerment, but there is little rigorous evidence to substantiate these claims. A systematic review by Crawford *et al.* (2002) showed that most investigations were descriptive case studies, usually written by project managers, and the authors concluded that there was insufficient data to demonstrate any advantage in terms of quality of life or satisfaction for patients involved in planning and developing services. Gott highlights the special issues for engaging palliative care patients and carers in planning services and in research. She reports on different levels of involvement from mere consultation to active participation in the design and analysis of user-led services and research studies.

Essentially, user involvement initiatives are about power. The active participation of patients, carers, the general public and voluntary organizations has the potential to redistribute power. The idealistic vision is that service users can truly engage in planning services that are responsive to their needs and concerns. But a more conservative, arguably realistic, view is that patients may become disillusioned if services are not seen to change, or that particular organizational views are privileged (e.g. the most well-resourced or special interest group). A cynical view is that users may be used to provide an illusion of democracy and representation that is merely tokenistic (Payne 2002).

Improving the care of patients near the end of life may or may not be associated with improving access to specialist palliative care services. In Chapter 5, Julia Addington-Hall draws comparisons between the organization and funding of services in the UK and the USA. She highlights how services have evolved in each country in rather different ways, which she largely attributes to different funding mechanisms and the extent to which there is public and professional support. This chapter complements the earlier historical analysis provided by David Clark.

Addington-Hall goes on to consider two special groups, those with diseases other than cancer (she describes them as non-cancer) and older people. They are not mutually exclusive groups, as older people are more likely to die of diseases other than cancer. She argues that while there is evidence to indicate bias in current referrals and the uptake of specialist palliative care services in the UK (this is less evident in the USA), it cannot be concluded that older people and those without cancer would necessarily benefit from additional services. Little research has examined the views of older people about the acceptability of palliative care, and the same lack of evidence of benefit is true for others.

There are several other groups of people who currently fail to access specialist palliative care services. These people may be socially disadvantaged, and some of the issues related to referral are dealt with in Part Two by Koffman (dealing with problems of access related to race and ethnicity) and Katz (dealing in more depth with services for older people and prisoners).

In Chapter 6, Vanessa Taylor focuses on the extent to which general hospitals provide palliative care. Virtually all patients with life-threatening conditions will have been diagnosed and treated in acute hospitals. For many patients, care in acute hospitals becomes a recurrent theme of their experience of illness, as they undergo initial treatment, recurrence and further episodes of investigation and therapy [see research by The (2002) highlighted at the beginning of this chapter].

Taylor's chapter is drawn from the British health care system and emphasizes the role of nurses in providing care. There are three main types of palliative care available in acute hospitals. First, general palliative care is delivered by all health and social care practitioners. Such care aims to ensure that all patients' needs for symptom control, emotional support and social care are recognized. If the patient's and/or family's needs are complex, they will require referral to specialist practitioners. The second level of provision comes from clinical nurse specialists and Taylor describes aspects of their role in detail. Third, some hospitals employ specialist palliative care practitioners from a number of disciplinary backgrounds and these may work together as a team. There is little evidence or agreement about the optimal skill mix of these teams, but at a minimum they comprise medical and nursing specialists in palliative care. Their expertise appears to be most in demand in relation to managing difficult symptoms and for psychosocial support. Less attention appears to have been directed to providing specialist services to enhance social functioning and to deal with existential concerns.

The term 'transition' means the movement from one state of being to another. In Chapter 7, Margaret O'Connor attends first to the experience of the person with a life-threatening condition and then at the response of health care policies and services. Life transitions can be regarded as normal. For example, menopause strictly refers to the point at which a woman ceases to menstruate and signifies the end of fertility. However, this biological description is compounded by complex psychological, social and cultural nuances. Similarly, O'Connor draws attention to the differing ways in which illness is understood and experienced. She presents stages of transition through illness and wellness, with differing outcomes including survival, which has been mainly researched in relation to those with cancer, and terminal decline. She explores some of the tensions in access to palliative care policy in Australia where assumptions are made about the stage of illness (end-stage versus throughout the illness trajectory), the types of diseases (cancer versus non-cancer) and the special needs of older people. These themes pick up issues dealt with by Addington-Hall in Chapter 5 on referral to palliative care. They are themes that will recur throughout this book.

In another of the recurring themes, communication, there has been a radical transformation in the practice of medicine and nursing in the last 30 years. According to Sullivan (2003: 1595), 'Bioethics has pointed to the importance of the patient's point of view in health care decisions through its call to respect patient autonomy. Facts known only by physicians need to be supplemented by values known only by patients.' In most Western countries, open disclosure of diagnosis and, to a lesser extent, prognosis is common practice for those with cancer and, to a lesser extent, other chronic life-threatening conditions. Patients are encouraged to take responsibility for their health and participate in medical decisions. Such decisions rely on a careful blending of the technical knowledge of health care professionals with the values, desires and expectations of patients. Gone are the days in which the role of the nurse was merely to 'reassure' the patient and collude in conspiracies of silence. Patient-centred styles of interaction and outcomes, such as quality of life and place of care preferences, are now regarded as desirable goals.

In Chapter 8, Nikki Jarrett and Sian Maslin-Prothero provide a broad overview of the communication literature, drawn predominantly from the UK context of care. They argue that patients and health professionals communicate in a complex matrix of understandings, misunderstandings, expectations and wishes. Drawing from a post-structuralist perspective, they demonstrate that language use does not merely reflect reality but serves to shape and define social realities. They argue that despite the growth in communication skills training, structural and organizational factors limit the transferability of desirable communication skills to everyday working environments. Sadly, complaints by patients and carers testify to continuing problems in communication practices in many health care institutions. An alternative strategy is, therefore, to empower patients to elicit the information and communication styles they desire. An initiative originally developed in the USA with people with chronic disease offers an opportunity for patients to be trained as 'expert patients'. As yet, there is little evidence about the efficacy of this model of improving communication in people with advanced and deteriorating conditions, where it may be anticipated that problems such as fatigue may seriously impact upon their willingness to engage in training or longer-term activities. To conclude, the principle of good communication which is responsive and respectful of patients' wishes is well established, but the practice of achieving this for all remains elusive.

In Chapter 9, Debbie Fitzsimmons and Sam Ahmedzai draw attention to the importance of assessment in health care. They start by examining the influence of nursing theories in shaping the assessments undertaken when admitting patients to hospital or hospices. It is only in the last 20 years or so that British nurses have conducted separate assessments of patients from medical 'clerking' procedures on admission to hospital. Nursing assessments initially arose as part of 'the nursing process', a systematic approach to documenting, planning and measuring outcomes of care, which focused on nursing outcomes not merely medical outcomes. These assessments were to be conducted in collaboration with patients who participated in goal-setting and defining achievable and desirable outcomes, thus individualizing the care delivered and the goals attained. While the rhetoric of individualized care remains, care plans are now frequently pre-prepared documents that relate to specific conditions or medical procedures.

A major critique by patients of hospital procedures is that they are repeatedly subjected to assessment by different health and social care professionals. Not only can this be perceived as very invasive, but it is exhausting for patients who are often required to volunteer the same information repeatedly. It is also very time-consuming for professionals in creating their own records and there is much overlap and redundancy of effort. Two initiatives have sought to address these concerns: one is for patients to hold their own heath care records and the other is to have interdisciplinary shared records such as that pioneered in the care of older people (Philp *et al.* 2001). Both of these may have a place in ensuring better transfer of information about patients across health and social care boundaries and between primary and secondary care providers (Payne *et al.* 2002).

In the remainder of their chapter, Fitzsimmons and Ahmedzai review the literature on the use of standardized measures of quality of life and measures of specific symptoms. They highlight the different approaches to quality-of-life assessment and consider their strengths and weaknesses in palliative care contexts.

References

Addington-Hall, J.M. and Higginson, I.J. (2001) *Palliative Care for Non-Cancer Patients*. Oxford: Oxford University Press.

Ajzen, I. (1991) The theory of planned behaviour. *Organizational Behavior and Human Decision Processes*, 50: 179–211.

American Psychiatric Association (1994) *Diagnostic and Statistical Manual of Mental Disorders*, 4th edn. Washington, DC: APA.

Barnard, D., Towers, A., Boston, P. and Lambrinidou, Y. (2000) *Crossing Over: Narratives of Palliative Care*. Oxford: Oxford University Press.

Becker, M.H. and Maiman, L.A. (1975) Sociobehavioural determinants of compliance with health and medical care recommendations. *Medical Care*, 13: 10–24.

Bem, D. (1972) Self perception theory, in L. Berkowitz (ed.) *Advances in Experimental Social Psychology*, Vol. 6. New York: Academic Press.

Blaxter, M. (1990) *Health and Lifestyle*. London: Heinemann.

Bowers, B.J. (1987) Inter-generational caregiving: adult caregivers and their ageing parents. *Advances in Nursing Science*, 9(2): 20–31.

British Heart Foundation (2001) Palliative care of heart failure, Factfile No. 5. London: BHF.

Buckley, J. (2002) Holism and a health-promoting approach to palliative care. *International Journal of Palliative Nursing*, 8(10): 505–8.

Bury, M. (1982) Chronic illness as biographical disruption. *Sociology of Health and Illness*, 4(2): 167–82.

Carlsson, M. and Hamrin, E. (1994) Psychological and psychosocial aspects of breast cancer treatment. *Cancer Nursing*, 17(5): 418–28.

Charmaz, K. (1991) *Good Days, Bad Days: The Self in Chronic Illness and Time.* New Brunswick, NJ: Rutger University Press.

Christakis, C.A. (1999) *Death, Foretold Prophecy and Prognosis in Medical Care.* London: University of Chicago Press.

Cobb, S. (1976) Social support as a moderator of life stress. *Psychosomatic Medicine*, 38(5): 300–14.

Corner, J., Halliday, D., Haviland, J. *et al.* (2003) Exploring nursing outcomes for patients with advanced cancer following interventions by Macmillan specialist palliative care nurses. *Journal of Advanced Nursing*, 41(6): 561–74.

Costain Schou, K. and Hewison, J. (1999) *Experiencing Cancer: Quality of Life in Treatment.* Buckingham: Open University Press.

Crawford, M., Rutter, D., Manley, C. *et al.* (2002) Systematic review of involving patients in the planning and development of health care. *British Medical Journal*, 325: 1263–9.

Crossley, M. (2000) *Introducing Narrative Psychology: Self, Trauma and the Construction of Meaning.* Buckingham: Open University Press.

Crossley, M. (2003) 'Let me explain': narrative emplotment and one patient's experience of oral cancer. *Social Science and Medicine*, 56: 439–48.

Del Vecchio Good, M., Munakata, T., Kobayashi, Y., Mattingly, C. and Good, B. (1994) Oncology and narrative time. *Social Science and Medicine*, 38: 855–62.

Denzin, N.K. (1997) *Interpretive Ethnography.* Thousand Oaks, CA: Sage.

Field, D. (1993) Social definitions of health and illness, in S. Taylor and D. Field (eds) *Sociology of Health and Health Care*, 2nd edn. Oxford: Blackwell Science.

Field, D. (2000) *What Do We Mean by 'Psychosocial'? Briefing 4.* London: National Council for Hospice and Specialist Palliative Care Services.

Field, D. and Copp, G. (1999) Communication and awareness about dying in the 1990s. *Palliative Medicine*, 13: 459–68.

Frank, A. (1995) *The Wounded Storyteller: Body, Illness and Ethics.* Chicago, IL: University of Chicago Press.

Freud, S. (1923) *The Ego and the Id.* Standard edition. London: Howarth Press.

Froggatt, K.A. (2001) Palliative care and nursing homes: where next? *Palliative Medicine*, 15: 42–8.

Froggatt, K.A., Poole, K. and Hoult, L. (2002) The provision of palliative care in nursing homes and residential care homes: a survey of clinical nurse specialist work. *Palliative Medicine*, 16: 481–7.

Giddens, A. (1976) *New Rules of Sociological Method: A Positive Critique of Interpretive Sociologies.* London: Hutchinson.

Giddens, A. (1998) *Sociology.* Cambridge: Polity Press.

Glaser, B.G. and Strauss, A.L. (1965) *Awareness of Dying.* New York: Adline.

Greenberger, H. and Litwin, H. (2003) Can burdened caregivers be effective facilitators of elder care-recipient health care? *Journal of Advanced Nursing*, 41(4): 332–41.

Greenhalgh, T. and Hurwitz, B. (1998) *Narrative Based Medicine*. London: British Medical Journal Books.

Gurowka, K.J. and Lightman, E. (1995) Supportive and unsupportive interactions as perceived by cancer patients. *Social Work in Health Care*, 21: 71–88.

Harrison, J., Maguire, P. and Pitceathly, C. (1995) Confiding in crisis: gender differences in pattern of confiding among cancer patients. *Social Science and Medicine*, 41(9): 1255–60.

Helman, C.G. (2000) *Culture, Health and Illness*, 4th edn. Oxford: Butterworth Heinemann.

Hinds, C. and Moyer, A. (1997) Support as experienced by patients with cancer during radiotherapy treatments. *Journal of Advanced Nursing*, 26: 371–9.

Hileman, J.W. and Lackey, N.R. (1990) Self-identified needs of patients with cancer at home and their home caregivers: a descriptive study. *Oncology Nursing Forum*, 17(6): 907–13.

Jones, G.Y. and Payne, S. (2000) Searching for safety signals: the experience of medical surveillance amongst men with testicular teratomas. *Psycho-Oncology*, 9: 385–95.

Kellehear, A. (1999) *Health Promoting Palliative Care*. Oxford: Oxford University Press.

Kelly, G. (1955) *A Theory of Personality – The Psychology of Personal Constructs*. New York: W.W. Norton.

Kleinman, A. (1980) *Patients and Healers in the Context of Culture*. Berkeley, CA: University of California Press.

Launer, J. (2003) Narrative-based medicine: a passing fad or a giant leap for general practice? (editorial). *British Journal of General Practice*, 53(2): 91–2.

Lawler, J. (1991) *Behind the Screens: Somology and the Problem of the Body*. London: Churchill Livingstone.

Lawler, J. (1997) *The Body in Nursing*. Melbourne, VIC: Churchill Livingstone.

Lawton, J. (2000) *The Dying Process: Patients' Experiences of Palliative Care*. London: Routledge.

Lloyd-Williams, M. and Payne, S. (2002) Can multi-disciplinary guidelines improve the palliation of symptoms in the terminal phase of dementia? *International Journal of Palliative Nursing*, 8(8): 370–5.

Lupton, D. (1994) *Medicine as Culture: Illness, Disease and the Body in Western Societies*. London: Sage.

Maslow, A.H. (1970) *Motivation and Personality*, 2nd edn. New York: Harper & Row.

May, C. (1992) Nursing work, nurses' knowledge and subjectification of the patient. *Sociology of Health and Illness*, 14: 472–87.

May, C. (1995) Patient autonomy and the politics of professional relationships. *Journal of Advanced Nursing*, 21(1): 83–7.

May, T. (1996) *Situating Social Theory*. Buckingham: Open University Press.

McCarthy, M., Lay, M. and Addington-Hall, J.M. (1996) Dying from heart disease. *Journal of the Royal College of Physicians*, 30: 325–8.

Neufeld, A. and Harrison, M.J. (2003) Unfulfilled expectations and negative interactions: non-support in the relationships of women caregivers. *Journal of Advanced Nursing*, 41(4): 323–31.

Nolan, M., Grant, G. and Keady, J. (1995) Developing a typology of family care: implications for nurses and other service providers. *Journal of Advanced Nursing*, 21: 256–65.

Nuland, S.B. (1994) *How We Die*. London: Chatto & Windus.

Payne, S. (2002) Are we using the users? (editorial). *International Journal of Palliative Nursing*, 8(5): 212.

Payne, S. and Ellis-Hill, C. (2001) *Chronic and Terminal Illness: New Perspectives on Caring and Carers*. Oxford: Oxford University Press.

Payne, S., Horn, S. and Relf, M. (1999) *Loss and Bereavement*. Buckingham: Open University Press.

Payne, S., Hardey, M. and Coleman, P. (2000) Interactions between nurses during handovers in elderly care. *Journal of Advanced Nursing*, 32(2): 277–85.

Payne, S., Jarrett, N., Wiles, R. and Field, D. (2002) Counselling strategies for bereaved people offered in primary care. *Counselling Psychology Quarterly*, 15(2): 161–77.

Petrie, K. and Weinman, J. (1997) *Perceptions of Health and Illness*. Amsterdam: Harwood Academic Press.

Philp, I., Newton, P., McKee, K.J. *et al.* (2001) Geriatric assessment in primary care: formulating best practice. *British Journal of Community Nursing*, 6(6): 290–5.

Prochaska, J.O. and DiClemente, C.C. (1983) Stages and process of self-change of smoking: toward an integrative model of change. *Journal of Consulting and Clinical Psychology*, 51: 390–5.

Radley, A. (1993) *Worlds of Illness: Biographical and Cultural Perspectives on Health and Disease*. London: Routledge.

Rogers, C. (1961) *On Becoming a Person: A Therapist's View of Psychotherapy*. London: Constable.

Rook, K.S. and Pietromonaco, P. (1987) Close relationships: ties that heal or ties that bind?, in W.H. Jones and D. Perlman (eds) *Advances in Personal Relationships: A Research Annual*. Greenwich, CT: JAI Press.

Seymour, J. (2001) *Critical Moments: Death and Dying in Intensive Care*. Buckingham: Open University Press.

Seymour, J.E., Clark, D. and Philp, I. (2001) Palliative care and geriatric medicine: shared concerns, shared challenges (editorial). *Palliative Medicine*, 15(4): 269–70.

Seymour, J.E., Gott, M., Bellamy, G., Clark, D. and Ahmedzai, S. (in press) Planning for the end of the life: the views of older people about advance statements. *Social Science and Medicine*.

Simmons, S. (1994) Social networks: their relevance to mental health nursing. *Journal of Advanced Nursing*, 19: 281–9.

Sudnow, D. (1967) *Passing On*. Englewood Cliffs, NJ: Prentice-Hall.

Sullivan, M. (2003) The new subjective medicine: taking the patient's point of view on health care and health. *Social Science and Medicine*, 56: 1595–604.

Taylor, C. (1989) *Sources of the Self: The Making of Modern Identity*. Cambridge: Cambridge University Press.

The, A.-M. (2002) *Palliative Care and Communication: Experiences in the Clinic*. Buckingham: Open University Press.

Williams, A. and Botti, M. (2002) Issues concerning the on-going care of patients with comorbidities in acute care and post-discharge in Australia: a literature review. *Journal of Advanced Nursing*, 40(2): 131–40.

History, gender and culture in the rise of palliative care

David Clark

As the work of palliative care expands around the world, there is a growing interest in understanding more about how this field of activity first began to develop in its modern form. This chapter draws on a programme of research that has been developing since the mid-1990s and is now recognized as a key source of information about the history of modern hospice and palliative care.[1] It explores how it was that in the nineteenth century a new interest in the care of the dying first began to emerge and describes some of the activities led by hospice pioneers at that time. It then goes on to analyse key developments taking place in the second half of the twentieth century that began to establish this work not just as the interest of religiously and philanthropically motivated individuals and groups, but as something that might be capable of finding a place within the wider systems of health and social care delivery. The history of modern palliative care is a short one, and many of those who have shaped it are still alive to tell their stories and to reflect on their experience. Learning from that history is a crucial way in which an increasingly specialized field can better understand its current dilemmas and also develop effective strategies for the future. But the modern field also has a pre-history and to make sense of that we must begin by looking back more than 150 years.

In many parts of Europe, North America and Australia, as the nineteenth century advanced, an epidemiological transition got underway that saw the beginnings of a shift in the dominant causes of death: from fatal infectious diseases of rapid progression to chronic and life-threatening diseases of longer duration. As this transition became more marked, the departure from life for many people became an extended and sometimes uneven process. Consequently, people called 'the dying' began to emerge more clearly as a social category and, over time, the most common place to end one's life began to shift from the domestic home to some form of institution. For the first time in history, special institutions were formed, often the work of religious orders or religiously motivated philanthropists, that were uniquely concerned with the care of dying people. At first, the influence of these 'hospices' and 'homes for the dying' was quite limited, scarcely capable of changing attitudes and practices more generally. They appeared in several countries through the late nineteenth and early twentieth centuries, but seemed to have little impact on the wider environment of care for dying people. In the second half of the twentieth century, however, major innovations did begin to take place, building on and developing some of the ideas that prevailed in the original religious and philanthropic homes. By this time a modern 'movement' was emerging: reformist in character, advocating new approaches to old experiences, and above all opening up a space in which the 'process of dying' could be newly problematized, shaped and moulded. Hospice care came to be defined in unprecedented terms, emphasizing 'quality of life', 'pain and symptom management' and 'psycho-social care'. In several countries, palliative medicine gained recognition as a specialty and advanced programmes of training developed, not only for physicians, but also for nurses, social workers and others involved in what came to be seen as the multidisciplinary activity of modern palliative care. During the last quarter of the twentieth century, and particularly in the 1990s, there was a steady growth in the number of services operating in this way, across countries and continents. In some of the more affluent nations, palliative care, by the start of the twenty-first century, had reached a stage of relative maturation, gaining a measure of recognition on the part of the public, the professions and policy makers. Yet in most resource-poor regions of the world, hospice and palliative care were still struggling to gain a foothold, seen as a low priority in settings where overall health care expenditure remained limited and where other social problems appeared more pressing. Over a relatively short period of time, the achievements made by palliative care protagonists reveal a line of development that can be traced back to nineteenth-century foundations. These were laid by nursing orders, philanthropic associations and voluntary medical practitioners. Now transformed into the guise of modern palliative care, the achievements and challenges take on a new character. They are accompanied by new ways of thinking and behaving towards dying members of society. Indeed, they seem capable of generating previously unimagined ways of experiencing illness, suffering and even mortality itself.

Nineteenth-century origins

The nineteenth century was a time of great hospital building, but it did little to foster concern for those at the end of life whose condition was beyond cure (Granshaw and Porter 1989). Here were the first signs of death as a medical failure. The dying were an unwelcome embarrassment in the new medical citadels, and so it was outside the 'mainstream' of medical practice that philanthropic and charitable endeavours led to the creation of special institutions, some of them called hospices, which sought to provide care and sanctuary to those nearing death. From the beginning of the nineteenth century, therefore, it is possible to identify certain important developments in the care of dying people, and several of which were led by women (Clark 2000).

The young widow and bereaved mother, Jeanne Garnier, together with others in similar circumstances, formed L'Association des Dames du Calvaire in Lyon, France, in 1842. The association opened a home for the dying the following year, which it was said was characterized by 'a respectful familiarity, an attitude of prayer and calm in the face of death' (quoted in Clark 2000: 51). Jeanne Garnier died in 1853, but her influence led to the foundation of six other establishments for the care of the dying between 1874 (in Paris) and 1899 (in New York). In both of these cities, modern-day palliative care services now exist which originate directly from the work of L'Association des Dames du Calvaire. Reflecting a sense of religious calling to her endeavours, Jeanne Garnier remarked in a memoir towards the end of her own life, 'J'ai fondée mon refuge avec cinquante francs; la providence a faire la reste'.

Mary Aikenhead was born in Cork, Ireland, in 1787. At the age of 25 she became Sister Mary Augustine and was established almost immediately as Superior of a new Order, the Irish Sisters of Charity, the first of its kind in Ireland to be uncloistered. The Order made plans to establish a hospital. Three of the sisters went to Paris to learn the work of the Hôpital Notre Dame de la Pitié. In Ireland they opened St Vincent's Hospital, Dublin, in 1834. Following many years of chronic illness, Mary Aikenhead died at nearby Harold's Cross, in 1858. Fulfilling an ambition which she had long held, the convent where Mary Aikenhead spent her final years became Our Lady's Hospice for the Dying in 1879. The Sisters of Charity followed it with others in Australia, England and Scotland, all of which still exist today and are run by the Order as modern palliative care units. One of these, St Joseph's Hospice, Hackney, in the impoverished East End of London, and established in 1905, has a particularly important place in the narrative of modern palliative care history (see below).

The first institutional home for the dying in England, however, was established by a Scot, Frances Davidson, in 1885, and was known as 'The Friedenheim; a place of peace for those at the end of life' (Humphreys 1999). It was opened in Mildmay Park, London, and was intended in particular for those with tuberculosis. Preference was given to those for whom mortal illness had reduced their circumstances and to whom the workhouse infirmary was a 'dreaded last resort' (Humphreys 1999: 48). Initially, the Friedenheim had eight beds, but in 1892 a move to new premises in South Hampstead provided accommodation for up to 35 patients. Admission was free, though there were private rooms for those who could afford to pay. Humphreys (1999) also describes another key development around this time with the establishment, also in London, of the Hostel of God, which was founded as a result of an appeal in *The Times* on Christmas Day 1891. The Anglican Sisters of St James' Servants of the Poor ran the home from 1892 to 1896, when the Sisters of St Margaret's of East Grinstead took over. In

1900, new premises were acquired on Clapham Common, with facilities for 36 patients. Trinity Hospice as it is now known, is no longer under the governance of a religious order, but continues to operate from premises in Clapham, and constitutes the longest established palliative care service in the UK.

In the USA, Rose Hawthorne, the daughter of Nathaniel Hawthorne, had experienced the death of a child and watched her friend, the poet Emma Lazarus, dying of cancer. In September 1896, on New York's Lower East Side, she opened what is said to be the first home in America for the free care of 'incurable and impoverished victims of cancer'.[2] The work met with 'countless hardships and almost universal distrust', but was part of the efforts of an organized group of women known as the Servants of Relief of Incurable Cancer, formed with Alice Huber, the daughter of a Kentucky physician. In 1900, when Rose Hawthorne's husband died, she took religious orders, under the title Mother Alphonsa, and formed an order known as the Dominican Sisters of Hawthorne. Following the establishment of St Rose's Hospice in Lower Manhattan, another home was founded at Rosary Hill, outside New York, followed by others in Philadelphia, Fall River, Atlanta, St Paul and Cleveland.

Against this background of institutional provision of specific homes for the dying, there is also evidence of small numbers of doctors and nurses who were showing a special interest in the care of the dying by the later decades of the nineteenth century. In 1890, Mrs Dacre Craven published her guide to district nurses and home nursing, which contained a chapter on 'the best positions for the dying according to their ailment' (Dacre Craven 1890). Four years later, Oswald Brown (1894) published his lecture to nurses on the care of the dying. He drew heavily on William Munk's (1887) work *Euthanasia*, which set out the case for medical treatment in aid of an easy death (and not for medicalized killing in the sense that the term 'euthanasia' subsequently came to connote). There were also the medical contributions of Herbert Snow on the use of opium and cocaine in the relief of suffering associated with advanced cancerous disease, which appeared in the *British Medical Journal* and elsewhere (Snow 1890a,b, 1896, 1897). It is unclear to what extent these writings had an influence in the institutional homes for the dying that were being created in this period. If they did have an effect, it was insufficient to set in train any broader movement of reform; for the time being these writers and the founders of the homes remained isolated from one another and lacking a synergy that could lead to more widespread change.

Although unknown to each other, Jeanne Garnier, Mary Aikenhead, Frances Davidson and Rose Hawthorne shared a common purpose in their concern for the care of the dying, and in particular the dying poor. Directly and indirectly they founded institutions that, a generation later, led to the development of other homes and hospices elsewhere. They also established base-camp for what was to follow, for their achievements created some of the pre-conditions for modern hospice and palliative care development. Humphreys (2001) has shown how these early hospices and homes for the dying reveal three sets of concerns: religious, philanthropic and moral. Such institutions placed a strong emphasis on the cure of the soul, even when the life of the body was diminishing. They drew on charitable endeavours and were often concerned to give succour to the poor and disadvantaged. They were not, however, places in which the medical or nursing care of the dying was of any real sophistication. Rooted in religious and philanthropic concerns that would diminish as the twentieth century advanced, the early homes for the dying represent the vital prologue to a period of subsequent development, which got underway in the decades after the Second World War.

A mid-twentieth-century sea-change

We know that from the middle of the twentieth century these early hospice founders were a key source of inspiration to Cicely Saunders as she set about her life's work to improve the care of dying people. Indeed, they influenced her clinical activities, her research and teaching, and the formation of St Christopher's Hospice in 1967. They were also a source of inspiration for her continuing leadership and inspiration to palliative care workers in many places (Clark 2001a). We also know that Cicely Saunders was acting as part of an international network of like-minded people, even from as early as 1958 when she published her first paper in *The St Thomas's Hospital Gazette*. This network covered North America, India and Ceylon, Australia, France, Switzerland, the Netherlands and communist Poland, and is revealed in her remarkable and extensive correspondence of the time (Clark 2002a). Indeed, it can be argued that the foundation of St Christopher's Hospice in London in 1967 by Cicely Saunders and her colleagues should be seen not as the beginning of the modern hospice movement, but rather as the conclusion to the first stage of its international development (Clark 1998).

Box 2.1

I am a doctor of medicine, having read this rather late in life after training first as a nurse and then as an almoner. I read medicine because I was so interested and challenged by the problems of patients dying of cancer, and have for the past twelve years had in mind the hope that I might be led to found a new Home for these patients . . . I am enclosing a reprint of some articles which I wrote for the 'Nursing Times' at their request last year, and which contain something of what I have learnt so far. I am also enclosing a scheme for a Home which I am trying to plan for at the moment.

Cicely Saunders to Olive Wyon, 4 March 1969

(Clark 2002a: 23)

By the late 1950s, the British National Health Service had been in existence for more than a decade; it formed part of a welfare state pledged to provide care 'from the cradle to the grave'. Yet the new health service had done nothing to promote the care of its dying patients. Instead, the thrust of policy was moving towards acute medicine and rehabilitation. Yes, there was increasing awareness of the demographic changes that would lead to far more elderly people in the population, but the consequences for their care, and in particular for those affected by malignant disease, received scant attention. Cicely Saunders was one of a handful of clinicians on both sides of the Atlantic who began to take a special interest in the care of the dying in this context.

It is also important to note that the most immediate audience for Cicely Saunders's writings was among nurses. Although she struggled to spawn medical interest in her work (Clark 1998; Faull and Nicholson 2003), nursing colleagues encouraged her, became involved in her plans and fostered the publication of her ideas. A series of six articles by Cicely Saunders that appeared in the *Nursing Times* in the autumn of 1959 provoked a huge written response from the readership, as well as an editorial in the *Daily Telegraph* (Clark 1997). The articles were among the first to elucidate a set of principles for the care of the dying that could be used as a guide to practice. Rooted in strong personal, religious and moral convictions, they also made compelling, if controversial, reading. The following year they were reproduced in a *Nursing Times* pamphlet (Saunders 1960a), *Care of the Dying*, and Cicely Saunders continued to write for the journal throughout the early 1960s. Similarly, in 1964, she was invited to contribute a piece to the *American Journal of Nursing* (Clark 2001b). When it appeared, the piece used case illustrations from St Joseph's Hospice to focus on nursing aspects of care, giving particular prominence to a major point of discussion at that time: the question of whether to reveal the patient's prognosis. Once again, the article produced a considerable postbag, and every nurse who wrote in from across the USA received a personal reply from the author.

Why were nurses so eager to read such material and how was it that these writings on terminal care found such resonances within nursing audiences? By the mid-twentieth century, important changes were occurring in Western medicine and health care. Specialization was advancing rapidly, new treatments were proliferating, and there was an increasing emphasis on cure and rehabilitation. At the same time, death in the hospital, rather than at home, was becoming the norm; and the dying patient or 'hopeless case' was often viewed as a failure of medical practice. In a series of famous lectures in the 1930s, the American physician and champion of nursing revisionism, Alfred Worcester, had noted: 'many doctors nowadays, when the death of their patients becomes imminent, seem to believe that it is quite proper to leave the dying in the care of the nurses and the sorrowing relatives. This shifting of responsibility is un-pardonable. And one of its results is that as less professional interest is taken in such service less is known about it' (Worcester 1935: 33). It seems that nurses bridled at such trends and observations. If Worcester thought it unpardonable that patients should be left in this way, nurses considered that they and their dying patients had been abandoned by their medical colleagues and indeed ignored by society. Nurses who had remained with the task of staying with their dying patients therefore found some endorsement and succour in the early writings of Cicely Saunders and indeed showed a willingness to contribute to the new thinking, even when doctors remained sceptical and doubting. It was as if in reading this new writing on a traditional aspect of nursing care, in some way the notion of nursing as a 'calling' was being rekindled: 'you have been a guiding light in helping me to discover what I have been searching for as a student nurse', observed one American correspondent (Clark 1998: 54).

An emerging specialization

Despite these concerns, some initiatives for improving care at the end of life did begin to gain a wider hearing from the early 1960s. In Britain, attention focused on the medical 'neglect' of the terminally ill; in the USA, a reaction to the medicalization of death began to take root. Four particular innovations can be identified (Clark 1999a). First, there was a shift within the professional literature of care of the dying, from idiosyncratic anecdote to systematic observation. New studies – by nurses, doctors, social workers and social scientists – provided evidence about the social and clinical aspects of dying in contemporary society. By the early 1960s, leading articles in *The Lancet* and *British Medical Journal* were drawing on the evidence of research to suggest ways in which terminal care could be promoted and arguments for euthanasia might be countered. Second, a new view of dying began to emerge that sought to foster concepts of dignity and meaning. Enormous scope was opened up here for refining ideas about the dying process and exploring the extent to which patients should and did know about their terminal condition. Third, an active rather than a passive approach to the care of the dying was promoted with increasing vigour. Within this, the fatalistic resignation of the doctor was supplanted by a determination to find new and imaginative ways to continue caring up to the end of life and, indeed, beyond it in the care of the bereaved. Fourth, a growing recognition of the interdependency of mental and physical distress created the potential for a more embodied notion of suffering, thus constituting a profound challenge to the body–mind dualism upon which so much medical practice of the period was predicated.

Box 2.2   Key innovations in care of the dying in the 1950s and 1960s

- Emergence of the first research studies
- A new approach to dignity and meaning in dying
- Active solutions to clinical problems
- Recognition of the interdependency of mental and physical suffering

As we have already observed, it was the work of Cicely Saunders, first developed in St Joseph's Hospice in Hackney, East London, that was to prove most consequential, for it was she that began to forge a peculiarly modern philosophy of terminal care. Through systematic attention to patient narratives, listening carefully to stories of illness, disease and suffering, she evolved the concept of 'total pain' (Clark 1999b). This view of pain moved beyond the physical to encompass the social, emotional, even spiritual aspects of suffering, captured so comprehensively by the patient who told her: 'All of me is wrong' (Saunders 1964: viii). But it was also linked to a hard-headed approach to pain management. Her message was simple: 'constant pain needs constant control' (Saunders 1960b: 17). Analgesics should be employed in a method of regular giving, which would ensure that pain was prevented in advance rather than alleviated once it had become established, and they should be used progressively, from mild to moderate to strong.

Even before the opening of St Christopher's Hospice in South London in 1967, it had become a source of inspiration to others and was also firmly established in an international network. The correspondence of Cicely Saunders shows clearly how it attracted the interests of senior academics and managers in American nursing, as well as those from many countries who were eager to develop their practical skills through work on the wards of the hospice (Clark 2002a). As the first 'modern' hospice, it sought to combine three key principles: excellent clinical care, education and research. It therefore differed significantly from the other homes for the dying which had preceded it and sought to establish itself as a centre of excellence in a new field of care. Its success was phenomenal and it soon became the stimulus for an expansive phase of hospice development, not only in Britain, but also around the world.

Growth and diversification in the later twentieth century: the global perspective

From the outset, ideas developed at St Christopher's were applied differently in other places and contexts. Within a decade it was accepted that the principles of hospice care could be practised in many settings: not only in specialist in-patient units, but also in home care and day care services. Similarly, hospital units and support teams were established that brought the new thinking about dying into the very heartlands of acute medicine. Modern hospice developments took place first in affluent countries, but in time they also gained a hold in poorer countries, often supported by mentoring and 'twinning' arrangements with more established hospices in the West. By the mid-1980s, a process of maturation was in evidence in some countries, but elsewhere growth was slow and a source of disappointment to palliative care activists.

Table 2.1 Pan-national associations and initiatives in hospice and palliative care

1973	International Association for the Study of Pain, founded Issaquah, Washington, USA
1976	First International Congress on the Care of the Terminally Ill, Montreal, Canada
1980	International Hospice Institute, became International Hospice Institute and College (1995) and International Association for Hospice and Palliative Care (1999)
1982	World Health Organization Cancer Pain Programme initiated
1988	European Association of Palliative Care founded in Milan, Italy
1990	Hospice Information Service, founded at St Christopher's Hospice, London, UK
1998	Poznan Declaration leads to the foundation of the Eastern and Central European Palliative Task Force (1999)
1999	Foundation for Hospices in Sub-Saharan Africa founded in USA
2000	Latin American Association of Palliative Care founded
2001	Asia Pacific Hospice Palliative Care Network founded
2002	UK Forum for Hospice and Palliative Care Worldwide founded by Help the Hospices

Pioneers of first-wave hospice development and some of their second-generation successors worked to promote their work in many countries of the world, building increasingly on international networks of support and collaboration. The International Association for the Study of Pain was founded by John Bonica and associates in 1973 at an interdisciplinary meeting of 300 specialists, held in Issaquah, Washington. By 1998 it had 55 chapters on six continents.[3] In 1976, the First International Congress on the Care of the Terminally Ill was held in Montreal, and organized every 2 years thereafter by Balfour Mount and colleagues. In 1980, Josefina Magno and others formed the International Hospice Institute; in 1995 it evolved into the International Hospice Institute and College, and in 1999 became the International Association for Hospice and Palliative Care (Woodruff *et al.* 2001; Bruera *et al.* 2002). In 1982, the World Health Organization Cancer Pain Programme began to develop, under the leadership of Jan Stjernswärd, and was to promulgate the three-step analgesic ladder for cancer pain relief (Swerdlow and Stjernswärd 1982), the influence of which quickly spread to dozens of countries. In 1988, the European Association for Palliative Care was formed in Milan, Italy, and Vittorio Ventafridda became its first President the following year (Blumhuber *et al.* 2002). In 1990, the Hospice Information Service, based at St Christopher's Hospice in London, began its newsletter, *Hospice Bulletin*, which quickly became a source of information on hospice innovation around the world (Saunders 2000). In 1999, the Eastern and Central European Palliative Task Force (ECEPT) came into being at a congress held in Geneva (Luczak and Kluziak 2001); building on the tenets of the Poznan Declaration (1999), it aimed to gather data on hospice and palliative care in the region, share experiences of achievements and obstacles, influence the institutions of government, set standards to meet local needs and raise awareness. The Foundation for Hospices in Sub-Saharan Africa was established in 1999 to serve hospice developments in the region (FHSSA 2002). In the new millennium, the year 2000 saw the creation of the Latin American Association of Palliative Care. In 2001, the Asia Pacific Hospice Palliative Care Network was founded, representing 14 countries (Goh 2002). Next came the UK Forum for Hospice and Palliative Care Worldwide, which became operational in 2002, with aims to coordinate the work of relevant groups in the UK, to support education, to advocate, to provide information and to raise funds (Richardson *et al.* 2002). A 1999 listing of palliative care organizations with a global perspective (Speck 1999) also includes British Aid for Hospices Abroad, Global Cancer Concern, the Hospice Education Institute and the WHO Collaborating Centre for Palliative Cancer Care, Oxford; other WHO collaborating centres have also been established in Milan, Wisconsin and Saitama.

In relation to services on the ground, according to the UK group Hospice Information,[4] it is estimated that in 2002 hospice or palliative care initiatives existed, or were under development on every continent of the world, in around 100 countries. The total number of hospice or palliative care initiatives was in excess of 8000 and these included in-patient units, hospital-based services, community-based teams, day care centres and other modes of delivery. Such a picture must be set against the stark realities of global need for palliative care at the beginning of the twenty-first century: 56 million deaths per year, with an estimated 60 per cent who could benefit from some form of palliative care (Stjernswärd and Clark 2003). A substantial literature on national developments in hospice and palliative care records important achievements and many developments in the face of adversity, together with a large agenda of 'unfinished business' (Stjernswärd and Clark 2003).

Hospice services in the USA grew dramatically from the founding organization in New Haven in 1974 to some 3000 providers by the end of the twentieth century. In 1982, a major milestone was the achievement of funding recognition for hospices under the Medicare programme. Several key developments occurred in the 1990s. National representative bodies appeared to take a more professionalized approach to their activities, giving greater emphasis to palliative care as a specialized field of activity (the National Hospice Association became the National Hospice and Palliative Care Association; the American Academy of Hospice Physicians became the American Academy of Hospice and Palliative Medicine). At the same time, two major foundations developed extensive programmes concerned with improving the culture of end-of-life care in American society (the Robert Wood Johnson Foundation created the Last Acts initiative; the Open Society Institute established the Project on Death in America). Meanwhile, in neighbouring Canada, where Balfour Mount first coined the term 'palliative care' in 1974 (Mount 1997), a Senate report in 2000 stated that no extension of palliative care provision had occurred in the previous 5 years, and set out recommendations for further development among the country's 600 services (Carstairs and Chochinov 2001). In Latin America, there was evidence of faltering progress, with palliative care services existing in seven countries, and the greatest amount of development in Argentina (de Lima 2001). A chief problem here, as in other developing regions, was the problem of poor opioid availability, an issue being addressed by the World Health Organization and highlighted in the 1994 Declaration of Florianopolis (Stjernswärd *et al.* 1995).

The first evidence of hospice developments in the Asia Pacific region came with a service for dying patients in Korea, at the Calvary Hospice of Kangung, established by the Catholic Sisters of the Little Company of Mary, in 1965; services had increased to 60 by 1999 (Chung 2000). In Japan, the first hospice was also Christian, established in the Yodogwa Christian Hospital in 1973; by the end of the century, the country had 80 in-patient units (Maruyama 1999). In Australia, the country that established the world's first chair in palliative care, commonwealth and state funds for palliative care increased steadily from 1980 and palliative medicine was recognized as a specialty in 2000; by 2002, there were 250 designated palliative care services (Hunt *et al.* 2002). Protocols for the WHO three-step analgesic ladder were first introduced into China in 1991 and there were said to be hundreds of palliative care services in urban areas by 2002 (Wang *et al.* 2002). In India, with one-sixth of the world's population, palliative care developments were again patchy, with only 100 services across the country by 2000 (Burn 2001) and with ongoing problems of opioid availability in some states (Joranson *et al.* 2002), but also with an outstanding demonstration project in Kerala reaching large numbers through out-patient clinics and home care visits (Rajagopal 2002).

The first hospice in Africa was founded in 1980, in Zimbabwe, and seems to have been largely modelled along British lines (Williams 2000); it continues to be the main source of palliative care in the country and efforts to influence the public health care system have been largely unsuccessful. By contrast, in Uganda, where a hospice was first founded in 1993, there is evidence of a widespread training programme, of impact upon government health policy in favour of opioid availability and recognition of palliative care as an essential clinical service (Jagwe 2002; Merriman 2002). The whole of Sub-Saharan Africa, however, faces a level of unprecedented palliative care need brought about by the epidemic of HIV/AIDS. Almost three-quarters of all cases of HIV infection in the world are found in this region, with 29.4 million out of a total of 42 million worldwide (Stjernswärd and Clark 2003).

In the former communist countries of Eastern Europe and Central Asia, there were few palliative care developments in the years of Soviet domination. Most initiatives can be traced to the early 1990s, after which many projects got underway. These have been documented in detail (Clark and Wright 2002) and show evidence of some service provision in 23 of 28 countries in the region. Poland and Russia have the most advanced programmes of palliative care, with considerable achievements also made in Romania and

Hungary. Nevertheless, in a region of over 400 million people, there were just 467 palliative care services in 2002, more than half of which were found in just one country, Poland.

Palliative care developments in Western Europe made rapid progress from the early 1980s, but by the late 1990s there were still striking differences in provision across different states (ten Have and Clark 2002). After the foundation of St Christopher's as the first modern hospice in England, in 1967, it was to be another 10 years before services began to appear elsewhere: in Sweden (1977), Italy (1980), Germany (1983), Spain (1984), Belgium (1985) and the Netherlands (1991). In all of these countries, the provision of palliative care has moved beyond isolated examples of pioneering services run by enthusiastic founders. Palliative care is being delivered in a variety of settings (domiciliary, quasi-domiciliary and institutional), though these are not given uniform priority everywhere.

Conclusions

Within the professional lifetime of the founders of the modern hospice movement, a remarkable proliferation of service provision and related activity had occurred. At the same time, the definition of hospice and palliative care came into sharper focus, with ongoing debates and discussions about the place of the care of those with advanced disease within the wider organization of health care systems in the modern world.

In the early decades of development, modern hospice and palliative care in the West had many of the qualities of a social movement supported by wider forces: consumerism and increasing discernment among the users of health and social care services; demographic trends that created substantial numbers of individuals able to volunteer their labour in local hospices; and greater affluence, which led to an increase in charitable giving. This movement may well have contributed to a new openness about death and bereavement that was in evidence in the late twentieth century (one of the first persons ever to be seen to die on television, for example, was in the care of an Irish 'hospice at home service'). Inspired by charismatic leadership, it was a movement that condemned the neglect of the dying in society, called for high-quality pain and symptom management for all who needed it, sought to reconstruct death as a natural phenomenon rather than a clinical failure, and marshalled practical and moral argument to oppose those in favour of euthanasia. Indeed, for Cicely Saunders and her followers, such work served as a measure of the very worth of our culture: 'A society which shuns the dying must have an incomplete philosophy' (Saunders 1961: 3).

At the same time, other interests were at work. In several countries, including Britain, Australia, Canada and the USA, professional recognition of this emerging area of expertise seemed desirable. Specialty recognition occurred first in Britain, in 1987, and was seen by some as a turning point in hospice history (James and Field 1992). It was part of a wider shift away from 'terminal' and 'hospice' care towards the concept of palliative care. Today, 'modernizers' claim that specialization, the integration of palliative care into the mainstream health system, and the development of an 'evidence-based' model of practice and organization are crucial to long-term viability. Yet others mourn the loss of early ideals and regret what they perceive to be an emphasis upon physical symptoms at the expense of psychosocial and spiritual concerns. In short, there have been assertions that forces of 'medicalization' and 'routinization' are at work, or even that the putative 'holism' of palliative care philosophy masks a new, more subtle form of surveillance of the dying and bereaved in modern society (Clark and Seymour 1999). Perhaps it is more helpful to see the rise of modern palliative care as creating and then colonizing a space somewhere between the hope of cure and the acceptance of death – a view of the response to life-threatening illness that is more consistent with the concerns and perspectives of patients in late modern culture (Clark 2002b).

By the end of the twentieth century, two forces for expansion were also clearly visible in the new specialty. First, there was the impetus to move palliative care further upstream in the disease progression, thereby seeking integration with curative and rehabilitation therapies and shifting the focus beyond terminal care and the final stages of life. Second, there was a growing interest in extending the benefits of palliative care to those with diseases other than cancer to make 'palliative care for all' a reality. The new specialty was therefore delicately poised. For some, such integration with the wider system was a *sine qua non* for success; for others, it marked the entry into a risky phase of new development in which early ideals might be compromised.

Hospice care and palliative care have a shared and brief history. The evolution of one into the other marks a transition, which, if successful, could ensure that the benefits of a model of care previously available to just a few people at the end of life will in time be extended to all who need it, regardless of diagnosis, stage of disease, social situation or means. As the field of palliative care matures, so too our knowledge of its history is deepening and widening. What emerges is a rich field of innovation, taking place in different forms in many varied settings. Out of this has emerged the potential not only to relieve individual suffering at the end of life, but also to transform the social dimensions of dying, death and bereavement in the modern world.

Notes

1   http://www.hospice-history.org.uk.
2   Sister Mary Eucharia (undated) The apostolate of Rose Hawthorne, pp. 46–9. Pamphlet article, source unknown.
3   http://www.library.ucla.edu/libraries/biomed/his/painexhibit/panel10.htm.
4   http://www.hospiceinformation.info/hospicesworldwide.asp.

References

Blumhuber, H., Kaasa, S. and de Conno, F. (2002) The European Association for Palliative Care. *Journal of Pain and Symptom Management*, 24(2): 124–7.

Brown, O. (1894) *On the Care of the Dying: A Lecture to Nurses*. London: George Allen.

Bruera, E., de Lima, L. and Woodruff, R. (2002) The International Association for Hospice and Palliative Care. *Journal of Pain and Symptom Management*, 24(2): 102–5.

Burn, G. (2001) A personal initiative to improve palliative care in India: ten years on. *Palliative Medicine*, 15: 159–62.

Carstairs, S. and Chochinov, H. (2001) Politics, palliation and Canadian progress in end-of-life care. *Journal of Palliative Medicine*, 4(3): 369–96.

Chung, Y. (2000) Palliative care in Korea: a nursing point of view. *Progress in Palliative Care*, 2000, 8(1): 12–16.

Clark, D. (1997) Someone to watch over me: Cicely Saunders and St Christopher's Hospice. *Nursing Times*, 26 August, pp. 50–1.

Clark, D. (1998) Originating a movement: Cicely Saunders and the Development of St Christopher's Hospice, 1957–67. *Mortality*, 3(1): 43–63.

Clark, D. (1999a) Cradle to the grave? Preconditions for the hospice movement in the UK, 1948–67. *Mortality*, 4(3): 225–47.

Clark, D. (1999b) 'Total pain', disciplinary power and the body in the work of Cicely Saunders 1958–67. *Social Science and Medicine*, 49(6): 727–36.

Clark, D. (2000) Palliative care history: ritual process. *European Journal of Palliative Care*, 7(2): 50–5.

Clark, D. (2001a) Religion, medicine and community in the early origins of St Christopher's Hospice. *Journal of Palliative Medicine*, 4(3): 353–60.

Clark, D. (2001b) A special relationship: Cicely Saunders, the United States and the early foundations of the modern hospice movement. *Illness, Crisis and Loss*, 9(1): 15–30.

Clark, D. (2002a) *Cicely Saunders, Founder of the Hospice Movement: Selected Letters 1959–1999*. Oxford: Oxford University Press.

Clark, D. (2002b) Between hope and acceptance: the medicalisation of dying. *British Medical Journal*, 324: 905–7.

Clark, D. and Seymour, J. (1999) *Reflections on Palliative Care*. Buckingham: Open University Press.

Clark, D. and Wright, M. (2002) *Transitions in End of Life Care: Hospice and Related Developments in Eastern Europe and Central Asia*. Buckingham: Open University Press.

Dacre Craven, F.S. (1890) *A Guide to District Nurses and Home Nursing*. London: Macmillan.

De Lima, L. (2001) Advances in palliative care in Latin America and the Caribbean: ongoing projects of the Pan American Health Association (PAHO). *Journal of Palliative Medicine*, 4(2): 228–31.

Faull, C. and Nicholson, A. (2003) Taking the myths out of the magic: establishing the use of opioids in the management of cancer pain, in C. Bushnell and M. Meldrum (eds) *Opioids, the Janus Drugs, and the Relief of Pain*. Seattle, WA: IASP Press.

Foundation for Hospices in Sub-Saharan Africa (2002) *Challenging Times*. Liverpool, NY: FHSSA.

Goh, C.R. (2002) The Asia Pacific Hospice Palliative Care Network: a network for individuals and organisations. *Journal of Pain and Symptom Management*, 24(2): 128–33.

Granshaw, L. and Porter, R. (1989) *The Hospital in History*. London: Routledge.

Humphreys, C. (1999) 'Undying Spirits': religion, medicine and institutional care of the dying 1878–1938. Unpublished PhD thesis, University of Sheffield.

Humphreys, C. (2001) 'Waiting for the last summons': the establishment of the first hospices in England 1878–1914. *Mortality*, 6(2): 146–66.

Hunt, R., Fazekas, B.S., Luke, C.G., Priest, K.R. and Roder, D.M. (2002) The coverage of cancer patients by designated palliative services: a population-based study, South Australia, 1999. *Palliative Medicine*, 16: 403–9.

Jagwe, J.G.M. (2002) The introduction of palliative care in Uganda. *Journal of Palliative Medicine*, 5(1): 160–3.

James, N. and Field, D. (1992) The routinisation of hospice. *Social Science and Medicine*, 34(12): 1363–75.

Joranson, D.E., Rajagopal, M.R. and Gilson, A.M. (2002) Improving access to opioid analgesics for palliative care in India. *Journal of Pain and Symptom Management*, 24(2): 152–9.

Luczak, J. and Kluziak, M. (2001) The formation of ECEPT (Eastern and Central Europe Palliative Task Force): a Polish initiative. *Palliative Medicine*, 15: 259–60.

Maruyama, T.C. (1999) *Hospice Care and Culture*. Aldershot: Ashgate.

Merriman, A. (2002) Uganda: current status of palliative care. *Journal of Pain and Symptom Management*, 24(2): 252–6.

Mount, B. (1997) The Royal Victoria Hospital Palliative Care Service: a Canadian experience, in C. Saunders and R. Kastenbaum (eds) *Hospice Care on the International Scene*. New York: Springer.

Munk, W. (1887) *Euthanasia: Or Medical Treatment in Aid of an Easy Death*. London: Longmans, Green & Co.

Poznan Declaration 1998 (1999) *European Journal of Palliative Care*, 6: 61–3.

Rajagopal, M.R. (2002) Kerala, India: status of cancer pain relief and palliative care. *Journal of Pain and Symptom Management*, 24(2): 191–3.

Richardson, H., Praill, D. and Jackson, A. (2002) The UK Forum for Hospice and Palliative Care Overseas. *European Journal of Palliative Care*, 9(2): 72–3.

Saunders, C. (1958) Dying of cancer. *St Thomas's Hospital Gazette*, 56(2): 37–47.

Saunders, C. (1960a) *Care of the Dying*. London: Nursing Times Reprint.

Saunders, C. (1960b) Drug treatment in the terminal stages of cancer. *Current Medicine and Drugs*, 1(1): 16–28.

Saunders, C. (1961) 'And from sudden death . . .'. *Frontier*, Winter, pp. 1–3.

Saunders, C. (1964) Care of patients suffering from terminal illness at St Joseph's Hospice, Hackney, London. *Nursing Mirror*, 14 February, pp. vii–x.

Saunders, C. (2000) Global developments and the Hospice Information Service (editorial). *Palliative Medicine*, 14: 1–2.

Snow, H. (1890a) *The Palliative Treatment of Incurable Cancer: With an Appendix on the Use of the Opium Pipe*. London: J. & A. Churchill.

Snow, H. (1890b) *On the Re-appearance (Recurrence) of Cancer After Apparent Extirpation, with Suggestions for its Prevention*. London: J. & A. Churchill.

Snow, H. (1896) Opium and cocaine in the treatment of cancerous disease. *British Medical Journal*, 19 September, pp. 718–19.

Snow, H. (1897) The opium–cocaine treatment of malignant disease (letter). *British Medical Journal*, 17 April, p. 1019.

Speck, P. (1999) Palliative care organisations with a global perspective. *Palliative Medicine*, 13: 69–74.

Stjernswärd, J. and Clark, D. (2003) Palliative care – a global perspective, in G. Hanks, D. Doyle, C. Calman and N. Cherny (eds) *Oxford Textbook of Palliative Medicine*, 3rd edn. Oxford: Oxford University Press.

Stjernswärd, J., Bruera, E., Joranson, D. *et al.* (1995) Opioid availability in Latin America: The Declaration of Florianopolis. *Journal of Pain and Symptom Management*, 10(3): 233–6.

Swerdlow, M. and Stjernswärd, J. (1982) Cancer pain relief – an urgent public health problem. *World Health Forum*, 3: 329.

ten Have, H. and Clark, D. (2002) *The Ethics of Palliative Care: European Perspectives*. Buckingham: Open University Press.

Wang, X.S., Yu, S., Gu, W. and Xu, G. (2002) China: status of pain and palliative care. *Journal of Pain and Symptom Management*, 24(2): 177–9.

Williams, S. (2000) Zimbabwe. *Palliative Medicine*, 14: 225–6.

Woodruff, R., Doyle, D., de Lima, L., Bruera, E. and Farr, W.C. (2001) The International Association for Hospice and Palliative Care (IAHPC): history, description and future direction. *Journal of Palliative Medicine*, 4(1): 5–7.

Worcester, A. (1935) *The Care of the Aged, the Dying and the Dead*. Springfield, IL: Charles C. Thomas.

3

What's in a name?

A concept analysis of key terms in palliative care nursing

Jane Seymour

This chapter focuses on the core concepts used to describe palliative care nursing. It explores the different meanings attached to these, their roots and their implications for current practice. In so doing, it draws upon literature from the fields of palliative care, nursing, feminist studies, sociology, history and ethics. In thinking about *which* concepts to discuss in this chapter, it seemed appropriate to seek some definitions or descriptions of 'palliative care nursing' and to attempt to identify the core concepts within these. In the UK, possibly the first introduction of the term 'palliative nursing' was in 1989 by a specialist interest group of the Royal College of Nursing, the Palliative Nursing Group. This group now represents specialist palliative care nurses in the UK, the majority of whom care for patients suffering from cancer. There has been extensive discussion of the role of clinical nurse specialists in palliative care (see, for example, Seymour *et al.* 2002), and it is not the intention of this chapter to review these debates, especially since most patients with palliative care needs are cared for by nurses who are not clinical nurse specialists. Nor is it my intention to analyse the meaning of 'palliative care', since this is addressed elsewhere in this book. Rather, this chapter looks at how palliative care nursing is described in the literature and what commonalities may be identified.

One of the clearest descriptions of palliative care nursing is provided by Lugton and Kindlen, who note:

> all life threatening illnesses – be they cancer, neurological, cardiac or respiratory disease – have implications for the physical, social, psychological and spiritual health for both the individual and their family. The role of palliative care nursing is therefore to assess needs in each of these areas and to plan, implement and evaluate appropriate interventions. It aims to improve the quality of life and to enable a dignified death.

(Lugton and Kindlen 1999: 2)

Lugton and Kindlen go on to note the importance of teamwork in palliative care nursing, observing that an overarching aim is to 'support patients and their families, wherever they may be – hospital, home or hospice' (p. 3). Clearly, the relief of suffering may be understood as the overarching role of the palliative care nurse (Morse and Johnson 1991), but within this key descriptors of the role of the nurse in palliative care can be identified. Research conducted during the 1990s in the USA produced the following:[1]

- 'support' and 'valuing' (Davis and O'Berle 1990, 1992);
- 'continuous knowing' (Dobratz 1990);
- 'fostering hope' (Herth 1990; Rittman *et al.* 1997);
- 'providing comfort' (Degner *et al.* 1991);
- 'providing empathy' (Raudonis 1993);
- 'being there' (Cohen and Sarter 1992; Steeves *et al.* 1994).

Since these early studies, research has been conducted outside the USA into the roles and aims of palliative care nursing. I have chosen to focus on three examples from different parts of the world, although I touch on related work in each case. In the UK, Luker *et al.* (2000) conducted interviews with 62 members of a district nursing team to determine which factors respondents believed contributed to good palliative care for patients under their care. 'Getting to know' the patient and the family emerged as an essential basis for good quality palliative care. This was achieved through spending time in patients' homes, adopting a friendly manner, paying attention to the importance of good quality communication, ensuring continuity of care and paying attention to individual needs beyond the purely physical. 'Getting to know' patients and their relatives and carers was contingent upon having time to build a good relationship with them and was aided by early referral to community nursing services. Drawing on the work of Radwin (1996), Luker *et al.* (2000) conclude that these elements constitute a model for palliative care nursing which closely resembles that 'espoused in "new nursing", which embraces a holistic approach to care and acknowledges the individuality of patients and the uniqueness of their needs' (p. 781).

Rasmussen *et al.* (1995) provide an interesting phenomenological study of 19 hospice nurses in Sweden who were asked to narrate their reasons for becoming hospice nurses, and their hopes for their future work in the field. The findings from this study mirror closely those outlined above. Thus nurses expressed an overarching concern with being able to provide a dignified death for dying patients[2] and spending time getting to know patients and their families was seen as essential. Nurses placed a priority on caring for the whole human being and believed that this was best achieved through the use of self and in the context of collaborative efforts to build a supportive and caring hospice environment.

A study in Australia by Kristjanson *et al.* (2001), which sought to describe how 20 palliative care nurses perceived good or bad deaths among their patients, highlighted that nurses prioritized patients' comfort and dignity, and made efforts to protect and enhance the relationships between patients and their families. Successful teamwork and good team communication was regarded as critical to achieving a good death. The importance of comfort during the terminal phase was highlighted in a study by Low and Payne (1996) of palliative care professionals' perceptions of good and bad deaths in the UK, and this was also a theme in hospice nurses' accounts of death reported by McNamara *et al.* (1994).

From this selective review, a number of concepts that have been used to define palliative nursing can be identified (see Box 3.1). Of these, 'teamwork', 'suffering', 'quality of life' and 'hope' have been written about extensively in the wider palliative care literature and beyond. This discussion, therefore, will turn shortly to the remaining concepts ('knowing the patient', 'dignity', 'comfort', 'empathy' and 'support'), which are less well analysed and which, arguably, are more closely linked to the areas of palliative care in which nurses claim to make a special, and perhaps unique, contribution. I want though, at this point, to pause for a moment and to extend the discussion beyond these individual concepts to the overarching concept of 'caring'. Of all concepts, 'caring' is perhaps the fundamental element of palliative care nursing. Yet it is relatively poorly articulated in the nursing literature. As this review of selected research shows, much attention has been directed at identifying *components* of palliative nursing care, rather than exploring what 'care' and 'caring' consist of.

Box 3.1   Key concepts associated with palliative care nursing

- 'Knowing the patient'
- Teamwork
- Dignity
- Comfort
- Empathy
- Support and 'supportive care'
- Hope
- Suffering
- Quality of life

Caring

The most detailed and critical analyses available of the concept of caring are in the field of feminist studies, which emerged in the early 1970s and 1980s. The important distinction between 'caring for' and 'caring about' is highlighted and the gendered aspects of informal care-giving are described and debated (Twigg 1993; Nolan *et al.* 1996). Davies (1995) presents a valuable overview of the overlaps between 'care-giving', 'carework' and 'professional care', observing that the 'fusion of labour and love is frustratingly diffuse,

[and] hard to capture by means of the usual apparatus of definition and measurement in the disciplines of psychology, sociology and social policy (p. 140). As Davies observes, while informal carers find it difficult to put into words exactly what is involved in care-giving, the physical tasks associated with it are readily discernible and therefore easy to evaluate. Similarly with the professional care-giving provided by nurses. However, 'caring', whether by informal carers or nurses, has other elements beyond physical 'care-giving' that are less well understood. Caring does not involve specific tasks but depends upon a quality and type of sustained relationship. This involves 'attending, physically, mentally and emotionally to the needs of another and giving commitment to the nurturance, growth and healing of another' (Davies 1995: 141). In palliative care nursing, opportunities for sustained relationships with patients are frequent and will often involve very high levels of emotion. For many palliative care nurses, the link between themselves and their patient will end only when that person dies, and this may occur many months, if not years, after their first meeting. A key issue for palliative care nurses, then, is how to contain powerful emotions while at the same time nurturing the type of caring relationship with their patients described by Davies.

Developing the work of Hochschild (1983), James (1989) employs the term 'emotional labour' to account for the manner in which hospice nurses manage emotions associated with caring in such a way as to allow themselves the 'space' to continue with their normal work routines and the demands of their particular working environment. Emotional labour, suggests James, acts as a form of regulation of emotional expression yet also, paradoxically, facilitates the emotional expression that is so necessary for the accomplishment of the caring that attends 'good' nursing. The chapter by Sanchia Aranda in this book, 'The cost of caring: surviving the culture of niceness, occupational stress and coping strategies', sheds further light on the emotional labour with which specialist palliative care nurses and the multidisciplinary team engage, suggesting that 'the capacity to maintain a balance between making a difference and accepting the limitations of what can be achieved requires a significant level of self and team awareness'.

An interesting example of the links between emotional labour and painstaking physical care-giving in a non-specialist palliative care setting is provided by Simpson (1997). Simpson describes how intensive care nurses use emotional expression as a means of overcoming 'the dehumanizing aspects of dying in a technological environment' (p. 189) and to allow the 're-connection' of patients with their families. Simpson argues that this process of re-connection, in which emotional expression and investment by nurses plays such an important role, underpins the breakdown of barriers between the dying person and his or her companions, *and* plays a central role in the development of trust between companions and clinical staff. Simpson implies that bodily care-giving, which she calls 'basic care', is an integral aspect of 're-connection' by which means nurses are able to prepare families for the death of the patient: 'Basic care was continued to ensure that the patient was well cared for, again as much for the benefit of the family as the patient. The nurses attempted to provide privacy for the family, to answer their questions and to "be there" for the family' (Simpson 1997: 195).

The link between 'care-giving' and 'caring' in intensive care has also been observed in a study of how intensive care nurses care for dying patients and their families:

> physical care and careful presentation of the body apparently becomes the means of affirming the individuality of the dying person. Such bodily attention appears to be central to nurses' attempts to portray to companions the social worth of dying people: individuals whom nurses have often never 'known' as conscious beings. Further, it becomes the means by which nurses themselves *relate to* their patients as subjective individuals and the way in which their relationships with patients' companions are sustained.
>
> (Seymour 2003: 333–4; emphasis in original)

Drawing on an account by Tisdale (1986), Bowden (1997) observes that part of the emotional labour of caring in nursing is learning how to 'tread lightly' between the opposite poles of 'burdensome emotional identification and that severance from the person in pain that creates a schism in the nurse's experience' (p. 112). Arguably, this is the essential moral and ethical problem that besets nurses working in palliative care, and one which is least adequately addressed. However, where the balance between these poles is successful, the emotional and physical acts of caring offer nurses the opportunity to protect and enhance the dignity of their patients and patients' families.

Dignity

'Dignity' is a concept applied very frequently to describe an idealized 'good death'. De Raeve (1996: 71), writing about the links between 'death with dignity' and 'good death', notes that we need to think carefully and reflectively about the term 'dignity' in order to move away from prevalent 'crude images' of the good death in which people are manoeuvred through predetermined 'stages'. She suggests that we consider 'dignity' in terms of its contribution as a quality or aspect of nursing care given to people who are seriously ill or dying, and whose sense of innate dignity or personal, spiritual and physical integrity may be under threat:

> what sense can be made of the idea of death with dignity? Could it escape the good death straitjacket by being construed not as a manner of dying but as a way of treating the dying? Dying and seriously ill people perhaps deserve to be treated with dignity in such a way as to try to preserve the dignity that they have and help them regain the sense of dignity that feels lost.
>
> (De Raeve 1996: 71)

If we accept De Raeve's observation, then it is necessary to consider what treating someone with dignity entails and what nursing practices maintain or compromise dignity. In a phenomenological study with patients and nurses in a hospital, Walsh and Kowanko (2002) show that nurses and patients agree on the key elements of dignity and the sorts of nursing care practices that support or detract from it (see Box 3.2). In both nurses' and patients' accounts in this study, the body, its treatment and its exposure were central themes, with maintenance of privacy being inextricably linked to perceptions of respect, consideration and personhood. Threats to dignity were perceived to emanate from a neglectful attitude to patients and their bodies; for example, where nurses forgot, or saw others forget, to extend ordinary everyday civilities to their patients (such as a greeting or polite request to enter a room) that are taken for granted outside of the health care system. Incursions of this type, which may seem relatively trivial, were seen to lead to more fundamental breaches of personhood, such as being left exposed to view, or not having one's permission asked before medical students witnessed embarrassing procedures, or having one's feelings disregarded.

Box 3.2 Elements of 'dignity' identified by nurses and patients (adapted from Walsh and Kowanko 2002)

Nurses' descriptions of dignity	Patients' descriptions of dignity
Privacy of the body	Not being exposed
Private space	Being treated with discretion
Consideration of emotions	Consideration
Giving time	Having time/not being rushed
The patient as a person	Being seen as a person
The body as an object	The body as an object
Showing respect	Being acknowledged
Giving control	Having time to decide
Advocacy	

Protection of dignity in the simple ways that Walsh and Kowanko (2002) describe is central to the palliative care approach (NCHSPCS 2001), and other recent studies confirm that the preservation of dignity is a prime issue for patients with palliative care needs and their carers. For example, Rogers *et al.* (2000) analysed the qualitative comments appended to questionnaires by 138 carers whose views were surveyed on the care their deceased relatives received in hospital during the last year of their lives. They found that, while overall ratings of satisfaction with services were good, specific sources of dissatisfaction related to feelings of being devalued, dehumanized or disempowered. A loss of dignity in relation to physical care needs was a prime cause of complaint and appeared to occur when 'bureaucratic imperatives appeared to override individual patients' needs' (Rogers *et al.* 2000: 771).

Picking up this theme of bureaucratic imperatives, Walsh and Kowanko (2002) note the powerful way in which structural and environmental influences make it hard for nurses to treat patients as people all of the time. They observe how the 'system', and how it militates against maintaining patients' and nurses' dignity, has been an enduring theme in commentaries about health and health care. Within these commentaries, objectification of the patient is seen as a strategy with which nurses engage to protect themselves from personal involvement in situations where they are relatively powerless to influence patients' treatment or inexorable progress through the bureaucracy of health care (see, for example, Menzies 1970). Maintaining patients' dignity is perhaps especially difficult in the context of the complex and paradoxical nature of demands facing contemporary health care professionals who have the responsibility for the treatment and care of dying people in an era of rapid change and scarce nursing resources. It is important to understand, therefore, as De Raeve (1996) observes, that preservation of dignity does not only depend on the type of social interaction nurses have with ill people and their carers. It also depends upon institutional structures, managerial cultures and social policies that allow nurses to value the work that they do and thus care for patients in ways that protects and enhances their dignity. To this extent, nurses who work in palliative care settings such as hospices are fortunate. Those aspects of patient care that are conducive to dignity are likely to be highly valued and nurses will frequently have been able to place emphasis on acquiring skills that help them to blend expert technical and physical aspects of nursing care and communication skills that are perceived to contribute to it.

Comfort

Comfort has been cited as a goal of nursing care for over a century and has been associated with 'surveillance, presence, empathy, touch and compassion as [a] critical component[s] of nursing care' (Walker 2002: 43). McIlveen and Morse (1995), in a content analysis of textbooks and articles written by nurses during the twentieth century, observe that while comfort as an aim of care has always been significant for nursing, the term has undergone various interpretations. In the early years of the twentieth century, 'comfort' denoted primarily physical strategies that contributed to physical and emotional comfort, such as the positioning or cleanliness of the patient. McIlveen and Morse (1995) note that during these early years there was a strong belief that the provision of comfort by physical care could enable patients to benefit more fully from their medical therapy. This link was strengthened when more medical treatments became available, through developments in pharmacology and improved understanding of how best to administer morphine to relieve severe pain. However, McIlveen and Morse (1995) state that, as a consequence of such developments, there was a trend for nursing interventions to be subordinated to, and dependent upon, medical techniques for relieving pain and suffering, with the relief of pain seen as of overarching importance. Between 1960 and the 1990s, improvements in nursing education and wider cultural changes produced an emphasis on the role of communication and psychological care strategies in comfort. In this way, nurses' comforting role became confirmed as far more than just that associated with medical treatments and physical care-giving:

> Expectations changed from the nurse merely cheering the patient up with diverting conversation, to direct discussion of the patient's condition (Knowles 1962) – a taboo in earlier days. Use of interpersonal and communication skills such as listening (Brogden 1966), reflecting and restating meaning (Craytor 1969), empathy (Brogden 1966) and expression of feelings (Knowles 1962) came in to use as part of comforting . . . this new attitude toward patient interaction seemed to reflect an involvement of patients in their own care, a change from the previous period when the nurse was expected to take responsibility away from the patient.
>
> (McIlveen and Morse 1995: 141–2)

It is within this context of wider changes in nursing and medical care that palliative nursing emerged and has been enabled to flourish, with its explicit emphasis on the combined importance of physical, emotional and spiritual comfort. Particular challenges are involved in bringing comfort to patients suffering from advanced disease and who may have symptoms that are difficult to control or severe emotional or existential distress. The provision of comfort by relieving or ameliorating such problems is a foundational principle of palliative care nursing, such that the term 'comfort care' has become synonymous with a wider cultural understanding of the transfer from care focused on cure to that focused on patient and family comfort as dying approaches. However, as Aranda (1998) notes, such an understanding rests on the assumption that full relief of symptoms and distress is possible, that patients *want* the measures necessary to provide this relief and that they regard nurses as well placed to be their 'comforters'.

With regard to the issue of the extent to which the relief of suffering is *possible*, the debates about the role of 'palliative' or 'terminal sedation' (Broeckaert and Nunez Olarte 2002), in which dying people in acute and enduring distress are kept deeply asleep until death occurs, are examples of one area where the amount of 'comfort' produced by palliative care practices is hotly disputed. A key debate is whether such a practice amounts to 'slow euthanasia' (Billings and Block 1996), or should rather be seen as part of the physician's responsibility not to abandon patients and their families to unrelieved suffering during dying (Quill and Byock 2000). Here we see a contrast between the intentions of palliative care to bring about a comfortable, easeful death and the hidden consequences of changing technologies such that the means to procure 'comfort' potentially becomes surrounded by moral and legal risks of an unprecedented nature.

Turning to the issue of whether patients *want* care that emphasizes comfort, while acknowledging that it is never an 'either–or' choice between comfort or interventionist treatment, there is some evidence both from the UK (Johnson *et al.* 1990) and the USA that some patients with palliative care needs reject care that emphasizes comfort rather than length of life, especially if they have little prognostic information on which to base their choice. In the USA, there is evidence from the SUPPORT study (Principal Investigators for the SUPPORT Project 1995), in which the care received by 9000 severely ill patients from five US hospitals was monitored, that many patients wanted high-technology interventions since they feared that the alternative of comfort care may lead to physicians giving up hope of cure prematurely. Nurses in palliative care will be centrally involved in such issues, and may often argue that they are best placed to make informed judgements about the 'best interests' of patients who can no longer speak for themselves. Critical care is one area where the role of the nurse in 'comfort care' is particularly visible. Puntillo notes that as patients approach death in intensive care:

> Critical care nurses play a major role in setting goals related to comfort care. They are unique health care providers for patients because they are frequently with patients for up to 12 hours each day or night. Generally, and optimally, they are in a position to care for a particular patient over a period of time and have learned to 'know' the patient and the patient's family. They are the major providers of comfort for critically ill patients at *all* times. Therefore it is imperative that critical care nurses advocate for when they believe, and the patient's conditions indicate, that comfort care should be the primary goal for this patient. Thus a primary nursing activity is to be present during team and family discussions of the patient. The nurses should be direct, clear and assertive in their communications with physicians and other health care providers.
>
> (Puntillo 2001: 151)

To this extent, we can see that 'comfort', in the sense of the focus and aims of care for people with palliative care needs, moves beyond what nurses can *do* for patients to become associated with how nurses interrelate and communicate with clinical colleagues and to what extent they are able (and allowed) to influence the character of care given to patients. 'Comfort' in this sense thus becomes bound up with issues of professional boundaries, professional power and 'team working'. As Puntillo notes, this may involve nurses making particular claims about expertise based on knowing the patient and his or her family. It may also resonate with nurses' feelings about the work that they do. Thus, Wurzbach (1996), in a study of 15 nurses working in long-term care, reports that the nurses' ability to provide comfort depended on their own feelings of 'moral comfort' with medical decisions about patients, the resources available to achieve care goals and the extent to which they felt able to act as patient advocates. To this extent, 'comfort' may be seen as a product of skilled nursing care together with the ability to access appropriate resources and to influence the decision-making process around individual patients: 'Many of these nurses described comfort as being both something they provide and something they feel when they believe they have met their practice ideal and the resident's needs' (Wurzbach 1996: 262).

Whether patients always *want* and *expect* nurses to be cast in the role of comforter, or advocate, and how they understand the proper role of nursing with regard to the these issues is not clear. Skilbeck and Payne (2003) draw together some evidence (e.g. von Essen and Sjoden 1991; Larsson *et al.* 1998) that suggests that patients' and nurses' views differ about the provision of emotional support, which is an important aspect of comforting, with patients more likely to place importance on nurses' technical skills and knowledge, abilities to provide reliable information and to anticipate needs than on their emotionally supportive interventions. Similarly, care-giving directed at comfort is believed to be more important than psycho-emotional care by the close families of terminally ill patients (Hull 1989), reflecting the link between 'caring' and 'care-giving' observed in intensive care and discussed above.

A useful concept for understanding the links between and fluctuating importance of the various aspects of comfort may be that of 'total comfort'. This term is used by Morse *et al.* (1994) to describe the myriad activities with which nurses engage when looking after severely ill patients, and how nurses can potentially help patients whose bodies may be irrevocably altered by illness and its treatments to adjust to living 'in the world in a new way without being dominated by [their] body' (p. 194). Developing the theme of the relationship between care-giving and caring, and effectively providing a definition of 'palliation', Morse *et al.* observe that nurses'

> sensitive comfort work . . . provides patients who are overwhelmed by the pain of fatigue, exhaustion and illness with the opportunity to forget (or at least to decrease their attention toward) their bodies and be connected to the world again in a familiar way, to be comfortable. Comfort, for patients, is the bridge to life and to living (Botoroff 1991). It is achieved when the provision of treatments and support provide opportunities to function as normally as possible . . . and the diseased or injured body becomes a body that functions with varying degrees of ease once again.
>
> (Morse *et al.* 1994: 194)

Knowing the patient

Tanner *et al.* (1993), writing about nursing knowledge, trace a development that takes place during the acquisition of nursing expertise. This results in the discourse of 'knowing the patient' and is defined as:

> a reference to how they [nurses] understood the patient, grasped the meaning of the situation for the patient, or recognized the need for a particular action. In expert nursing practice this kind of knowing is very different from the formalized, explicit, decontextualized data-based

knowledge that constitutes formal assessments, yet it is central to skilled nursing judgment.

(Tanner *et al.* 1993: 73)

As May (1995) observes, threaded throughout the debates in the nursing literature about 'knowing the patient' is an assumption that this is an essential prerequisite for 'providing nursing care in a more enlightened and humane way' (p. 83). Drawing on Armstrong (e.g. 1987), May charts how nursing has reconstructed the meaning of patienthood: from a passive object of medical attention to a person with a valid experience of illness and the ability to engage actively with health care professionals in addressing that experience. This has had certain consequences for nursing practices, with enquiries into the 'private' world and character of the patient, involvement and an emphasis on protecting and nurturing patient autonomy becoming prerequisites for good care (May 1995: 84). As observed above, 'knowing' has, in this way, become bound inextricably with 'caring' and 'comfort' and 'emotional labour' in nursing discourse. May poses some critical questions about this discourse, noting that where it is used in a idealistic and unrealistic manner, it risks being seen as a set of prescriptive demands on nurses: demands that can never be achieved. May further argues that, although there is good evidence that patients' value nurses who make an effort to treat them as persons, such discourse fails to deal with the possibility of resistance:

> what if the patient does not see him/herself as an active collaborator, partner in care, or as an expert in his/her own health, or fails to see the realm of the psychosocial as one into which the nurse is legitimately entitled to intrude? Such a patient may actively resist the operation of the new nursing, and is easily categorised as non-compliant and maladaptive.
>
> (May 1995: 86)

Clearly, May's argument stands as a corrective to some of the more extreme elements in the nursing literature, and as a valuable reminder that nurses have no automatic rights of entry to patients' private thoughts and experiences. Arguably, however, his anxieties obscure the importance of understanding what occurs between nurses and their patients during 'nursing', how each perceive this, what aspects of that interaction are helpful or unhelpful, and in which contexts. In drawing our attention to how critical this issue is to palliative nursing, Lawler uses the metaphor of the 'captive' to describe the relationship between nurse and patient:

> The patient is captive in a dysfunctional and/or sick body or with an embodied problem and the nurse is captive with the patient, often for hours or days on end, or until death occurs. As captives, their worlds are necessarily brought together and focused on immediate concerns and on ways in which experiences can be endured and transcended. It is possible to understand some of these experiences, both for the patient and the nurse, within the conceptual and discursive space of captivity about

which we know little except so far as it relates to matters over which the state presides.

(Lawler 2002: 170)

What Lawler seems to be saying here, and indeed goes on to explain by way of drawing on her earlier work (Lawler 1991), is that nursing suffers from a 'gap' in understanding this 'captivity', and the relationships it engenders between nurse and patient, because nursing borrows from disciplines in which an emphasis is placed upon observable, material reality rather than felt, lived reality. This creates a disjuncture between 'the felt' and 'the seen', which nurses have little or no language to explain. As a result, the lived reality of nursing, in which feelings, emotions *and the doing of* nursing are most important, risks becoming subordinate to efforts to regulate and control nursing work according to concerns with 'cost-effectiveness' and 'efficiency' and with measured and objective assessment of the outcomes of nursing. Lawler gives the example of contrasting interpretations of what is occurring when nurses talk with patients. This could be seen by an observer as a potentially wasteful use of their employment, since it merely 'passes time' with patients.[3] Alternatively, for patients, 'talk' may be an essential part of their therapeutic environment, no less important than the drugs and other medical interventions of which they may be in receipt. The problem for nurses in communicating the value of nursing acts such as 'talk' is that

> much of nurses' business is like women's business – it is taken for granted, it is storied, it is grounded in experiential knowing . . . The knowledges of nursing itself are to be found in practising nursing, reflecting on it, and coming to understand ways of being which inhere in the relationships between nurse, patient and contexts in which nursing occurs.

(Lawler 2002: 185)

Lawler's work draws our attention to the need to develop the means to articulate what it means to 'know' the patient and to study the complexity of that state, with its risks and benefits for both nurses and patients. Palliative nursing is in a ideal position to take a lead in this, since it is in the fortunate position of being located within a wider discourse of palliative care in which the quality of the relationship between nurse and patient is seen as a critical element, and in which much is made of the unique contribution of nursing to the work of the palliative care team. Efforts are discernible in the palliative care literature to define the personal contribution that palliative care practitioners make when caring for their patients. Thus, for example, Macleod (2001) describes how a practitioner 'listens, responds and relates to the patient as a unique individual, attempting to understand the other's needs and feelings . . . Care can begin when one individual enters the life world of another person and attempts to understand what it is like to be that person' (p. 1720). Macleod draws on a seminal paper by Peabody (1927), who was himself terminally ill at the time he was writing, to explain how essential this 'personal offering' is to the whole project of caring for dying people. Most interestingly, Macleod observes that Peabody describes 'getting to know the patient' as an essential aspect of the 'art' of medicine, and empathy as an essential prerequisite of this.

Empathy

Empathy is an essential prerequisite for 'treading lightly' (Tisdale 1986; Bowden 1997) between emotional over-identification and depersonalized under-identification. Wiseman (1996), in a concept analysis of empathy, notes that the term was first introduced as a translation of the German word *einfuhling*: 'feeling into'. Clearly, then, empathy involves emotion and most critically it involves accessing the emotions of others. Goldie (1999) suggests that there are five ways of thinking about others' emotions, of which empathy is one:

- Understanding and explaining the emotions of others.
- Emotional contagion: 'catching' the emotions of others.
- Empathy: imagining the emotional experiences of others from the inside.
- 'In-his-shoes' imagining of another's situation.
- Sympathy: recognizing another's emotions and having feelings of distress about them.

Goldie distinguishes between 'empathy' and 'in his shoes imagining', which are at first sight similar, in the following way:

> Their distinctness is reflected in the fact that in-his-shoes imagining, unlike empathy, involves . . . having a mixture of my own characterization and some of his; empathy, if successful, does not involve any aspect of me in this sense, for empathic understanding is a way of gaining a deeper understanding of what it is like for him.
>
> (Goldie 1999: 398)

Goldie likens empathy to the imagining of a story, or narrative, about another. He calls this 'acting in the head' (p. 397). Goldie alerts us to the central importance of 'imagination' and the reflexive use of self in empathic understanding, while making it clear that this type of understanding does not necessarily involve the requirement to feel as the other person feels.

Wiseman (1996) summarizes a body of literature about empathy, concluding that in practical terms empathy means to: see the world as others see it; be non-judgemental; be able to understand another's feelings; be able to communicate that understanding. She observes that empathy is a crucial skill for nursing practice and all helping relationships and, echoing Goldie, points out that self-awareness is an essential prerequisite for the development of empathy. Hope-Stone and Mills (2001) conducted an interesting study in which 14 nurses were interviewed about their interpretation of empathy, the conditions which they perceived influenced empathy, and their beliefs about how empathy is established in nursing. Their findings show how 'empathy' was seen to be linked tightly to 'knowing the patient' and that this was believed to be best achieved through a combination of personal and professional experience. A useful distinction was made between 'sympathy' and 'empathic helping'. This suggests that empathy can be expressed through the care-giving acts of nurses and goes beyond any need for words. Seven nurses believed that empathy was a skill that could be taught, although the remaining seven believed that it was a quality dependent upon intuition and experience. In a discussion that echoes the references made above to the influence of environment and resources on nursing care, Hope-Stone and Mills report that their respondents perceived that a conducive environment for expressing empathy was essential: quiet, space and an organization of work to allow continuity of care were seen as especially important. Risks and benefits were seen to be associated with empathy: it was recognized that the requirement to be empathic could result in feelings of increased stress and vulnerability for nurses and patients. At the same time, the expression of empathy was described as an integral part of their job satisfaction. From conducting the interviews, Hope-Stone and Mills observe that their respondents found great difficulty in conceptualizing and verbally expressing the meaning of empathy, and thus had difficulty in describing or identifying empathic behaviours. These problems are another example of the problem discussed above of communicating to others the value and skills of nursing in ways that move beyond a superficial description of observable behaviours. Such communication is essential if education in palliative care is to develop further and nurses are to define confidently what their particular role and contribution is to the palliative care team.

Support and 'supportive care'

In a study of Macmillan nursing in the UK, the use of the term 'support' was a central feature in nurses' accounts of their patient care role (Skilbeck and Seymour 2002). Exploration of what this term meant to post holders elicited descriptors such as 'social care', 'listening', 'talking', 'reassurance', 'help' and 'advice' in the context of spending time with patients and their families. Importantly, Macmillan nurses perceived their ability to enact a supportive role to depend on both their relationships with individual consultants, cancer site-specific nurses and non-specialist staff, and their ability to take a 'softly-softly' approach in their negotiations with these individuals. This study shows that support and its provision has dimensions that relate to both the dyad of the nurse–patient relationship and to the more diffuse aspects of team organization and interaction. Skilbeck and Payne (2003) explore these issues in more detail in a paper which looks at 'emotional support' in specialist palliative care nursing. Skilbeck and Payne identify 'communication skills' and 'emotional labour' to be integral to the success-

ful provision of emotional support, but note the pervasive loose and interchangeable use of terms such as emotional care and support, psychological
care and support, and psychosocial care and support. Moreover, they
note that the meaning of these terms depends heavily on the theoretical
perspective within which they are placed.

One reason for further defining the nature of support is the evidence
that many patients are referred to palliative care nurses for 'support' with
little or no indication of the expectations attached to this (Skilbeck *et al.*
2002). There are profound implications for refining referral criteria and
exploring the processes associated with giving support and how these
relate to the outcomes of care as understood by patients and their carers.
Somewhat more clearly defined is the term 'supportive care'.

Supportive care

In the context of cancer care, a coordinated European activity funded by the
European Community and facilitated by the European Organization for
Research and Treatment of Cancer (EORTC) Pain and Symptom Control
Task Force, has led to the agreement of the following definition for support-
ive care in cancer treatment:

> Supportive care for cancer patients is the multi professional attention to
> the individual's overall physical, psychosocial, spiritual and cultural
> needs, and should be available at all stages of the illness, for patients of
> all ages, and regardless of the current intention of any anti-cancer
> treatment.

(Ahmedzai *et al.* 2001: 1)

In the UK, an alternative definition put forward by the National Council for
Hospice and Specialist Palliative Care Services has been adopted by policy
makers:[4]

> helps the patient and their family to cope with cancer and treatment of it
> – from pre-diagnosis, through the process of diagnosis and treatment, to
> cure, continuing illness or death and into bereavement. It helps the
> patient maximise the benefits of treatment and to live as well as possible
> with the effects of the disease. It is given equal priority alongside
> diagnosis and treatment.

(NCHSPCS 2002: 3)

Of course, framing 'supportive care' within the remit of cancer care in this
way marginalizes its potential contribution to the care of people with diseases other than cancer. Another problem with both these definitions is that
they differ little from the definitions of palliative care discussed elsewhere in
this book. Examination of the NHS Cancer Plan in the UK (Department of
Health 2000) is helpful, in so far as it discusses the elements of a planned
supportive care strategy in the context of evidence that cancer patients place
high priority on: being treated with humanity, dignity and respect; good
communication; clear information; symptom control; and psychological

support (see also Cancerlink 2000). Mechanisms for addressing these priorities are outlined in the Cancer Plan, with special note being made of the need for coordination across professional boundaries, for education programmes for specialist and non-specialist staff, and support groups where patients and their carers can share experiences and channel their opinions to service providers. Interestingly, in the Cancer Plan, palliative care is discussed as if it is one element of the support network that should be made available by cancer patients. While this may be puzzling, it draws attention to interdependency of palliative and acute cancer care, and to the need to understand palliative care as a modality of care that exists side by side with others and which takes greater or lesser importance depending on the stage of disease and the preferences and concerns of the patient. Furthermore, understanding palliative care in this way may be helpful when trying to develop new models of palliative care for patients with diseases other than cancer, where it is likely that indirect education, support and partnership between specialities will be critical to success (NCHSPCS 2002: 12–13), and within which the role of the nurse may be critical (Seymour *et al.* 2002).

Conclusions

In this chapter I have tried, somewhat ambitiously, to provide an analytical commentary on some selected key concepts in palliative care nursing: concepts often located and hidden in the 'taken-for-granted' world of the caring work with which nurses engage. Defining and exploring these is arguably a first step towards identifying the complex outcomes associated with palliative care nursing; and towards identifying more clearly a distinctive educational and research agenda for palliative care nursing. This is important so that nurses of all levels can recognize and articulate their worth, and support their colleagues to do so. Thus my intention throughout has been to celebrate, through critical commentary, the role of the nurse in the delivery of excellent multidisciplinary care to patients with palliative care needs and their families.

I will leave you with some key points that emerge from the chapter:

- Within palliative nursing, it is possible to identify key elements: teamwork; the relief of suffering; the promotion of quality of life and hope; knowing the patient; and the promotion of dignity, comfort and support.

- Ideas about 'caring' and care-giving' are central to palliative nursing. A key issue is how to contain powerful emotions while engaging in caring. 'Emotional labour' is a useful way of thinking about how this is done.

- Dignity is a concept often associated with the 'good death' and relates to respect for persons and their bodies. Institutional structures and cultures are as critical to the preservation of dignity as individual nurse–patient relationships.

- Comfort has been a goal of nursing care for over a century: which nursing practices contribute to comfort, and how these are perceived by patients in the context of changing expectations of medical technology, are under-examined.

- Contemporary analyses of 'knowing the patient' remind us that little is known about the nurse–patient relationship, and the risks and benefits that surround it.

- Empathy is an essential prerequisite for palliative nursing. An empathic stance is learnt partly through experience and but is also a skill that can be acquired through education.

- Supportive care encompasses palliative care, and is debated within at the level of UK policy largely in relation to the care and treatment of patients with cancer. New models of supportive and palliative care for patients with diseases other than cancer need to be developed.

Notes

1 Most, but not all, of the references listed here are cited by Lugton and Kindlen (1999: 14–16).
2 Ramussen *et al.* (1995) use the term 'guest' rather than 'patient'. I have used the term 'patient' throughout for the sake of clarity and consistency.
3 Here Lawler references a report by Reeve (1993) on 'Quality assurance in Australian hospitals'.
4 In particular, this definition forms the basis of the *Guidance on Cancer Services: Improving Supportive and Palliative Care for Adults with Cancer*, published as a consultation document in 2002 by the National Institute for Clinical Excellence (NICE). This institute was set up as a Special Health Authority for England and Wales on 1 April 1999. It is part of the National Health Service and its role is to provide patients, health professionals and the public with authoritative, robust and reliable guidance on current 'best practice'. See the NICE website: http://www.nice.org.uk.

References

Ahmedzai, S.H., Lubbe, A. and Van den Eynden, B. (2001) *Towards a European Standard for Supportive Care of Cancer Patients: A Coordinated Activity Funded by DGV*. Final Unpublished Report for EC on behalf of the EORTC Pain and Symptom Control Task Force.

Aranda, S. (1998) Palliative care principles: masking the complexity of practice, in J. Parker and S. Aranda (eds) *Palliative Care: Explorations and Challenges*. Sydney, NSW: McClennan & Petty.

Armstrong, D. (1987) Theoretical tensions in biopyschosocial medicine. *Social Science and Medicine*, 25: 1213–18.

Billings, J.A. and Block, S.D. (1996) Slow euthanasia. *Journal of Palliative Care*, 12(4): 21–30.

Botoroff, J.L. (1991) The meaning of comfort: the lived experience of being comforted by a nurse. *Phenomenology and Pedagogy*, 9: 237–52.

Bowden, P. (1997) *Caring: Gender Sensitive Ethics*. London: Routledge.

Broeckaert, B. and Nunez-Olarte, J.M. (2002) Sedation in palliative care: facts and concepts, in H. ten Have and D. Clark (eds) *The Ethics of Palliative Care: European Perspectives*. Buckingham: Open University Press.

Brogden, S. (1966) Nursing a dyspnoeic patient. *Canadian Nurse*, 62(4): 29–31.

Cancerlink (2000) *Cancer Supportive Care Services Strategy: Users' Priorities and Perspectives*. London: Cancerlink.

Cohen, M.Z. and Sarter, B. (1992) Love and work: oncology nurses' view of the meaning of their work. *Oncology Nursing Forum*, 19(10): 1481–6.

Craytor, J. (1969) Talking with persons who have cancer. *American Journal of Nursing*, 69: 744–8.

Davies, C. (1995) *Gender and the Professional Predicament in Nursing*. Buckingham: Open University Press.

Davis, B. and O'Berle, K. (1990) Dimensions of the supportive role of the nurse in palliative care. *Oncology Nursing Forum*, 17: 87–94.

Davis, B. and O'Berle, K. (1992) Support and caring: exploring the concepts. *Oncology Nursing Forum*, 19: 763–7.

Degner, L.F., Gow, C.M. and Thompson, L.A. (1991) Critical nursing behaviours in care for the dying. *Cancer Nursing*, 14: 246–53.

Department of Health (2000) *The NHS Cancer Plan: A Plan for Investment, A Plan for Reform*. London: HMSO.

de Raeve, L. (1996) Dignity and integrity at the end of life. *International Journal of Palliative Care Nursing*, 2(2): 71–6.

Dobratz, M.C. (1990) Hospice nursing: present perspectives and future directions. *Cancer Nursing*, 13: 116–22.

Goldie, P. (1999) How we think of others' emotions. *Mind and Language*, 14(4): 394–423.

Herth, K. (1990) Fostering hope in terminally ill people. *Journal of Advanced Nursing*, 15: 1250–9.

Hochschild, A. (1983) *The Managed Heart*. Berkeley, CA: University of California Press.

Hope-Stone, L.D. and Mills, B. (2001) Developing empathy to improve patient care: a pilot study of cancer nurses. *International Journal of Palliative Nursing*, 7(3): 146–50.

Hull, M.M. (1989) Family needs and supportive behaviours during terminal cancer: a review. *Oncology Nursing Forum*, 16: 787–92.

James, N. (1989) Emotional labour: skill and work in the social regulation of feelings. *Sociological Review*, 37: 15–42.

Johnson, I.S., Rogers, C., Biswas, B. and Ahmedzai, S. (1990) What do hospices do? A survey of hospices in the United Kingdom and Ireland. *British Medical Journal*, 300: 791–3.

Knowles, L. (1962) How our behaviour affects patient care. *Canadian Nurse*, 58(1): 30–3.

Kristjanson, L.J., McPhee, I., Pickstock, S. *et al.* (2001) Palliative care nurses' perceptions of good and bad deaths and care expectations: a qualitative analysis. *International Journal of Palliative Care Nursing*, 7(3): 129–39.

Larsson, G., Widmark, V., Lampic, C., von Essen, L. and Sjoden, P. (1998) Cancer patient and staff ratings of the importance of caring behaviours and their relations to patient anxiety and depression. *Journal of Advanced Nursing*, 27: 855–64.

Lawler, J. (1991) *Behind the Screens: Nursing, Somology and the Problem of the Body*. Melbourne, VIC: Churchill Livingstone.

Lawler, J. (2002) Knowing the body and embodiment: methodologies, discourses and nursing, in A.M. Rafferty and M. Traynor (eds) *Exemplary Research for Nursing and Midwifery*. London: Routledge.

Low, J. and Payne, S. (1996) The good and bad death perceptions of health professionals working in palliative care. *European Journal of Cancer Care*, 5: 237–41.

Lugton, J. and Kindlen, M. (eds) (1999) *Palliative Care: The Nursing Role*. Edinburgh: Churchill Livingstone.

Luker, K.A., Austin, L., Caress, A. and Hallett, C.E. (2000) The importance of 'knowing the patient': community nurses' constructions of quality in providing palliative care. *Journal of Advanced Nursing*, 31(4): 775–82.

Macleod, R.D. (2001) On reflection: doctors learning to care for people who are dying. *Social Science and Medicine*, 52(11): 1719–27.

May, C. (1995) Patient autonomy and the politics of professional relationships. *Journal of Advanced Nursing*, 21(1): 83–7.

McIlveen, K.H. and Morse, J.M. (1995) The role of comfort in nursing care: 1900–1980. *Clinical Nursing Research*, 4(2): 127–48.

McNamara, B., Waddell, C. and Colvin, M. (1994) The institutionalisation of the good death. *Social Science and Medicine*, 39: 1501–8.

Menzies, I. (1970) *The Functioning of Social Systems as a Defence Against Anxiety* (reprint of Tavistock Pamphlet No. 3). London: Tavistock Institute.

Morse, J.M. and Johnson, J.L. (1991) *The Illness Experience: Dimensions of Suffering*. Newbury Park, CA: Sage.

Morse, J.M., Botoroff, J.L. and Hutchinson, S. (1994) The phenomenology of comfort. *Journal of Advanced Nursing*, 20: 189–95.

National Council for Hospice and Specialist Palliative Care Services (2001) *What Do We Mean by Palliative Care? A Discussion Paper*. Briefing, No. 9, May. London: NCHSPCS.

National Council for Hospice and Specialist Palliative Care Services (2002) *Information Exchange*, No. 36, September. London: NCHSPCS.

Nolan, M., Grant, G. and Keady, J. (1996) *Understanding Family Care*. Buckingham: Open University Press.

Peabody, F.W. (1927) The care of the patient. *Journal of the American Medical Association*, 252: 813–18.

Principal Investigators for the SUPPORT Project (1995) A controlled trial to improve care for seriously ill hospitalized patients: the study to understand prognoses and preferences for outcomes and risks of treatment (SUPPORT). *Journal of the American Medical Association*, 174: 1591–8.

Puntillo, K.A. (2001) The role of critical care nurses in providing and managing end of life care, in J. Randall-Curtis and G.D. Rubenfeld (eds) *Managing Death in the Intensive Care Unit: The Transition from Cure to Comfort*. Oxford: Oxford University Press.

Quill, T.E. and Byock, I.R. (2000) Responding to intractable terminal suffering: the role of terminal sedation and voluntary refusal of food and fluids. *Annals of Internal Medicine*, 132(5): 408–14.

Radwin, L.E. (1996) 'Knowing the patient': a review of research on an emerging concept. *Journal of Advanced Nursing*, 23: 1142–6.

Rasmussen, B.H., Norberg, A. and Sandman, P.O. (1995) Stories about becoming a hospice nurse: reasons, expectations, hopes and concerns. *Cancer Nursing*, 18(5): 344–54.

Raudonis, B.M. (1993) The meaning and impact of empathic relationships in hospice nursing. *Cancer Nursing*, 16: 304–9.

Rittman, M., Paige, P., Rivera, J., Sutphin, L. and Godown, I. (1997) Phenomenological study of nurses caring for dying patients. *Cancer Nursing*, 20(2): 115–19.

Rogers, A., Karlsen, S. and Addington-Hall, J. (2000) 'All the services were excellent. It is when the human element comes in that things go wrong': dissatisfaction with hospital care in the last year of life. *Journal of Advanced Nursing*, 31(4): 768–74.

Seymour, J.E. (2003) Caring for dying people in critical care, in M. O'Connor and S. Aranda (eds) *Palliative Care Nursing: A Guide to Practice*. Melbourne, VIC: Ausmed.

Seymour, J.E., Clark, D., Hughes, P. *et al.* (2002) Clinical nurse specialists in palliative care. Part 3: Issues for the Macmillan nurse role. *Palliative Medicine*, 16: 386–94.

Simpson, S.H. (1997) Reconnecting: the experiences of nurses caring for hopelessly ill patients in intensive care. *Intensive and Critical Care Nursing*, 13: 189–97.

Skilbeck, J. and Payne, S. (2003) Emotional support and the role of clinical nurse specialists in palliative care. *Journal of Advanced Nursing*, 43(5): 521–30.

Skilbeck, J. and Seymour, J.E. (2002) Meeting complex needs: an analysis of Macmillan nurses' work with patients. *International Journal of Palliative Nursing*, 8: 574–82.

Skilbeck, J., Corner, J., Bath, P. *et al.* (2002) Clinical nurse specialists in palliative care. Part 1: A description of the Macmillan nurse caseload. *Palliative Medicine*, 16(4): 285–96.

Steeves, R., Cohen, M.Z. and Wise, C.T. (1994) An analysis of critical incidents describing the essence of oncology nursing. *Oncology Nursing Forum Supplement*, 218: 19–25.

Tanner, C.A., Benner, P. and Chelsa, C. (1993) The phenomenology of knowing the patient. *IMAGE: Journal of Nursing Scholarship*, 25: 273–80.

Tisdale, S. (1986) *The Sorcerer's Apprentice: Tales of the Modern Hospital*. New York: McGraw-Hill.

Twigg, J. (ed.) (1993) *Informal Care in Europe*. Proceedings of a Conference held in York. York: Social Policy Research Unit, University of York.

von Essen, L. and Sjoden, P.O. (1991) The importance of nurse caring behaviours as perceived by Swedish hospital patients and nursing staff. *International Journal of Nursing Studies*, 28: 267–81.

Walker, A.C. (2002) Safety and comfort work of nurses glimpsed through patient narratives. *International Journal of Nursing Practice*, 8(1): 42–8.

Walsh, K. and Kowanko, I. (2002) Nurses' and patients' perceptions of dignity. *International Journal of Nursing Practice*, 8: 143–51.

Wiseman, T. (1996) A concept analysis of empathy. *Journal of Advanced Nursing*, 23(6): 1162–7.

Wurzbach, M.E. (1996) Comfort and nurses' moral choices. *Journal of Advanced Nursing*, 24(2): 260–4.

4

User involvement and palliative care

Rhetoric or reality?

Merryn Gott

User involvement in health services research and development has been almost universally adopted as a 'good thing'. In the UK, the Department of Health, for example, has underlined their commitment to involving users in this way by appointing a Director of Patient Experience and Public Involvement (Department of Health 2002). Furthermore, demonstrating how users will be involved in the research process is increasingly necessary to secure research funding.[1] The drive to promote user involvement has now reached palliative care services, with the National Council for Hospice and Specialist Palliative Care Services arguing that user involvement 'can enrich the principles and practices of palliative care' (NCHSPCS 2000: 1). Indeed, on the face of it, palliative care appears to have much to be gained from an approach that purports to place those with direct experience of using health services at the centre of priority setting and shaping practice. Moreover, user involvement appears to be consistent with the tenets of modern palliative care, evolving as they have done from a movement that grew by listening to provide a voice for the voiceless (Saunders, quoted by Oliviere 1999).

The rhetoric of user involvement is certainly persuasive. As Harrison and Mort (1998) acknowledge, 'being in favour of ... more user involvement is rather like being against sin; at a rhetorical level, it is hard to find disagreement' (p. 66). However, problems arise when translating the rhetoric of user involvement into reality. Indeed, although an agenda of user involvement in UK health service development has been espoused for over a decade, progress in implementing this policy 'has been patchy' (Rhodes and Nocon 1998). Similarly, user involvement 'in NHS research is not fiction, but it appears to be at an early stage of implementation, with few researchers confident about carrying it out' (Telford *et al.* 2002: 97). Making the jump from rhetoric to reality poses particular challenges within palliative care, where the users whose involvement is sought may be especially vulnerable. If user involvement is to become a feature of palliative care research and service development, there is a need to address the specific context of palliative care while also learning from experiences in other areas. These have shown that, at its best, user involvement can be an effective means of developing services and research programmes that are truly people-centred; at its worst, it can waste users' time by merely serving to legitimize previously determined professional agendas. This is a particular issue for people in receipt of palliative care services, for whom time is likely to be at a premium.

In this chapter, I argue that although the principles of user involvement are both admirable and, in many instances, desirable, involving users effectively involves critically examining mechanisms of involvement and desired outcomes. Several questions have to be addressed at the outset. Who are the users? What do we mean by involvement? Do they want to be involved? Are they in a position to be involved? What if the views of user and professional conflict? How can the success of user involvement be measured? I will address these questions and argue that the ethics and practicalities of pursuing an agenda of user involvement within palliative care require careful thought. The potential benefits of this approach must not only be conceived of in professional terms, but also from the perspective of users themselves. The practical obstacles that may impede an agenda of user involvement developing must be weighed against the need to ensure that the voices of people at the end of their lives are heard.

Who are the users?

Although there is an ongoing debate as to which terminology most appropriately describes the group(s) of people whose 'involvement' is being sought, little attention has been paid to how the 'users' themselves would prefer to be known. Indeed, the terminology adopted by the National Health Service (NHS), which currently favours the term 'consumer' rather than 'user', is largely professionally determined and, ironically for an approach that purports to place those in receipt of services at the centre of decision making, a wider consultation appears not to have been undertaken. Telford *et al.* (2002), for example, identified a professional preference for the term 'consumer' in a recent scoping exercise and therefore advocate this as the terminology of choice, arguing that it is consistent with UK health policy documents. This choice is not merely a matter of semantics, as the definitions adopted reflect wider philosophical understandings. For NHS policy documents to come down on the side of 'consumers', for example, would be expected given the trend towards NHS consumerist health policies over the last two decades. This use of language indicates support for a market-led system where choices are driven by commercial or economic factors. Herein lies the opposition to the use of the term 'consumer' both by some professionals, who see it as attributing health services with similar characteristics to supermarkets (Telford *et al.* 2002), and also some service users. For example, we know that people who have had cancer 'do not see themselves as customers or consumers; health and social care are not commodities to them' (Gott *et al.* 2000: 1).

The term 'user' has been described as exemplifying an approach stressing democratization and empowerment, in which 'users' are able to make their 'voices' heard within a system enabling their participation (Saltman 1994). Opposition to this term has been voiced due to its association with substance misuse and client groups who are disadvantaged in some way (e.g. wheelchair users) (Herxheimer and Goodacre 1999). However, it still appears to more fully embody what user involvement in a palliative care context would hope to achieve, although it is important to acknowledge that this conceptual debate is one with which palliative care needs to engage further. This debate needs to include users themselves, not only to ensure that shared understandings are developed, but also because of the recognition that defining the key concepts of user involvement and, notably, deciding on the body of participants to be involved in decision making, can be the most important means of exercising power within the whole process (Drake 2002).

So, within a palliative care context, who are our 'users'? The National Council for Hospice and Specialist Care Services defines palliative care 'users' as follows: people with life-threatening illnesses and conditions; their families, partners and friends; and people who become bereaved (NCHSPCS 2000). These groups will be the main focus of this chapter. However, overall, it could be argued that this definition may not go far enough. For example, the NHS Executive (1998), which has adopted the term 'consumer' rather than 'user': 'define consumers as patients and potential patients, carers, organisations representing consumers' interests, members of the public who are targets of health promotion campaigns and groups asking for research because they believe they have been exposed to potentially harmful circumstances, products or services' (p. 3). If this more far-reaching definition is applied to palliative care, it is apparent that many more groups of people can be included under this umbrella term of 'user'. People with a family history of a particular life-threatening illness or condition, for example, may perceive themselves as potential users of palliative care services and, therefore, have a vested interest in how those services develop. Many older people think about, and have concerns about death – in particular, the nature of dying – and welcome the opportunity to reflect on these and make recommendations as to how experiences at the end of life can be improved (Seymour *et al.* 2002). If adopting an extreme position, it could be argued that everyone is a potential user of palliative care services and may have views about these. For example, debates around the ethics of euthanasia are ones in which the wider public need to be involved (although it is recognized that 'public involvement' is not the same as that of 'user involvement' and that perspectives change when the transition to 'patient' is made). Finally, various 'professionals' – both individuals and organizations – may see themselves as user-advocates and may want to help promote the user voice. These can include voluntary organizations and charities mobilized around a particular condition, for example

Macmillan Cancer Relief, or a particular social group, for example Age Concern. Organizations such as the UK Association of Palliative Medicine may similarly cast themselves in this role, although their own professional interests must also be acknowledged.

Indeed, it is not my intention to imply that the interests and concerns of these various groups of people are the same, even though they could all be lumped together under the umbrella term 'users'. It is rather to draw attention to the fact that the term 'user' can imply a simple homogeneity, when this is highly unlikely to exist. All of these various groups will have different needs and perspectives. Patients and carers, for example, can both be users of palliative care services, but in very different capacities. There is an ongoing debate about the role that 'professionals' should play in promoting the user agenda; the ability of professionals to adequately represent users has been hotly disputed within the disability movement, for example (Drake 1999). Even within the apparently straightforward 'patient' group, wide heterogeneity exists – the experiences and needs of people with terminal cancer, for example, will differ from those of people with end-stage heart failure and those recently diagnosed with multiple sclerosis. Although some people with palliative care needs will have access to specialist palliative care services, the majority will not (Eve and Higginson 2000), which is another reason why a narrow definition of 'user' is not appropriate within palliative care. A diversity of experiences and attitudes also exists along socio-demographic lines, including ethnicity, age and gender. Indeed, being a palliative care 'user' is no more likely to infer commonality than being a 'cancer patient' or an 'older person'.

Even at this very preliminary stage of thinking about user involvement, therefore, things may not be as straightforward as would first appear. Indeed, it is apparent that, as with all aspects of user involvement, no one model will fit all. If 'user involvement' is sought as a means of improving a hospice day care service, for example, then the views of someone with direct experience of using this service are likely to be sought. If the aim is to explore the ethical dimensions of euthanasia, it might be more appropriate to adopt a wider definition of the 'user'. As such, it is impossible to be prescriptive in defining the 'users', but rather at a practical level to try and involve those whose input is most relevant to the circumstances of a particular agenda or project. Whether these users themselves will welcome invitations to be involved in this way is another matter and will be addressed below.

Involvement and the issue of power

'Involvement' is another term that can be understood in different ways and it is not my intention here to revisit these debates (for a thorough conceptual overview of the term 'user involvement' with reference to palliative care, see Small and Rhodes 2000; with reference to cancer care, see Gott *et al.* 2000,

2002). To summarize, the multiple meanings of involvement relate not just to the activities the users undertake, but ultimately to the amount of power they are able to wield in the decision-making process. Arnstein's (1969) spectrum or 'ladder' of participation is widely cited in the user involvement literature with his recognition that 'involvement' can range from tokenism to extensive democratic power sharing and genuine collaboration. Hamilton-Gurney (1993), for example, builds on this model to propose the following three-stage hierarchy: *involvement*, a loose umbrella term describing when users are brought into the decision-making process at an individual level; *consultation*, where the user perspective is more intentionally targeted; and *participation*, a more active process where users work in 'partnership' with professionals. A similar three-level model has been proposed within research, using slightly different terminology (Consumers in NHS Research Support Unit 2000): *consultation*, where users are consulted, but do not have any power in decision making; *collaboration*, where an ongoing partnership between researchers and users exists throughout the research process; and *user control*, where users design, undertake and disseminate research findings.

Each of these conceptual models raises different challenges for both users and 'professionals'. Central to these is the question of power and, as Carter and Beresford (2000) acknowledge, this means that user involvement 'is complicated, confusing and highly political . . . conflict, duplicity and possible heartache are never too far away' (p. 10). Users may be loath to be involved if they have no real power to make decisions and effect change (Gott *et al.* 2000). However, Poulton (1999) notes that 'as yet professionals seem unable to contemplate sharing their knowledge and power with the people they serve' (p. 1294), with many being sceptical about the value of user involvement. Resolving tensions such as these lies at the heart of developing effective user involvement initiatives, as explored in more detail below.

The potential of user involvement in palliative care

As Small (1999) has identified, involvement – both at the level of the individual and that of the wider public – has a long history within the hospice movement. He quotes a key figure in the UK hospice movement:

> I think the original hospice world promoted itself as a response, as indeed it was to some extent, a response to public demand, to need, to things that were wrong. This was a protest movement, but it was a look at things and saying, 'God, things could be better, you know we have got a little section of people here at the most painful, critical, heart breaking time of their lives, and they are being badly looked after, what are we going to do about this thing'.
>
> (Small 1999: 296)

Alongside this public impetus to improve care for the dying are the personal stories of individual service users, instrumental to Cicely Saunders in her conceptualization and subsequent development of the hospice movement (Saunders 2002).

Listening and responding to the unique voice of the service user is still central to palliative care philosophy and there is no doubt that, both within research and service development, this needs to be given priority. No-one would dispute the fact that palliative care services must be responsive to the people that use them and that palliative care research must be relevant, either directly or potentially, to users' day-to-day experiences. However, existing evidence indicates that this may not always be the case. For example, Raynes *et al.* (2001) note that, within palliative care, 'relatively few studies have directly sought the views and values of patients, their carers or relatives' (p. 170). Where these views have been sought, the potential to improve services has been identified – for example, a focus group study with terminally ill cancer patients identified a need to improve the provision of practical help with daily living, as well as to provide additional information about a range of issues (Raynes *et al.* 2001).

A particular debate in which the voices of people with palliative care needs are notable by their absence relates to the provision of specialist palliative care services beyond their traditional remit of cancer. Although this debate has been ongoing both within and outside of specialist palliative care for several years, it has been largely professionally driven and little is known of the wishes of patients without cancer and, in particular, their willingness to use services associated with cancer and death (Field and Addington-Hall 1999). However, acceptability to this group must be acknowledged as crucial to the success or otherwise of extending access to specialist palliative care and any attempt to involve users in this debate must be welcomed.

Although we know little about the research priorities of people using palliative care services, evidence from other areas of health care highlights that these are likely not always to accord with professional agendas. Users involved in prioritizing research areas for the NHS Health Technology Assessment Programme, for example, tended to 'highlight issues about patients' views, social contexts, information and support needs, long term outcomes, and dissemination of research', whereas professional referees 'tended to focus on more scientific and economic aspects of the work'.[2] Within palliative care, it can be argued that user input may be vital to ensuring that we are measuring the right thing in the right way. In randomized controlled trials, for example, traditional end-points such as survival become less appropriate and need to be weighed against more subjective measures such as quality of life. Involving users in deciding outcome measures could, therefore, be very valuable.

The challenges of user involvement in palliative care

The first challenge when addressing the role of user involvement in palliative care is to identify whether this is a policy that users themselves find acceptable. Indeed, currently, the user involvement agenda within health and social care is predominantly professionally driven, at least outside of those areas where it originally evolved (most notably mental health and learning disability). Within palliative care, we know little of how positively this policy is viewed or whether it is something that people with palliative care needs are willing, or feel able, to engage with. A recent seminar exploring the potential for user involvement within palliative care, and including a significant number of direct users of palliative care services, found support for developing a user involvement agenda (Beresford *et al.* 2000). One service user with HIV identified that: 'Somehow we've got to be asked and we've got to be listened to' (Beresford *et al.* 2000: 5). However, little work like this is currently being undertaken and it is imperative that we know more about how users feel about involvement in research and service delivery before this agenda is taken forward. If user involvement is merely a professionally driven policy, not only would this appear to negate its intrinsic value, but it would also run the risk of 'using the users' (Payne 2002).

This is not to say that all professionals welcome user involvement. Although we know little about professional opinion within palliative care, resistance has been documented in other areas of health and social care. Some of the concerns that professionals have expressed in relation to user involvement have revolved around representativeness, fears that users will not fully understand the complexities of research and service development, worries about users having biased views and/or basing these upon individual rather than collective experience, concerns that users may have unrealistic expectations and fears that involving users will require more time and resources than are available (Boote *et al.* 2002; Gott *et al.* 2000). Finally, and maybe most critically, some professionals have expressed concerns that user involvement can diminish their power to make decisions and maintain control over the research or service development process (McFadyen and Farrington 1997). Indeed, a study in which users were involved in the research process to the extent that they conducted interviews, led the researchers to express considerable anxiety about their lack of control over the quality of the data and, therefore, the overall validity of the study (Elliott *et al.* 2002). For researchers who adopt a positivist stance to research, user involvement is also likely to pose epistemological problems given that positivism is underpinned by the notion that 'knowledge can be developed "at a distance" from consumers, who are treated as passive suppliers of data' (Boote *et al.* 2002: 6).

Resolving tension between user and professional perspectives must lie at the heart of developing effective user involvement initiatives, although this issue is rarely openly acknowledged. When such tensions arise, they also do so in a situation where users are already likely to be inherently less powerful – the doctor–patient relationship is certainly not an equal one. These power imbalances that exist within the culture of health care can be compounded if users are involved in discussions where their own health care provider is present. In particular, they may be worried that disagreeing with the professional may jeopardize their current or future care, or that they will not be consulted again if they 'rock the boat' (Gott *et al.* 2000: 26). Moreover, even though such user–professional tensions are known to have been resolved over time as trust develops, time may not be a resource that is always readily available within palliative care.

Therefore, although the user voice has potential value for palliative care as a whole, translating this rhetoric into reality is likely to be highly complex. Examples of how this can be achieved from other areas of health and social care are also limited, as the current literature on user involvement is heavily weighted in favour of – often unsubstantiated – opinion rather than practical examples. Written accounts of actual user involvement in research, for example, remain scarce, leading one commentator to acknowledge that 'the challenge now is to conduct research to identify whether their [user] involvement leads to actual, rather than merely perceived, benefits for research processes and output' (Hanley *et al.* 2001: 522). Similarly, at a service development level, the agenda of user involvement has been slow in translating from policy to practice. A survey of user involvement in cancer services in one region in England, for example, found that although this agenda was promoted by the Calman-Hine Report, the pace of establishing specific initiatives of involvement had been slow (Gott *et al.* 2000).

Even where user involvement initiatives are up and running, these are rarely evaluated and criteria to measure 'successful' involvement remain to be developed. Appropriate methods of evaluation must first elucidate what users actually contribute to the research or service development process and then identify how this 'added-value' can be measured (Boote *et al.* 2002). Such an evaluation would invariably be complex, giving due consideration to both the process of user involvement and the eventual outcome. Furthermore, it must capture the perspectives of all stakeholders, both user and professional. Indeed, to date, when evaluations of user involvement have been undertaken, they have tended to concentrate on the professional rather than the user perspective. For example, two recent surveys of user involvement focused on the experiences of lead investigators and did not capture the perspectives of the users who had been involved (Hanley *et al.* 2001; Telford *et al.* 2002). Therefore, although the investigators' experiences of involving users were generally positive, it is premature to advocate involvement from these findings and is certainly too early to claim that 'involvement seems likely to improve the relevance to consumers of the questions addressed and the results obtained' (Hanley *et al.* 2001: 519).

What's in it for the user?

The question remains, therefore, of 'what is in it for the user?' Indeed, although one of the arguments for promoting user involvement, particularly within the political non-consumerist models of involvement, has been that users have the potential to derive therapeutic benefit from such initiatives, few data exist either to support or refute this position. Moreover, although some authors claim that user involvement can empower users, making them feel confident, competent and in control (Liddle 1991), others argue that there 'is a fine line between involving and empowering people on the one hand, and exploiting their labour and expertise on the other' (Elliot *et al.* 2002: 175). This issue is crucial for palliative care to address and reconcile given the uniquely vulnerable circumstances of some of our 'users'.

Indeed, for user involvement in palliative care to be an ethically sound proposition, the risks and benefits of involvement must be explored. Similar consideration needs to be given to the ethics of user involvement, as has been given to the ethics of conducting research within palliative care. The first ethical principle of medical research expounded in the Declaration of Helsinki[3] states that: 'Considerations related to participants' well-being take priority over the interests of science and society. Risks of participation for the individual must never outweigh the benefits'. This leads on to the question of what the experience of user involvement is like for the user and, in particular, to what we know about the risk–benefit ratio within this context.

In terms of benefit, it is unlikely that the direct users of palliative care services, namely people who are dying, will benefit personally from any improvements in services that derive from policy and research development they are involved with. Therefore, it is the potential for therapeutic benefit to derive from involvement in the decision-making process that requires further attention. Existing evidence to support this position, however, is mainly small-scale or anecdotal, although individual accounts indicate that, for some people at least, it may have this potential. Members of the Fife User Panel, for example, who constituted frail, housebound older people, were largely positive about their involvement in an advocacy project that was aimed at influencing local services: 'That's been one of the best things that has ever happened to me, is getting to go there so that I could voice my opinions on things and say to them what I think. I feel, you feel you are getting somewhere by doing that and being able to do it, whereas before I couldn't' (quoted in Barnes and Walker 1996: 388). Similar accounts by users are reported elsewhere, for example on the Cancerlink website: 'Since I've been on the committee, I feel that people are beginning to really listen to me and value what I know about cancer.'[4]

However, it must not be assumed, as many currently appear to, that user involvement will necessarily bring direct benefit to those users who participate. At one level, it is immediately apparent that individual variations will occur – for example, what is empowering for one person may not be for another. However, although again the empirical data are limited, there are published examples of cases where user involvement has not proved a positive experience from the perspective of users. One study of an involvement initiative, for example, found increased stress among users when learning about problems that existed and the lack of easy solutions for these (Gray *et al.* 1995). Involvement can also be a frustrating process: As one user involved in cancer service development stated: 'I'm still waiting to see some positive evidence to come back to show that they've [providers] acted on something we've said' (Gott *et al.* 2000: 22). Similarly, an individual user may well find sitting on a research steering committee an intimidating and potentially disempowering experience, particularly if they have not received adequate information or appropriate training to do so.

It may be that some of the negative experiences reported by both users and professionals result from failures in planning and execution of user involvement programmes that could be rectified. However, as identified above, it is similarly apparent that what is a positive experience for one person may not be for another. It is therefore very important that users never feel under any obligation to 'fit into' a professionally driven user involvement agenda. This potential for user involvement to become coercive has been recognized by Small and Rhodes (2000) as a particular challenge for palliative care:

> Problems arise where opportunity is translated into obligation and user involvement comes to be regarded as a condition of receipt of services and, more widely, of responsible citizenship. An expectation that people will co-operate in a programme of user involvement moves from an agenda of empowerment to one of moral coercion. This form of coercion may be especially inappropriate when people are approaching the ends of their lives, have little time left to them and may have alternative goals to which they wish to devote their remaining energies.
>
> (Small and Rhodes 2000: 216)

This issue of time has been acknowledged elsewhere as a potential barrier to involving users who have life-limiting illness or who are older. As an older participant in a user involvement initiative identified, how time is spent can become more significant in the context of life-limiting illness and/or older age: 'We need to stress the issue of urgency' (member of Steering Group of Older People's Programme: quoted in Carter and Beresford 2000: 19). When time is at a premium, priorities can also change. There is no doubt that, for many people who may not have long to live, becoming involved in a research or service development project would be seen as much less important than spending time with family and friends. However, effective involvement can be time-consuming. To be fully involved in all decision making requires involvement over the length of a project (or projects) and may additionally involve receiving training before the project begins and time spent involved in dissemination afterwards. It is for these reasons that the usual term of membership on the NHS Health Technology Assessment consumer panel is 4 years (see Hanley *et al.* 2001). For most direct users of palliative care services, this would be a commitment they would be unable to fulfil.

A further challenge when initiating user involvement with people with life-limiting illnesses is that they may not want to think ahead to when their condition might have deteriorated. This is exemplified by the following account from a man with motor neurone disease: 'I didn't really want to know to what extent the disease could develop. I need to be able to cope with it as it developed and not be worrying what might, or might not happen two years down the road. That's how I have looked at it' (quoted in Small and Rhodes 2000: 141). However, many palliative care initiatives address issues relevant to the last few months of life, issues that people who have not reached that stage of their illness may find difficult to consider, while people at that stage of their illness may be too unwell to comment. Conceptualizing palliative care needs in advance can also prove problematic – attitudes and needs change over the progression of a disease and may be hard to predict.

A desire not to think about disease progression may also mitigate against membership of a user group, as this is likely to involve mixing with people at different disease stages. Although most user groups are for cancer sufferers, some do exist for a range of other conditions and operate both locally and nationally. Although they have been criticized for being unrepresentative of the entire user population (Beresford and Campbell 1994) and of being led by politically motivated activists (Harrison *et al.* 1992), they currently remain the main route through which users are recruited to participate in user involvement initiatives (Gott *et al.* 2000). Moreover, users have reported the benefits of collective as opposed to individual involvement: 'One of the great strengths of a group is that people feel more able to express concerns than they do individually. It can also be quite intimidating . . . when you are trying to ask things and you are not sure whether it is a particularly clever thing to say' (quoted in Gott *et al.* 2000: 15). This has significant implications for user involvement in palliative care. First, there are few user groups for people with more advanced disease (although a user group for people with secondary cancer has recently been reported: McLeod 1999). Second, not only may people with advanced disease be too unwell to travel to group meetings, but they may also not want to mix with people whose condition is more advanced than their own for the reasons discussed above. This popular mechanism of involving users may, therefore, not be feasible within a palliative care context.

Models of user involvement in palliative care

So we know a little of what may be unlikely to work within palliative care, but little about what would constitute 'best practice' in user involvement within this context. As noted above, there are few evaluated models to borrow from other areas of health and social care, although previous experience and exploratory research has identified factors that support effective involvement at a practical level, including providing training for users and ensuring that involvement does not bring any financial penalties with it (see

Gott *et al.* 2000). However, it is apparent that there will never be one model to fit all. Modes of involvement need both to be responsive to specific circumstances and highly flexible. Thornton (2000) has also identified that 'many conventional methods of getting people's views are dull and unrewarding for those who take part' (p. 10). Innovative methods of involvement with older people have been developed using drama (Toffaleti 1997), 'letter-writing circles' (Thornton 2000) and telephone discussion groups (as evaluated by Thornton and Tozer 1995). Such techniques also seem appropriate within palliative care given the importance of making involvement a rewarding experience for users.

Outreach initiatives are also likely to be useful when people may be too ill to travel to regular meetings, or would not want to be involved in this way. Such initiatives may be particularly appropriate to access the views of more excluded groups within society, for example older people, people of a non-heterosexual orientation and those from Black and ethnic minority groups.

Conclusions

In this chapter, I have explored the potential for developing an agenda of user involvement within palliative care. The philosophy of involvement is both consistent with the principles of palliative care and has the potential to improve the relevance and responsiveness of current research and practice. However, to date user involvement in health and social care remains more rhetoric than reality, reflecting the complexities of practical implementation. For palliative care, additional challenges in pursuing an agenda of user involvement exist and a key issue to address remains the experience of involvement from a user perspective.

There is a danger that palliative care will get swept along by the convincing rhetoric of user involvement without fully considering the practical implications. Therefore, before promoting user involvement as the 'next big thing', it is important for researchers, health and social care professionals and 'users' to engage in a debate as to whether and how involvement should be implemented within palliative care. There are risks for palliative care in not having this debate. It could mean that we fail to learn from the positive aspects of user involvement policy and ignore the need to ensure the voices of palliative care users are heard. It could also mean that we miss out in other ways, given that user involvement has become a significant feature of mainstream health and social care. Demonstrating user involvement is increasingly becoming a prerequisite to securing research funding. Furthermore, with competing claims on finite NHS resources, the onus is upon all areas of health and social care, including palliative care, to show how services measure up to the aspirations and experiences of its users (Department of Health 2002). As O'Rourke has identified, within this context 'less articulate and poorly organised' users may be marginalized.[5] The challenge now is therefore to critically consider both the rhetoric and reality of user involvement within palliative care and develop effective and appropriate mechanisms to ensure that involvement is a positive and rewarding experience both for our 'users' and for palliative care as a whole.

Notes

1 See, for example, NHS Executive Research and Development Programme (http://www.nhstrent.users.netlink.co.uk/trentrd.html) and Economic and Social Research Council (2002) *The ESRC's Research Priorities Policy on User Engagement* (http://www.esrc.ac.uk/esrccontent/research funding/usereng.asp).
2 Oliver, S. (1998) Developing consumer involvement in the NHS R&D HTA programme: a needs and feasibility study (http://www.hta.nhsweb.nhs.uk/consrept.htm): accessed 11 November 2002.
3 World Medical Association (2000) *Ethical Principles for Medical Research Involving Human Subjects* (The Declaration of Helsinki). Adopted by the 52nd WMA General Assembly, Edinburgh, UK, October 2000.
4 See the Macmillan Cancer Relief website (http://www.cancerlink.org).
5 O'Rourke, A. (2002) Public involvement: threat or opportunity (http://www.shef.ac.uk/uni/projects/wrp/cgptinv.htm).

References

Arnstein, S.R. (1969) A ladder of citizen participation. *Journal of the American Institute of Planners*, 35: 368–71.
Barnes, M. and Walker, A. (1996) Consumerism versus empowerment: a principled approach to the involvement of older service users. *Policy and Practice*, 24(4): 375–93.
Beresford, P. and Campbell, J. (1994) Disabled people, service users, user involvement and representation. *Disability and Society*, 9: 315–25.
Beresford, P., Broughton, F., Croft, S, *et al.* (2000) *Palliative Care: Developing User Involvement, Improving Quality*. Summary Report. London: Brunel University.
Boote, J., Telford, R. and Cooper, C. (2002) Consumer involvement in health research: a review and research agenda. *Health Policy*, 61(2): 213–36.
Carter, T. and Beresford, P. (2000) *Age and Change: Models of Involvement for Older People*. York: York Press.
Consumers in NHS Research Support Unit (2000) *Involving Consumers in Research and Development in the NHS: Briefing Notes for Researchers*. Winchester: Consumers in NHS Research Support Unit.
Department of Health (2002) New director of patient experience and public involvement appointed, *Press Release* (Reference 2002/0210). London: Department of Health.
Drake, R.F. (1999) *Understanding Disability Policies*. London: Macmillan.
Drake, R.F. (2002) Disabled people, voluntary organisations and participation in policy making. *Policy and Politics*, 30(3): 373–85.
Elliott, E., Watson, A.J. and Harries, U. (2002) Harnessing expertise: involving peer interviewers in qualitative research with hard-to-reach populations. *Health Expectations*, 5: 172–8.

Eve, A. and Higginson, I.J. (2000) Minimum dataset activity for hospice and hospital palliative care services in the UK 1997/98. *Palliative Medicine*, 14(5): 395–404.

Field, D. and Addington-Hall, J. (1999) Extending specialist palliative care to all? *Social Science and Medicine*, 48(9): 1271–80.

Gott, M., Stevens, T., Small, N. and Ahmedzai, S.H. (2000) *User Involvement in Cancer Care: Exclusion and Empowerment*. Bristol: Policy Press.

Gott, M., Stevens, T., Small, N. and Ahmedzai, S.H. (2002) User involvement in cancer care. *British Journal of Clinical Governance*, 7(2): 81–5.

Gray, R., Fitch, M., Greenberg, M. and Shapiro, S. (1995) Consumer participation in cancer service planning. *Journal of Palliative Care*, 11(4): 27–33.

Hamilton-Gurney, B. (1993) *Public Participation in Healthcare Decision Making*. Cambridge: Health Services Research Group, University of Cambridge.

Hanley, B., Truesdale, A., King, A., Elbourne, D. and Chalmers, I. (2001) Involving consumers in designing, conducting and interpreting randomised controlled trials: questionnaire survey. *British Medical Journal*, 322(7285): 519–23.

Harrison, S. and Mort, M. (1998) Which champions, which people? Public involvement in health care as a technology of legitimisation. *Social Policy and Administration*, 32(1): 60–70.

Harrison, S., Hunter, D., Marnock, G. and Pollitt, C. (1992) *Just Managing: Power and Culture in the National Health Service*. London: Macmillan.

Herxheimer, A. and Goodacre, H. (1999) Who are you, and who are we? Looking through some key words. *Health Expectations*, 2: 3–6.

Liddle, B. (1991) *Caring Principles: Personal Service Initiative Guidelines*. Sheffield: Trent Regional Health Authority.

McFadyen, J. and Farrington, A. (1997) User and carer participation in the NHS. *British Journal of Health Care Management*, 3(5): 260–4.

McLeod, E. (1999) Self-help support groups in secondary breast cancer – a new UK initiative. *European Journal of Palliative Care*, 6(3): 103–5.

NHS Executive (1998) *Research: What's in it for Consumers?* London: Department of Health.

National Council for Hospice and Specialist Palliative Care Services (2000) Our lives, not our illness: user involvement in palliative care, *Briefing*, No. 6. London: NCHSPCS.

Oliviere, D. (1999) Cicely Suanders interview for the *VIth Congress of the European Association for Palliative Care*, September, Geneva.

Payne, S. (2002) Are we using the users? (editorial) *International Journal of Palliative Nursing*, 8(5): 212.

Poulton, B. (1999) User involvement in identifying health needs and shaping and evaluating services: is it being realised? *Journal of Advanced Nursing*, 30(6): 1289–96.

Raynes, N.V., Leach, J.M., Rawlings, B. and Bryson, R.J. (2001) Using focus groups to seek the views of patients dying from cancer about the care they receive. *Health Expectations*, 3: 169–75.

Rhodes, P. and Nocon, A. (1998) User involvement and the NHS reforms. *Health Expectations*, 1(2): 73–81.

Saltman, R.B. (1994) Patient choice and patient empowerment in Northern European health systems – a conceptual framework. *International Journal of Health Services*, 24(2): 201–29.

Saunders, C. (2002) Keeping the balance. *European Journal of Palliative Care*, 9(1): 4.

Seymour, J., Bellamy, G., Gott, M., Clark, D. and Ahmedzai, S.H. (2002) Using focus groups to explore older people's attitudes to end of life care. *Ageing and Society*, 22(4): 415–26.

Small, N. (1999) The modern hospice movement: 'Bright lights sparkling' or 'a bit of heaven for the few'?, in J. Bornat, R. Perks, P. Thompson and J. Walmsley (eds) *Oral History, Health and Welfare*. London: Routledge.

Small, N. and Rhodes, P. (2000) *Too Ill to Talk? User Involvement in Palliative Care*. London: Routledge.

Telford, R., Beverley, C.A., Cooper, C. and Boote, J.D. (2002) Consumer involvement in health research: fact or fiction? *British Journal of Clinical Governance*, 7(2): 92–103.

Thornton, P. (2000) *Older People Speaking Out: Developing Opportunities for Influence*. York: Joseph Rowntree Foundation.

Thornton, P. and Tozer, R. (1995) *Having a Say in Change: Older People and Community Care*. Community Care into Practice Series. York: Joseph Rowntree Foundation and Community Care.

Toffaleti, C. (1997) *The Older People's Initiative: Giving Older People a Say – Acting Locally to Improve Housing Choices*. Manchester: Greater Manchester Centre for Voluntary Organization.

5

Referral patterns and access to specialist palliative care

Julia Addington-Hall

In this chapter, I present evidence on the availability of specialist palliative care services and on who accesses them. I draw primarily, but not exclusively, on data from the UK. The appropriateness or otherwise of these services focusing primarily on cancer patients is discussed, as is the question of whether older people are disadvantaged in terms of access to these services. Variations in access to specialist palliative care by social class and ethnic group are not considered here as they are discussed elsewhere in this book.

Availability of specialist palliative care

Access to health services is determined both by availability and eligibility. The availability of specialist palliative care services in the UK has increased considerably over the past 20 years. In 1990, there were 124 in-patient units, 277 community palliative care teams and more than 40 hospital palliative care teams (St Christopher's Information Service 1990). By 2002, this had risen to 209, 338 and 325, respectively.[1] New forms of specialist palliative care service have also developed, for example hospice day care, of which there were 245 in 2002, and hospice at home services, providing 24-hour nursing care for limited periods, of which there were 70.

Much of the development of these services has taken place outside of the National Health Service (NHS), although the NHS is playing an increasing role in the provision of these services, particularly of community and hospital palliative care services. However, although there are 56 in-patient units funded and managed by the NHS, most are independent and receive on average 35 per cent of their funding from the NHS, the rest coming from local fund-raising and charitable contributions. These services have been initiated by local enthusiasts in response to local perceived need, rather than resulting from local or national health care planning. This has given them the freedom to expand and to develop new initiatives without having to compete with all other forms of health care for limited NHS funding. The reliance on non-NHS funding sources can threaten the financial viability of services, however, particularly in a time of reduced charitable giving and economic recession. Independent hospices in the UK are therefore campaigning for a larger contribution to their running costs from the NHS. Their success in achieving this, together with the state of the national economy, will impact on the availability of palliative care services, particularly in-patient care, across the UK.

Two national charities have played a significant role in increasing specialist palliative care in the UK: Macmillan Cancer Relief, which has provided initial funding and continued educational support for many palliative care nursing, medical and social work posts, has contributed to the costs of buildings and funded innovative services; and Marie Curie Cancer Care, which funds ten specialist palliative care in-patient units as well as providing night-sitting services. Lunt and Hillier observed in 1981 that the development of services by local groups in response to local need had led to considerable regional variations in services, with most being in the relatively affluent south. Macmillan Cancer Relief played an important role in funding services in less affluent areas and in reducing inequalities in service provision (Lunt 1985).

Despite this, and the increasing role played in the 1990s by local health authorities in assessing need for palliative care and developing local strategies (Clark *et al.* 1995), inequalities in the availability of specialist palliative care persist. In 1999, the Department of Health commissioned two surveys to provide a picture of the current level of provision for palliative care and health authority views about the need for such services (National Council of Hospice and Specialist Palliative Care Services 2000). The results identified widely differing volumes of service between regions, and even greater discrepancies at health authority level. The conclusion was that the differing levels of provision were unlikely to reflect differing levels of need. The government has used the New Opportunities Fund, money generated by the National Lottery, to fund new initiatives in palliative care aimed at reducing inequalities in provision. Given the major role played by local charities in both funding and running specialist palliative care services in the UK, unequal access to this care across the UK is likely to continue. Access to palliative care is not only therefore determined by the characteristics of the individual and the 'match' between these and eligibility criteria for palliative care (discussed below), but by local availability of these services.

This highlights how access to specialist palliative care cannot be fully explained by the criteria for eligibility developed by services themselves. Instead, the organization and funding of health care systems and the relationship of palliative care to these play a major role. Theoretically, access to this care in the UK might have been expected to be better if it had developed within the NHS via centralized planning, although the current debate about the 'postcode lottery' of health care in the UK and the development of national bodies such as the National Institute for Clinical Excellence aimed explicitly at reducing inequalities suggest that this would not have eliminated all local variations in care provision.

The influence of funding mechanisms on the availability of palliative care is illustrated by the example of the USA, where the Medicare hospice benefit was approved by the Health Care Financial Administration in 1983. This was designed specifically to increase access to hospice programmes and has enabled hospice programmes to grow on the basis of a predictable income flow. About 60 per cent of hospice patients are covered by the benefit (Field and Cassel 1997). Patients certified as having a life expectancy of 6 months or less and who waiver the right to standard Medicare benefits for curative treatments are eligible for the benefit, which provides a *per diem* payment. This covers short in-patient stays (provided these do not exceed 20 per cent of the total hospice care days for the hospice) and a variety of medical and non-medical services at home. The benefit has influenced not only the speed of growth of hospice programmes but also their characteristics: services are expected to use volunteers and to limit in-patient care, while patients have to have a predictable prognosis and usually to have informal carers to share in the care. The characteristics of patients receiving hospice care in the USA differ in a number of ways from those of hospice patients in the UK: they are much more likely to have a diagnosis other than cancer, to be closer to death, to be at home rather than an in-patient and to be in a nursing home. The benefit's availability has encouraged an entrepreneurial approach to the provision of hospices, with expansion into new markets (such as nursing homes and non-cancer patients) and the development of for-profit hospice chains. Initial enthusiasm for this benefit has changed in some quarters to opposition to the ways it constrains and shapes hospice provision.

As these examples illustrate, the availability of specialist palliative care services is largely determined by the health care system of the country in question and the level of health care funding. A third element is the political will to support these services. Palliative care has to compete with many other deserving recipients of the 'health pound', and its success or otherwise in gaining political support is an important determinant of the funding it receives and therefore of service availability. In many countries, including the UK and the USA, innovative services have been initiated by local supporters, but achieving acceptance within the health care system and political support are important if existing services are to be sustained and new services are to be developed. Italy and Canada are both examples of successful sustained attempts to gain political support and the impact of doing so on service provision, although, as with the Medicare benefit in the USA, the initial champions and initiators of palliative care do not always like the consequences of gaining political support and becoming more 'mainstream' within national health care provision (Toscani 2002).

The availability of specialist palliative care thus varies between and across countries depending on the health care system, health care funding and both political and public support for these services. Access to the available services is determined by eligibility criteria, both explicit and implicit, which are themselves determined by beliefs about the purpose and benefits of palliative care. These are considered in the remainder of this chapter.

Access to specialist palliative care

Most people who receive care from hospice and specialist palliative care services have a diagnosis of cancer: in 2000–2001, 95 per cent of patients receiving palliative care had cancer.[2] In the UK at least, specialist palliative care is largely synonymous with cancer care, in particular terminal cancer care.

This is not surprising given that a strong desire to improve care for dying cancer patients provided much of the motivation for founding St Christopher's Hospice, usually regarded as the first modern hospice, and accounts for the rapid uptake of the ideas developed by its founder, Dame Cicely Saunders. The number of people who died from cancer increased rapidly in the twentieth century as better public health and the development of effective treatments such as antibiotics led to a decline in the number of deaths from infectious diseases. The same period saw the development of modern, scientific medicine with its emphasis on cure rather than care, and the concomitant growth in hospital provision and utilization. Glaser and Strauss, in their seminal work in the 1960s (Glaser and Strauss 1965, 1968), observed how dying cancer patients were often ignored, kept in the dark about their prognosis and isolated in hospitals, particularly by medical staff. Dame Cicely's own observation while a medical almoner or social worker of the neglect and poor symptom control experienced by these patients in hospitals had earlier led her to undertake medical training to find ways to improve their care. The picture of poor communication with health professionals, of inadequate support and of distressing, uncontrolled symptoms was reinforced by the results of surveys of patients nursed at home (Marie Curie Memorial Foundation 1952), cared for in terminal care homes (Hughes 1960) and dying in hospital (Hinton 1963). Dying from cancer in the 1950s and 1960s could often be an appalling experience for patients and their families (as, of course, it can still be today in the absence of effective palliative care). The groundswell of public and professional support which made possible the opening of St Christopher's Hospice in 1967 and which fuelled the rapid spread of the hospice movement is evidence of widespread dissatisfaction with the care these patients received.

The growth of hospice and specialist palliative care has led to improvements in the care that can be offered to terminally ill cancer patients and their families. Cancer pain can now be controlled in the majority of patients, and effective therapies are available – or are being developed – for other distressing symptoms (Doyle *et al.* 1998). Dame Cicely's concept of 'total pain' embraces psychological, social and spiritual as well as physical distress (Clark 1999), and expertise has also been developed in addressing these aspects of the patient's experience. Dame Cicely Saunders has argued that much less progress would have been made if hospices had from the beginning been open to all dying patients, regardless of diagnosis (personal communication). The initial focus of hospice services on terminal cancer care can therefore be explained by the overwhelming needs of these patients, and by a desire to focus on one group to make rapid progress in, for example, symptom control. Rapid progress in the understanding and treatment of pain at this time was also important.

From its inception, however, the relevance has been recognized of the principles and practice of hospice care to patients dying from other diseases. For example, Dame Cicely Saunders and Dr Mary Baines from St Christopher's Hospice wrote in 1983 that 'many of the symptoms to be treated and much of the general management will be relevant to other situations . . . Terminal care should not only be a part of oncology but of geriatric medicine, neurology, general practice and throughout medicine' (p. 2). The hope – and expectation – was that other medical specialties would take on the task of developing services specific to and appropriate for 'their' terminally ill patients. There is little evidence that this has happened in terms of service provision, although occasional publications have recognized the needs of dying patients (Graham and Livesley 1983; Wilkes 1984; Volicer 1986).

Some non-cancer patients have been cared for by hospice and specialist palliative care services. For example, St Christopher's Hospice initially provided care for some long-term chronically ill patients such as those with multiple sclerosis or motor neurone disease, mirroring the practice of St Joseph's Hospice where Dame Cicely had previously worked. It continues to care for motor neurone patients, as do other services.

Challenges to the focus on cancer: AIDS/HIV

The focus of specialist palliative care services on terminal cancer care has been challenged, particularly in the past decade. The inception of the AIDS/HIV epidemic in the 1980s meant that there were growing numbers of predominately young terminally ill patients who, like cancer patients, experienced distressing physical, psychological, social and spiritual problems, compounded by the fear and stigma associated with an AIDS diagnosis. There was considerable debate as to whether these patients' needs could best be met within existing hospice and specialist palliative care services, or whether new AIDS/HIV-specific services needed to be developed. Initially, specific services were developed, in part because of the availability of ring-fenced funds for AIDS/HIV services. The characteristics of people with AIDS in the UK have, however, changed, with a growth in the proportion of sufferers who are women and who come from sub-Saharan Africa. These clients may not feel comfortable in services developed primarily for gay men and, because of the stigma attached to AIDS, may prefer to access generic services. This demographic shift, together with removal of ring-fenced funding and the decline in AIDS-related mortality due to use of the triple therapies, has led to increased use of generic hospice services and a decline in the availability of AIDS-specific services.

NHS reforms

Changes to the organization of the NHS in the early 1990s also resulted in challenges to the focus of specialist palliative care services on cancer. District health authorities no longer managed patients directly, but instead were made responsible for assessing the need of their resident population for health care, and then purchasing (later commissioning) care from local health service providers to meet these needs. This led to interest in needs assessment, accompanied in palliative care by increasing recognition that cancer patients are not alone in needing palliative care. An expert report to the Department of Health in 1992 from the Standing Medical Advisory Committee and the Standing Nursing and Midwifery Advisory Committees on the Principles and Provision of Palliative Care (1992) recommended that 'all patients needing them should have access to palliative care services. Although often referred to as equating with terminal cancer care, it is important to recognise that similar services are appropriate and should be developed for patients dying from other diseases' (p. 28). Here the emphasis is on separate services being developed for patients with conditions other than cancer, which is consistent with the approach adopted by the hospice movement since its inception. However, in 1996 an NHS Executive letter to health authorities stated that

> purchasers are asked to ensure that provision of care with a palliative approach is included in all contracts of service for those with cancer and other life-threatening diseases . . . although this letter is focused on services for cancer patients, it applies equally for patients with other life threatening conditions, including AIDS, neurological conditions, and cardiac and respiratory failure.

This uses a model of palliative care that distinguishes between the palliative care approach, the responsibility of all health care providers, and specialist palliative care (NHS Executive 1996). It does not explicitly require either that separate services should be provided for non-cancer patients or that they should have increased access to existing specialist services, but it does re-define the boundaries of palliative care to include non-cancer patients. This is reflected in the epidemiologically based needs assessment for palliative care (Higginson 1997) that provided estimates of the number of people per 1,000,000 population with cancer, progressive non-malignant disease and HIV/AIDS who may need palliative care. In 2000, the National Service Framework for Cardiac Disease (Department of Health 2000a) reflected this boundary shift and, indeed, took it further by stating that patients with severe heart failure should have access to specialist palliative care services.

Political changes in the NHS, first producing the purchaser/provider split and fuelling the development of needs assessments, and then commissioning national service frameworks, have been influential in changing the rhetoric of palliative care to include non-cancer as well as cancer patients.

Non-cancer palliative care needs

Stating that palliative care should be provided on the basis of need is not in itself, however, sufficient to produce an increase in the numbers of non-cancer patients accessing specialist palliative care services. These patients may not have physical, psychological, social or spiritual needs at the end of life, and thus may not require these services. Some evidence that this is not the case comes from the increasing body of research into the palliative care needs of non-cancer patients. For example, the Regional Study of Care for the Dying, a large population-based interview study of bereaved relatives of a representative sample of deaths in England in 1990 (Addington-Hall and McCarthy 1995; McCarthy *et al.* 1997a), found that people who died from heart disease were reported to have experienced a wide range of symptoms, which were frequently distressing and often lasted more than 6 months, and which were associated with a decreased quality of life. Half were thought to have known they were dying: most worked it out for themselves, a situation similar to cancer in the 1960s (McCarthy *et al.* 1996, 1997b). Other papers from the study highlighted the experiences of people who died from respiratory disease, stroke or dementia (Addington-Hall *et al.* 1995; McCarthy *et al.* 1997a; Edmonds *et al.* 2001). At the same time, evidence was emerging from a large US study, the SUPPORT study, of the poor quality of life, uncontrolled symptoms and inadequate communication of people dying from conditions such as severe heart failure, chronic obstructive pulmonary disease (COPD) and cirrhosis of the liver (Lynn *et al.* 1997b). Other studies have been reported more recently expanding on and refining these findings (see Addington-Hall and Higginson 2001). Although many questions remain unanswered, there is growing evidence that many people who die from causes other than cancer need in their last weeks and months of life better symptom control, more psychological and spiritual support, more open communication with health professionals, and more support for their families.

Establishing that some non-cancer patients have similar problems at the end of life as cancer patients is not in itself, however, sufficient to establish a *need* for specialist palliative care provision beyond cancer. According to the definition of need adopted in the influential publications on epidemiologically based needs assessment (Stevens and Raftery 1997), it is necessary to establish that someone will benefit from a health care intervention before describing them as needing that service. Evidence that cancer patients benefit from specialist palliative care services is sparse (Bosanquet and Salisbury 1999) and that for non-cancer patients even sparser, particularly beyond HIV/AIDS and neurological conditions (for a review, see Addington-Hall and Higginson 2001). Specialist palliative care services need to add to this evidence base by evaluating the impact of their care on non-cancer patients, and demonstration projects incorporating evaluation are needed of new innovative palliative care services for these patients. It is not self-evident that they will want or benefit from services developed primarily for cancer patients, and it is important to establish the costs and benefits of specialist palliative care outside cancer if harm to patients is to be avoided and resources are to be used efficiently.

Use of palliative care services by non-cancer patients

The lack of evidence that specialist palliative care services benefit non-cancer patients may explain in part why in the UK the proportion of patients using these services who do not have cancer is rising slowly, if at all. This differs from the USA, where the proportion of hospice patients in 1995 who had a diagnosis other than cancer was 40 per cent, with 6 per cent having heart-related diagnoses, 4 per cent AIDS, 2 per cent Alzheimer's disease and 27 per cent other diagnoses. Differences between the two countries illustrate the impact that funding systems have on access to palliative care, and it has been hypothesized that the number of non-cancer patients served by specialist palliative care services in the UK would rise more swiftly if additional funding was available. The Medicare hospice benefit has served this role in the USA, as discussed above, while ring-fenced funding for HIV/AIDS was important in encouraging the development of palliative care for these patients in the 1990s. Existing specialist palliative care services in the UK depend heavily on charitable fund-raising, much of it explicitly directed to the care of terminally ill cancer patients. Within the NHS, the National Cancer Plan, the development of supportive and palliative care guidelines by the National Institute of Clinical Excellence (NICE) and increased funding for cancer research and service provision (Department of Health 2000b),[3] have again focused attention on cancer. Even if specialist palliative care services are shown to benefit non-cancer patients, demonstrating need will not be sufficient to increase access – the question of who will fund care for these patients will also need to be addressed.

Funding is not the only barrier to existing specialist palliative care services caring for non-cancer patients (Field and Addington-Hall 1999). An important difference between cancer and non-cancer is the difficulty in judging prognosis and thus in identifying suitable candidates for palliative care. For example, the SUPPORT study used multivariate computer models based on clinical and biochemical indices to predict prognosis. On the day before death, lung cancer patients were estimated to have less than a 5 per cent chance of surviving for 2 months, while chronic heart failure patients had a more than 40 per cent chance (Lynn *et al.* 1997a). This causes several problems. For example, palliative care services are concerned about providing care for patients who may survive for months or years, limiting the care they can offer other patients. Heart failure patients may never be viewed by their clinicians as 'dying' or having a limited prognosis, and they may consequently (and perhaps correctly) continue to receive intensive medical care until they die. Prognostic uncertainty is a barrier to many non-cancer patients receiving palliative care until very close to death (as in the American hospice experience) or at all. Innovative models of care are needed such as, for example, offering one-off consultations, short-term interventions with the possibility of re-referral if new problems develop, or 'full' palliative care depending on the complexity of the patient's problems (George and Sykes 1997).

Many nurses and doctors in palliative care have mainly worked and trained in cancer patient care and may rightly be concerned about whether they have the skills to care for other patient groups. As has happened with AIDS/HIV patient care, they may need to work in partnership with colleagues in, for example, cardiology or health care for the elderly. Encouraging and facilitating health professionals from backgrounds other than cancer to train and work in palliative care will also be important.

A final barrier to non-cancer patients accessing specialist palliative care services is the image of these services and their acceptability to, for example, patients with heart failure or chronic respiratory diseases. Cancer patients can be reluctant to accept referrals to hospices or other services because of their association with dying. Changes in terminology from 'hospice' to 'palliative care', in eligibility criteria to include patients earlier in the disease trajectory, and in patterns of service delivery (including joint clinics with oncologists in hospitals) will all help to attract earlier referrals for terminally ill cancer patients, and to overcome the anxieties cancer patients and their families may have about accessing this care. Cancer, however, still has a close association with death and dying in the public imagination. Heart failure, like other chronic diseases, does not. The shock of being referred to a palliative care service may be even greater in these patients and needs very careful explanation. The acceptability of these services to non-cancer patients is largely unknown, and may represent a major challenge to increasing access for them. Again, innovative patterns of service provision with, for example, hospital and community palliative care teams working closely with the growing numbers of heart failure nurses (Blue *et al.* 2001) will be needed.

In summary, specialist palliative care provision in the UK is primarily used by cancer patients, with some AIDS/HIV and motor neurone disease patients also receiving care. The higher proportion of non-cancer patients in American hospice programmes shows that the focus on cancer is not inevitable. There is growing evidence of palliative care needs among patients with chronic progressive diseases such as chronic heart failure and COPD, although there is little evidence that specialist palliative care services benefit these patients. There are barriers to increasing access for non-cancer patients, including funding, the difficulty of identifying appropriate candidates because of prognostic uncertainty, the putative lack of appropriate skills among palliative care professionals, and unanswered questions about the acceptability of these services to non-cancer patients. Innovation and trial-and-error, accompanied by both summative and formative evaluations, will be needed to adapt palliative care to the needs of non-cancer patients and to the settings where they currently receive care.

Improving access for non-cancer patients will not just – or, perhaps, even primarily – mean opening the doors of existing services to these patients, but will require adaptations to these services as well as the development of new services. It will require a close partnership between palliative care and other specialities, particularly health care for the elderly (including nursing homes) given the ageing population and the higher incidence of chronic, progressive conditions in older people (Lye and Donnellan 2000). Indeed, discussing access for non-cancer patients to palliative care services without considering access issues for older people, including older cancer patients, is to over-simplify the issues. The access of older people to specialist palliative care services is therefore considered in the next section.

Older people's access to palliative care

Causes of death vary significantly with age. While overall rates of heart disease remain fairly stable across age groups (unlike chronic heart failure rates, which increase with age: Lye and Donnellan 2000), the proportion of deaths from stroke increase from 5 per cent in those aged under 65 to 13 per cent in those aged 85 or over. Dementia accounts for less than 1 per cent of deaths in the youngest age group, compared with nearly 10 per cent in the oldest age group. The proportion of cancer deaths decreases significantly with age, from 37 per cent in those who die before age 65 to 12 per cent in those who survived to at least 85. This has led to the suggestion that age is the crucial factor in determining how people with cancer differ from non-cancer patients (Seale 1991a). While this is true when the proportion of deaths from each cause is considered, the total number of deaths increases with age. This means that the number of people aged 75 or older who die from cancer does not differ much from the number who die from it before the age of 75: 63,049 versus 70,397 in England and Wales in 1999. Cancer and non-cancer patients differ at the end of life in a number of ways, includ-ing the pattern and severity of symptoms and their dependency levels (Addington-Hall and Karlsen 1999). This is true of patients under 65 as well as of older patients, and it is therefore not helpful to see age as the main difference between cancer and non-cancer patients. It risks obscuring the needs of younger non-cancer patients and of older cancer patients. Never-theless, in terms of numbers, the limited access to specialist palliative care services for non-cancer patients has a greater impact on older people who die than it does on younger people. This is compounded by evidence that older cancer patients access specialist palliative care services less frequently than younger patients, at least in the UK.

Older terminally ill cancer patients are less likely to access hospice in-patient care than younger patients. In the Regional Study of Care for the Dying, patients under the age of 85 years at death were almost three times (2.82) more likely to have been admitted to a hospice than those over this age (Addington-Hall *et al.* 1998). Differences in site of cancer, dependency levels and reported symptoms were controlled for statistically and do not explain this finding. In health districts with a lower than average number of hospice beds, patients under the age of 65 were significantly more likely to access hospice care than those over this age. Other studies have reported similar findings (Hunt and McCaul 1996; Eve and Higginson 2000; Grande *et al.* 2002).

Why might older cancer patients be less likely than younger ones to access in-patient hospice care? Hospices – or those making referrals – may be focusing a scarce resource on patients they believe to be most at need. Nursing homes may be an acceptable alternative for older people unable to remain at home, but be considered less suitable for younger patients who are therefore admitted to a hospice instead. This apparent use of in-patient hospices to provide care for younger patients who can no longer cope at home is out of step with the increasing emphasis of many UK hospices on short-term admissions to alleviate difficult physical or psychological symptoms. The Regional Study of Care for the Dying, which took place in 1990–91, may not reflect the current situation, particularly given the rise of specialist palliative care units. It also cannot fully explain the evidence of age-related differences in access to specialist palliative care services, as the same pattern is found in community palliative care services.

Grande *et al.* (1998) reviewed the evidence and concluded that having a primary carer (particularly one who was not 'too old', male or employed), being female and from a high social economic group were associated with high hospice home-care usage, while being older, having long-term care requirements or haemotological cancer were associated with low usage. In the Regional Study of Care for the Dying, ten factors were found to independently predict community specialist palliative care use in the last year of life (Addington-Hall and Altmann 2000). Factors significantly associated with increased use were requiring assistance with dressing/undressing, needing help at night, having constipation, experiencing vomiting/nausea, being mentally confused, having breast cancer and being under the age of 75 years. In contrast, having a lymphatic/haemotological cancer, a brain tumour and being dependent on others for help with self-care for more than 1 year were associated with decreased use. The use of community specialist palliative care nurses to provide expertise in symptom control and to support families of patients who are dependent or have symptom control problems is consistent with the aims of palliative care. It is more difficult to argue that the age differential in use of these services is appropriate.

Why might being older affect access to these services? Again, older individuals may be seen – or see themselves – as being less in need of the expert support provided by specialist palliative care services. There is some evidence that they experience less symptom distress than younger patients (Degner and Sloan 1995) but the evidence is not conclusive. The similarities in how pain is experienced by younger and older people may be more apparent than the differences. The requirements for pain management in a geriatric hospice population appear to be similar to those of younger patients with advanced cancer, with some two-thirds of both groups experiencing pain (Stein and Miech 1993). Older people may be at increased risk of experiencing uncontrolled pain, with health professionals failing to detect or treat their pain, perhaps because of beliefs that it is less of a problem in this population. On admission nurses are almost twice as likely to miss pain from a problem list with older patients than with their younger counterparts. A seminal study of pain management in a large population of older patients with cancer concluded that daily pain is prevalent and often goes untreated (Bernabei *et al.* 1998). More information is needed on how the prevalence, perception and control of symptoms varies with age, but the limited available evidence suggests that the relative under-utilization of specialist palliative care services in older people cannot be wholly explained by these factors, although health professional beliefs about symptom experience at different ages may play an important role.

Specialist palliative care includes psychological and spiritual support as well as the control of physical symptoms. Do older people need this type of support less than younger patients? Older cancer patients are thought to be less troubled by a cancer diagnosis than younger people (Harrison and Maguire 1995) and are believed to be more accepting of death (Feifel and Branscomb 1973). Lower rates of death anxiety have indeed been reported for older people in some studies; however, the evidence for this being a general characteristic of older age remains equivocal (Wagner and Lorion 1984). Some, perhaps many, older people do find it less difficult to face death than their younger counterparts. However, this is not true of all older people and some may benefit from the expertise of specialist palliative care teams in helping them to come to terms with their own mortality and to make some sense of their lives. Their families may also benefit from the care and continuing support these teams provide: although younger families with children have particularly acute social and psychological need, the devastation experienced by many older spouses and their adult children and the physical consequences of care-giving in older people with their own health problems should not be overlooked.

People who are admitted to a hospice in the last year of life are more likely than other cancer patients to have cancer alone recorded as cause of death on their death certificate (Seale 1991b). Older cancer patients are likely to have co-morbidities, such as musculoskeletal, respiratory and circulatory conditions, and this may contribute to their under-utilization of specialist palliative care services. As discussed above, these services focus on patients for whom the consequences of cancer are the main problem, and who are often relatively unfamiliar with the management of other conditions. The higher incidence of dementia may also reduce hospice usage in the UK (but to a lesser extent in the USA; Hanrahan *et al.* 2001), as these services are reluctant or unable to care for patients with severe mental health problems (Addington-Hall 2000).

There is little evidence with which to address the question of whether the focus on cancer patients who have limited or no co-morbidities is appropriate or whether it discriminates against older people. A patient's age conveys little or no information about the needs of that individual, however much information it conveys about the needs of the total population of people of that age. Patients need to be assessed as individuals and to have their eligibility for specialist palliative care determined on the basis of this assessment, not on the basis of their chronological age.

This discussion presupposes that the age differential in access to specialist palliative care is a consequence solely of the admission policies and practices of these services. These are important, but the attitudes of those making referrals and of the patients themselves are also important in determining access to specialist palliative care. Hinton (1994) reported that age differentials were evident in referrals to a palliative care community service, but not in referrals from that service to an in-patient hospice. Health professionals caring for these patients may not make referrals to specialist palliative care if they perceive the referral as being unlikely to be accepted, if they underestimate the patient's physical, psychological or spiritual needs, or if they (perhaps rightly) consider themselves to have superior skills in the management of the patient. They may also be caring for patients in a setting with limited access to palliative care services. Further research is needed to explore the attitudes of referrers to palliative care for older people, and to explore the attitudes of older people themselves. Many older people spend at least some time in a nursing home and current efforts in the UK and elsewhere to improve palliative care in these settings are therefore important (Maddocks and Parker 2001).

Conclusions

Access to specialist palliative care services is determined primarily by availability. This varies between and across countries depending on the health care system, health care funding and both political and public support for these services. Access to the available services is determined by eligibility criteria, both explicit and implicit, which are themselves determined by beliefs about the purpose and benefits of palliative care.

Older people are more likely than younger people to die from causes other than cancer and to have a number of co-morbidities alongside cancer. They are therefore disproportionately affected by the focus of specialist palliative care on cancer. Even those who die from cancer are less likely to access specialist palliative care than younger patients with similar dependency and symptoms. There is limited research evidence to justify either the focus on cancer or the age-related differentials in access to these services.

The evidence on palliative care needs in non-cancer supports the argument that many of these patients have unmet palliative care needs, but there is almost no evidence that they would benefit from specialist palliative care interventions. Establishing benefit is an essential stage in establishing need for specialist palliative care beyond cancer, and innovative research and audit studies are needed to build the evidence base. Evidence is also lacking on older people's attitudes to specialist palliative care, their needs at the end of life and the reasons why older cancer patients are referred to these services less often than younger patients. Again, further research is needed. Access to specialist palliative care for non-cancer patients and for older people are closely related issues and should not be considered in isolation.

The literature on access to these services illustrates the importance of assessing each individual's need for palliative care rather than making judgements based implicitly or explicitly on the basis of their age or diagnosis. This, however, presumes that 'palliative care needs' are easily defined and identified. The debate elsewhere in this book on definitions of palliative care shows that they are not. There will continue to be local and national variations in access to specialist palliative care, and there also needs to be continued reflection and debate about whether these variations are justified or are a consequence of stereotypical views of levels of palliative care need among different demographic and diagnostic groups.

- Specialist palliative care availability varies between and across countries depending on the health care system, health care funding and both political and public support for these services.

- Access to the available services is determined by eligibility criteria, both explicit and implicit, which are themselves determined by beliefs about the purpose and benefits of palliative care.

- Palliative care in most, but not all, settings is focused on the care of terminally ill cancer patients. Patients dying from HIV/AIDS or from motor neurone disease often also access this care.

- In the UK, there has been a shift in the rhetoric of palliative care away from a focus on cancer and towards access being determined by need, not diagnosis.

- There is increasing evidence that people who die from other chronic and progressive conditions have physical, psychological, social and spiritual problems in the last weeks or months of life. It is not yet known whether specialist palliative care can address these problems successfully.

- Until there is evidence that specialist palliative care benefits non-cancer patients, they cannot be said conclusively to have palliative care needs. Making access depend on need rather than diagnosis will not, therefore, necessarily change the characteristics of those receiving care.

- Barriers to extending specialist palliative care beyond cancer include a lack of funding, difficulties identifying suitable candidates because of prognostic uncertainty, a lack of skills in non-cancer conditions among specialist palliative care health professionals, and a lack of evidence that non-cancer patients would find referral to these services acceptable.

- Older people with cancer access specialist palliative care services less often than younger people with similar problems. This age differential may be justified: there is some limited evidence that older people need less help to face death and have fewer symptom control problems. Older people need to have their palliative care needs assessed individually and not predetermined from their age or diagnosis.

- Cancer in older people often co-exists with other chronic and progressive conditions. The lack of familiarity of many specialist palliative care services with these conditions may explain in part the under-representation of older cancer patients in these services.
- Differences between countries in the characteristics of patients receiving palliative care demonstrate that specialist palliative care services need not be focused on cancer or primarily serve younger patients.
- There will continue to be local and national variations in access to specialist palliative care, and there also needs to be continued reflection and debate about whether these variations are justified or are a consequence of stereotypical views of levels of palliative care need among different demographic and diagnostic groups.

Notes

1   See Hospice Information Service (2002) UK hospice and palliative care units January 2002 (http://www.hospiceinformation.info/factsandfigures/ukhospice).
2   Ibid.
3   See National Institute for Clinical Excellence (2003) Supportive and palliative care (http://www.nice.org.uk/cat.asp?c=20102).

References

Addington-Hall, J.M. (2000) *Positive Partnerships: Palliative Care for Adults with Severe Mental Health Problems*. Occasional Paper No. 17. London: National Council for Hospices and Specialist Palliative Care Services/Scottish Partnership Agency for Palliative and Cancer Care.

Addington-Hall, J.M. and Altmann, D. (2000) Which terminally ill cancer patients receive care from community specialist palliative care nurses? *Journal of Advanced Nursing*, 32: 799–806.

Addington-Hall, J.M. and Higginson, I.J. (2001) *Palliative Care for Non-Cancer Patients*. Oxford: Oxford University Press.

Addington-Hall, J.M. and Karlsen, S. (1999) Age is not the crucial factor in determining how the palliative care needs of people who die from cancer differ from those of people who die from other causes. *Journal of Palliative Care*, 15: 13–19.

Addington-Hall, J.M. and McCarthy, M. (1995) The Regional Study of Care for the Dying: methods and sample characteristics. *Palliative Medicine*, 9: 27–35.

Addington-Hall, J.M., Lay, M., Altmann, D. and McCarthy, M. (1995) Symptom control, communication with health professionals, and hospital care of stroke patients in the last year of life as reported by surviving family, friends and officials. *Stroke*, 26: 2242–8.

Addington-Hall, J.M., Altmann, D. and McCarthy, M. (1998) Who gets hospice in-patient care? *Social Science and Medicine*, 46: 1011–16.

Bernabei, R., Gambassi, G., Lapane, K. *et al.* (1998) Management of pain in elderly patients with cancer. SAGE Study Group: Systematic Assessment of Geriatric Drug Use via Epidemiology. *Journal of the American Medical Association*, 279: 1877–82.

Blue, L., Lang, E., McMurray, J.J. *et al.* (2001) Randomised controlled trial of specialist nurse intervention in heart failure. *British Medical Journal*, 323: 715–18.

Bosanquet, N. and Salisbury, C. (1999) *Providing a Palliative Care Service: Towards an Evidence Base*. Oxford: Oxford University Press.

Clark, D. (1999) 'Total pain', disciplinary power and the body in the work of Cicely Saunders, 1958–1967. *Social Science and Medicine*, 49: 727–36.

Clark, D., Neale, B. and Heather, P. (1995) Contracting for palliative care. *Social Science and Medicine*, 40: 1193–202.

Degner, L.F. and Sloan, J.A. (1995) Symptom distress in newly diagnosed ambulatory cancer patients and as a predictor of survival in lung cancer. *Journal of Pain and Symptom Management*, 10: 423–31.

Department of Health (2000a) *National Service Framework for Coronary Heart Disease*. London: Department of Health.

Department of Health (2000b) *The NHS Cancer Plan: A Plan for Investment, A Plan of Reform*. London: Department of Health.

Doyle, D., Hanks, W.C. and MacDonald, N. (1998) *Oxford Textbook of Palliative Medicine*, 2nd edn. Oxford: Oxford University Press.

Edmonds, P., Karlsen, S. and Addington-Hall, J.M. (2001) Quality of care in the last year of life: a comparison of lung cancer and COPD patients. *Palliative Medicine*, 15: 287–95.

Eve, A. and Higginson, I.J. (2000) Minimum dataset activity for hospice and hospital palliative care services in the UK 1997/98. *Palliative Medicine*, 14(5): 395–404.

Feifel, H. and Branscomb, A.B. (1973) Who's afraid of death? *Journal of Abnormal Psychology*, 81(3): 282–8.

Field, D. and Addington-Hall, J. (1999) Extending specialist palliative care to all? *Social Science and Medicine*, 48: 1271–80.

Field, M.J. and Cassel, C.K. (1997) *Approaching Death: Improving Care at the End of Life*. The Committee on Care at the End of Life, Division of Health Care Services, Institute of Medicine. Washington, DC: National Academy Press.

George, R. and Sykes, J. (1997) Beyond cancer? in D. Clark, J. Hockley and S. Ahmedzai (eds) *New Themes in Palliative Care*. Buckingham: Open University Press.

Glaser, B.G. and Strauss, A.L. (1965) *Awareness of Dying*. Chicago, IL: Aldine.

Glaser, B.G. and Strauss, A.L. (1968) *Time for Dying*. Chicago, IL: Aldine.

Graham, H. and Livesley, B. (1983) Dying as a diagnosis: difficulties of communication and management in elderly patients. *The Lancet*, 2, 670–2.

Grande, G., Todd, C. and Addington-Hall, J.M. (1998) Variables related to place of death and access to home care services: are certain patient groups at a disadvantage? *Social Science and Medicine*, 47: 565–79.

Grande, G.E., McKerral, A. and Todd, C.J. (2002) Which cancer patients are referred to hospital at home for palliative care? *Palliative Medicine*, 16: 115–23.

Hanrahan, P., Luchins, D.J. and Murphy, K. (2001) Palliative care for patients with dementia, in J.M. Addington-Hall and I.J. Higginson (eds) *Palliative Care for Non-Cancer Patients*. Oxford: Oxford University Press.

Harrison, J. and Maguire, P. (1995) Influence of age on psychological adjustment to cancer. *Psycho-Oncology*, 4: 33–8.

Higginson, I.J. (ed.) (1997) *Health Care Needs Assessment: Palliative and Terminal Care*. Health Care Needs Assessment, 2nd Series. Oxford: Radcliffe Medical Press.

Hinton, J. (1963) The physical and mental distress of the dying. *Quarterly Journal of Medicine*, 32: 1–21.

Hinton, J. (1994) Which patients with terminal cancer are admitted from home care? *Palliative Medicine*, 8: 197–210.

Hughes, H.L.G. (1960) *Peace at the Last*. London: Gulbenkian Foundation.

Hunt, R. and McCaul, K. (1996) A population-based study of the coverage of cancer patients by hospice services. *Palliative Medicine*, 10: 5–12.

Lunt, B. (1985) Terminal cancer care services: recent changes in regional inequalities in Great Britain. *Social Science and Medicine*, 20: 753–9.

Lunt, B. and Hillier, R. (1981) Terminal care: present services and future priorities. *British Medical Journal*, 283: 595–8.

Lye, M. and Donnellan, C. (2000) Heart disease in the elderly. *Heart*, 84: 560–6.

Lynn, J., Harrell, F. Jr., Cohn, F. *et al.* (1997a) Prognoses of seriously ill hospitalised patients on the days before death: implications for patient care and public policy. *New Horizons*, 5: 56–61.

Lynn, J., Teno, J.M., Phillips, R.S. *et al.* (1997b) Perceptions by family members of the dying experience of older and seriously ill patients. *Annals of Internal Medicine*, 126: 97–106.

Maddocks, I. and Parker, D. (2001) Palliative care in nursing homes, in J.M. Addington-Hall and I.J. Higginson (eds) *Palliative Care for Non-Cancer Patients*. Oxford: Oxford University Press.

Marie Curie Memorial Foundation (1952) *Report on a National Survey Concerning Patients Nursed at Home*. London: Marie Curie Memorial Foundation.

McCarthy, M., Lay, M. and Addington-Hall, J.M. (1996) Dying from heart disease. *Journal of the Royal College of Physicians of London*, 30: 325–8.

McCarthy, M., Addington-Hall, J.M. and Altmann, D. (1997a) The experience of dying with dementia: a retrospective survey. *International Journal of Geriatric Psychiatry*, 12: 404–9.

McCarthy, M., Addington-Hall, J.M. and Lay, M. (1997b) Communication and choice in dying from heart disease. *Journal of the Royal Society of Medicine*, 90: 128–31.

National Council of Hospice and Specialist Palliative Care Services (2000) *The Palliative Care Survey 1999*. London: NCHSPCS.

NHS Executive (1996) *A Policy Framework for Commissioning Cancer Services: Palliative Care Services*. EL(96)85. London: NHS Executive.

Saunders, C. and Baines, M. (1983) *Living with Dying: The Management of Terminal Disease*. Oxford: Oxford University Press.

Seale, C. (1991a) Death from cancer and death from other causes: the relevance of the hospice approach. *Palliative Medicine*, 5: 12–19.

Seale, C. (1991b) A comparison of hospice and conventional care. *Social Science and Medicine*, 32: 147–52.

St Christopher's Hospice Information Service (1990) *Directory of Hospice and Specialist Palliative Care Services in the UK and the Republic of Ireland*. London: St Christopher's Hospice Information Service.

Standing Medical Advisory Committee and the Standing Nursing and Midwifery Advisory Committees (1992) *The Principles and Provision of Palliative Care.* London: SMAC/SNMAC.

Stein, W.M. and Miech, R.P. (1993) Cancer pain in the elderly hospice patient. *Journal of Pain and Symptom Management,* 8: 474–82.

Stevens, A. and Raftery, J. (1997) Introduction, in I.J. Higginson (ed.) *Health Care Needs Assessment: Palliative and Terminal Care.* Health Care Needs Assessment, 2nd Series. Oxford: Radcliffe Medical Press.

Toscani, F. (2002) Palliative care in Italy: accident or miracle? *Palliative Medicine,* 16: 177–8.

Volicer, L. (1986) Need for hospice approach to treatment of patients with advanced progressive dementia. *Journal of the American Geriatrics Society,* 34: 655–8.

Wagner, K.D. and Lorion, R.P. (1984) Correlates of death anxiety in elderly persons. *Journal of Clinical Psychology,* 40: 1235–41.

Wilkes, E. (1984) Dying now. *Lancet,* 1: 950–2.

6

Acute hospital care

Vanessa Taylor

From its origins outside mainstream health care in the 'hospice movement', palliative care is re-emerging as an integrated part of mainstream health care delivery (NCHSPCS 1996; Llamas *et al.* 2001), with the acute hospital setting playing a dominant role in the provision of care for patients with palliative care needs. Some authors have questioned the transferability of palliative care to the acute hospital setting. The benefits of palliative care are described as being context-specific, particularly with regard to the caring relationships and collegial commitment of team members in a hospice setting, which may not be as effective when transferred to the acute care setting (Rumbold 1998). Furthermore, the biomedical approach of acute hospitals is considered to over-emphasize the medical and physical aspects of care in the delivery of palliative care (Rumbold 1998; Street 1998). Hospice care is, however, not accessible to everyone (NCHSPCS 2000) and nurses on wards within the hospital setting continue to have responsibility for a significant number of patients with palliative care needs and their families. In general, as many as 90 per cent of people may need some in-patient hospital care in their last year of life and 55 per cent of all deaths in the UK occur in hospital (Ramirez *et al.* 1998). This suggests that there is a need for skilled and compassionate palliative care for patients with palliative care needs within the hospital setting whatever challenges this environment may pose.

In this chapter, I focus on the provision of general and specialist palliative care services within the hospital setting and the challenges faced by nurses when attempting to integrate the principles and practices of palliative care in this setting. General palliative care is described as a vital and integrated part of the routine clinical practice delivered by the usual professional carers of the patient and family with low to moderate complexity of palliative care need. Specialist palliative care services are provided by professional carers who specialize in palliative care for patients and their families with moderate to high complexity of palliative care need (NCHSPCS 2002). The chapter is divided into four sections. First, I examine the prevalence of patients with palliative care needs within the hospital setting. Next, I examine the experiences of patients with palliative care needs and their families of being cared for within this setting. Then I identify the challenges faced by qualified nurses when attempting to integrate the philosophy of palliative care and provide general palliative care in this setting. Finally, I look at the role of, and challenges for, specialist palliative care nurses within the hospital setting.

Palliative care needs in the acute hospital setting

The influence of wider changes in health and social policy is recognized as having a significant effect on the development of palliative care services (Clark *et al.* 2000). Indeed, for people with cancer, contemporary health policy within the UK may be viewed as influencing a broadening of the provision of palliative care services and attempting to reduce inequities in the availability of specialist palliative care services.

Traditionally, the major emphasis of palliative care has been the care of patients with advanced cancer. More recently, however, health policy has emphasized the importance of access to specialist palliative care services for cancer patients from diagnosis onwards (Department of Health 1995, 2000a). Palliative care has, therefore, extended beyond its original focus on terminal care to acknowledge the needs of those who have been recently diagnosed with cancer and those who are not going to die imminently. Furthermore, in recognition of an inequity of service provision across the UK, National Health Service (NHS) palliative care for patients with cancer has become a priority for the government, with additional monies available to support service provision, for education for district nurses and for projects aimed at widening access to palliative care (Department of Health 2000a). The British Government's goal is to set standards and monitor cancer service delivery, seeking to ensure that all cancer patients have access to specialist palliative care services when needed, achieved through a coordinated approach between the NHS and voluntary palliative care services (Department of Health 2000a).

The acute hospital is, for many patients, the place where the majority of investigations, treatment, follow-up, and palliative and terminal care following a diagnosis of cancer are provided. A large proportion of patients receive their diagnosis of cancer within the hospital setting (Cancer Relief Macmillan Fund 1991). Subsequently, patients may attend or be admitted to an acute general hospital for treatment of the disease, management of complications or emergencies, investigation of a suspected recurrence of their cancer, for follow-up or to die. Difficulties of symptom control, rapid deterioration of some patients, and physical and emotional exhaustion of carers have been identified as the major reasons why people die in hospital (Dunlop and Hockley 1998). Multi-professional palliative care support may be introduced to patients and families at the diagnostic phase, alongside curative or life-prolonging treatment, as well as during disease progression and the terminal phase of the patient's illness (Gott *et al.* 2001). This broad inclusive definition of palliative care has, therefore, the potential for many more patients with cancer in the acute hospital to be viewed as being eligible for palliative care (Gott *et al.* 2001).

The NHS Cancer Plan (Department of Health 2000a) addresses the palliative care needs of patients with cancer while ignoring those of patients with other life-limiting illnesses. There has, however, been a realization by the British Government, demonstrated in the national service frameworks for heart disease and older people, that palliative care should be an important and integral part of patient care. This government position endorses the view of the National Council for Hospice and Specialist Palliative Care Services (NCHSPCS) that the principles of palliative care apply equally to patients with diseases other than cancer (Addington-Hall 1998; NCHSPCS 2002). These diseases, while not amenable to curative treatment, may have a prognosis of months or years (McCarthy *et al.* 1996; Addington-Hall 1998; Skilbeck *et al.* 1998; Higginson and Addington-Hall 1999). This includes patients with neurological diseases, AIDS, chronic cardiovascular disease, chronic respiratory disease (Higginson 1993), renal failure, cerebrovascular accident and dementia (Dharmasena and Forbes 2001). These patients may also be diagnosed, managed and cared for within the acute hospital setting and have palliative care needs that may benefit from general and specialist palliative care services. The adoption of such an inclusive definition for palliative care raises the question of the number of patients with palliative care needs within the hospital setting who may require general and/or specialist palliative care services.

Recent studies have demonstrated that between 5 and 23 per cent of patients in hospital have palliative care needs. Skilbeck *et al.* (1999) surveyed nurses in one NHS Trust. They found that approximately 5 per cent of the hospital population of 1200 patients were considered to be suitable for some form of specialist palliative care. Twenty-five per cent of the identified patients were described as terminally ill, 60 per cent were viewed as having palliative care needs and 15 per cent were seen as meeting both criteria. Patients were cared for across a variety of clinical settings, including medical and elderly (49 per cent), cardiothoracic (18 per cent), general surgery (15 per cent), renal (11 per cent), obstetrics and gynaecology (4 per cent), orthopaedics (1 per cent) and burns and plastics (1 per cent) (Skilbeck *et al.* 1999). Similarly, Gott *et al.* (2001) identified the proportion of in-patients at one acute hospital considered by the nursing and medical staff to have palliative care needs during a 1-week period. Overall, 23 per cent of the total in-patient population of 452 were identified as having palliative care needs and/or being terminally ill, although only approximately half had a primary cancer diagnosis. Non-cancer diagnoses included neuromuscular disorders (11 per cent), respiratory disease (9 per cent) and cardiovascular disease (8 per cent). Eleven per cent of the patients identified with palliative care needs were described as being suitable for referral to a specialist palliative care bed.

The study by Gott *et al.* (2001) differed from that of Skilbeck *et al.* (1999) in that Gott and co-workers sought the views of both medical and nursing staff and utilized a broader, more inclusive definition of palliative care. This perhaps reflects the higher proportion of patients identified with palliative care needs. Interestingly, this study revealed a low level of agreement between nursing and medical staff as to which patients had palliative care needs, with nurses more likely than medical staff to identify patients with non-cancer diagnoses as having palliative care needs. This may reflect nurses' greater recognition of the psychosocial aspects of palliative care, while doctors may be more influenced by the medical diagnoses when making such an assessment (Gott *et al.* 2001). Although these studies illustrated the prevalence of patients with palliative care needs within the hospital setting, the range of physical and psychosocial needs experienced by the non-cancer patients have been demonstrated to be at least as severe as for those with cancer (Anderson *et al.* 2001; Edmonds *et al.* 2001).

For those attempting to manage and deliver general and specialist palliative care services within hospitals, these studies provide a helpful indication of the need for service provision and the range of palliative care needs experienced by patients with life-limiting illnesses. A model of service delivery was, therefore, developed by the NCHSPCS to meet these needs. In recognizing the palliative care needs of both cancer patients and patients with non-malignant diseases within the hospital setting, the document *Palliative Care in the Hospital Setting* (NCHSPCS 1996) recommended that the palliative care approach should be an integral part of all clinical practice and should be available to all patients with life-threatening illness, supported by a multidisciplinary hospital palliative care team and integrated with community-based specialist palliative care services and primary health care teams. The term 'palliative care approach' has, more recently, been redefined as general palliative care (NCHSPCS 2002). Nevertheless, the assumptions underpinning this position are that the philosophy and practice of palliative care can be transferred from the traditional hospice setting to the hospital environment and that health professionals are able to deliver general palliative care. The realization of this vision for palliative care within the hospital setting has proved – and continues to prove – challenging, as discussed below.

Patient and family experiences of palliative care in the acute hospital setting

Research in the UK in the 1980s documented deficiencies in the care of those dying in the hospital setting. Staff working in acute hospital settings were described as ineffective in the care of dying patients, with poor communication leading to inadequate support for relatives and patients (Field 1989). In addition, nurses have been shown to respond to the demands of caring for the dying by withdrawal and shying away from death (Morris

1988). A study of deaths in two hospitals in Scotland provided graphic descriptions of people dying in the acute sector in the 1980s (Mills *et al.* 1994). These studies reflected provision of care before the recommendations of the NCHSPCS for hospital-based palliative care services.

Nevertheless, more recent studies continue to highlight the difficulties experienced by patients with palliative care needs and their families within hospital. Rogers *et al.* (2000) reported on the findings of a post-bereavement survey of people who registered a cancer death during 1996–97. The survey aimed to investigate the sources of dissatisfaction with hospital care in the last year of life. While care given by hospital doctors and nurses was rated as 'excellent' or 'good', respondents expressed dissatisfaction with a number of aspects of care arising from a sense of being 'devalued', dehumanized' or 'disempowered'. These sources of dissatisfaction related to instances where the patients or respondents felt that their individual needs or wishes were not given priority or credence (Rogers *et al.* 2000). The findings indicated that the principles of palliative care had yet to be incorporated into the care of the terminally ill in hospital.

Similar sources of dissatisfaction were identified by Dunne and Sullivan (2000), who sought to gain insight into the lived experiences of families who journeyed with their relative through the palliative phase of cancer as in-patients within the acute hospital setting without a specialist palliative care service. The analysis of the interviews undertaken with eight relatives suggested that the acute hospital environment had many shortcomings as a place to deliver palliative care, with the environment described as rushed and lacking in privacy, with patients being moved around the ward as dictated by the needs for acute beds. In addition, family members described feeling isolated and helpless as a result of not being involved in the care of their relative, seeing their relatives in pain (which was poorly managed) and the unsatisfactory level of communication with health professionals in the hospital setting. Dunne and Sullivan (2000) concluded that, despite the advances in palliative care, the acute hospital setting did not appear to have made significant changes for families and patients during the palliative phase of their illness.

These studies provide an insight into the more recent experiences of palliative care for patients with cancer and their relatives within the acute hospital setting, and highlight the gap between the vision of the NCHSPCS recommendations and the reality of palliative care. The environment and the culture of care within the acute hospital setting is criticized together with the skills of the health care professionals to communicate effectively with patients and their families and manage patients' symptoms. This raises concerns about the experiences of patients with palliative care needs arising from other life-limiting illnesses. Regrettably, the care provided by hospitals has been subject to more criticism than any other model of palliative care, with consumers preferring hospice care for the non-clinical aspects of humaneness, the ability of the staff to reduce anxiety and the supportive nursing care (Wilkinson *et al.* 1999). It would appear that the need to achieve a supportive environment within the hospital setting is as important as good symptom control in the delivery of palliative care, and hospitals have yet to make the necessary improvements for patients and their families.

It is important, therefore, that these criticisms are discussed and examined within clinical teams, including specialist palliative care services in hospitals, as well as at an organizational level, if change is to be effective and improvements are to be made to patients' and families' experiences. While changes to the physical environment may not be feasible, energies may be directed at identifying and addressing the issues that challenge health care professionals' abilities to provide general and specialist palliative care in this setting. Some challenges faced by nurses attempting to provide general palliative care within this setting have been identified and are explored next.

Challenges to nurses of providing general palliative care within the acute hospital setting

In the provision of palliative care, it has been suggested that good hospital practice should include the principle that nurses spend time with, and be available for, patients and their families, discussing and planning care within a multidisciplinary team framework (Wilson-Barnett and Richardson 1993). Implicit within this statement is a partnership approach, with a requirement for open and honest communication with the patient, their relatives and between members of the health care team, and the acquisition of appropriate knowledge. Such ideology is central to the nursing philosophy of individualized care, which embraces a holistic approach and active patient participation in care, with a retreat from the biomedical approach (Trnobranski 1994). Similarities between the philosophy and principles of palliative care and individualized nursing care are, therefore, evident. Nevertheless, for nurses, the process of reintegrating palliative care, which largely developed as a marginal activity outside of the NHS in small and often charitable organizations, into the culture of the NHS hospital is not without difficulty.

As nurses are at the forefront of general palliative care delivery within the hospital setting, exploring their experiences may help to uncover why the quality of care for patients with palliative care needs and their families within this setting attracts such criticism. Few studies have, however, focused on discovering the opinions of qualified nurses regarding the provision of care to patients with palliative care needs within the acute hospital setting.

Two studies (Taylor 1995; McDonnell *et al.* 2002) demonstrated the difficulties faced by qualified nurses in the delivery of general palliative care within the hospital setting and go some way to explain the criticisms raised by patients and families. These studies, despite being undertaken 7 years apart, revealed very similar findings. Taylor (1995) interviewed ten qualified nurses (clinical grades D–G) to uncover their experiences of providing continuing care to adult patients with cancer on an acute surgical unit within a district general hospital in south-east England. The hospital Trust had an established multiprofessional specialist palliative care team that included five clinical nurse specialists, two part-time social workers, a part-time staff grade medical doctor and a part-time clinical psychologist. In contrast, McDonnell *et al.* (2002) surveyed 263 nurses representing 18 wards in four district general hospitals in Northern Ireland. Access to specialist palliative care medical staff was available for half the respondents, while access to a specialist palliative care nurse was available for two-thirds of respondents. These studies demonstrated that nurses, with limited education in the principles of palliative care, inexperienced and unsupported in its practices, including the development of teamworking skills, were attempting to provide palliative care in a setting whose culture and context was viewed as being at odds with the philosophy of palliative care (Taylor 1995; McDonnell *et al.* 2002).

The limited access to palliative care education by nurses highlighted in these studies was reinforced by a recent survey (Lloyd-Williams and Field 2002) that identified the extent of teaching that nurses received during their pre-registration undergraduate education. The study revealed that diploma students received a mean of 7.8 hours, while degree students received a mean of 12.2 hours. These figures compare unfavourably with a mean of 20 hours available to undergraduate medical students in the UK (Lloyd-Williams and Field 2002). Furthermore, following registration, nurses practising within the hospital setting reported having limited opportunities to attend education events about cancer and/or palliative care, impeded by staff shortages and a lack of recognition by managers of the need for these types of education within this environment (Taylor 1995). This lack of pre- and post-registration preparation about cancer and/or palliative care for nurses is, therefore, a cause for concern if the vision for the provision of general palliative care for patients with palliative care needs, regardless of diagnosis, is to be realized within the hospital setting. Support by senior managers to include palliative care study days into mandatory programmes for health care staff has been identified as a valuable strategy for reducing the 'fire-fighting' role of Macmillan nurses and achieving more appropriate referrals to hospital teams (Seymour *et al.* 2002).

Other difficulties experienced by nurses providing palliative care in hospitals include problems with multidisciplinary teamworking (Taylor 1995; McDonnell *et al.* 2002). In particular, nurses have been shown to have minimal involvement in the decision-making processes about patients' care and treatment (Taylor 1995) and to perceive a lack of advice from medical colleagues (McDonnell *et al.* 2002). Communicating with patients can also prove challenging, as nurses have limited time to develop a rapport with patients and families and many report feeling ill-prepared to deal with the informational needs of patients (Taylor 1995) and the psychosocial needs of patients' relatives (Taylor 1995; McDonnell *et al.* 2002). Nurses have described feeling isolated and unsupported by medical staff and ancillary staff (McDonnell *et al.* 2002), although this was provided by specialist palliative care services (Taylor 1995; McDonnell *et al.* 2002).

The difficulties of teamworking may highlight the effects of organizational culture and professional socialization on the provision of care.

Nurses, attempting to implement the good hospital practice (Wilson-Barnett and Richardson 1993) described above within this environment, face a challenge to overcome the effect of health care policy and organizational restructuring of the NHS (Department of Health 1997) as well as the professional socialization of other colleagues, especially doctors. Organizational restructuring has shifted the emphasis in the provision of health care, with hospitals becoming places where acute, intensive, short-stay treatment is provided (James and Field 1992), exploiting advances in medical technology that enable many investigations, treatments and conditions to be managed on a day or short-stay in-patient basis (Department of Health 1997). Yet, at the same time, documents such as *The NHS Plan* (Department of Health 2000b) and the national service frameworks, including *The Cancer Plan* (Department of Health 2000a), may be viewed as raising users' and providers' expectations about the individualized and high standard of care they should expect. Nurses, working within hospital settings, may, therefore, have difficulty reconciling the competing demands evident within these policy documents. While patients may benefit from shorter in-patient stays, for those with palliative care needs this may limit the time available to discuss their diagnosis, treatment and the psychosocial impact of the disease and its treatment, resulting in the feelings of isolation and dissatisfaction identified by Dunne and Sullivan (2000) and Rogers *et al.* (2000). Furthermore, as demonstrated by Taylor (1995) and McDonnell *et al.* (2002), nurses can feel isolated and frustrated about their abilities and opportunities to provide palliative care, having to rely on specialist nurses to meet the psychosocial needs of patients and families.

Equally, professional socialization, the hierarchical tradition where the doctor has total authority, issues of 'ownership' of the patient and debates about 'who is the expert?' are considered to be barriers to establishing the collaborative practice necessary for palliative care within this setting (Coyle 1997). The focus of medical care on curing disease may lead to death being perceived as a failure, resulting in dying patients and their families being marginalized and their needs being unrecognized and unmet in the mainstream health care context (Llamas *et al.* 2001). Taylor (1995) and McDonnell *et al.* (2002) have demonstrated, however, that nurses are aware of the needs of patients requiring palliative care and their families and attempt to provide the best service that they can, while acknowledging that provision of care could be improved. It would appear, therefore, that needs are identified but difficulties arise in meeting these needs.

The culture and philosophy of task-orientated care within hospitals may, therefore, be considered at odds with the holistic and individualized care of patients with palliative care needs, influencing the way in which care is provided (McDonnell *et al.* 2002). McDonnell *et al.* (2002) demonstrated that everyday work pressures undermined nurses' abilities to provide palliative care and time constraints acted as a barrier to nurses developing an effective rapport with dying patients and their families. Furthermore, nurses were required to prioritize physical care over psychosocial needs, with an average of three minutes per patient per shift being estimated as the time available to devote to the psychological care of all patients (McDonnell *et al.* 2002). It is, therefore, perhaps unsurprising that emotional care for patients and for relatives represent 57 and 20 per cent, respectively, of reasons for referral to specialist palliative care (Macmillan) nursing services (Skilbeck and Seymour 2002).

Key recommendations from these studies to help improve the quality of general palliative care to patients and their families include the need to develop strategies to improve accessibility to cancer and/or palliative care education, both intraprofessional and interprofessional, and the need for valuing and developing collaborative working in clinical teams, with recognition and support from specialist palliative care services and service managers (Taylor 1995; McDonnell *et al.* 2002).

The support provided by specialist palliative care nurses appeared significant in the provision of general palliative care in these studies. The role of nurse specialist is currently evolving to meet the demands of contemporary health care policy and professional regulation (Department of Health 2000a; UKCC 2002). Specialist palliative care nurses, therefore, face a number of challenges in providing specialist services within the hospital setting.

Challenges to nurses of providing specialist palliative care within the acute hospital setting

The need to improve the care of the dying in the acute hospital setting resulted in the growth of hospital-based specialist palliative care services (Hockley 1992). In England, the first hospital palliative care team was established in 1976 at St Thomas' Hospital, London. In 2000–2001, within the UK, there were 100 hospital support nurses and 221 hospital support teams (Hospice Information Service 2002). The publication *Palliative Care in the Hospital Setting* (NCHSPCS 1996) made several recommendations for the development of specialist palliative care services, including:

- The hospital palliative care team should be a multidisciplinary group of full-time, part-time and attached staff and have a range of complementary skills.

- There should be clear understanding between the hospital palliative care team, referring clinicians and patients as to the advisory nature of the relationship between the team and the primary hospital carers.

The recommendations identified by the NCHSPCS (1996) are described as underpinning the provision of specialist palliative care services within the acute hospital setting (Pitcher and Davis 2001). More recently, the role of specialist palliative care services has been redefined as that provided by professional carers who specialize in palliative care for patients and their families with moderate to high complexity of palliative care need. This definition focuses on the clinical role of professionals working within such services. For nurses, however, the specialist palliative care role (sometimes referred to as Macmillan nurse) is often associated with the clinical nurse specialist, who has five areas of responsibility: clinical practice, consultation services, leadership, teaching and research (Webber 1997). The role of clinical nurse specialist requires specialist palliative care nurses, therefore, to influence patient care through indirect or direct services (Skilbeck and Seymour 2002). Indirect services focus on empowering professional colleagues to deliver general palliative care through education, support and advice (Skilbeck and Seymour 2002). In addition, the strategic development of services and practice may be achieved through research and leadership activities. In contrast, direct services involve the assessment and delivery of patient care and is reserved for those patients and families with complex needs (Skilbeck and Seymour 2002). Specialist palliative care nurses face challenges in terms of these five areas of responsibility, as discussed below.

Clinician/educator

An important aim of the hospital-based specialist palliative care service, including specialist palliative care nurses, is to improve the generic palliative care skills throughout the hospital by example and education (Pitcher and Davis 2001). Education may be provided both formally through the organization of study days or informally within the clinical setting as part of clinical care. Dowell (2002) recommends that specialist input can be used as a learning experience by junior staff, enabling new skills and knowledge to be acquired through observation and discussion. Furthermore, the involvement of specialist palliative care services may provide support for ward staff in the provision of general palliative care and strengthen relationships to help alter practice and improve patient outcomes. The relationship between the hospital specialist palliative care team and other health care professionals is, therefore, considered to be vital to the successful integration of general palliative care in the acute hospital setting (Pitcher and Davis 2001).

The provision of education has, however, been described as a source of conflict and ambiguity by Macmillan nurses (Seymour *et al.* 2002). Although these nurses view education as the key to developing the assessment skills of staff and ensuring that patients with palliative care needs are identified, Seymour *et al.* (2002) highlighted that many feel constrained in their attempts to provide formal education because of a lack of resources and a constant demand to provide direct patient care. Equally, informal education was recognized as a strategy for reducing dependency on specialist nurses by empowering others rather than taking over patient care (Seymour *et al.* 2002). For hospital staff, however, the pressure of ward work meant that acquired skills could not be put into practice and required specialist nurses to become substitutes for inexperienced nurses and doctors (McDonnell *et al.* 2002; Seymour *et al.* 2002). Indeed, Skilbeck and Seymour (2002) reported that Macmillan nurses spent an average of 56.3 per cent of their time on activities related to direct patient care, with 10.9 per cent of time on formal or informal education. It appears, therefore, that the concerns raised about the potential for specialist nurses to deskill ward nurses (Marshall and Luffingham 1998; Jack *et al.* 2002) may be challenged.

Referral to specialist palliative care services, it may be argued, should be dependent on the skills, knowledge and experience of the ward teams, with specialist palliative care services providing support and advice once the complexity of a patient's needs exceeds the level of knowledge, skill and experience of the ward staff. It appears, however, that the demands of the hospital ward may lead staff to routinely call the specialist nurse when difficulties arise (Seymour *et al.* 2002), preventing ward staff from developing their clinical skills in general palliative care. This reliance on specialist nurses to fill in means that ward nurses may disempower and deskill themselves (Ibbotson 1999). It may be argued, therefore, that the organizational culture within hospitals must support specialist palliative care nurses to deliver formal and informal education to ward nurses and provide a clinical structure that enables ward nurses to apply this learning in practice, thus allaying the concerns of managers and specialists about deskilling and the criticism that specialist nurses 'take over' (Jack *et al.* 2002). In addition, this would enable specialist nurses to address the other aspects of their role that are assuming increasing prominence as a result of the redefining of palliative care.

Clinician/consultant

A further challenge for specialist nurses is the impact of current health policy on the organization and delivery of specialist services for all patients with palliative care needs within the hospital setting. In attempting to meet the palliative care needs of patients with life-limiting illnesses other than cancer, concerns have been raised about the potential number of referrals, the lack of resources and funding, and the potential for dilution of existing cancer services (Wallwork 2000). In addition, concerns about the professional knowledge and skills of specialist palliative care nurses to meet the needs of non-cancer patients have been raised by both members of specialist palliative care services and hospital staff (Addington-Hall 1998; Dharmasena and Forbes 2001). Addington-Hall (1998) argues, however, that a lack of knowledge may not be a barrier to providing palliative care for all if staff work in cooperation with those familiar with non-malignant diseases. This approach would also allow expertise to develop (Addington-Hall 1998).

Dharmasena and Forbes (2001) identified that, while physicians would consider referring patients with non-malignant disease to a specialist palliative care service, the majority favoured a form of shared care or one-off advice as a way of ensuring that patients did not feel abandoned by a consultant with whom they may have established an important therapeutic relationship over many years (Dharmasena and Forbes 2001). It would appear, therefore, that specialist palliative care nurses will have to negotiate their role within these clinical teams, including its boundaries, particularly as other nurse specialist roles for disease-specific groups or conditions are developing. In addition, specialist palliative care nurses need to recognize the appropriateness and limitations of their knowledge base in palliative care for patients with a range of life-limiting illnesses. Similar issues related to co-working between generic specialist palliative care nurses and site-specific cancer nurses have been raised in the delivery of specialist palliative care services for cancer patients, as problems of role overlap and role confusion within organizations have emerged (Seymour *et al.* 2002).

The current changes to the focus of palliative care are, it would appear, posing significant challenges for specialist palliative care nurses within hospitals in terms of negotiating their role within clinical teams for patients with a range of life-limiting illnesses. In addition, generic specialist palliative care nurses are having to negotiate role boundaries with tumour site-specific nurses usually on an individual basis. The role of generic specialist palliative care nurses within the hospital setting may, therefore, require review and redefinition as the boundaries between specialist nursing roles become increasingly blurred and the opportunities for role confusion and conflict for patients and other health care professionals are heightened.

Leader

As well as the possibility of needing to redefine the generic specialist palliative care nursing role, Clark *et al.* (2002) suggest that the British Government's agenda for cancer, palliative care and supportive care services poses a challenge for specialist palliative care nurses in determining the future development of the services they offer within hospital and community settings. It would appear that specialist nurses may be increasingly pressured to spend more time on strategic issues focused on the development and delivery of specialist palliative care services by managers who view the nurse's role as moving beyond being patient-centred to that of service development and education (Seymour *et al.* 2002). Clark *et al.* (2002), however, have gone further and have suggested that a complete reconfiguration of services may be necessary to achieve the type of teamworking required for the higher level integration of work with the range of teams providing palliative care.

It would appear, therefore, that if specialist palliative care nurses are to have a voice, there is a need to become more actively engaged in the leadership aspect of their role to influence and shape the development of their role and the delivery of specialist palliative care services within the organization. The demand to substitute for inexperienced ward staff may, however, impede this as hospitals struggle to achieve the vision of general palliative care.

Research, audit and service evaluation

Hospital-based specialist palliative care nurses appear to have a significant role to play in improving the quality of palliative care within the hospital setting for patients with cancer and other life-limiting illnesses. Services have to justify their existence in more than purely humanitarian terms (Clark *et al.* 1997) as, at the heart of the British Government's drive to modernize health care, is a commitment to quality, person-centred health services based on evidence (Department of Health 1997). Evidence is beginning to emerge of the impact of hospital palliative care teams on the care of hospitalized patients, with statistically significant improvements in symptoms being demonstrated following input by a multi-professional hospital palliative care team (Edmonds *et al.* 1998). More recently, a systematic literature review of 13 studies indicated a small positive effect of the hospital palliative care team in improving the care for patients or families at the end of life by reducing time in hospital, improving prescribing practices and symptom management. Difficulties were, however, acknowledged in undertaking this review due to a paucity of good evaluation studies (Higginson *et al.* 2002). Recommendations, therefore, were made for evaluation studies that compare different models of hospital-based teams. Furthermore, the use of standardized outcome measures was suggested to assess patients' pain, symptoms, carer outcomes, the effect on professionals and overall hospital service (Higginson *et al.* 2002). Similarly, Fakhoury (1998) noted that, in palliative care, no comprehensive research has focused on identifying relevant dimensions of satisfaction for the care of terminally ill patients, which, for dying patients in hospital, may include concerns related to physical surroundings, accessibility and availability of staff, and continuity of care. Fakhoury (1998) concluded that multidimensional models of satisfaction with palliative care that would evaluate care delivered, taking account of carers' and patients' aspirations and experiences, were needed if professionals were to have accurate assessments of satisfaction with palliative care services.

It would appear, therefore, that specialist palliative care nurses, together with other members of the hospital-based specialist team, need to evaluate the service provided through audit and/or research to determine the dimensions of quality and satisfaction of patients with palliative care needs, their families and health care professionals. The findings may then inform the development of clinical practice and service delivery within the hospital setting.

The introduction and evaluation of care pathways in many hospitals can potentially provide some objective evidence of the effect of specialist palliative care services on patient care throughout a hospital (Higginson *et al.* 2002). Integrated care pathways are defined as determining locally agreed multidisciplinary practice, based on guidelines and evidence for a specific patient group. The pathway forms all or part of the clinical record, documents the care given and facilitates the evaluation of outcomes to allow continuous improvement in quality (Riley 1998). Care pathways, therefore, enable the incorporation of research evidence and 'best practice' into a structured framework (Wigfield and Boon 1996).

Within palliative care, the evaluation of care pathways is emerging. While the development and implementation of an integrated care pathway has been described as labour-intensive (Fowell *et al.* 2002), pioneering work at Liverpool in the development and implementation of an integrated care pathway in palliative care demonstrated that outcome-based practice, improvement in clinical practice and continuing evaluation were possible (Ellershaw *et al.* 1997). More recently, Fowell *et al.* (2002) reported the Wales-wide implementation of an integrated care pathway for the last two days of life and discussed the value of variance reports within integrated pathways in identifying problematic aspects of palliative care provision across a range of settings. In addition, care pathways have been described as a strategy for addressing issues of co-working between specialist nurses (Seymour *et al.* 2002). It would appear, therefore, that the use of integrated care pathways across statutory and voluntary sectors on a large scale may help in benchmarking and quality monitoring palliative care and contribute to raising the standard of general palliative care within hospital settings.

The challenges to specialist palliative care nurses identified above raise issues about how nurses are prepared to undertake these roles and the support required from service managers and professional colleagues to develop general and specialist palliative care services within the hospital setting. Currently, for specialist palliative care nurses in hospitals, it would appear that support and attention need to be directed towards the culture in which general palliative care is being provided, focusing on teamworking and enabling ward nurses to develop and apply their knowledge and skills in palliative care. Such an investment has the potential to reduce the current tension between the need to substitute for inexperienced ward staff and the increasing demands to develop other aspects of the specialist nursing role. In addition, it should enable specialist palliative care support to be more widely available and a climate to develop in which specialist palliative care nursing can flourish (Seymour *et al.* 2002).

Conclusions

Despite concerns about the milieu of the setting, the hospital has a significant role in the provision of palliative care for patients with cancer and other life-limiting illnesses and their families throughout the disease trajectory. Studies have highlighted the poor experiences of patients and families, with criticisms raised about the context and culture of care within the hospital setting. Furthermore, the experiences of qualified nurses caring for patients on wards have revealed the challenges faced when attempting to provide general palliative care. Nurses with limited education in the principles of palliative care and inexperienced in its practice attempt to provide palliative care in a setting where the acute, short-stay and biomedical culture is at odds with the philosophy of palliative care. Hospital-based specialist palliative care teams, therefore, have a significant role to play in supporting and educating general staff about the philosophy, principles and skills of palliative care and there is tentative evidence that such teams are having a positive impact on patient outcomes. Specialist palliative care nurses, however, face a number of challenges. In particular, specialist nurses face a tension between their clinical workload, which may involve substituting for inexperienced ward staff who have limited time to develop their knowledge and skills in palliative care, and focusing on the strategic aspects of their role. There is a need, therefore, for specialist palliative care nurses to be proactive and encourage open discussion of these issues within clinical teams and the organization so that strategies can be developed that may assist in raising the standard of general palliative care within the hospital setting and are demonstrable through the evaluation of service delivery.

The apparent lack of education about palliative care in pre-registration undergraduate nurse education and the limited access to post-registration education highlight the need for national guidance to standardize pre-registration undergraduate nursing education and to coordinate post-registration education in palliative care, utilizing a range of teaching and learning methods, to improve accessibility for nurses. This, together with the requirement for ongoing professional development and support within the clinical environment, may serve to improve nurses' knowledge, understanding and practice of general palliative care.

The acute hospital setting poses significant challenges for the delivery of palliative care, yet as Llamas *et al.* (2001) assert, there is a moral imperative to ensure that the care of dying patients in acute settings is optimized within the limitations of the environment. This applies equally to any patient with palliative care needs and their family in the acute hospital at any stage of the disease trajectory. Although improvements have been achieved, further work is needed if the vision set out by the British Government and the National Council for Hospice and Specialist Palliative Care Services for general and specialist palliative care is to become a reality within the hospital setting. Identifying the challenges and encouraging discussion of these is a step in that direction.

| References

Addington-Hall, J.M. (1998) *Reaching Out: Specialist Palliative Care for Adults with Non-Malignant Disease.* London: NCHSPCS.

Anderson, H., Ward, C., Eardley, A. *et al.* (2001) The concerns of patients under palliative care and a heart failure clinic are not being met. *Palliative Medicine*, 15: 279–86.

Cancer Relief Macmillan Fund (1991) *The Experience of a Cancer Diagnosis.* Unpublished Research Report. London: Cancer Relief Macmillan Fund.

Clark, D., Malson, H., Small, N. *et al.* (1997) Half full or half empty? The impact of health reform on palliative care services in the UK, in D. Clark, J. Hockley and S. Ahmedzai (eds) *New Themes in Palliative Care.* Buckingham: Oxford University Press.

Clark, D., ten Have, H. and Janssens, R. (2000) Common threads? Palliative care service developments in seven European countries. *Palliative Medicine*, 14: 479–90.

Clark, D., Seymour, J., Douglas, H. *et al.* (2002) Clinical nurse specialists in palliative care. Part 2: Explaining diversity in the organization and costs of Macmillan nursing services. *Palliative Medicine*, 16: 375–85.

Coyle, N. (1997) Interdisciplinary collaboration in hospital palliative care: chimera or goal? *Palliative Medicine*, 11: 265–6.

Department of Health (1995) *A Policy Framework for Commissioning Cancer Services.* A Report by the Expert Advisory Group on Cancer to the Chief Medical Officers of England and Wales. London: Department of Health.

Department of Health (1997) *The New NHS: Modern, Dependable.* London: Department of Health.

Department of Health (2000a) *The Cancer Plan.* London: Department of Health.

Department of Health (2000b) *The NHS Plan.* London: Department of Health.

Dharmasena, H.P. and Forbes, K. (2001) Palliative care for patients with non-malignant disease: will hospital physicians refer? *Palliative Medicine*, 15: 413–18.

Dowell, L. (2002) Multiprofessional palliative care in a general hospital: education and training needs. *International Journal of Palliative Nursing*, 8(6): 294–303.

Dunlop, R.J. and Hockley, J.M. (1998) *Hospital-Based Palliative Care Teams: The Hospital–Hospice Interface*, 2nd edn. Oxford: Oxford University Press.

Dunne, K. and Sullivan, K. (2000) Family experiences of palliative care in the acute hospital setting. *International Journal of Palliative Nursing*, 6(4): 170–8.

Edmonds, P.M., Stuttaford, J.M., Penny, J., Lynch, A.M. and Chamberlain, J. (1998) Do hospital palliative care teams improve symptom control? Use of a modified STAS as an evaluation tool. *Palliative Medicine*, 12: 345–51.

Edmonds, P., Karlsen, S., Khan, S. and Addington-Hall, J. (2001) A comparison of the palliative care needs of patients dying from chronic respiratory diseases and lung cancer. *Palliative Medicine*, 15: 287–95.

Ellershaw, J., Foster, A., Murphy, D., Shea, T. and Overill, S. (1997) Developing an integrated care pathway for the dying patient. *European Journal of Palliative Care*, 4(6): 203–7.

Fakhoury, W.K.H. (1998) Satisfaction with palliative care: what should we be aware of? *International Journal of Nursing Studies*, 35: 171–6.

Field, D. (1989) *Nursing the Dying.* London: Tavistock/Routledge.

Fowell, A., Finlay, I., Johnstone, R. and Minto, L. (2002) An integrated care pathway for the last two days of life: Wales-wide benchmarking in palliative care. *International Journal of Palliative Nursing*, 8(12): 566–73.

Gott, C.M., Ahmedzai, S.H. and Wood, C. (2001) How many inpatients at an acute hospital have palliative care needs? Comparing the perspectives of medical and nursing staff. *Palliative Medicine*, 15: 451–60.

Higginson, I.J. (1993) Palliative care: a review of past trends and future directions. *Journal of Public Health Medicine*, 15: 3–8.

Higginson, I.J. and Addington-Hall, J.M. (1999) Palliative care needs to be provided on basis of need rather than diagnosis. *British Medical Journal*, 318: 123.

Higginson, I.J., Finlay, I., Goodwin, D.M. *et al.* (2002) Do hospital-based palliative care teams improve care for patients or families at the end of life? *Journal of Pain and Symptom Management*, 23(2): 96–106.

Hockley, J.M. (1992) Role of the hospital support team. *British Journal of Hospital Medicine*, 48: 250–3.

Hospice Information Service (2002) *Directory of Hospices and Palliative Care Services.* London: Hospice Information Service.

Ibbotson, K. (1999) The role of the clinical nurse specialist: a study. *Nursing Standard*, 14(9): 35–8.

Jack, B., Oldham, J. and Williams, A. (2002) Do hospital-based palliative care clinical nurse specialists de-skill general staff? *International Journal of Palliative Nursing*, 8(7): 336–40.

James, N. and Field, D. (1992) The routinization of hospice: charisma and bureaucratization. *Social Science and Medicine*, 34(12): 1363–75.

Llamas, K.J., Pickhaver, A.M. and Piller, N.B. (2001) Mainstreaming palliative care for cancer patients in the acute hospital setting. *Palliative Medicine*, 15: 207–12.

Lloyd-Williams, M. and Field, D. (2002) Are undergraduate nurses taught palliative care during their training? *Nurse Education Today*, 22: 589–92.

Marshall, Z. and Luffingham, N. (1998) Specialist nursing: does the specialist nurse enhance or deskill the general nurse? *British Journal of Nursing*, 7(11): 758–62.

McCarthy, M., Lay, M. and Addington-Hall, J.M. (1996) Dying from heart disease: symptoms and hospital care in the last year of life reported by informal carers. *Journal of the Royal College of Physicians*, 30: 325–8.

McDonnell, M., Johnston, G., Gallagher, A.G. and McGlade, K. (2002) Palliative care in district general hospitals: the nurse's perspective. *International Journal of Palliative Nursing*, 8(4): 169–75.

Mills, M., Davies, T.O. and Macrae, W.A. (1994) Care of dying patients in hospital. *British Medical Journal*, 309: 583–6.

Morris, E. (1988) A pain of separation. *Nursing Times*, 84(35): 54–7.

National Council for Hospice and Specialist Palliative Care Services (1996) *Palliative Care in the Hospital Setting.* Occasional Paper No. 10. London: NCHSPCS.

National Council for Hospice and Specialist Palliative Care Services (2000) *The Palliative Care Survey 1999.* London: NCHSPCS.

National Council for Hospice and Specialist Palliative Care Services (2002) *Definitions of Supportive and Palliative Care.* London: NCHSPCS.

Pitcher, P. and Davis, C. (2001) Palliative care in the hospital setting for patients with non-malignant disease, in J.M. Addington-Hall and I.J. Higginson (eds) *Palliative Care for Non-Cancer Patients.* Oxford: Oxford University Press.

Ramirez, A., Addington-Hall, J.M. and Richards, M. (1998) ABC of palliative care: the carers. *British Medical Journal*, 316: 208–11.

Riley, K. (1998) *Definitions of Care Pathways.* National Pathway Association Autumn Newsletter No. 2.

Rogers, A., Karlsen, S. and Addington-Hall, J.M. (2000) 'All the services were excellent. It was when the human element comes in that things go wrong': dissatisfaction with hospital care in the last year of life. *Journal of Advanced Nursing*, 31(4): 768–74.

Rumbold, B.D. (1998) Implications of mainstreaming hospice into palliative care services, in J. Parker and S. Aranda (eds) *Palliative Care: Explorations and Challenges.* Sydney, NSW: Maclennan & Petty.

Seymour, J., Clark, D., Hughes, P. *et al.* (2002) Clinical nurse specialists in palliative care. Part 3: Issues for the Macmillan nurse role. *Palliative Medicine*, 16: 386–94.

Skilbeck, J. and Seymour, J. (2002) Meeting complex needs: an analysis of Macmillan nurses' work with patients. *International Journal of Palliative Nursing*, 8(12): 574–82.

Skilbeck, J., Mott, L., Page, H. *et al.* (1998) Palliative care in chronic obstructive airways disease: a needs assessment. *Palliative Medicine*, 12: 245–54.

Skilbeck, J., Small, N. and Ahmedzai, S.H. (1999) Nurses' perceptions of specialist palliative care in an acute hospital. *International Journal of Palliative Nursing*, 5(3): 110–15.

Street, A. (1998) Competing discourses within palliative care, in J. Parker and S. Aranda (eds) *Palliative Care: Explorations and Challenges*. Sydney, NSW: Maclennan & Petty.

Taylor, V.A. (1995) Nurses' experiences of providing continuing care for patients with cancer in the acute surgical setting of a district general hospital. Unpublished MSc thesis, University of Surrey.

Trnobranski, P.H. (1994) Nurse–patient negotiation: assumption or reality. *Journal of Advanced Nursing*, 19: 733–7.

United Kingdom Central Council for Nursing, Midwifery and Health Visiting (2002) *Report of the Higher Level of Practice Pilot and Project*. London: UKCC.

Wallwork, L. (2000) Palliative care in non-malignant disease: a pragmatic response. *International Journal of Palliative Nursing*, 6(4): 186–91.

Webber, J. (1997) *The Evolving Role of the Macmillan Nurse*. London: Macmillan Cancer Relief.

Wigfield, A. and Boon, E. (1996) Critical care pathway development: the way forward. *British Journal of Nursing*, 5(12): 732–5.

Wilkinson, E.K., Salisbury, C., Bosanquet, N. *et al.* (1999) Patient and carer preferences for, and satisfaction with, specialist models of palliative care: a systematic literature review. *Palliative Medicine*, 13: 197–216.

Wilson-Barnett, J. and Richardson, A. (1993) Nursing research and palliative care, in D. Doyle, G.W.C. Hanks and N. MacDonald (eds) *Oxford Textbook of Palliative Medicine*. Oxford: Oxford Medical Publications.

7

Transitions in status from wellness to illness, illness to wellness

Coping with recurrence and remission

Margaret O'Connor

A view of illness that incorporates the whole illness experience –from beginning to end –may be difficult for a health practitioner to grasp. The reasons for this may be many and varied: from the inability of the ill person to retell their whole story, to the busyness of the health professional, preventing them from grasping nothing more than the presenting issue.

Contemporary dying emphasizes the individual and their personal experience (Mellor 1993), and what emerges is an individual response to the particular challenges of the illness journey. But illness should not be regarded as a unique transition for the individual, since similar developmental experiences occur throughout the life span, in response to life's movements and challenges.

In this chapter, an emphasis is placed on understanding the illness journey as part of life's transitions, with similar characteristics to other journeys made in life. This requires a longitudinal view of illness along the illness trajectory, rather than as a series of events. Health professionals, therefore, should endeavour to gain insight into the whole narrative of a person's illness –to seek an understanding of the ups and downs that are inherent in the illness experience and its impact on the person. This requires a different perspective than the myopic immediacy of a particular health care encounter and also means that illness, and its associated life problems, should be viewed as an inherent part of the person's whole life narrative. In palliative care practice, with its philosophy of care of the total person, this perspective is especially pertinent. In that sense, it is the transition response that is important rather than a focus on the outcome –further illness or survival.

Sociological views of illness

Illness as a sociological phenomenon, needs to be understood within a framework that encompasses issues such as the sequestration of the dying experience from everyday life (Giddens 1991), the lack of involvement of the community in death (Elias 1985), the medicalization of illness and dying (Giddens 1991) and the lack of meaning and answers to existential problems like illness and death (Giddens 1991; Mellor 1993).

Gaining a balanced understanding of life-threatening illness appears to be a problem for many societies, perhaps because it confronts observers with the lack of security in their own lives. Lack of meaning and lack of answers to existential problems are distinctive of contemporary societies in the writings of Giddens (1991) and Mellor (1993). Death ultimately represents the absence of meaning, and issues for which there is a lack of meaning and control become private, invisible and individualized. Giddens (1991) suggests that death is 'the moment at which human control over human existence finds an outer limit' (p. 162).

The medicalization of illness means that most people make the health care system (the hospital, the general practitioner or the specialist) their main focus of support, reducing the importance of communal and family care, as well as the opportunity for expanding societal understandings of illness and dying. Frank (1995) suggests that the 'modern experience of illness begins when popular experience is overtaken by technical expertise' (p. 5); thus illness assumes a life of its own with a language, setting and behaviours that are different from the culture of family and neighbourhood. The relationship between institutional supports and the individual experience of illness is what Giddens (1991) describes as one of the distinctive features of modernity, making the connections between 'globalising influences' and 'personal dispositions' (p. 1).

If illness, particularly chronic illness, is hidden from the community, then advances in treatment and care may be less visible. If chronic illness is compounded by age, then it is even less accessible as a communal issue. Perhaps some of the appeal of palliative care discourse and practice is that within this system of care, choice, control and involvement in decision making are visible, in contrast to other aspects of the health care system where people often feel overwhelmed and disempowered by language and technology. Similarly, living wills, euthanasia and advanced directives may be seen as attempts at exercising tangible control over choices during the illness experience, as well as at the end of life, and serve to open the subject of dying to wider communal scrutiny (Giddens 1991).

Australian society, as in many other parts of the world, is an increasingly rich multicultural fabric. The rituals of illness, death and grieving that particular cultural groups bring with them often serve as a tangible reminder of what has been left behind, as well as a way of binding the group together in a common language. This, in turn, has contributed to broadening cultural discourses in these areas. Efforts to understand and incorporate particular cultural rituals into mainstream health care have become an ongoing challenge in balancing a variety of needs within a dominant Anglo-Irish view of the world as in Australia. For example, many cultural groups value care for their ill family member in the home setting, regarding institutionalization as abandonment, while others regard hospital as the place where the best care will be received. And Australians are just beginning to understand the particular sensitivities that surround the care of the original inhabitants of their country – the increased percentages of chronic illness and subsequent early death; the collective grief at their loss of culture, family and homeland; and the fragility of a cultural group that regards each indigenous death as a family death (O'Connor 2001).

Illness and death create insecurity in people and are an affront to the dominant belief that life can be predicted and controlled. In the face of this lack of control, religion may present a comforting framework for understanding life's journey, illness, death, suffering and an afterlife. Berger (1969) began a sociological debate many years ago, arguing that secularization has arisen because of a declining immediacy of death. Modern practices ensure that care and dying occur out of sight, mainly in an institution, which reduces the community's involvement in the event (Corr *et al.* 1999). Additionally, if illness and dying and accompanying disability occur in old age, as well as in an institution, they are doubly invisible to the communal gaze. With these experiences being less visible and less part of the community's fabric, they may become less feared. In traditionally conservative religious terms, less fear means a declining hold of religion on everyday behaviour, as preparation for an afterlife (Griffin and Tobin 1997).

Like most Western societies, economic rationalism remains the persistent discourse in most current Australian Government policy, and this places a cost on all activities in health care. Many religious discourses, Christianity in particular, stand in contrast in valuing the sacredness and dignity of all human life at whatever stage that life is. The value of the life is inherent simply in its living, at whatever limited level that may be, without a demand for productivity to establish self-worth. Within this value system, those people in the community with chronic illnesses are valued at whatever stage of life and disability they find themselves. This is one justification for the Churches being involved in caring for the sick, the dying and the aged (O'Connor 2001).

Thus, contemporary secular society presents a picture of a culturally diverse community with different faiths and no faiths, as well as individual expectations and experiences of illness, dying and death. This demands flexibility about views of illness and end-of-life rituals that respects these different traditions. A religious ritual may simply be a familiar comforting ritual, inseparable from the cultural experience of the individual and having little to do with the expression of, or identification with, the particular belief system. It is not uncommon in death rituals in Australia to find a civil celebrant performing the rituals, a civilian role under the auspice of local government and therefore not bound by traditional rubrics of particular religious traditions. The interpretation of rituals by this sort of person may, in turn, accentuate the uniqueness of each person's dying and grieving experiences. The experience of illness and death has now well and truly been situated as an individual experience within the medical domain, with the mass media as the interpreter of experiences of illness, dying and death.

Views of illness

Seeking understanding of the meaning of illness from *inside* the person's experience necessarily involves taking a longitudinal view of things, like when the illness began, how the person understands their illness, how it affects them, what adaptations they have made – in other words, listening to their narrative. Narrative, or telling the story of illness, as suggested by Frank (1995), transforms the dominant cultural image of illness as being a passive experience into a strengthened experience of shared vulnerability. Frank suggests that stories heal by creating empathetic bonds between the teller and the listener, thus widening the 'circle of shared experience' (p. xii). The gathering of these stories of individual experience, as opposed to seeking one common and dominant cultural experience, may assist others in understanding the illness journey, as well as supporting the disparate post-modern view of illness and death (Seale 1998).

This understanding of the individual's broad experience offers the health professional a different world-view from that which concentrates on the current clinical manifestation of disease, a view that is particularly pertinent in the practice of palliative care. In encounters with those for whom we care, it may be expedient to filter all information that is extraneous to the presenting clinical issue. However, this approach risks a limited view of the person's individual response to their illness and the immediacy of its impact on their lives. Kleinman graphically notes that

> illness becomes embodied in a particular life trajectory, environed in a concrete life world. Acting like a sponge, illness soaks up personal and social significance from the world of the sick person. Unlike cultural meanings of illness that carry significance *to* the sick person, this intimate type of meaning transfers vital significance from the person's life to the illness experience.
>
> (Kleinman 1988: 31)

A longitudinal view of illness affords a different understanding of the impact of illness on a person's life. This may be particularly pertinent if the person is older and/or has an uncertain diagnosis or prognosis. Instead of considering the different aspects that make up the total person – physical, social, spiritual, emotional, cultural – this view takes account of the person's whole experience of life, situating illness as part of that experience, which will necessarily involve all aspects of the person. In viewing illness this way, transition then becomes a phase along that trajectory – be it from health to illness, illness to further illness, or illness to remission or cure.

A view of illness that encompasses the total journey also needs to encompass the understanding of the chronic characteristics of illness, rather than a series of unrelated acute episodes. The presence of chronic illness in the community is increasing, if only because of advances in health technology and because people are living longer. Field and Cassell (1997) note that in countries like the USA most people die of chronic illness. They suggest that 'many people are fearful that a combination of old age and modern medicine will inflict on them a dying that is more protracted and in some ways more difficult than it would have been a few decades ago' (p. 14). Many types of illness, including cancer, once treated with the goal of seeking a cure (and death was regarded as almost inevitable but nevertheless a failure when it occurred) are now targeted with treatments aimed at enabling people to live longer and to experience periods of remission. Thus, people are *living* with their illnesses, with the associated issues of treatment and lifestyle limitations, not necessarily *dying* from them.

Chronic illness may manifest in many forms – sudden or insidious onset, with episodic symptoms or remission, various trajectories and perhaps with the presence of co-morbidities. Lubkin graphically describes the difference between acute and chronic illness:

> Acute illness may be compared with an unexpected visitor who leaves one's house after a short stay . . . Chronic illness on the other hand, announces plans to visit for an indefinite stay and gradually becomes part of the household. Although this guest is a welcome alternative to death, the illness provides a mixed blessing to the host household and to society at large. In addition, the illness frequently becomes attached to the person's identity.
>
> (Lubkin 1990: 4)

Many people who would benefit from palliative care, particularly in services that take prognosis-based referrals, will have illnesses with the characteristics of chronicity. This becomes an issue of perception for health carers, in terms of whether those with long prognoses are considered suitable to receive palliative care, or whether their illness profile is too uncertain.

Curtin and Lubkin (1990) note that health care carers often view chronic illness negatively, as increasing disability and deterioration leading to death. This perception is reflective of community attitudes, which are challenged by these reminders of illness and death. McNamara (2001), however, states that if the cultural and social dimensions of death can be addressed, then it can be more readily embraced in all its aspects. In contrast, those people who have chronic illness may not necessarily take on these negative perceptions, but learn to live with their limitations in developing a meaningful life. Illness, then, assumes a place in the way the individual perceives himself or herself, thus balancing an understanding of chronic illness that goes beyond the traditional disease focus.

Transition

> passage . . . change from one place or state to another.
>
> (*Oxford English Dictionary* 1972)

By its very definition, a transition is a dynamic experience – that is, it involves movement and change within the person. Transitions are part of life's journey and the term 'transition' is familiar in developmental theory, especially in the writing of Erikson (1968) and the anthropological theories of van Gennep (1960). Van Gennep, in particular, regarded modern transitions as akin to primitive rites of passage involving three phases: separation (a time of being separate from the community), transition (a time of being neither part of the old nor part of the new) and aggregation (becoming accepted into the community with new status).

Bridges (1996) writes about the commonality of the transition experience whatever its causes. The background to understanding transition theory, as applied to the illness experience, is grounded in the natural transition phases that all people experience in life. Bridges suggests that rather than identifying periods of specific change in life (e.g. the mid-life crisis), adulthood is an at-once continuous process that 'unfolds its promise in a rhythm of expansion and contraction, change and stability' (p. 42). At the start of all experiences of transition is the need to facilitate the 'letting go' (p. 12). Bridges describes this as a most difficult and ambiguous task of beginning the transition process because, at heart, one is surprised to 'discover that some part of us is still holding on to what we used to be'. This is especially pertinent if change has not been sought – for example, when illness occurs – with the implication that the person has little control over such events.

Stages of transition

There are three distinct phases in transition: endings, the neutral zone and new beginnings (Bridges 1996). An analogy that illustrates the journey through transition is when a person jumps off a diving board into the water – the transition phase of change is the stage between having left the diving board, but not having hit the water. The sense is that one has left what was, but not landed in what is to come.

Endings

Transition may begin with an inner sense of dissatisfaction with life or an external occurrence, like illness, that creates a disturbance, a 'lack of fit' with one's previously settled life. Disenchantment with life can often be a precipitating factor, when a person finds they need to let go of their preciously held assumptions about themselves and life. This creates disorientation, the loss of meaning in life and a consequent fear of the emptiness created. This is described as 'diss-identification' (Bridges 1996: 96); that is, not being able to identify *oneself* anymore. This may be most readily seen externally through changes in social roles, especially work, or when illness necessitates an inability to perform certain roles. The 'in-between-ness' of the endings of transition is characterized by the letting go described above, but also by an inability to draw on familiar patterns of behaviour and psychological supports, because they do not work or are no longer appropriate. The onset of illness can be an unfamiliar experience for the individual, creating uncertainty in the previously familiar patterns of life.

Letting go involves not looking back at what was familiar, but looking forward, 'developing new skills for negotiating the perilous passage across the "nowhere" that separates the old life situation from the new' (Bridges 1996: 14). Part of the confusion of transition is not facing new beginnings, but the loss of what has gone before, which previously composed a generally satisfying life, but is now of little use in the movement forward. Because illness is most often an unexpected and unfamiliar experience in life, the individual may find little in their previous life that will assist them in moving forward; Bridges (1996) suggests that the old self can actually stand in the way of the journey of transition.

One way to assist an individual in the illness transition, to understand their response to letting go, is to recall other experiences of transition in their life that are not necessarily illness related. Even developmental experiences of letting go, shared by all as we grow from one stage of life to another, can provide the individual with insight into their own pattern of response to letting go – from fully grappling with the challenge of change to a response arising from anxiety and fear.

Endings often begin with something going wrong in a person's life. This may be the loss of a job, a change in a relationship (e.g. divorce) or the diagnosis of an illness. All of these involve loss for the person and, in that sense, will evoke the same feelings as death – especially grief in reaction to the losses.

Endings in transition should not be regarded as either positive or negative, but a neutral experience. This can, however, be interpreted either negatively – of being 'in a hole' – or as a positive opportunity of stopping and examining the taken-for-granted pattern of one's life and even experimenting with different or new behaviours. Endings may occur throughout the illness trajectory, but especially at diagnosis, when one begins to grapple with its meaning, marking the beginning of a distinctive journey. Other triggers include ending a treatment cycle, when one is declared to be in remission or when disease recurs, because each of these events demands a re-thinking of what was before in order to move into the future.

The neutral zone

Bridges (1996) describes this stage as akin to crossing the street. Once having stepped off the footpath we want to reach the other side as quickly as possible, not pause in the middle. In relation to transitions, one might wonder why one crossed the road in the first place, or regret crossing the road at all, because of the sense of 'lostness' and waiting that is created. This stage may be quite uncomfortable and is characterized by the person wishing to be alone – a time of retreat and thinking. Priorities and values may shift in response to reflection on the endings that have been grappled with. This phase takes its place from ancient primitive communities, when a person in transition (e.g. from childhood to manhood) would withdraw from their everyday activities, spending time alone (van Gennep 1960). Van Gennep used the word *luminaire* to describe this state of being in between – between the inside and the outside, a waiting time, between what was before and what is to come. This period can be experienced as chaos, a time when one's familiar life patterns and personal supports do not appear to work any more. In the illness experience, this time of waiting can be experienced when one receives a new diagnosis; also when the person grapples with the implications of recurrence or remission, or when someone is recovering from illness but is not fully recovered. Neutral time is meant to be temporary and, when one has accomplished the tasks of separation, life must be resumed – however, it is now differently shaped.

New beginnings

New beginnings only start when the endings have been completed and the neutral zone has been negotiated. In Bridge's observations of people in transition over many years, he describes beginnings as starting with a vague idea, an image or an impression. It appears to be a time of starting life again, perhaps in fulfilment of long-held dreams, or of changing direction in work or lifestyle. Some people may use the illness experience as the impetus for creating long yearned-for changes in their lives. This involves taking risks, returning from the isolation of the neutral time, to grapple with what life now offers: 'Endings and beginnings, with emptiness and germination in between. That is the shape of the transition periods in our lives . . . the same process is going on continuously in our lives' (Bridges 1996: 150).

Beginnings during the illness trajectory are experienced when a person has negotiated a treatment regime, when active treatment is ceased and when a period of remission is begun. For some people, beginnings may involve the realization that life will be shortened if treatment has not succeeded; thus the challenge is to use the remaining time as they wish. One may also begin to consider oneself a cancer survivor if treatment has been successful and one may start to negotiate life with a changed outlook or values.

In relation to the applications of illness transition theory in clinical encounters, Bridges suggests that one way to assist an individual to understand their current response is to assist them to recall other experiences of transition in their life. Even in the experience of maturing from one age of life to another: How did they respond? Did they find this life-movement difficult, easy, challenging, exciting? Can the person recall what episodes in life represented an important transition, and do they know why? Reflective questions such as these may assist the individual with their transition issues in relation to their current illness.

Surviving

Because of routine screening systems based in public health policy, early detection and more effective treatment, increasing numbers of people with a diagnosis of cancer consider themselves to be cancer survivors. Seeking a definition of a cancer survivor is difficult, since there is a subjective sense to this status, as well as a changing understanding, depending on different phases of illness and treatment. Frank (1995) uses the term 'remission society' to describe those people who, though not considered cured of their illness, are nevertheless well. Mullen (1985) used the term 'seasons of survival' to connote that survival is cyclical and that it is not uniquely attached to a cured state. He described three states of survival: acute, extended and permanent.

Little *et al.* (2001) have undertaken significant work on survival, contrasting the inspirational literature about individual resilience with that of the difficulty of being a survivor. The difficulties of finding oneself as a survivor are compounded at a communal level, since Little *et al.* (2001) suggest that the discourse on survival is under-developed. Discourse needs to draw on the thematic commonalities of this state as described by individuals, thus providing a framework and articulation of the experience, for others to understand. Individual survivor difficulties also arise because the person is unable to completely move beyond the neutral or liminal stage to new beginnings. This is why when listening to their narrative survivors describe their illness experience as integral to their identity, especially in relation to their vulnerability to the possibility of recurrence and the subsequent impact on all aspects of their social life.

In developing a discourse of survivorship, Little *et al.* suggest several important factors:

- the way we construct our identities and the multiple selves we express in our relationships;
- some of the categories of the survival experience, including vulnerability, disempowerment, the need to preserve 'face', the need for approval and the pressure survivors feel to pay something back for their survival;
- the nature of extreme experience and the effect it has on identity.

(Little *et al.* 2001: 18)

Little *et al.* argue that personal identity, understood simply as 'the core of our being in the world' (p. 19), is essential to understanding the way that surviving occurs. Narrative, as described earlier, provides a means for understanding the person's identity, through examining aspects of illness like the chronology of events, their interpretation of the meaning of illness and the subsequent construction of their sense of self.

A distinctive part of identity is the continuity of memory, which among other things serves to construct the individual's narrative of illness (Little *et al.* 2002). And an aspect of memory that is important in understanding survival is described by Little *et al.* as 'future memory' (p. 171). Future memory involves the individual imagining looking back at stages of life that are yet to occur – a young man with a poor prognosis imagining himself as a grandfather, for example, and placing a value on what he anticipates that experience to mean. Little and co-workers argue the significance of this loss is that it arises from the meaning that we apply to the expectations of a predictable life span. The discontinuities in narratives reflect discontinuity in identity, if these anticipated life experiences are important aspects of the individual's identity.

Coming to terms with one's identity as a survivor may take considerable time, with many people remaining in the neutral or liminal phase. In the process of becoming a survivor, the individual may experience anger, restlessness, alienation and dislocation, and Little *et al.* (2002) suggest that this is because continuity of identity has been interrupted, impaired or alienated. If the community narrowly interprets survival to mean cure, there is an underlying expectation that survival means that the person's life will return to 'normal' – relationships will be resumed, work will re-commence and the patterns of life will be restored. Making sense of their survivor status means that the person:

> reviews the life lived thus far, and must choose what kind of life to live hereafter, what kind of 'future memory' to construct. The sense of continuity is of central importance in the experience of survivorship, whatever adaptive direction is taken.
>
> (Little *et al.* 2002: 176)

Some work has addressed the difficulties experienced by cancer survivors in their return to normal life, in particular their working life. Spelten *et al.* (2002) undertook a search of the literature on the return-to-work experiences of cancer survivors, finding a lack of systematic research had been undertaken in this area. They suggest that return-to-work rates vary considerably, with factors like a supportive work environment facilitating ease of return. Visible cancers (e.g. head and neck) were found to disadvantage the person's return to the workplace, but age was not found to be a factor. Bradley and Bednarek (2002) looked specifically at the employment patterns of survivors, regarding this as an important issue, since once treatment is completed the broad impact of the person with cancer is a social one, affecting their families as well as their work life. Their results appear promising – people diagnosed with cancer while employed tended to remain employed, even if they needed time away for treatment. Most employers were accommodating, particularly if the illness involved disability. Bradley and Bednarek (2002) postulate: 'Perhaps maintaining their employment after diagnosis is entangled with access to comprehensive health insurance and treatment, as well as psychological reasons such as empowerment and the ability to maintain a sense of control' (p. 197).

A new beginning for the survivor is a challenge, made all the more difficult because of a lack of communal discourse about survival. Some survivors may be regarded as fortunate or 'lucky' to be alive, when others have died; others may remain in dependency relationships adopted during the illness. The beginning phase of transition, however, challenges the person beyond old roles and expectations, to develop a new identity, new values, altered relationships and social roles (Little *et al.* 2001). These adaptations may be difficult, simply because of the ever-presence of the illness experience as integral to identity and the sense that, at some level, many people never move beyond the neutral (liminal) stage, remaining caught in a partial adaptation.

Little *et al.* (2001) suggest that the most important help one can give to a survivor is to assist in the development of a discourse of survival, helping that person to articulate their own narrative. Individual narratives will contribute to the development of a communally understood framework for articulating the experience, thus legitimizing the survivor state.

Recurrence

If the period of transition turns into the person needing to face an early death, Davies *et al.* (1995) suggest that change is integral – in one's social life, relationships, family life and work, as well as in roles and responsibilities. There is considerable literature that suggests that while the prospect of an untimely death is distressing for people to consider, what causes more distress is the process of dying – the prospect of dependency, a slow decline and social disengagement (Pollard 1999; Pollard *et al.* 1999; Lawton 2000). A major task at this stage of life is searching for meaning – to put the experience 'in context and endure the turmoil'; 'connecting with their inner and spiritual selves, connecting with others or with nature' (Davies *et al.* 1995: 43).

Day-to-day living becomes the important concern and the goal of each day may change as the impact of disease progression is felt. Literature describes this phase as one where discussion about the transition to palliative care may be appropriate (Pollard *et al.* 1999). There may, however, be confusion in the person's mind about what this transition means, because of disagreements between health professionals about the goal of care, the false dichotomizing of palliative care and treatment for cure, and ambiguous language. Continuous conversations with different members of the health care team at this stage of the person's disease may assist in clarifying care goals and who might be the most appropriate person to offer such care. Ideally, the transition from active treatment to palliative care should occur over a period of time, involving the person and other decision makers at every step. Health professionals may find themselves acting as 'coaches' in facilitating the person in this journey and in assisting them to express uncertainties, to gain as much information as they need and to adjust to their changing circumstances (Aranda and Kelso 1997).

Implications for palliative care policy

Given the general hidden-ness of death in post-modern societies, it is not surprising that connections between palliative care and policy remain under-developed. Smith (2000) notes that in Australia, 'palliative care is a low profile small area of health provision which has a big theoretical following but this does not translate into support or involvement' (p. 307). Early palliative care policy development in Australia traditionally emphasized care for people with cancer diseases, with funding loosely tied to referrals being diagnosis- and/or prognosis-based. The National Strategy for Palliative Care in Australia (Commonwealth Department of Health and Aged Care 1998) still assumed that those in receipt of palliative care would mostly have cancer, although note is made of people with a shortened life expectancy from illnesses like motor neurone disease, HIV/AIDS and end-stage respiratory, cardiac, renal and liver disease. Similarly, the Calman-Hine Report (1995) in the UK suggested extending palliative care services to people who do not necessarily have a terminal prognosis. While in Australia palliative care is still described as being for 'those who are dying' (Commonwealth Department of Health and Aged Care 2000: 5), note is also made that this may range from hours or days to weeks or months of episodic and less intensive care. Thus, as in other places in the world, Australian policy documents *suggest* that palliative care is offered for all in need of such care, with the implication that care models are flexible and responsive.

However, anecdotal evidence points to limitations in access, especially for those with lengthy or uncertain prognoses and for older people living in residential aged care, in need of palliative care. So, with its emphasis on 'cost efficient ... home based, low technology services' (Commonwealth Department of Health and Aged Care 2000: 3), the concepts of transition and chronic illness in the illness trajectory are contradictory. In a policy sense, some illnesses may have a predictable progression that is more readily attached to a funding formula. Others will have a less certain progression of chronic illness with episodic needs for health care interventions. Transitions are difficult to accommodate within a policy framework, which is ultimately a tool that provides direction about who is eligible to receive service and to place a cost on that service.

If people are living longer with the chronic nature of illness, and require the support of palliative care services at varying stages, then it is important to consider the issue of consumer involvement in palliative care policy development. Finding ways to empower the consumer voice during times of transition may indeed be a challenge, if only because of the all-consuming individual agendas of such transitions (see Chapter 4). However, Small and

Rhodes (2000) argue the importance of user involvement to both enhance quality of service and to promote empowerment and legitimacy of service. Within a societal context that increasingly values the individual experience of end-of-life care and dying

> it is important to consider the needs of those people who have lived with complex physical conditions who are now in the final stages of life. While all around them the nature of service delivery changes, they, and their carers, are faced with many challenges as to how they might live this last part of their lives and how the services they receive might best meet their requirements.
>
> (Small and Rhodes 2000: 59)

Emerging issues

The view of illness

This chapter is premised on a longitudinal view of the illness experience, which values the total illness narrative – from diagnosis to survival or death. This stands in contradiction to the currently promoted funding systems noted above, as well as the emerging work (e.g. casemix) that seeks to further tie the illness trajectory to funding levels. Thus, more thinking is required from policy makers in understanding the needs of the terminally ill along the illness trajectory that promotes flexible care systems and recognizes changing needs over a sometimes lengthy period of time.

If we accept this longitudinal view of illness, which also encompasses the understanding of chronic illness, then palliative care policy based on prognosis or diagnosis will not meet needs. Although this view of palliative care has been known to be inadequate for many years, much work is still required to expand the application of the expertise of palliative care to those people with non-cancer diseases or lengthy or uncertain prognoses.

Care of the older person

In particular, in the residential aged environment, caring for a terminally ill person is a relatively common experience, which with our ageing communities will only become more common. However, Palliative Care Australia, in a discussion paper released in 1999, note the difficulties in translating the principles of palliative care into the aged care environment, in particular those of caring for both the terminally ill person and their family using the interdisciplinary approach. Other issues noted were the staffing skill mix, the educational needs of staff, the burden of staff stress and the facility's budget, the availability of expertise in low care settings, and the lack of resident choice of general practitioner who may or may not have skills in palliative care. Komaromy *et al.* (2000) report being surprised by the lack of familiarity of staff with palliative care, in the nursing homes they surveyed, and a consequent lack of knowledge of what palliative care can achieve or, indeed, where to access such expertise. The predictable result was less than optimal terminal care in these homes.

Despite these difficulties, and because of the belief that palliative care ought to be available to all people wherever they live, there needs to be an ongoing commitment to seek ways in which palliative care expertise can be made available to those residents who need it, within aged care facilities. In comparison, the National Council for Hospice and Specialist Palliative Care Services in the UK has recommended that hospices should offer nursing and respite care for older people rather than being limited to their current restrictive practices (Clark and Seymour 1999).

Content of clinical conversations

This chapter has suggested that health professionals need to understand the illness experience of people as a story, not as a series of unrelated events. An open-ended style of questioning will be more likely to elicit the story, but may also require an open-ended appointment time; however, clinicians need to find the balance between the essential clinical information and seeking broader understandings from the person. In particular, the way clinicians understand the illness trajectory, chronic illness, recurrence and survival will impact on the person's understandings. Clinicians need to undertake their own reflective exploration of their role as 'coaches' in their encounters with those in their care.

Conclusions

The individualizing of many of life's experiences, including illness and death, has become a distinctive pattern in contemporary life. Understanding the individual's experience of what occurs in their own illness narrative is an essential part of palliative care. The individual's encounter with health professionals may occur anywhere along a trajectory of illness – where the person may be grappling with diagnosis or burdensome treatment, with recurrence or with what it means to be a survivor. Health professionals need to have an understanding of the transition stages that underlie all these experiences. Individuals will be empowered in their own personal narrative by being connected to the shared discourses of illness, recurrence and survival.

References

Aranda, S. and Kelso, J. (1997) The nurse as coach in care of the dying. *Contemporary Nurse*, 6: 117–22.

Berger, P. (1969) *The Social Reality of Religion*. London: Faber.

Bradley, C.J. and Bednarek, H.L. (2002) Employment patterns of long-term cancer survivors. *Psycho-Oncology*, 11: 188–98.

Bridges, W. (1996) *Transitions: Making Sense of Life's Changes*. London: Redwood Books.

Calman, K. and Hine, D. (1995) *A Policy Framework for Commissioning Cancer Services*. London: Department of Health and Welsh Office.

Clark, D. and Seymour, J. (1999) *Reflections on Palliative Care*. Buckingham: Open University Press.

Commonwealth Department of Health and Aged Care (1998) *Background for a National Strategy for Palliative Care in Australia*. Publications approval number 4066. Canberra, ACT: Commonwealth of Australia.

Commonwealth Department of Health and Aged Care (2000) *National Palliative Care Strategy: A National Framework for Palliative Care Service Development*. Publications approval number 4065. Canberra, ACT: Commonwealth of Australia.

Corr, C.A., Doka, K.J. and Kastenbaum, R. (1999) Dying and its interpreters: a review of selected literature and some comments on the state of the field. *Omega*, 39(4): 239–59.

Curtin, C. and Lubkin, I.M. (1990) What is chronicity?, in I.M. Lubkin (ed.) *Chronic Illness: Impact and Interventions*, 2nd edn. Boston, MA: Jones & Bartlett.

Davies, B., Reimer, J.C., Brown, P. and Martens, N. (1995) *Fading Away: The Experience of Transition in Families with Terminal Illness*. New York: Baywood.

Elias, N. (1985) *The Loneliness of the Dying*. Oxford: Blackwell.

Erikson, E. (1968) *Identity, Youth and Crisis*. New York: W.W. Norton.

Field, M.J. and Cassell, C.K. (eds) (1997) *Approaching Death: Improving Care at the End of Life*. Washington, DC: National Academy Press.

Frank, A.W. (1995) *The Wounded Storyteller: Body, Illness and Ethics*. London: University of Chicago Press.

Giddens, A. (1991) *Modernity and Self-identity: Self and Society in the Late Modern Age*. Stanford, CA: Stanford University Press.

Griffin, G.M. and Tobin, D. (1997) *In the Midst of Life: The Australian Response to Death*. Melbourne, VIC: Melbourne University Press.

Kleinman, A. (1988) Personal and social meanings of illness, in *The Illness Narratives: Suffering, Healing and the Human Condition*. New York: Basic Books.

Komaromy, C., Sidell, M. and Katz, J. (2000) The quality of terminal care in residential and nursing homes. *International Journal of Palliative Nursing*, 6(4): 192–200.

Lawton, J. (2000) *The Dying Process: Patients' Experiences of Palliative Care*. London: Routledge.

Little, M., Paul, K., Jordens, C. and Sayers, E.-J. (2001) *Surviving Survival: Life After Cancer*. Sydney, NSW: Choice Books.

Little, M., Paul, K., Jordens, C.F.C. and Sayers, E.-J. (2002) Survivorship and discourses of identity. *Psycho-Oncology*, 11: 170–8.

Lubkin, I.M. (ed.) (1990) *Chronic Illness: Impact and Interventions*, 2nd edn. Boston, MA: Jones & Bartlett.

McNamara, B. (2001) *Fragile Lives: Death, Dying and Care*. Sydney, NSW: Allen & Unwin.

Mellor, P. (1993) Death in high-modernity: the contemporary presence and absence of death, in D. Clark (ed.) *The Sociology of Death: Theory, Culture, Practice*. Oxford: Blackwell.

Mullen, F. (1985) Seasons of survival: reflections of a physician with cancer. *New England Journal of Medicine*, 313: 270–3.

O'Connor, M. (2001) The veils of death: understanding dying in residential aged care. Unpublished thesis, La Trobe University, Melbourne, VIC.

Palliative Care Australia (1999) *Palliative Care in Aged Care Facilities*. Discussion Paper. Canberra, ACT: Palliative Care Australia.

Pollard, A., Cairns, J. and Rosenthal, M. (1999) Transitions in living and dying: defining palliative care, in S. Aranda and M. O'Connor (eds) *Palliative Care Nursing: A Guide to Practice*. Melbourne, VIC: Ausmed Publications.

Pollard, B. (1999) *The Principles of Palliative Care: An Introduction*. Newcastle, NSW: Copy Centre.

Seale, C. (1998) *Constructing Death: The Sociology of Dying and Bereavement*. Cambridge: Cambridge University Press.

Small, N. and Rhodes, P. (2000) *Too Ill to Talk? User Involvement and Palliative Care*. London: Routledge.

Smith, M. (2000) Death, health policy and palliative care, in A. Kellehear (ed.) *Death and Dying in Australia*. Melbourne, VIC: Oxford University Press.

Spelten, E.R., Sprangers, M.A.G. and Verbeek, J.H.A. (2002) Factors reported to influence the return to work of cancer survivors: a literature review. *Psycho-Oncology*, 11: 124–31.

van Gennep, A. (1960) *Rites of Passage* (translated by M.B. Vizedom and G. Chaffee). Chicago, IL: University of Chicago Press.

8

Communication, the patient and the palliative care team

Nikki Jarrett and Sian Maslin-Prothero

Effective communication in palliative care would be the goal of most health care workers; these skills are assumed to be innate in the caring professions but the evidence can be contrary. In this chapter, we explore the topic of communication in palliative care and the skills involved in this activity (see Box 8.1). We introduce the literature relating to communication within the health care setting with an emphasis on palliative care, and examine ways in which communication skills may be developed to gain more from the experiences encountered both personally and professionally. We discuss being partners in care with our patients and examine current issues such as the role of the 'expert patient'.

Box 8.1   Key Issues

- Review of current literature
  - ○ Communication in the palliative care setting
  - ○ Research into communication between health professionals and patients
    - ■ Research evaluating communication
    - ■ Research recognizing the social nature of interaction
- Inter- and intra-professional communication
- Explore the user and carer perspective
- Identify the important aspects for health care practitioners

---

Communication in the palliative care setting

Communication is the process of exchanging thoughts or information between individuals (*Merriman-Webster's Collegiate Dictionary* 2002). It is usually accomplished by using language:

- Verbal – which can be spoken, written, word processed, printed or displayed on a screen.

- Non-verbal – this usually transmits attitudes and beliefs through gestures, facial expressions or body language (Brooker 2002).

Whichever process is used, the communicator must be able to express their ideas effectively because patients and their carers are depending on health and social care professionals to convey information specific to their individual care. Therefore, effective communication is essential within palliative care (Wallace 2001), while ineffective communication is a source of complaint for many patients and their carers (Chan and Woodruff 1997).

Palliative care patients require information to manage their diagnosis and cope with the disease (Sawyer 2000), and to address their specific needs (Ronaldson and Devery 2001). The skill lies with the health care professional's ability to identify the information requirements of each individual and to communicate the options available to them, so that each individual receives the information they require and participate at a level that suits their requirements. Maguire (1999) argues that most cancer patients want to know their diagnosis, prognosis, possible treatment options and relevant side-effects, and that only a minority prefer not to know. Problems arise when there is a discrepancy between what the patient wants to hear and the content of the information given and the way the health care professional delivers information.

Health care professionals acknowledge their need for continuing professional development, especially in communicating with dying patients and their relatives (Samaroo 1996). Cooley (2000) points out that although many nurses may consider that their communication skills are insufficient when delivering palliative care, all nurses possess social communication skills that can provide the basis for building other interpersonal and communication skills. Exploring the literature identifies many studies relating to 'communication in health care settings'; however, these are often descriptive or opinion papers, reiterating the importance of quality communication and information giving. Much of this literature is from the developed world and published by nurses; there is little research examining aspects of communication specifically within the palliative care setting.

The issue of inadequate communication does not only arise in cancer palliative care, Addington-Hall and co-workers' (1995) survey of friends and relatives of 237 patients who died from cerebral vascular accidents in 1990 revealed that two-fifths had been unable to get all the information they had wanted about the patient's condition; the authors concluded that symptom control, psychosocial support and communication between health professionals and patients and their families all required improvement. This view is reinforced and supported by others (Clark *et al.* 2000; Payne 2002).

The importance of good communication in palliative care

There is a considerable amount of literature devoted to the importance of communication and counselling skills between health care professionals and patients. Even when the main focus of attention is not on communication, it is frequently referred to in the recommendations as something that needs improvement. Patients also have high hopes and expect health professionals in specialist palliative care settings to be able to provide psychological and emotional support through excellent communication as well as possess expertise in symptom control (Jarrett *et al.* 1999b). It would appear that patients are well aware when a health care professional is not able to deal with particular issues adequately or comfortably, as an excerpt from an interview with a patient with cancer reveals (see Box 8.2).

Box 8.2   Research findings: example of a patient judging health professionals' communication ability

'I think I'm in tune enough to know (. . .) you know (. . .) when I'm on to a loser so I wouldn't attempt that sort of conversation where I didn't feel it was going to help so I think I can probably pick up the vibes you know here is someone who would be helpful and who wouldn't.'

(Jarrett 1996: 92)

Jarrett argues that the maintenance of 'comfortable', non-threatening conversations between a nurse and a patient may be a 'guiding principle' for both patients and nurses, as they probably form part of their everyday interactions (Jarrett 1996). It is desirable, however, to have health care professionals who are able to communicate at the deeper levels with their patients if this is what the patients wish.

Fisher (2002) argues that professionals working in palliative care need to address the following three key areas when communicating with patients:

- the importance of assessment skills;
- being skilled at responding to the patients' needs and feelings such as reflecting back, facilitating emotional expression, drawing out, holding strong emotions such as anger and sadness; and
- dealing with their needs for information and to have their questions answered.

It could be argued that this is good practice required in any setting, not just a requirement for palliative care patients. As detailed elsewhere in this book, however, palliative care patients do have specific and extra needs that can make their communication needs more profound and their situations more complex.

In the UK, the National Institute for Clinical Excellence[1] has commissioned a guidance document; this will provide guidance on best practice in supportive and palliative care for all cancers. The areas covered by the guidelines will include evidence-based recommendations for supportive care networks, information delivery and communication, inter-professional communication, symptom control and access to specialist palliative care, community supportive care, complementary therapies, models of psychological care, social inclusion, users' and carers' needs, social care and meaning and belief. It aims to underpin the development of a supportive and palliative care strategy.

Research on communication between health care professionals and patients

It has been argued that research on communication between patients and health care professionals can be divided into three main types based on the research approach taken (Jarrett 1996): descriptive, skills-oriented and social interaction. *Descriptive* research on communication tends to describe the types and topics of the interaction. For example, Bond's (1978) study in one radiotherapy department identified that much of the nurse–patient interaction related to treatment, symptoms and social topics. Conversations about home life, the future, diagnosis or prognosis were limited. This kind of research tended to focus on what was talked about in terms of broad topic areas and for how long each interaction lasted. With the advent of more sophisticated recording devices, researchers of communication in the health care setting have been able to take a more detailed look at the interactions between patients and health care professionals and what is actually being said and how. Two general types of research approach appear to prevail – *skills-oriented* and *social interaction* – and these are discussed in the following two sections.

Research evaluating communication skills

Skills-oriented communication research focuses on the health care professional's communication skills and evaluates their performance. A good example of this is the study by Wilkinson (1991) of communication between nurses and patients with cancer on six wards. Wilkinson distinguished between the different skills of nurses and suggested that not all nurses lacked communication skills and blocked patients from discussing their concerns, as some previous studies appeared to indicate (e.g. Bond 1978; Clark 1982). Wilkinson demonstrated that some nurses were predominately 'blockers' of patients' concerns using strategies such as 'informing' or 'ignoring'; through the use of blocking mechanisms, these nurses were able to protect themselves, and patients, from anguish created when discussing any psychological issues. Other nurses, termed 'facilitators', were more able to encourage and elicit patients' concerns. Interestingly, key factors in determining the communication style of the nurses were found to be the ward in which they worked because of the ethos created by the charge nurse, the nurses' attitudes to death and their religious beliefs, rather than any specific communication skills training received.

Research recognizing the social nature of interaction

Jarrett and Payne (1995) identified that much previous research in communication neglected the important contribution of the patient within interactions; they suggested that by investigating communication as isolated excerpts of talk, research frequently neglects the social and contextual factors that play a part in an ongoing relationship between two individuals.

Another example of research that sees communication within the cancer care setting as a two-way social interaction is the work of Lanceley (1995, 1999). Lanceley's (1999) investigation of the emotional content of talk between nurses and cancer patients demonstrates that talk with emotional content is frequent and collaboratively produced. Patients appeared to be active in this and expressed their feelings openly, as well as covertly using metaphors and symbolic language. Lanceley (1999) reveals the impact upon the nurses of hearing the patients' distress. Hunt (1989, 1991) examined the interactions between patients and relatives and the community specialist palliative care nurses visiting them at home. She argued that all the participants in the interactions jointly created the informal friendly nature of conversations, such as commenting on photographs, including the conversation that occurs when a nurse enters or leaves the house.

Within palliative care, it is important that health care professionals maintain a feeling of hope with patients and their families that is realistic and not false (Penson 2000). The concept of maintaining hope or some optimism in the cancer and palliative care setting can be used to illustrate this social interaction approach to communication in more detail. Perakyla's (1991) description of the 'hope work' performed by staff and patients within the hospital setting in Finland as the patient approached death is an important contribution to the literature. Perakyla described three variations of 'hope work', as shown in Box 8.3. Perakyla emphasizes the significance of this skill and the competence required by health care workers when caring for seriously ill patients, knowing when and where they need to intervene with the three different types of 'hope work'. An important feature of the work is how the patient is viewed as an active contributor to this interactional practice; the health care professional is not solely responsible for creating and maintaining the hopeful side to verbal interactions.

This is similar to findings from Jarrett and Payne's study (2000), who

---

Box 8.3 Research findings: 'hope work' (after Perakyla 1991)

- *Curative hope work*: where the patient is defined as 'getting better'
- *Palliative hope work*: where the patient is described as 'feeling better'
- *Past recovery*: where the hope is dismantled and the patient is past recovery

describe the creation of a largely optimistic and cheerful nature to conversations in the cancer care context investigated. Examples of some of the ways the optimistic nature of the conversations appear to be maintained are listed in Box 8.4.

'Self-comparison' is when a patient compares himself or herself with another patient. This appeared to be a common feature and an important way in which patients learn from fellow patients. Patients were found to observe and comment on the stoicism and bravery of other patients and it is likely that individuals may learn how to behave as patients in the cancer and palliative care setting. Comparing oneself with others or 'social comparison' (Ashby Wills 1981) is a familiar characteristic of social behaviour. In the

Box 8.4 Research findings: examples of ways nurses and patients created cheerful and optimistic nature to their conversations together (Jarrett and Payne 2000)

- Searching for positive statements: this involves finding a positive aspect about what is being discussed and focusing attention on it
- 'Self-comparison': this includes acknowledging that other patients have more distressing, disfiguring or harder treatments or cancer to endure and so in comparison the patient is luckier
- Emphasizing 'individual differences' and how the patient could do much better than another patient with the same disease because people respond differently, thus avoiding the risks associated with self-comparison
- 'Optimistic knowledge': this involves focusing on the positive element of the information being delivered or focusing on areas where the message can be more positive, such as concentrating on more controllable symptoms sometimes at the expense of those harder to be positive about
- 'Reframing' or 'minimizing' events and emphasizing the routine, expected side of events, such as 'feeling a bit nauseous, but that's quite normal'
- The 'clinical uncertainty' associated with medicine generally means that even when the statistical chances for a patient appear poor, the patient and health professional can emphasize the uncertainty surrounding this and how every one is different in how they respond to treatments, so it is still possible to maintain hope

context of cancer patients (Jarrett and Payne 2000), it appeared to enable the patient to feel luckier or better off than fellow patients. The excerpt from an interview with a patient in Box 8.5 illustrates this.

Box 8.5   Research findings: an example of a patient employing self-comparison

'so far so good I haven't had quite so much damage done to me bodily wise or nausea reaction as our friend over here for example [indicating patient in next bed] . . . he's suffered badly you know. . . . But you know I haven't suffered anywhere nearly as badly.'

(Jarrett and Payne 2000: 85)

Self-comparison is quite a risky strategy if patients compare themselves with someone with the same illness who is deteriorating or dying. Consequently, the strategy of emphasizing 'individual differences' appeared to be very important in ensuring that the patient received the positive benefits of this strategy without highlighting their potential future deterioration.

Box 8.6 provides an excerpt from a conversation between a patient newly

---

Box 8.6   Example excerpt of conversation illustrating the use of 'individual differences' within nurse-patient conversation

1	Nurse:	. . . and I think those are the sort of reassurance
2		you need (.)
3	Patient:	did you know {name}? she was over here last April
4		(.)
5	Nurse:	N-no (.) April I actually wasn't here then
6	Patient:	oh you won't [well] she has both her breast removed
7	Nurse:	[no]
8		yes (.)
9		[that's a there are different types of cancer]
10	Patient:	[( )] she's a nursing sister]
11	Nurse:	and some cancer actually is renowned for (.)
12		affecting both breasts (.) um and it has even been
13		known for the two breasts to be removed
14		[at the] same time because of that (.) u:m but]
15	Patient	[what]
16		had her's done at different times
17	Nurse:	yes (2)
18		[[but never judge] your own case
19	Patient:	[[( )]
20	Nurse:	by someone [else's either] (.)
21	Patient:	[oh no I know]
22	Nurse:	u:m again as I say everybody is so individual . . .

(Nurse 006 and Patient 027; Jarrett and Payne 2000: 85–6)

diagnosed with breast cancer and a nurse. The nurse indicates that it is sometimes reassuring to hear about other patients who are doing well (line 1). The patient introduces another patient (line 3), but this patient has had a double mastectomy and it is interesting to note how the nurse emphasizes that the patient must not compare herself with another patient (lines 18–22) and the patient demonstrates an awareness of this by saying 'oh no I know' (line 21).

Researchers taking the above perspective argue that both patient and health professional were *active* in these *jointly* produced and constructed conversations, and that the conversation was not produced entirely by the professional with the patient taking a largely passive role. The concept of conversation being a two-way interaction is not new within the communication literature, but appears to have been largely neglected in the health care literature, which has focused so closely on describing the nature of the interaction and then measuring the quality of the communication skill produced by the health care professional.

Communication and decision making

The extent to which individuals want to be involved in decision making varies. Cassileth *et al.* (1982) indicated that it is younger and well-educated people who most wish to be involved in the decision-making process. Others have suggested that a patient's role in decision making is based on the seriousness of their illness – the more serious the illness, the less involved they want to be (Thompson *et al.* 1993). Some research has examined patient preferences for communication within cancer, but less so in palliative care. Yet there is a body of evidence to suggest that patients do not perceive that they have a role to play in the decision-making process, or choose to adopt a passive role, reinforcing the power and status of health professionals because of their assumed knowledge, expertise and social standing (Cassileth *et al.* 1980; Strull *et al.* 1984; Tobias 1988; Sutherland *et al.* 1989; Degner and Sloane 1992). The attitudes and expectations of both health care professionals and patients have changed; clinicians tend to be less paternalistic about what should or should not be disclosed to patients in their care, and patients tend to be more, although not necessarily better, informed about disease and treatment options through the media (Kiley 2002). The expectation is now greater for health professionals to involve patients in the decision-making process (Bond and Thomas 1992).

In the UK, there has been a change in policy to include the patient's perspective in health care provision, beginning with *The Patient's Charter* (Department of Health 1991) through to the creation by the National Institute for Clinical Excellence (NICE) of a Citizens' Council, where the public are invited to give their views on the work of NICE, which can be used to inform recommendations for care and treatment. Within these there is an assumption that all patients should be provided with as much information as possible and given the time to consider the facts in order that they can arrive at an informed decision. This assumes that all patients have the same ability to understand information before making an informed decision about their treatment, and that clinicians are willing and able to communicate with patients and their families (Maslin-Prothero 2000).

Degner *et al.* (1997) explored the information needs and decisional preferences of 1012 women with breast cancer in oncology clinics. They found that 22 per cent preferred to take the lead, 34 per cent wanted the clinician to make the decision and 44 per cent wanted to share the decision. The researchers found that less than half of these women achieved their preferred level of control. Miller and Managan (1983, cited in Maguire 1999) referred to two groups of patients: information seekers ('monitors') who try to find out as much information as possible, and the avoiders of information ('blunters') who put up barriers to information provided. Patients' information needs vary during the course of their illness, they use different coping mechanisms and it becomes the responsibility of the multidisciplinary team to identify which one each patient is presenting.

Bruera and co-workers' (2001) study of patient preferences for decision making and communication within Canadian cancer care is interesting, because it reveals that gender and age do not have a significant impact on patient preferences. Most (63 per cent) of the 78 patients preferred a shared approach with the physician. Importantly, a substantial minority preferred either taking the active role themselves (20 per cent) or being passive and allowing the physician to make the decision (17 per cent). The studies reviewed suggest that patients' willingness to be involved in decision making varies considerably. It is the duty of the clinician to determine how much patients want to be involved, regardless of their disease status (Degner *et al.* 1997; Maguire 1999). This appears to be associated with health care professionals' ability to communicate effectively with patients and vice versa (Fallowfield *et al.* 1998; Maguire 1999). Barriers to effective communication exist on both sides. Patients may be reluctant to disclose what they are feeling about their diagnosis and treatment options and how these might affect their life – they believe that health care professionals are not interested in their concerns. On the other hand, many health carer workers are concerned about patients asking difficult questions and displaying strong emotions, plus the difficulty of explaining complex information. Therefore, an individualized approach when dealing with patients and their preferences for involvement in their care decisions appears to be the most appropriate course of action and health care workers must not assume that they can predict the views of a patient.

Training and education

The need to provide training in communication and counselling skills for health professionals working within cancer and palliative care is a common theme in the literature (Faulkner *et al.* 1991). Evaluations of communication skills training programmes in palliative care are usually positive (Faulkner 1992; MacLeod *et al.* 1994) and have led to the production of guidelines on how to communicate with patients (Faulkner and Regnard 1994). Bowles *et al.* (2001) describe the evaluation of a communication skills training programme employing some training in solution-focused brief therapy. This is a time-limited, practical, problem-solving approach drawn from counselling that aims to deal with a client's presenting problems. Bowles *et al.* indicated that the techniques may be a 'useful, cost effective approach to the training of communication skills' (p. 347).

Several studies aimed at improving the communication skills of health professionals have been undertaken (e.g. Maguire *et al.* 1984; Maguire 1990, 1999; Fallowfield *et al.* 1998), yet the skills taught and developed in workshops are often lost within 3–12 months of completing the course (Corner and Wilson-Barnett 1992; Heaven and Maguire 1996). Wilkinson *et al.* (1998, 1999, 2002) have argued that following an integrated communication skills programme delivered to nurses, these skills can be maintained over time.

Counselling patients with cancer is not just about nurses having good communication skills; effective counselling for patients requires appropriate training, which has cost, time and emotional implications for members of staff (Potter 1996). Particular routes or guidelines have been prescribed for professionals to follow when dealing with difficult topic areas, for example when handling difficult questions (Faulkner and Regnard 1994). A great deal has been published about the importance of communication and counselling skills training. It would appear, however, that skills acquired in simulated interactions based in the classroom or prescribed verbal activities suggested in a flow diagram (see Box 8.7), may sometimes be difficult to apply in the clinical setting.

Inter- and intra-professional communication in palliative care settings

An important feature of communication is that it involves everyone involved in the care of the patient as well as the patient themselves. There has been an increasing recognition of the role inter- and intra-professional communication plays in health care settings and the palliative care setting. Problems with communication across the different locations of care and the different people involved can have a profound impact on patients' and their carers' experience of care. A study examining the perceptions and experiences of terminally ill patients in the community indicated that patients and their carers were often confused about the variety of health and social care professionals involved in their care, especially their different roles, areas of expertise and power (Jarrett *et al.* 1999a).

The chronic nature of cancer and other life-threatening diseases has meant that ensuring continuity of care – with the variety of health and social

---

Box 8.7 Summary of training and education

- There has been a tendency in communication research to:

  ○ describe communication between health professionals, usually nurses or doctors, as deficient in quality and quantity; and

  ○ to lay the blame for this firmly with the health professional, consequently viewing the patient as merely the passive recipient of communication.

- There has been an emphasis on training health professionals in communication skills, but skills learnt in the classroom do not always transfer easily to the clinical setting.

- Research taking the perspective of viewing interaction as social and contextual might also argue that:

  ○ the patient is active in contributing to this feature of health-related conversation;

  ○ some patients are experienced recipients of health-related communication.

Acknowledging, and also aiming to increase, the expertise and role of patients in their health care management largely through the medium of communication has been advocated.

However:

- Health care professionals may need to consider different patients' desires for certain types of interaction, for example:

  ○ patients may be influenced by contextual and environmental determinants, their beliefs or previous experiences about what constitutes appropriate communication in the health care setting;

  ○ patients may have views about whom is appropriate to talk to about certain issues and may be able to judge the abilities of different individuals or professional groups to cope with issues effectively.

---

care professionals, services and locations of care involved – is a huge challenge. Factors identified as being barriers to successful continuity and coordination of care include:

- Territoriality, such as problems surrounding domains of responsibility and locations of care delivery.

- Reimbursement issues, for example issues related to who is paying for care and particular budgets.

- Minimal collaboration across agencies.

- Inadequate communication between different health and social care professionals (Beddar and Aikin 1994).

Many agencies are involved in providing palliative care. A seamless, integrated service is one in which services meet an individual's need, are coordinated, and integrated across the health and social care system. In a seamless service:

- Organizational boundaries do not get in the way of care for patients, but it is clear who is responsible and accountable for their care at all times.
- The planning and contracting process supports practical working arrangements.
- Roles and responsibilities are clearly defined.
- Multi-professional teams come together to provide high-quality services for patients that make the best use of the specialist skills and experience of the staff involved.
- All staff are trained to work in multi-professional teams, and there is support in working across organizational boundaries (Department of Health 1996).

Developing an integrated service also depends on effective partnerships across the boundary of primary and secondary care. As more treatment and care is carried out in the home or local community, the role of secondary care professionals continues to evolve as they work together with the primary health care team, ensuring that patients receive integrated care that draws the best from both sectors.

The idea of interdisciplinary education is seen as an important factor in improving the communication and teamworking between the various health professionals (Ruebling *et al.* 2000). Koffman (2001) identified the growth in multi-professional educational programmes in palliative care and indicated that the evidence of benefits for patients and their carers through the delivery of palliative care is positive but also limited.

There is some evidence that communication problems can exist between different health professionals or across different locations of care delivery or management. Research investigating the communication needs and satisfaction of primary care physicians following letters sent about palliative radiotherapy from a radiation oncologist (Barnes *et al.* 2000) found that although most primary care physicians were satisfied with the information sent, they felt that unnecessary information was included while essential information was missing. Barnes and colleagues argued for an improvement in communication between these two professional groups.

An Australian study by Street and Blackford (2001) investigated communication between general practitioners and nurses. Through interviews and focus groups with 40 palliative care nurses working in the community, hospices or hospital settings, the following issues were highlighted as problems: the means of transferring information; networking; case management; multiple service providers; a lack of standardized documentation; and formal client-tracking systems. These all impeded positive communication between the two professional groups. Blackford and Street (2001) also reported upon the role of the palliative care nurse consultant in enabling continuity of care across the health care services by improving communication strategies and creating new networks. It appears that a professional role, which provides care or consultancy across several different care settings, such as the community and the hospital, may have a key role in ensuring continuity of care (Clark *et al.* 2000).

Health care professionals emphasize the importance of good inter- and intra-professional communication, particularly in the palliative care setting, although little is known about the perceptions of, and impact upon, patients themselves. Recent research has examined the perceptions and experiences of patients receiving specialist palliative care services and the communication among the various health and social care professionals involved in their care (Jarrett and Latter 2003). This ongoing study conducts in-depth interviews with 22 patients receiving specialist palliative care from two specialist palliative care units/hospices in the south of England. Initial findings indicate that for many patients in the palliative care setting, many different health and social care professionals can be involved in their care, often spread over a variety of geographical locations in the community, general hospital and specialist palliative care settings. Overall perceptions of inter- and intra-professional communication were positive, but a minority of patients felt there was sometimes a lack of organization and co-ordination, with some patients or family carers feeling they had to be quite proactive to ensure adequate communication and continuity of care across the various locations.

The patient and carer perspective

Patient involvement

Over the last decade in the UK there has been a growth in the number of policy initiatives calling for user participation in the planning and development of health and social services at local, regional and national level (Department of Health 1991, 1997a,b, 1998a,b,c, 1999b, 2000b; NHS Executive 1996, 1998; Welsh Office 1998). Permeating all these policy documents is an emphasis on the role of users in determining, shaping and evaluating services through the identification of health needs, and the chance to make choices about their own health care (see Chapter 4).

The emphasis has been on shaping the health and social care system around the needs of patients. The National Health Service (NHS) has to develop partnerships and cooperation at all levels of care – between patients, their carers and families, and NHS staff – to ensure a patient-centred service (Department of Health 2000b). It is important to evaluate the effectiveness of services from a user perspective, including an annual national survey of user experience (Department of Health 1997a). Health care professionals are increasingly being required to demonstrate that their care is patient sensitive and needs led; Smith (1997: 1059) describes this change 'as the balance of power in the doctor–patient relationship shift[ing] towards the patient'.

Patients' preferences for participation vary widely, with some patients choosing to play an active role and others a passive role (Waterworth and Luker 1990; Degner *et al.* 1997; Maguire 1999). Patient experiences are enhanced when there is evidence of staff–patient communication, patient involvement in decision making, the provision of clear and relevant information, and sufficient opportunity for questions and expressions of concern (Degner and Sloane 1992; Hack *et al.* 1994; Maslin 1994; Degner *et al.* 1997; Fallowfield *et al.* 1998).

The expert patient

The concept of the 'expert patient' (Department of Health 2001a) is very relevant to many patients with palliative care needs. Often by the time the patient reaches the palliative care setting they, and their family or lay-carers, are very experienced and familiar with health care environments, the drugs, the jargon and the different personnel and services involved in their care. Patients with palliative care needs have the potential to become 'confident partners with professionals in their care' (Department of Health 2001a: 13). The changing needs of the palliative care patient, as they move through the dying trajectory, mean that they might need extra support in maintaining their involvement.

In England and Wales, national service frameworks[2] have been developed to improve health, reduce inequalities and raise the quality of care through placing the patient at the centre of care. These standards have been developed with the assistance of an external reference group, which includes clinicians, scientists, epidemiologists, managers, voluntary organizations, patients and carers. Several national service frameworks have been produced – *Mental Health, Cancer* and *Older People* (Department of Health (1999a, 2000a, 2001b) – with more proposed. These appear to be targeting specific patient populations. They are relevant to many palliative care patients and their carers. The standards have been set by the National Institute for Clinical Excellence, an external reference group, will be delivered by clinical governance, and monitored by the Commission for Health Improvement, the Performance Assessment Framework and the National Commission for Public and Patient Involvement.

The approach to communication that views it as a social interaction, albeit within a professional health care setting, sees the patient as equal to the researcher and the health or social care professional. Within the interaction, both health professional and patient can potentially be seen as an 'expert' or skilled at communicating. Even though the health professional may have access to greater knowledge in some domains, patients are also experts about how they feel and what has happened to them and, importantly, what they wish to talk about or topics they feel able to deal with. As already discussed, they may have notions about who it is appropriate to talk to about certain issues, have witnessed and learned from the behaviour of other patients and their previous interactions. The interest is not just the verbal contribution made by the patient during specific interactions, but also of interest are the patients' views and experiences of communication.

The term 'patients' perspective', as used by Benz (2001), is in itself a label that suggests a divide between the 'care-giver' and the 'care-receiver'. This divide is quite traditional in the literature on communication as well as other areas within the palliative care field. The expertise and knowledge of the patient are recognized, but so to is the need to facilitate patients to be able to take on the role of partner in their care. The suggestion is to run workshops and train patients with the skills they need to be able to contribute effectively in the management of their care and to self-manage their symptoms; this has been implemented successfully with some chronic diseases, such as arthritis, depression and multiple sclerosis. The Department of Health (2001a) concluded that these self-management programmes resulted in 'tangible benefits', including: reduced severity of symptoms; significant decrease in pain; improved life control and activity; and improved resourcefulness and life satisfaction. If this approach is applied to the palliative care setting, then a possible solution might be to offer patients with life-threatening diseases training to prepare them to take a more active role in their own care or as patient advocates or representatives of other patients in the palliative care phase.

There is some evidence to suggest that seriously ill patients do wish to be involved with end-of-life decision making (Heyland *et al.* 2000), although some of the issues surrounding the end-of-life event in the intensive care unit, for example, can be very complex (Bowman 2000). The experiences of 16 palliative care patients revealed that although the choices and involvement in medical decisions appeared straightforward on the surface, the unpredictable nature of palliative care and the deliberations and trade-offs required meant that the process of patient involvement was not simple (Bottorff *et al.* 1998).

Key issues for consideration

It can be argued that it is important for research and theory investigating the communication between health and social care professionals and patients to acknowledge that the patient may not be the passive recipient of so-called good skilled communication or poor communication from the professional, but that they may also be contributing to the interaction. What might follow from this is the notion that part of the 'expert patient' is one who is skilled at initiating and manoeuvring a conversation that satisfies their needs.

Placing the patient at the centre of research, policy and professional education is vital, but not necessarily straightforward. Small and Rhodes (2000) discuss the role and importance of user involvement within palliative care focusing upon three life-threatening diseases: cystic fibrosis, multiple sclerosis and motor neurone disease. As they highlight, there is an assumption that user involvement is easy to achieve, but this is not always the case and not everyone concerned might welcome it. Developments in communications and information technology will have an important role to play so that the necessary information about patients and their care, and about the organization of services, is readily accessible to those who need it.

The risks associated with a move *beyond* recognizing the existing role and right of patients to participate equally in the management of their care and the communication and decision making involved in this are summarized in Box 8.8.

Box 8.8   Potential risks associated with the expert patient

- There is a potential risk that when communication breaks down, the blame is placed with the patient rather than the health or social care professional.
- Advocacy and patient representatives may be selected or self-selecting and this risks only a certain type of patient/person taking on these roles.
- Patients receiving palliative care are frequently debilitated and fatigued and may have cognitive impairment or other symptoms that may impede their ability to contribute at the level they would wish:

  - this risks patients' level of functioning being used as an excuse for not involving certain groups of patients;
  - it is also important to consider whether all patients wish to be involved despite health policy initiatives (Small and Rhodes 2000).

- Training and facilitating patients has cost implications, both financially and in terms of time.

One of the keys to effective communication in palliative care is multidisciplinary teamwork (Trueman 2001). The answer to improving the communication skills of multidisciplinary teams may lie in introducing the relevance and skills of communication to health care professionals earlier in their initial education and training, as well as at postgraduate level (Cockburn *et al.* 1998; Doyal and Gillon 1998). These subjects exist in the curricula, but there is a long lead-in time until these health care professionals are in a position to make a difference. There has been growth in shared interprofessional learning; central funding in England has been given to four universities to lead the development of multi-professional pre-registration education across nursing, allied health professions and medicine. In these pilot sites, health professionals will share learning in core subjects such as communications and health and social care principles with the aim of developing new ways of working (Department of Health 2002).

Conclusions

This chapter links closely with others in this book (see, for example, Chapter 4) and has reminded the reader about the importance of effective communication in the palliative care setting. We have provided a brief overview of communication and have reviewed the current literature in relation to communication in the palliative care setting, including research into communication between health professionals and patients, inter- and intra-professional communication, and exploring the user and carer perspective. Some examples have been offered as an illustration of communication in the palliative care setting. Communication as a skill requires constant attention and development if we are to be effective in the delivery of care to palliative care patients and their relatives, a skill that is taken for granted and assumed.

Notes

1   See NICE (2002) Scope for the development of service configuration guidance on supportive and palliative care (http://www.nice.org.uk/article.asp?a=30530). Accessed 20 December 2002.
2   See the National Service frameworks home page (http://www.doh.gov.uk/nsf/nsfhome.htm).

References

Addington-Hall, J., Lay, M., Altmann, D. and McCarthy, M. (1995) Symptom control, communication with health professionals, and hospital care of stroke patients in the last year of life as reported by surviving family, friends, and officials. *Stroke*, 26(12): 2242–8.

Ashby Wills, T. (1981) Downward comparison principle in social psychology. *Psychological Bulletin*, 90(2): 245–71.

Barnes, E.A., Hanson, J., Neumann, C.M., Nekolaichuk, C.L. and Bruera, E. (2000) Communication between primary care physicians and radiation oncologists regarding patients with cancer treated with palliative radiotherapy. *Journal of Clinical Oncology*, 18(15): 2902–7.

Beddar, S.M. and Aikin, J.L. (1994) Continuity of care: a challenge for ambulatory oncology nursing. *Seminars in Oncology Nursing*, 10(4): 254–63.

Benz, C. (2001) Patients' perspectives, in J.M. Addington-Hall and I.J. Higginson (eds) *Palliative Care for Non-Cancer Patients*. Oxford: Oxford University Press.

Blackford, J. and Street, A. (2001) The role of the palliative care nurse in promoting continuity of end-of-life care. *International Journal of Palliative Nursing*, 7(6): 273–8.

Bond, S. (1978) Processes of communication about cancer in a radiotherapy department. Unpublished PhD thesis. University of Edinburgh.

Bond, S. and Thomas, L. (1992) Measuring patients' satisfaction with nursing care. *Journal of Advanced Nursing*, 17: 52–63.

Bottorff, J.L., Steele, R., Davies, B. *et al.* (1998) Striving for balance: palliative care patients' experiences of making everyday choices. *Journal of Palliative Care*, 14(1): 7–17.

Bowles, N., Mackintosh, C. and Torn, A. (2001) Nurses' communication skills: an evaluation of the impact of solution focussed communication training. *Journal of Advanced Nursing*, 36(3): 347–54.

Bowman, K.W. (2000) Communication, negotiation, and mediation: dealing with conflict in end-of-life decisions. *Journal of Palliative Care*, 16: S17–S23.

Brooker, C. (ed.) (2002) *Churchill Livingstone's Dictionary of Nursing*, 18th edn. Edinburgh: Churchill Livingstone.

Bruera, E., Sweeney, C., Calder, K., Palmer, L. and Benisch-Tolley, S. (2001) Patient preferences versus physician perceptions of treatment decisions in cancer care. *Journal of Clinical Oncology*, 19(11): 2883–5.

Cassileth, B.R., Zupkis, R.V., Sutton-Smith, R. and Marsh, V. (1980) Information and participation preferences of hospitalised adult cancer patients. *Annals of Internal Medicine*, 92: 832–6.

Cassileth, B.R., Lusk, E.J., Miller, D.S. and Hurwitz, S. (1982) Attitudes towards clinical trials among patients and the public. *Journal of the American Medical Association*, 248(8): 968–70.

Chan, A. and Woodruff, R.K. (1997) Communicating with patients with advanced cancer. *Journal of Palliative Care*, 13(3): 29–33.

Clark, D., Hughes, P., Marples, R. *et al.* (2000) Experiences, outcomes and costs of Macmillan nursing: the patient's perspective. *Palliative Medicine*, 14: 343.

Clark, J.L. (1982) Nurse–patient verbal interaction: an analysis of recorded conversations in selected surgical wards. Unpublished PhD thesis, Chelsea College, University of London.

Cockburn, J., Redman, S. and Kricker, A. (1998) Should women take part in clinical trials for breast cancer? Issues and some solutions. *Journal of Clinical Oncology*, 16(1): 1354–62.

Cooley, D. (2000) Professional nurse study: communication skills in palliative care. *Professional Nurse*, 15(9): 603–5.

Corner, J. and Wilson-Barnett, J. (1992) The newly registered nurse and the cancer patient: an educational evaluation. *International Journal of Nursing Studies*, 29(2): 177–90.

Degner, L.F. and Sloane, J.A. (1992) Decision-making during serious illness: what role do patients really want to play? *Journal of Clinical Epidemiology*, 45: 941–50.

Degner, L.F., Kristjanon, L.J. and Bowman, L.D. *et al.* (1997) Information needs and decisional preferences in women with breast cancer. *Journal of the American Medical Association*, 233: 1485–91.

Department of Health (1991) *The Patient's Charter*. London: HMSO.

Department of Health (1996) *The National Health Service: A Service with Ambitions*. London: HMSO.

Department of Health (1997a) *The new NHS: Modern, Dependable*. London: The Stationery Office.

Department of Health (1997b) *The Caldicott Committee: Report on the Review of Patient-Identifiable Information*. London: Department of Health.

Department of Health (1998a) *A First Class Service*. London: The Stationery Office.

Department of Health (1998b) *Our Healthier Nation: A Contract for Health*. London: The Stationery Office.

Department of Health (1998c) *Health in Partnership: Patient, Carer and Public Involvement in Health Care Decision Making*. London: Department of Health.

Department of Health (1999a) *National Service Framework for Mental Health*. London: The Stationery Office.

Department of Health (1999b) *Patient and Public Involvement in the New NHS*. London: Department of Health.

Department of Health (2000a) *The NHS Cancer Plan*. London: The Stationery Office.

Department of Health (2000b) *The NHS Plan: A Plan for Investment, A Plan for Reform*. London: The Stationery Office.

Department of Health (2001a) *The Expert Patient: A New Approach to Chronic Disease Management for the 21st Century*. London: Department of Health.

Department of Health (2001b) *National Service Framework for Older People*. London: The Stationery Office.

Department of Health (2002) *Joint Training for Health Professionals*. Press Release, 14 February, London: Department of Health.

Doyal, L. and Gillon, R. (1998) Medical ethics and law as a core subject in medical education. *British Medical Journal*, 316: 1623–4.

Fallowfield, L., Jenkins, V., Brennan, C. *et al.* (1998) Attitudes of patients to randomised clinical trials of cancer therapy. *European Journal of Cancer*, 34(10): 1554–9.

Faulkner, A. (1992) The evaluation of training programmes for communication skills in palliative care. *Journal of Cancer Care*, 1(2): 75–8.

Faulkner, A. and Regnard, C. (1994) Handling difficult questions in palliative care – a flow diagram. *Palliative Medicine*, 8(3): 245–50.

Faulkner, A., Webb, P. and Maguire, P. (1991) Communication and counselling skills: educating health professionals working in cancer and palliative care. *Patient Education and Counselling*, 18(1): 3–7.

Fisher, M. (2002) Emotional pain and eliciting concerns, in J. Penson and R.A. Fisher (eds) *Palliative Care for People with Cancer*, 3rd edn. Malta: Arnold.

Hack, T.F., Degner, L.F. and Dyck, D.G. (1994) Relationship between preferences for decisional control and illness information among women with breast cancer: a quantitative and qualitative analysis. *Social Science and Medicine*, 39: 279–89.

Heaven, C.M. and Maguire, P. (1996) Training hospice nurses to elicit patients' concerns. *Journal of Advanced Nursing*, 23: 280–6.

Heyland, D.K., Tranmer, J. and Feldman-Stewart, D. (2000) End of life decision making in the seriously ill hospitalised patient: an organizing framework and results of a preliminary study. *Journal of Palliative Care*, 16: S31–S39.

Hunt, M. (1989) Dying at home: its basic 'ordinariness' displayed in patients', relatives' and nurses' talk. Unpublished PhD thesis, Goldsmiths College, University of London.

Hunt, M. (1991) Being friendly and informal: reflected in nurses', terminally ill patients' and relatives' conversations at home. *Journal of Advanced Nursing*, 16: 929–38.

Jarrett, N. (1996) Comfortable conversations: communication in the cancer care context. Unpublished PhD thesis, University of Southampton.

Jarrett, N. and Latter, S. (2003) *Towards Effective Inter-Professional Education and Practice: Patients' Perceptions of Inter- and Intra-Professional Communication in the Palliative Care Setting*. Unpublished report to HOPE, Wessex Medical Trust. University of Southampton: School of Nursing and Midwifery.

Jarrett, N. and Payne, S. (1995) A selective review of the literature on nurse–patient communication: has the patient's contribution been neglected? *Journal of Advanced Nursing*, 22: 72–8.

Jarrett, N. and Payne, S. (2000) Creating and maintaining 'optimism' in cancer care communication. *International Journal of Nursing Studies*, 37: 81–90.

Jarrett, N., Payne, S. and Wiles, R. (1999a) Terminally ill patients' and lay-carers' perceptions and experiences of community-based services. *Journal of Advanced Nursing*, 29(2): 476–83.

Jarrett, N., Payne, S., Turner, P. and Hillier, R. (1999b) 'Someone to talk to' and 'pain control': what people expect from a specialist palliative care team. *Palliative Medicine*, 13: 139–44.

Kiley, R. (2002) Finding health information on the internet: health consumers, in P. Richardson (ed.) *A Guide to Medical Publishing and Writing*. Dinton: Quay Books.

Koffman, J. (2001) Multiprofessional palliative care education: past challenges, future issues. *Journal of Palliative Care*, 17(2): 86–92.

Lanceley, A. (1995) Emotional disclosure between cancer patients and nurses, in A. Richardson and J. Wilson-Barnett (eds) *Nursing Research in Cancer Care*. Glasgow: Scutari Press.

Lanceley, A. (1999) The patient and nurse in emotion-talk and cancer: 'the tempest in my mind'. Unpublished PhD thesis, King's College, University of London.

MacLeod, R., Nash, A. and Charny, M. (1994) Evaluating palliative care education. *European Journal of Cancer Care*, 3(4): 163–8.

Maguire, G.P., Goldberg, D.P., Hobson, R.J. *et al.* (1984) Evaluating the teaching of a method of psychotherapy. *British Journal of Psychotherapy*, 144: 575–80.

Maguire, P.J. (1990) Can communication skills be taught? *British Journal of Hospital Medicine*, 43: 215–16.

Maguire, P. (1999) Improving communication with cancer patients. *European Journal of Cancer*, 35(10): 1415–22.

Maslin, A.M. (1994) A survey of the opinions of 'informed consent' of women currently involved in clinical trials within a breast unit. *European Journal of Cancer Care*, 3: 153–62.

Maslin-Prothero, S.E. (2000) Factors affecting recruitment to breast cancer clinical trials: an examination of the British Association of Surgical Oncology II trial and the International Breast Cancer Intervention Study. Unpublished PhD thesis, University of Nottingham.

NHS Executive (1996) *Patient Partnership: Building a Collaborative Strategy*. Leeds: NHS Executive.

NHS Executive, Institute of Health Services Management and NHS Confederation (1998) *In the Public Interest: Developing a Strategy for Public Participation in the NHS*. Leeds: NHS Executive Quality and Consumers Branch.

Payne, S. (2002) Information needs of patients and their families. *European Journal of Palliative Care*, 9(3): 112–14.

Penson, J. (2000) A hope is not a promise: fostering hope within palliative care. *International Journal of Palliative Nursing*, 6(2): 94–8.

Perakyla, A. (1991) Hope work in the care of seriously ill patients. *Qualitative Health Research*, 1(4): 407–33.

Potter, F. (1996) Counselling in cancer care. *Professional Nurse*, 12(3): 191–2.

Ronaldson, S. and Devery, K. (2001) The experience of transition to palliative care services: perspectives of patients and nurses. *International Journal of Palliative Nursing*, 7(4): 171–7.

Ruebling, I., Lavin, M.A., Banks, R. *et al.* (2000) Facilitating factors for, barriers to, and outcomes of interdisciplinary education projects in the health sciences. *Journal of Allied Health*, 29(3): 165–70.

Samaroo, B. (1996) Assessing palliative care educational needs of physicians and nurses: results of a survey. *Journal of Palliative Care*, 12(2): 20–2.

Sawyer, H. (2000) Meeting the information needs of cancer patients. *Professional Nurse*, 15(4): 244–7.

Small, N. and Rhodes, P. (2000) *Too Ill to Talk? User Involvement in Palliative Care*. London: Routledge.

Smith, R. (1997) Informed consent: the intricacies. *British Medical Journal*, 314: 1059–60.

Street, A. and Blackford, J. (2001) Communication issues for the interdisciplinary community palliative care team. *Journal of Clinical Nursing*, 10(5): 643–50.

Strull, M., Bernard, L. and Gerald, C. (1984) Do patients want to participate in medical decision making? *Journal of the American Medical Association*, 252: 2990–4.

Sutherland, H.J., Llewellyn-Thomas, H.A., Lockwood, G.A., Trichler, D.L. and Till, J.E. (1989) Cancer patients, their desire for information and participation in treatment decisions. *Journal of the Royal Society of Medicine*, 83: 260–3.

Thompson, S.C., Pitts, J.S. and Schwankovsky, C. (1993) Preferences for involvement in medical decision-making: situational and demographic influences. *Patient Education and Counselling*, 22: 133–40.

Tobias, J.S. (1988) Informed consent and controlled trials. *The Lancet*, **ii**: 1194.

Trueman, I. (2001) Specialist palliative care in the UK: its future and the effects of NHS reforms. *International Journal of Palliative Nursing*, 7(4): 198–203.

Wallace, P.R. (2001) Improving palliative care through effective communication. *International Journal of Palliative Nursing*, 7(2): 86–90.

Waterworth, S. and Luker, K. (1990) Reluctant collaborators: do patients want to be involved in decisions concerning care? *Journal of Advanced Nursing*, 15: 971–6.

Welsh Office (1998) *Putting Patients First*. Cardiff: Welsh Office.

Wilkinson, S. (1991) Factors which influence how nurses communicate with cancer patients. *Journal of Advanced Nursing*, 16(6): 677–88.

Wilkinson, S., Roberts, A. and Aldridge, J. (1998) Nurse–patient communication in palliative care: an evaluation of a communication skills programme. *Palliative Medicine*, 12: 13–22.

Wilkinson, S., Bailey, K., Aldridge, J. and Roberts, A. (1999) A longitudinal evaluation of a communication skills programme. *Palliative Medicine*, 13: 341–8.

Wilkinson, S., Gambles, M. and Roberts, A. (2002) The essence of cancer care: the impact of training on nurses' ability to communicate effectively. *Journal of Advanced Nursing*, 40(6): 731.

9

Approaches to assessment in palliative care

Deborah Fitzsimmons and Sam H. Ahmedzai

With the establishment of clinical governance and evidence-based practice, there is a need and demand for relevant and rigorous assessment of the outcomes of care on the patient experience. In recent years, there has been considerable debate within the literature as to what are the most important and relevant outcomes upon which to assess patient experience in palliative care, and what are appropriate methods to assess these outcomes of care. In this chapter, we review the current perspectives of patient-based outcome assessments in palliative care and reflect critically upon their application to palliative care nursing practice.

The purpose of assessment in palliative care

Assessment of the patient and family is viewed as of central importance to the multidisciplinary management of the patient with palliative care needs. To undertake an assessment, the palliative care nurse needs to be equipped with an in-depth knowledge base of the impact of advanced illness on the patient and family, and have skills in recognizing potential and actual health needs of patients and their families. Once a thorough assessment is undertaken, the nurse, in collaboration with the multidisciplinary team, can plan and implement appropriate care. The goals or outcomes of this care provision can then be evaluated. This is often done by evaluating the impact of care on patient-based outcomes such as symptom relief and quality of life. Several fundamental concepts underpin this practice (see Box 9.1).

Assessment is the first stage of the 'nursing process', which was devised to provide a more systematic approach to the provision of nursing care (Yura and Walsh 1967). It is important to recognize, however, that assessment is not a discrete step in the provision of nursing care but a dynamic process. In palliative care, patients' health needs can change rapidly,

> **Box 9.1**   Fundamental concepts that underpin nursing assessment in palliative care
>
> - Dynamic
> - Individualized
> - Patient- and family-centred
> - Holistic
> - Therapeutic
> - Sensitive and appropriate to patient/family needs
> - Comprehensive
> - Contextual
> - Provides reliable and valid information
> - Evidence-based
> - Focused upon process and outcomes of care

requiring the nurse to be sensitive, flexible and creative, based on assessment of an individual's ongoing needs. Furthermore, nursing assessment should go beyond assessment of symptoms, functional status and other physical problems associated with terminal illness. Recognition of the complexity and differences in each individual's experience of palliative care is dependent on an assessment process that allows the wider context of patients' social, emotional, cultural and spiritual needs to be explored fully.

In defining the nursing process, the World Health Organization (1977) emphasizes the application of effective problem solving and decision making in synergy with caring activities in a systematic manner to the assessment, planning, implementation and evaluation of care. However, the nursing process does not inform the nurse about what to assess, what the aim or purpose of assessment should be, or how care should be implemented or evaluated (Schoeber 1998). Often, frameworks or models of care are used to assist the nurse to understand and interpret the purpose and nature of nursing assessment. The choice of which model to use will be influenced by a number of factors. At an individual level, this will include the needs of the individual patient and also the values and beliefs of the individual nurse making the assessment. This choice will also be shaped by broader consideration of the needs of the wider group or population of patients, the values and beliefs of the health care team, the philosophy of the care environment and the resources available (Schoeber 1998). Current research evidence and policy may also be influential in this choice.

The medical model of assessment

A medical model approach to assessment has many traditions within health care. The assessment is aimed predominantly at identifying the pathological causes of patients' problems, focusing on the signs and symptoms of disease and the impact of illness upon patient functioning. The goal of nursing assessment within this context is to make a diagnosis, usually described in terms of a particular disease state or condition.

Nursing models of assessment

Specific nursing models of care have been developed to assist understanding of the nature and complexity of nursing. Often derived from theoretical perspectives of nursing, these models of care have provided a knowledge base on ways to understand the nature of people and their health-related needs (Aggleton and Chambers 2000).

A key feature of all models is the emphasis on a structured and directed approach to assessment, although the perspectives drawn upon in undertaking the nursing assessment will vary according to the model used. In contrast to the medical model, emphasis is placed on the whole person whose state of health, rather than their disease process, requires nursing intervention (Christenson and Kenney 1995). A number of nursing models have been described in the literature and several texts and papers are devoted to this subject (see Aggleton and Chambers 2000), but it is beyond the scope of this chapter to give an in-depth critique of the usefulness of these models within palliative care. In brief, these models usually outline the methods and process of assessment but differ in the emphasis and content of the assessment, depending on the theoretical perspective taken. For example, using Roper and co-workers' (1986) Activities of Daily Living, the nurse assesses all or some of the 12 daily activities identified, working with the patient to identify individual needs.

All these models allow assessment to be approached in a systematic, problem-solving manner and provide analysis of care. Nursing models provide a focus and clarity to the nursing assessment and provide a means to understand the theoretical approach taken to nursing assessment. Such theories have made significant contributions to our understanding of the nature of nursing assessment.

There are, however, some limitations in using nursing models of assessment as a sole means to identify appropriate patient-based outcomes in palliative care. First, they are usually used by nurses for nurses – they are not widely used or known by other members of the multidisciplinary team. Crucially, patients and their carers will had little, if any, knowledge of these approaches to assessment, and much of the language (e.g. adaptation, open systems, pattern appraisal) will have little meaning to those outside the discipline of nursing. Second, because they are theoretical models, there has been limited evaluation of whether they are valid or reliable methods of undertaking nursing assessment. Third, the emphasis of assessment in this context is often on the process of care rather than the consideration of the outcomes of palliative care. There is disparity in the documentation of assessment, which precludes comparison or evaluation of care across centres, units, settings or indeed across individual nurses – the 'robustness or rigour' of such assessment approaches can be questioned. One of the criticisms of nursing has been the lack of rigour in outcome assessment or the link between the process of nursing care and its impact on relevant health outcomes (Richardson and Maynard 1997).

Assessment and evaluation in palliative care

To understand the argument for more structured approaches to nursing assessment in palliative care, there is a need to consider further what the purpose of assessment is, and to place nursing assessment in the wider context of assessment in palliative care. One of the main purposes of assessment, it is argued, is to allow identification of individual patients' needs or problems in order to set appropriate and achievable goals or outcomes. Once care is planned and implemented, we then evaluate the success or otherwise of this care – that is, how effective our care has been in meeting the intended outcomes. Within palliative care, the focus is on ensuring that these outcomes reflect the individual, are achievable and can be delivered effectively. There is an intrinsic link between what we decide are the outcomes of care and how we assess what the objectives of care should be.

Assessment and evaluation in palliative care can also be looked at from a broader perspective than the individual patient and family. Evidence of the effectiveness of interventions, treatments or services is becoming increasingly important in palliative care. To evaluate effectiveness requires the selection of what are the most important and relevant outcomes that reflect the specific objectives of the intervention or service. This allows the evaluation and development of effective and efficacious palliative care services (Hearn and Higginson 2001). They can be used to demonstrate the value of nursing interventions or services, including symptom management (Bredin *et al.* 1999), needs assessments (Morasso *et al.* 1999) and models of palliative care delivery (Edmonds *et al.* 1998; Hearn and Higginson 1998; Tierney *et al.* 1998; Goodwin *et al.* 2003).

Historically, evaluation relied for the most part on the intuition and subjective assessment of health professionals who, it was assumed, were capable of assessing the intended objectives and success of treatment (Jenkinson 1997). Much of this relied upon the clinical interview, which still remains a central aspect of the role of the health professional.

The changing context of health care delivery, such as the emergence of evidence-based practice and clinical governance, has resulted in a move away from this approach to a more scientifically rigorous approach to evaluation of new services and interventions. In terms of assessment, this has resulted in considerable interest in the development of valid and reliable assessments of patient-based outcomes, the majority of which use a structured measurement-oriented approach to patient-based outcome assessment in palliative care.

What should be assessed?

A definition of health outcomes is 'a change in patients' current and future health status that can be attributed to antecedent health care' (Donabedian 1985). Traditionally, the focus within health care has been on the assessment of objective, clinically based measures such as length of survival, toxicity from treatments and indicators of physical performance. However, in the last 25 years, there has been a move towards considering the impact of health and illness on the patient, illustrated by the considerable interest in patient-based assessment of health outcomes, including symptom relief, psychological well-being, quality of life and satisfaction with care. Within palliative care, there is increasing recognition that obtaining such information using structured assessments is of paramount importance (O'Boyle and Waldron 1997; Richards and Ramirez 1997).

What areas should be covered in a patient-based outcome assessment for use in palliative care?

There is a bewildering array of patient-based outcome assessments within the palliative care literature. One of the most confusing aspects when first encountering this area of literature is that there is no definition as to what exactly is our outcome of concern – this can be illustrated with the concept of quality of life. Although many definitions exist, there is still no definitive terminology. To some extent, this reflects the diversity of instruments and assessment systems (Fitzpatrick *et al.* 1998). Some patient-based outcome assessments will focus on one particular symptom (e.g. pain) or be very broad, focusing on general aspects of patients' health and quality of life. Assessments of, for example, subjective health, performance status, functioning and well-being, are often referred to in the literature as assessing quality of life. This has resulted in confusion and ambiguity (Muldoon *et al.* 1998), which makes it difficult for the health professional to make an informed decision on which assessment to choose. However, there is consensus in the literature that an appropriate assessment of health outcomes should, ideally, reflect the individual, multidimensional and contextual nature of patient experience.

The individual nature of patient-based outcome assessment

There are different perspectives on how health outcomes are viewed. For example, the clinician may consider health experiences from a disease perspective, the health economist from a utilitarianism perspective, and the sociologist from the gap between achievement and expectations (Fitzpatrick *et al.* 1998). However, it is worthwhile considering that what we think as health professionals is important to patients may not be the same as what patients perceive. Assessment of health outcomes is essentially a subjective assessment that is ideally made by the individuals themselves. Also, patients will attach different weights to each of the areas they feel are most important to them; for example, one patient may view having no pain as most important to their quality of life, whereas another patient (with a very similar disease state) may view being able to spend time with family and friends as most important. Studies have consistently demonstrated differences in perception between patients' and professionals' ratings of quality of life (Bernheim *et al.* 1987; Sprangers and Aaronson 1992; Marquart-Moulin *et al.* 1997; Fitzsimmons *et al.* 1999). It is generally accepted that any assessment of quality of life should be made, wherever possible, by the patient (Aaronson 1990; Fallowfield 1990; Addington-Hall and Kalra 2001; Bowling 2001). Therefore, measures of patient-based outcome assessment should share a common characteristic of summarizing the judgements people make to describe their experience of health and illness (Carr and Higginson 2001).

The multi-dimensional nature of patient-based outcome assessments

The experience of health and the impact of illness on quality of life is multidimensional – that is, it is an amalgamation of several key areas or domains of a person's life (Fallowfield 1990; Bowling 2001). Assessments of patient-based outcomes are usually divided into several broad domains (Table 9.1). Assessment instruments that purport to measure health outcomes will usually cover one or more of these domains. However, for many of these instruments, the focus has been predominantly upon disease symptoms, physical functioning and psychosocial well-being. Important domains such as economic and social status, happiness and spirituality are often not covered (Berzon 1998). This has been debated in the literature. Cohen *et al.* (1996) note that existential concerns are very important to people with life-threatening illness, but are not covered in measures of quality of life. Further work is needed to understand how spirituality can contribute to a more comprehensive assessment of health outcomes and quality of life (Efficace and Marrone 2002).

There are two important facts when considering these domains of patient-based outcomes. First, they are not discrete domains. For example, the psychological well-being of a person can have a considerable impact on their physical functioning and social well-being. Second, there is no hierarchy to these domains. A criticism of past approaches to patient-based outcome assessment in health care is that it has tended to give precedence to the domain of physical functioning and symptoms, whereas from the

Table 9.1   Common domains often covered in patient-based outcome assessments

Domain	Examples
Disease symptoms and treatment-related side-effects	Pain Fatigue Dyspnoea Appetite Nausea and vomiting Constipation
Physical functioning	Mobility Self-care activities (e.g. washing/dressing) Activities of daily living (e.g. household chores, meal preparation) Physical activity Disability
Psychological well-being	Depression Anxiety Adjustment to illness Coping Fear Self-esteem Body image Life satisfaction
Cognitive	Confusion Memory loss Concentration
Social	Personal relationships Ability to carry out hobbies and interests Sexuality Social isolation
Occupational	Work activities Financial status
Satisfaction with care	Information and communication Support from health professionals
Global assessments	Global health Global quality of life

psychosocial perspective the domains of psychological and social functioning are considered most important (Fallowfield 1990). Therefore, it is imperative that when choosing an assessment for use in palliative care, there has been careful consideration of which outcome you are most interested in assessing or best practice – which outcomes are most relevant to your patient.

The contextual nature of patient-based outcome assessments

Judgements of the outcomes of health are complex, varying not only between individuals but also within individuals depending on timing and circumstances: the issue of context is an important consideration in the assessment of health outcomes. As often seen in practice, patients with apparently similar disease, health status and prognosis may have very different perceptions of their quality of life. One of the most complex observations in patients' perception of their health and quality of life is the phenomenon of 'response shift'. The concept of response shift was initially developed by Golembiewski *et al.* (1976), who explored the measurement of change in relation to subjective assessment. Within quality of life research, Schwartz and Sprangers (1999) have considered response shift as an important mediator in a patient's adaptation to illness and consequent impact on their perception during a longitudinal assessment of changes in quality of life scores. Some studies (Breetvelt and Van Dam 1991; Wisloff *et al.* 1996) have reported that even with apparently life-threatening illness, patients report either stable quality of life throughout their illness trajectory or that their quality of life is not inferior to that of patients with less severe disease. What is lacking, however, is knowledge and understanding of the impact of terminal disease and the subsequent changes (or not) on patients' interpretation of their quality of life and health outcomes.

Recently, Carr *et al.* (2001) developed a model of quality of life in which the evaluation of health-related quality of life is determined between experiences and expectations, whereby the judgement is the gap between our expectations of health and our experience of it. This approach highlights that the relationship between symptoms and health outcomes is not simple or direct. This was observed in an earlier study (Fitzsimmons *et al.* 1999), in which a direct (linear) relationship between symptoms and quality of life in patients with pancreatic cancer was not portrayed by patients (i.e. the greater the symptomology, the greater the impact on patients' quality of life). Rather, this relationship was influenced by the success or otherwise of coping strategies that were important in shaping the impact of symptom perception on quality of life. The use of particular coping strategies themselves was context-dependent, with factors such as culture, previous illness experience and social support important in overall perception of health-related quality of life. There is evidence to suggest that, in cancer patients, factors such as perceived social support, existential issues and satisfaction with care can assume the same or greater importance as issues related to symptoms or physical functioning (Cohen *et al.* 1996; Wan *et al.* 1997; Sahey *et al.* 2000). Within palliative care, further exploration of the impact of such factors on judgement of health outcomes is required.

Areas of patient-based outcome assessments utilized in palliative care

There are several structured assessments that have been reported within the palliative care literature, and a comprehensive review is beyond the scope of this chapter. A systematic review of outcome measures used in palliative care for advanced cancer patients can be found in Hearn and Higginson (2001). For the purposes of this chapter, we will consider some of the most common assessments of symptoms, psychological morbidity, quality of life and other structured assessments specifically designed for use within palliative care.

Symptom assessment

The assessment of symptoms in palliative care has long been an integral part of nursing assessment, with increasing emphasis within the nursing literature on symptom documentation (Sitza *et al.* 1995, Williams *et al.* 2001). There has been a move towards the development of more structured approaches to symptom assessment. Three of the most popular instruments cited in palliative care literature are the Rotterdam Symptom Checklist (de Haes *et al.* 1990), the Edmonton Symptom Assessment Schedule (Bruera *et al.* 1991) and the Symptom Distress Scale (McCorkle and Young 1978). These offer different approaches to structured assessment. The Rotterdam Symptom Checklist is a 38-item scale designed for patient self-completion, which measures physical and psychological symptoms using a 4-point Likert scale. Initially developed for cancer patients, its use in more advanced disease has been queried. The Edmonton Symptom Assessment Schedule comprises nine visual analogue scales on which patients rate symptoms along a 100-mm line. Further work on its validity and reliability is required (Hearn and Higginson 2001). The Symptom Distress Scale was developed for cancer and heart disease. It is self-administered using a 5-point Likert scale to assess 13 global symptoms. A comprehensive review of symptom assessment in palliative care is provided by Roberts and Bird (2001).

Although it is well established that assessment of symptoms is important, what is ambiguous in the literature is the definition of what a symptom is and what the best approach to assessment is. Symptom assessment is often concerned with the completion of checklists where the prevalence of each particular symptom is recorded, with some having been developed for patient self-completion. However, many of the approaches purported to assess symptoms have been designed for completion by the clinician. One of the other limitations of current approaches to symptom assessment is that they neglect the subjective nature of symptom perception or the disruption brought to daily life. This has been illustrated by work on the symptoms of fatigue (Krishnasamy 2000) and dyspnoea (O'Driscoll *et al.* 1999), which demonstrates the subjective interpretation of symptom experience and the variance in how patients cope with symptoms on a daily basis. Also, much work has assessed symptoms at discrete points in time rather than looking at the cumulative effects of symptoms and treatments on all aspects of a person's life. This may be especially relevant for the patient with palliative care needs. The interplay between different symptoms has been identified as important in shaping experience (Richardson and Ream 1997). For example, a patient who has nausea and vomiting may also experience loss of appetite, taste changes, fatigue, weight loss and muscle weakness; their ability to function may also be affected, such as their ability to carry out daily activities. This may also have an indirect impact on other aspects such as social functioning, self-esteem and satisfaction with life and, consequently, may impact on patients' experiences.

Psychological morbidity

The assessment of psychological morbidity in palliative care has been developed from traditional approaches used in general psychiatry. Three main assessment approaches are used: a directed interview approach; single questions using a categorical or linear analogue scale; or structured instruments. Regarding structured instruments, a systematic review of depression in advanced disease identified the most common instrument used to be the Hospital Anxiety and Depression Scale (Zigmond and Snaith 1983; Hotopf *et al.* 2002). This instrument, which has been used widely in many fields of health care, consists of 14 questions relating to traits of anxiety and depression. The validity and reliability of this instrument is well established and it can be used in screening for anxiety and depression in the community (Kramer 1999). However, its performance in advanced disease has been questioned in in-patients (Urch *et al.* 1998).

Fairly recently, the Edinburgh Depression Scale, originally developed to assess post-natal depression, has been used with reasonable success (Lloyd Williams *et al.* 2001). Cognitive impairment is purported to be an area of concern in palliative care, but this poses some specific difficulties due to the complexity of reasons for cognitive impairment; for example, is it due to the disease process itself or a consequence of treatment or medication? The problems have been illustrated by Greilish (2000) when critiquing a commonly used instrument, the Mini-Mental State Questionnaire. Although this has shown good reliability and validity, its limitations are perceived to be a loss of dignity and lack of consideration of pre-morbid ability and intelligence. Radbruch *et al.* (2000) warn of the problem of cognitive impairment in patients with advanced illness, and suggest that assessments should be in the form of a simple categorical scale or where possible be administered by an interviewer. Common to all assessments is the need for further evaluation of their use in palliative care patients, and the impact of cognitive impairment on completion.

▌Quality of life

A number of different approaches to the measurement of (health-related) quality of life exist, ranging from generic measures of health through to the use of a single index of quality of life (see Table 9.2). All have their advantages and disadvantages when used in palliative care.

Several studies have compared quality of life measures for use in palliative care. These include a comparison of the McGill Quality of Life Questionnaire and Patient Evaluated Problem Scores (PEPS)

Table 9.2 Selection of types of quality of life instruments available

Type of quality of life instrument	Examples	Advantages	Disadvantages
Generic	SF-36 (Ware *et al.* 1993)	• Used across a broad range of populations • Allows cross-study comparisons • Widely tested for validity and reliability • Normative data often available • Used widely • Short version often available	• Lack of specificity • Lack of responsiveness to changes over time • Emphasis on functional status
Disease-specific (e.g. cancer)	EORTC QLQ-C30 (Aaronson *et al.* 1993)	• Covers important issues for particular disease • Responsive to changes over time • Relevant to patient • Used in clinical trials	• Lack of cross-study comparisons • Lack of normative data • Emphasis on symptoms and functioning
Dimension-specific	McGill Pain Questionnaire (Melzack 1975) HADS (Zigmond and Snaith 1983)	• Detailed coverage of domain of interest • Used across a range of patient populations • Cross-study comparison • Used as screening tools	• Not primarily designed as outcome measures • Does not capture multidimensional aspect of quality of life
Individual	SEIQOL (O'Boyle *et al.* 1993)	• Captures individual perception • Content validity • Responsive to changes in individuals across time	• Trained interviewer administered • Not tested in many patient populations • Validity and reliability requires further assessment

(Pratheepawanit *et al.* 1999), the Missoula-Vitas quality of life index (Byock and Merriman 1998), a review of selected measures compared to problems recorded in patients' medical records (Stromgren *et al.* 2002) and the use of single question assessments (Edwards *et al.* 1997). Bibliographic reviews of quality of life assessments in palliative care are available (e.g. Donnelly 2000; Massaro 2000), with a systematic review currently in progress (Paz *et al.* 2003). These have all highlighted the variety and disparity in approaches taken to quality of life assessment, with no 'gold standard' approach. Two of the most common assessment methods cited in the palliative care literature are the European Organization for Research and Treatment of Cancer QLQ-C30 (Aaronson *et al.* 1993) and the McGill Quality of Life Questionnaire (Cohen *et al.* 1997). The QLQ-C30 comprises a 30-item questionnaire with a number of scales and single items that assess symptoms, functioning and global health/quality of life. This core questionnaire can be supplemented with other disease-specific assessments. It is now the most established quality of life assessment in cancer patients; however, its use needs further evaluation, with difficulties seen in trying to adapt it for use in palliative care. The McGill Quality of Life Questionnaire was developed in advanced cancer populations and measures overall quality of life. An existential domain is incorporated alongside symptoms, physical and psychological well-being and support.

An individualized assessment of quality of life has been developed for use in palliative care. The Schedule for Evaluation of Individual Quality of Life uses a psychological approach to quality of life, which allows patients to weight the most important areas of life to them. It has been shown to be appropriate for use in palliative care populations (Hickey *et al.* 1996), although it has been criticized for being too long and difficult for patients to complete (Ahmedzai *et al.* 1994).

Satisfaction with care

Evaluation of patient and carer satisfaction with care has been used widely within palliative care, with national studies undertaken to assess patients' satisfaction (e.g. Department of Health 2002). In a recent review of the literature, Aspinal *et al.* (2003) identified 56 relevant studies purporting to assess satisfaction with palliative care. Assessment methods include qualitative interviews (e.g. McLoughlin 2002), 'one-off' questionnaires that have been used specifically for particular studies or audits, and specifically designed measures that have been validated for use in several palliative care populations (e.g. FAMCARE; Ringdal *et al.* 2003). Several systematic reviews of a variety of palliative care services (specialist palliative care teams: Hearn and Higginson 1998; Higginson *et al.* 2003; specialist models of palliative care: Wilkinson *et al.* 1999; general practitioner models of palliative care: Mitchell 2002) have demonstrated the importance of patient and carer satisfaction as key outcome measures for demonstrating the effectiveness of palliative care services.

In their review, Aspinal *et al.* (2003) highlight the methodological and practical limitations of assessing satisfaction within the context of palliative care. Such measures may not truly reflect the perspectives of patients and carers. In parallel with many outcome measures in palliative care, there is a lack of theoretical underpinning of what 'satisfaction' means to the patient and family with palliative care needs. The disparity in definitions has resulted in a number of approaches to its assessment, limiting our ability to make meaningful comparisons between different studies of palliative care. The potential bias of proxy assessments of satisfaction and undertaking retrospective assessments of satisfaction have been highlighted. In their review, Aspinal *et al.* (2003) identify the consensus that provision of information, staff competence and pain control are important for satisfaction. However, the influence of other factors, such as symptom perception, psychological morbidity and social support, has been largely overlooked in satisfaction measurement, together with the impact of other variables such as age, ethnicity and geographical access to palliative care services. Further work is needed to provide a better understanding of the concept of satisfaction and the most appropriate methods of assessment in relation to palliative care.

Other outcome assessments used in palliative care

Specific instruments have been developed for use within palliative care that incorporate a combination of appropriate outcomes, such as symptoms, quality of life and quality of care. The Support Team Assessment Schedule (Higginson and McCarthy 1993) was developed to assess the effectiveness of palliative care on patients' lives using a 5-point Likert scale. However, professionals rather than patients usually complete this instrument. The Palliative Outcome Scale (Hearn and Higginson 1999) was designed to be a core measure of health outcomes in palliative care. It has shown adequate validity and reliability and is currently being evaluated and used in a number of studies.

Is there a need for specific patient-based outcome assessment to evaluate nursing care?

An interesting area for debate is whether current patient-based outcome assessments are appropriate and relevant in the evaluation of nursing care. Relatively little recent work on the development of patient-based outcome assessments has been undertaken from a nursing perspective. However, earlier work highlighted the possible relationship between quality of nursing care and its impact on patients' evaluation of quality of life (Glaus 1993).

With the focus on evaluation of advanced practice and specialist roles and models of care delivery, it is imperative that evaluation of these should use assessment measures that reflect the 'true' impact of nursing care on health outcomes for patients. Unfortunately, it is difficult to define concisely what this value is (Annells and Koch 2001). Corner *et al.* (2002) argue that despite a major expansion in specialist nursing posts, little is known about the impact of these services and little consideration has been given to how their effectiveness might be assessed. One limitation of current outcome measures, in particular those for patient satisfaction and quality of life, is findings that are not easily linked to service development needs. There is a need for further work on how best to capture the impact of nursing care on health outcome. Here, broad areas of health outcomes, such as symptom experience, self-management, coping, enhancing independence and quality of life, may be the most relevant.

Choosing an appropriate patient-based outcome assessment for use in palliative care

The choice of which assessment approach to use will be determined primarily by which aspect of the patient experience is to be assessed. This appears logical, but in much of the literature there is no consideration of whether the measure selected reflects the actual outcome of choice. For example, Gill and Feinstein (1994), in a review focusing on the use of quality of life instruments, found that only 11 per cent of studies included a satisfactory definition of the outcome they were purporting to measure and provided justification as to the choice of instrument selected. Within palliative care, outcome measures require the measurement of aspects that reflect the specific goals of palliative care (Hearn and Higginson 2001). These may focus on a particular aspect such as symptom palliation, improving psychological morbidity, quality of care and quality of life, or a combination of these outcomes.

The rationale for which instrument to use should be based on evidence of its scientific rigour rather than its purported popularity, or an 'anything goes' attitude. It should not be assumed that an instrument used in one context (for example, as an outcome measure in a clinical trial) can be used directly in another (for example, in clinical audit). It is imperative that in selecting a suitable outcome measure, the health professional considers carefully the properties of the instrument. Much of this consideration will relate to assessment of the appropriateness, reliability and validity of the instrument. This information is usually derived from (ideally systematic) reviews or by undertaking and reviewing previous studies in which the instrument has been used. Many of the more established outcome measures will have key papers written about them that outline their development and provide evidence of their validity and reliability. Several reviews and texts (see Hearn and Higginson 1997; Fitzpatrick *et al.* 1998; Muldoon *et al.* 1998; Bowling

2001; Kaasa and Loge 2002; Robinson *et al.* 2003) explore the criteria for selecting a patient-based outcome assessment. A summary of these criteria is provided in Box 9.2.

Box 9.2 Criteria for selecting a patient-based outcome assessment

- Is the content appropriate for use in your particular palliative care setting (consider patient population and setting)?
- Does the content reflect (address) the particular areas of health outcomes that you are interested in assessing?
- Does the instrument reflect (address) the most relevant areas of health outcomes for the patient?
- Has the assessment been specifically designed or adapted for use in palliative care?
- Is there evidence of the reliability (i.e. ability to produce results that are reproducible and internally consistent) of the assessment within a palliative care population/setting?
- Is there evidence of the validity (i.e. ability to assess what it purports to assess) of the assessment?
- Can the assessment detect changes over time (i.e. responsiveness) – is there evidence of appropriate time-frames for assessment in palliative care?
- Is the assessment easy to score, analyse and interpret?
- Is the assessment easy to administer?
- Can the assessment be used with proxies?

Who should assess the experience of palliative care?

As already discussed, ideally an individual should assess their own experience. However, within the context of palliative care, it is sometimes difficult to obtain the perspective of the patient. In such circumstances, the logical consequence would be to obtain a proxy assessment. The methodological and practical difficulties of this have been discussed widely in the literature. In summarizing the evidence, Addington-Hall and Kalra (2001) report that the advantages of proxy responders (e.g. care-givers or health professionals) include moderate agreement usually between patients and proxies and proxies are almost as good at detecting changes over time, and can provide useful information on the more concrete, observable aspects of quality of life. The disadvantages reported include the overestimation of some aspects of quality of life and the changing priorities of patients over time. For example, Horton (2002) found that although there was good agreement between nurses and patients with advanced cancer with respect to symptom control and pain, there were important differences in anxiety scores, personal thoughts, practical matters and information received. In comparing scores from the Edmonton Symptom Assessment System, Nekolaichuk *et al.*

(1999) observed that, even over time, there were still differences between health professionals' and patients' scores of symptom intensity. The importance of understanding the context of patients' experiences should be acknowledged when interpreting the results of such assessments.

Also of crucial importance to assessment in palliative care are the needs of care-givers. It is becoming increasingly clear that decisions regarding care should be based on evaluation of patient outcome in the context of the effects upon those around them (Sulch and Kalra 2003). Many of the assessments developed focus on the burden placed on care-givers.

The clinical application of structured assessments of patient-based outcomes in palliative care

Despite the interest in developing structured patient-based outcome assessments for use in palliative care, there is relatively little evidence at present for their use in clinical practice. To date, most of the focus has been on the use of these assessment methods as part of research studies, predominantly clinical trials, which evaluate the effectiveness of new drug therapies such as chemotherapeutic agents in patients with advanced cancer. It is now widely agreed that in the assessment of any new therapeutic agent for use in palliative care populations, quality of life assessment must be an end-point of concern (Kaasa and Loge 2002).

Assessment of patient-based outcomes has also been used in the evaluation of new models of care or service provision in palliative care. Goodwin *et al.* (2003) examined the effectiveness of day care using the McGill Quality of Life Questionnaire and Palliative Outcomes Scale, with no differences in day care and routine services being reported. However, the authors suggest that this failure to detect any significant differences was in part related to the insensitivity of the instruments. In a systematic review of the effectiveness of specialist care within palliative care, Hearn and Higginson (1998) illustrated the popularity of health outcome assessments but also the heterogeneity and breadth of such assessments, including symptom control, patient and family satisfaction with care, place of death, psychosocial well-being and quality of life. This makes it difficult to provide any definitive answer to whether specialist care improves the patient experience. There is a need for consistency in the way assessments are used so that studies can be rigorously compared in the future. It should also be acknowledged that much previous work within palliative care has been weighted towards advanced cancer; further consideration of the experiences of patients with non-malignant diseases is urgently required.

In terms of clinical practice, there has been little exploration of the use of these assessments in health care in general. Higginson and Carr (2001) suggest eight potential uses of quality of life measures in routine clinical practice, including a role in screening for potential problems, clinical decision making, monitoring the response to treatment and clinical audit.

However, there are a number of aspects to patient-based outcome assessment that need to be overcome (Kaasa and Loge 2002). A summary of current methodological difficulties is provided in Box 9.3. One of the main practical difficulties, discussed by Higginson and Carr (2001), is that many of these assessments were primarily designed to evaluate groups or populations of patients; therefore, difficulties are encountered when trying to explain what the significance of any changes mean to the individual patient and family. For many of these assessments, analysis and interpretation of findings relies on understanding fairly complex statistics. Furthermore, how these assessments can be integrated into routine practice and audit needs to be examined. Of great importance is appropriate training in the use of such assessment methods.

The ethical dilemmas surrounding the use of these assessments require careful consideration. One of the main areas for debate is in claiming that we can measure, for example, quality of life, from which can be inferred that we can make a definite impact on patients' quality of life, where as many areas that are important in patients' evaluation of quality of life may be outside the remit of health care (Feinstein 1992). Higginson and Carr (2001) highlight that trying to measure aspects such as quality of life has 'over-medicalized' these aspects of patients' lives. This creates a paradox, as the original intention of many of the authors of these assessments was primarily to develop a way of incorporating the holistic aspects of patients' experiences into the evaluation of health care and, therefore, to move away from the traditional medical model approach. Clearly, much work is needed on the potential uses of assessments in routine practice.

Box 9.3 Summary of current dilemmas in patient-based outcome assessment in palliative care

- Lack of agreement on which aspects of health outcomes are most relevant in palliative care
- Disparity in assessments used
- Lack of evaluation of assessments developed for use in other populations
- Current assessment not appropriate for palliative care populations (e.g. too long, irrelevant items, time between assessments too long)
- Drop out of patients and missing data
- Assessments focusing upon negative attributes of health rather than positive benefits of palliative care
- Failure to capture individual patient perception
- Complexity in completing assessments
- Concerns about the value of proxy assessments
- Focus on symptoms and functioning – lack of consideration of other aspects such as spirituality, quality of care
- Appropriate methods to score, analyse and interpret data from assessments

Conclusions

Undertaking assessment is common to all health care professionals in palliative care. Within nursing, this has traditionally centred on systematic but largely unstructured approaches, often incorporating a nursing model of care. Structured assessments of patient-based outcomes have an important role in the evaluation of palliative care. However, further research is needed in this area to address some of the limitations of current assessments and how they can be used in practice. In particular, for evaluating the effectiveness of nursing care, there is a need to consider further what the outcomes of our care are for patients and their families and to develop or adapt existing approaches to assessments that are able to address these areas of concern, from both a patient and family perspective. Developing appropriate assessments that are valid and reliable but which also provide clinically useful information is crucial to ensuring that the evaluation of our care is based on relevant and rigorous evidence.

References

Aaronson, N.K. (1990) Quality of life research in cancer clinical trials: a need for common rules language. *Oncology*, 4: 59–66.

Aaronson, N.K., Ahmedzai, S., Bergman, B. *et al.* (1993) The European Organisation for Research and Treatment of Cancer QLQ-C30: a quality of life instrument for use in international clinical trials in oncology. *Journal of the National Cancer Institute*, 85: 365–76.

Addington-Hall, J. and Kalra, L. (2001) Who should measure quality of life? *British Medical Journal*, 322: 1417–20.

Aggleton, P. and Chalmers, H. (2000) *Nursing Models and Nursing Practice*, 2nd edn. London: Macmillan.

Ahmedzai, S.H., Arrasas, J.I., Eisemann, M. *et al.* (1994) Development of an appropriate quality of life measure for palliative care, *Quality of Life Research*, 3: 57–64.

Annells, M. and Koch, T. (2001) 'The real stuff': implications for nursing of assessing and measuring a terminally ill person's quality of life. *Journal of Clinical Nursing*, 10: 806–12.

Aspinal, F., Addington-Hall, J., Hughes, R. *et al.* (2003) Using satisfaction to measure the quality of palliative care: a review of the literature. *Journal of Advanced Nursing*, 42(4): 324–39.

Bernheim, J.L., Ledure, G., Souris, M. and Razavi, D. (1987) Differences in perception of disease and treatment between cancer patients and their physicians, in N.K. Aaronson and J. Beckham (eds) *The Quality of Life of Cancer Patients*. New York: Raven Press.

Berzon, R.A. (1998) Understanding and using health-related quality of life instruments within clinical research studies, in M.J. Staquet, R.D. Hays and P.M. Fayers (eds) *Quality of Life Assessment in Clinical Trials: Methods and Practice*. Oxford: Oxford Medical.

Bowling, A. (2001) *Measuring Disease*, 2nd edn. Buckingham: Open University Press.

Bredin, M., Corner, J., Krishnasamy, M. *et al.* (1999) Multicentre randomised controlled trial of nursing intervention for breathlessness in patients with lung cancer. *British Medical Journal*, 318: 901–4.

Breetvelt, I.S. and Van Dam, F.S.A.M. (1991) Underreporting by cancer patients: the case of response shift. *Social Science and Medicine*, 32: 981–7.

Bruera, E., Kuehn, N., Miller, M. *et al.* (1991) The Edmonton Symptom Assessment System (ESAS): a simple method for assessment of palliative care patients. *Journal of Palliative Care*, 7(2): 6–9.

Byock, I.R. and Merriman, M.P. (1998) Measuring quality of life for patients with terminal illness: the Missoula-VITAS quality of life index. *Palliative Medicine*, 12: 231–44.

Carr, A.J. and Higginson, I.J. (2001) Are quality of life measures patient centred? *British Medical Journal*, 322: 1357–60.

Carr, A.J., Gibson, B. and Robinson, P.G. (2001) Measuring quality of life: is quality of life determined by expectations or experience? *British Medical Journal*, 322: 1240–3.

Christenson, P. and Kenney, J. (1995) *Nursing Process: Application of Conceptual Models*, 4th edn. St Louis, MO: C.V. Mosby.

Cohen, S.R., Mount, B.M., Tomas, J.J. *et al.* (1996) Existential well being is an important determinant of quality of life: evidence from the McGill quality of life questionnaire. *Cancer*, 77: 576–86.

Cohen, S.R., Mount, B.M., Bruera, E. *et al.* (1997) Validity of the McGill Quality of Life Questionnaire in the palliative care setting: a multi-centre Canadian study demonstrating the importance of the existential domain. *Palliative Medicine*, 11: 3–20.

Corner, J., Clark, D. and Normand, C. (2002) Evaluating the work of clinical nurse specialists in palliative care. *Palliative Medicine*, 16: 275–7.

de Haes, J.C.J.M., van Knippenberg, F.C. and Neijt, J.P. (1990) Measuring psychological and physical distress in cancer patients: structure and application of the Rotterdam Symptom Checklist. *British Journal of Cancer*, 62: 1034–8.

Department of Health (2002) *National Survey of NHS Patients Cancer National Overview 1999/2000*. London: The Stationery Office.

Donabedian, A. (1985) *Explorations in Quality Assessment and Monitoring*. Ann Arbor, MI: Health Administration Press.

Donnelly, S. (2000) Quality of life assessment in advanced cancer. *Current Oncology Reports*, 2(4): 338–42.

Edmonds, P.M., Stuttaford, J.M., Penny, J. *et al.* (1998) Do hospital palliative care teams improve symptom control? Use of a modified STAS as an evaluation tool. *Palliative Medicine*, 13: 345–51.

Edwards, A., Livingstone, H. and Daley, A. (1997) Single-question assessment of quality of life. *Palliative Medicine*, 11(4): 325–6.

Efficace, F. and Marrone, R. (2002) Spiritual issues and quality of life assessment in cancer care. *Death Studies*, 26: 743–56.

Fallowfield, L. (1990) *The Quality of Life: The Missing Measurement in Health Care*. London: Souvenir Press.

Feinstein, A.R. (1992) Benefits and obstacles for development of health status assessment measures in clinical settings. *Medical Care*, 30(suppl.): 50.

Fitzpatrick, R., Davey, C., Buxton, M.J. and Jones, D.R. (1998) Evaluating patient-based outcome measures for use in clinical trials. *Health Technology Assessment*, 2: 14.

Fitzsimmons, D., George, S., Payne, S.A. *et al.* (1999) Quality of life in pancreatic cancer: differences in perception between health professionals and patients. *Psycho-Oncology*, 35: 939–41.

Gill, T.M. and Feinstein, A.R. (1994) A critical appraisal of quality of life measurements. *Journal of the American Medical Association*, 272: 619–26.

Glaus, A. (1993) Quality of life – a measure of the quality of nursing care? *Support Care Cancer*, 1: 119–23.

Golembiewski, R.T., Billingsley, K. and Yeager, S. (1976) Measuring change and persistence in human affairs: types of change generated by OD designs. *Journal of Applied Behavioural Sciences*, 12: 133–57.

Goodwin, D.M., Higginson, I., Myers, K., Douglas, H.R. and Normand, C.E. (2003) Effectiveness of palliative day care in improving pain, symptom control and quality of life. *Journal of Pain and Symptom Management*, 25: 202–12.

Grealish, L. (2000) Mini-mental state questionnaire: problems with its use in palliative care. *International Journal of Palliative Nursing*, 6: 288–302.

Hearn, J. and Higginson, I.J. (1997) Outcome measures in palliative care for advanced cancer patients: a review. *Journal of Public Health Medicine*, 19: 193–9.

Hearn, J. and Higginson, I.J. (1998) Do specialist palliative care teams improve outcomes for cancer patients? A systematic literature review. *Palliative Medicine*, 12(5): 317–32.

Hearn, J. and Higginson, I.J. (2001) Outcome measures in palliative care for advanced cancer patients: a review, in D. Field, D. Clark, J. Corner and C. Davis (eds) *Researching Palliative Care*. Buckingham: Open University Press.

Hearn, J. and Higginson, I.J. (on behalf of the Palliative Care Core Audit Project Advisory Group) (1999). Development and validation of a core outcome measure for palliative care: the palliative care outcome scale. *Quality in Health Care*, 8(4): 219–27.

Hickey, A., Bury, G., O'Boyle, C.A. *et al.* (1996) A new short form individual quality of life measure (SEIQOL-DW): application in a cohort of individuals with HIV/AIDS. *British Medical Journal*, 313: 29–33.

Higginson, I.J. and Carr, A.J. (2001) Measuring quality of life: using quality of life measures in the clinical setting. *British Medical Journal*, 322: 1297–300.

Higginson, I.J. and McCarthy, M. (1993) Validity of the support team assessment schedule: do staff ratings reflect those made by patients or their families. *Palliative Medicine*, 7: 219–28.

Higginson, I.J., Finlay, I.G. and Goodwin, D.M. (2003) Is there evidence that palliative care teams alter end-of-life experiences of patients and their caregivers? *Journal of Pain and Symptom Management*, 25(2): 150–68.

Horton, R. (2002) Differences in assessment of symptoms and quality of life between patients with advanced cancer and their specialist palliative care nurses in a home care setting. *Palliative Medicine*, 16: 488–94.

Hotopf, M., Chidgey, J., Addington-Hall, J. and Lan, L.K. (2002) Depression in advanced disease: a systematic review. Part 1: Prevalence and case findings. *Palliative Medicine*, 16(2): 81–97.

Jenkinson, C. (1997) Assessment and evaluation of health and medical care: an introduction and overview, in C. Jenkinson (ed.) *Assessment and Evaluation of Health and Medical Care: A Methods Text*. Buckingham: Open University Press.

Kaasa, S. and Loge, J.H. (2002) Quality-of-life assessment in palliative care. *Lancet Oncology*, 3: 175–82.

Kramer, J.A. (1999) Use of the Hospital Anxiety and Depression Scale in the assessment of depression in patients with inoperable lung cancer. *Palliative Medicine*, 13: 353–4.

Krishnasamy, M. (2000) Fatigue in advanced cancer – meaning before measurement? *International Journal of Nursing Studies*, 37: 401–14.

Lloyd-Williams, M., Friedman, T. and Rudd, N. (2001) An analysis of the validity of the Hospital Anxiety and Depression Scale as a screening tool in patients with advanced metastatic cancer. *Journal of Pain and Symptom Management*, 22: 990–6.

Marquart-Moulin, G., Viens, P., Bouscary, M.L. *et al.* (1997) Discordance between physicians' estimations and breast cancer patients' self-assessment of side-effects of chemotherapy: an issue for quality of care. *British Journal of Cancer*, 76: 1640–5.

Massaro, T. (2000) Instruments for assessing quality of life in palliative care settings. *Journal of Palliative Nursing*, 6(9): 429–33.

McCorkle, R. and Young, K. (1978) Development of a symptom distress scale. *Cancer Nursing*, 1: 373–8.

McLoughlin, P.A. (2002) Community specialist palliative care: experiences of patients and carers. *International Journal of Palliative Nursing*, 8(7): 344–53.

Melzack, R. (1975) The McGill pain questionnaire: major properties and scoring methods. *Pain*, 1: 277–99.

Mitchell, G.K. (2002) How well do general practitioners deliver palliative care? A systematic review. *Palliative Medicine*, 16(6): 457–64.

Morasso, G., Capelli, M., Viterbori, P. *et al.* (1999) Psychological and symptom distress in terminal cancer patients with met and unmet needs. *Journal of Pain and Symptom Management*, 17: 402–9.

Muldoon, M.F., Barger, S.D., Flory, J.D. and Manuck, S.B. (1998) What are quality of life measurements measuring? *British Medical Journal*, 316: 542–5.

Nekolaichuk, C.L., Bruera, E., Spachynski, K. *et al.* (1999) A comparison of patient and proxy symptom assessments in advanced cancer patients. *Palliative Medicine*, 13(4): 311–23.

O'Boyle, C.A. and Waldron, D. (1997) Quality of life issues in palliative medicine. *Journal of Neurology*, 244: S18–S25.

O'Boyle, C.A., McGee, H.M., Hickey, A. *et al.* (1993) *The Schedule for the Evaluation of Individual Quality of Life (SEIQoL): Administration Manual.* Dublin: Royal College of Surgeons in Ireland.

O'Driscoll, M., Corner, J. and Bailey, C. (1999) The experience of breathlessness in lung cancer. *European Journal of Cancer Care*, 8: 37–43.

Paz, S., Fitzsimmons, D., Hendry, F. *et al.* (on behalf of the Association for Palliative Medicine) (2003). Measuring quality of life in palliative care: a systematic review. Communication to the *European Association of Palliative Care Conference*, The Netherlands, April.

Pratheepawanit, N., Salek, M.S. and Finlay, I.G. (1999) The applicability of quality-of-life assessment in palliative care: comparing two quality-of-life measures. *Palliative Medicine*, 13: 325–34.

Radbruch, L., Sabatowski, R., Loick, G. *et al.* (2000) Cognitive impairment and its influence on pain and symptom assessment in a palliative care unit: development of a minimal documentation system. *Palliative Medicine*, 14: 266–76.

Richards, M.A. and Ramirez, A.J. (1997) Quality of life: the main outcome measure of palliative care. *Palliative Medicine*, 11(2): 89–92.

Richardson, A. and Ream, E.K. (1997) Self-care behaviours initiated by chemotherapy patients in response to fatigue. *International Journal of Nursing Studies*, 34: 35–43.

Richardson, G. and Maynard, A. (1997) *Fewer Doctors? More Nurses? A Review of the Knowledge Base of Nurse–Doctor Substitution*. Report 135. York: University of York.

Ringdal, G.I., Jordroy, M.S. and Kaasa, S. (2003) Measuring quality of palliative care: psychometric properties of the FAMCARE scale. *Quality of Life Research*, 12(2): 167–76.

Roberts, A. and Bird, A. (2001) Assessment of symptoms, in S. Kinghorn and R. Gamlin (eds) *Palliative Nursing Bringing Comfort and Hope*. London: Ballière Tindall.

Robinson, P.G., Carr, A.J. and Higginson, I.J. (2003) How to choose a quality of life measure, in A.J. Carr, I.J. Higginson and P.G. Robinson (eds) *Quality of Life*. London: British Medical Journal Books.

Roper, N., Logan, W. and Tierney, A. (1986) *The Elements of Nursing*, 4th edn. London: Churchill Livingstone.

Sahey, T.B., Gray, R.E. and Fitch, M. (2000) A qualitative study of patient perspectives on colorectal cancer. *Cancer Practice*, 8: 38–44.

Schoeber, J. (1998) Nursing: issues for effective practice, in S. Hinchliff, S. Norman and J. Schoeber (eds) *Nursing Practice and Health Care: A Foundation Text*, 3rd edn. London: Arnold.

Schwartz, C.E. and Sprangers, M.A.G. (1999) Methodological approaches for assessing response shift in longitudinal health-related quality of life research. *Social Science and Medicine*, 48: 1531–48.

Sitza, J., Hughes, J. and Sobrido, L. (1995) A study of patients' experiences of side-effects associated with chemotherapy: pilot stage report. *International Journal of Nursing Studies*, 32: 580–600.

Sprangers, M.A. and Aaronson, N.K. (1992) The role of health care providers and significant others in evaluating the quality of life of patients with chronic disease: a review. *Journal of Clinical Epidemiology*, 45: 743–60.

Stromgren, A.S., Groenvold, M., Pedersen, L., Olsen, A.K. and Sjogren, P. (2002) Symptomatology of cancer patients in palliative care: content validation of self-assessment questionnaires against medical records. *European Journal of Cancer*, 38: 788–94.

Sulch, D. and Kalra, L. (2003) Quality of life in caregivers, in A.J. Carr, I.J. Higginson and P.G. Robinson (eds) *Quality of Life*. London: British Medical Journal Books.

Tierney, R.M., Horton, S.M., Hannan, T.J. *et al.* (1998) Relationships between symptom relief, quality of life and satisfaction with hospice care. *Palliative Medicine*, 12(5): 333–44.

Urch, C.E., Chamberlain, J. and Field, G. (1998) The drawback of the Hospital Anxiety and Depression Scale in the assessment of depression in hospice in-patients. *Palliative Medicine*, 12: 395–96.

Wan, G.J., Counte, M.A. and Cella, D.F. (1997) The influence of personal expectations on cancer patients' reports on health-related quality of life. *Psycho-Oncology*, 6: 1–11.

Ware, J.E., Snow, K., Kosinski, M. and Gandek, B. (1993) *Health Survey: Manual and Interpretation Guide*. Boston, MA: Medical Outcomes Trust.

Wilkinson, E.K., Salisbury, C. and Bosanquet, N. (1999) Patient and carer preference for, and satisfaction with, specialist models of palliative care: a systematic literature review. *Palliative Medicine*, 13(3): 197–216.

Williams, P.D., Ducey, K.A., Sears, A.M. *et al.* (2001) Treatment type and symptom severity among oncology patients by self-report. *International Journal Nursing Studies*, 38: 359–67.

Wisloff, F., Eika, S., Hippe, E. *et al.* (1996) Measurement of health-related quality of life in multiple myeloma. *British Journal of Haematology*, 92: 604–13.

World Health Organization (1977) *The Nursing Process Report on the First Meeting of a Technical Advisory Group*. Geneva: WHO.

Yura, H. and Walsh, M. (1967) *The Nursing Process*. Norwalk, NJ: Appleton-Century-Crofts.

Zigmond, A. and Snaith, R.P. (1983) The hospital anxiety and depression scale. *Acta Psychiatrica Scandinavica*, 67: 361–70.

PART TWO

Transitions into the terminal phase

10

Overview

Jane Seymour and Christine Ingleton

Death is both a fact of life and a mystery: we cannot report back once we have gone through the process of dying; we cannot evaluate the care that we were given or suggest ways in which it might have been done better. Although dying is regarded as one of the most critical stages of life, the quality of the experience of dying very largely depends upon others. At a societal level, value is placed on a humane approach to dying: there is a desire to serve people well when they die, in ways that protect their dignity and give comfort to them and their companions when they most need it. However, the way in which these aims are achieved has been radically transformed over the last century. Until the fairly recent past, death was something that took place at home within the family. There may not have been much that could be done to relieve physical suffering, but people knew how to manage death and how to behave around a dying person, who was embraced as part of the family unit and ministered to by relatives, friends and loved ones. A religious leader may have been called, and perhaps a doctor, but they would not be central figures in this scene (Ariès 1981). Moreover, death was a frequent visitor across the generations, not something that tends to happen primarily to older people as in modern society. Nowadays, in spite of efforts to the contrary, death at home is less common than institutional death. Even when death does occur at home, it tends to be overseen by technical and clinical 'experts'. Modern dying has some particular features that can make caring for dying people difficult:

- Clinical technologies and the potential of new treatments to offset death have made a diagnosis of dying difficult and the process of dying much longer than it used to be. Not recognizing imminent death means that some people die in pain and distress which could otherwise be relieved.

- Clinical training in the twentieth century has tended to encourage the view that death is a failure and has, to some extent, prioritized bodily or physical care rather than spiritual, social or family care, which may be just as or even more important to the dying person.

- The management of modern dying is fraught with ethical difficulties: poor understanding of ethics and law at the end of life can make good care at the end of life difficult to achieve.

Hospice and palliative care has, it might be argued, become synonymous with 'good death'. As Clark and Seymour (1999) note, this concept stands now not only as a 'symbolic critique' (McNamara 1997: 3) of medicalized, institutionalized death, but also as a central point of reference for popular expectations of dying and of standards of care at the time of death. These are, however, expectations that remain unfulfilled for the vast majority of the dying population across the world. Of the 54 million deaths that occur annually, 46 million take place in the low- and middle-income countries of the world (Singer 2000), meaning that there are fundamental inequalities in state-provided health and social care that the dying receive and in the resources that their family carers are able to mobilize in delivering care to them. In spite of these inequalities, it is now recognized that, ideally, we should all be able to expect a death that involves privacy, dignity, good quality care in comfortable surroundings, adequate pain relief and appropriate support (General Medical Council 2002). This translates into a number of propositions:

- Care for those approaching death is an integral and important part of health care. Care for the dying should involve and respect patients and those close to them.

- Care at the end of life depends upon health care professionals having strong interpersonal skills, clinical knowledge and is informed by ethical understanding and personal and professional values and experience.

- Good care for dying people is a team endeavour and depends as much on the organization of health care as it does on individuals.

- Nurses have special responsibilities in caring for dying people, since they most commonly have closest contact with the seriously and terminally ill.

In this chapter, we examine some of these important issues about death and dying, focusing in particular on: processes leading to the definition of dying; ethical issues encountered during clinical practice in end-of-life care; evidence about the experience of dying in different cultures and settings of care; and nursing care during dying. The chapter draws on research studies and 'critical cases' throughout.

Defining dying

Field, writing in 1996, argued that 'modern' dying is characterized by what Glaser and Strauss called a 'status passage' (Glaser and Strauss 1965, cited in Field 1996), in which there are four major characteristics: first, dying is linked to a medical definition of terminal disease; second, dying is linked to a loss of activities and social roles, with little or no new activities; third, there is little prior socialization to the role; and fourth, there are few 'rites of passage' to signal the person's transition to the dying role. Here, we focus on the first of these, the medical definition of dying. This is also examined in Chapter 22. Here, we look especially closely at the consequences that flow from the peculiarly modern problem of *defining* dying.

Medical definitions of dying

With advances in medical technology, diseases that are potentially life-threatening can be diagnosed at an early stage even to the point of identifying a genetic predisposition to developing such a disease in the future, where none may yet exist. Our awareness of our mortality is, as a result (at an intellectual level at least) highly developed (for a fuller discussion, see Chapter 25). For example, many of us will be aware of familial dispositions to particular types of chronic disease that could contribute to our eventual demise, and many of us spend a great deal of energy in trying to minimize such risks through attention to diet, weight control, screening opportunities and other similar devices. Yet, ironically, receiving a medical diagnosis of *dying* as a result of chronic disease is perhaps less likely now than at any time hitherto. Bauman (1992) identified two strategies which are employed by developed societies to ward off 'the problem' of death that result from the technical abilities that we now possess to diagnose disease. One strategy attempts to 'deconstruct' death into individual problems of health and disease that we conceive of as potentially soluble, given adequate knowledge, resources, effort and time. In this strategy, the problem of death becomes contained by the specific medical explanation of its cause; for example, cardiac arrhythmias at the late stages of heart disease may be dealt with as discrete problems rather than as indicators of any more general movement towards death. Thus we have a situation in which disease detection is highly developed, but the definition of dying is highly complex because of the extensive attempts made to defer, through a search for 'cure', any manifestations of dying (Lofland 1978; Bauman 1992). Even when it is recognized that death is a likely outcome of disease, widespread access to life-supporting interventions (such as artificial feeding or chemotherapy) may radically transform the life expectancy of some dying people from the few days or weeks usually associated with a terminal disease to the several months or years more often associated with a chronic disease (Jennett 1995). Questions about the withdrawal or withholding of life-supporting interventions (Hopkins 1997), and arguments about the best way in which to break the news to patients that dying may be inevitable, give rise to intense debate and ethical conjecture. Nicholas Christakis, a physician and sociologist, examined how doctors 'prognosticate' in cases of life-limiting and terminal illness. Christakis's thesis is that of the three main tasks of the physician – diagnosis, treatment and prognosis – the last was neglected during the twentieth century. This means that care and treatment options for people facing life-limiting illness are not always assessed, planned and evaluated appropriately. Christakis's observations are paralleled closely by those of Ellershaw and Ward (2003), who link quality of end-of-life care to the 'diagnosis of dying':

> In order to care for dying patients it is essential to 'diagnose dying'. However, diagnosing dying is often a complex process. In a hospital setting, where the culture is often focused on 'cure', continuation of invasive procedures, investigations, and treatments may be pursued at the expense of the comfort of the patient. There is sometimes a reluctance to make the diagnosis of dying if any hope of improvement exists and even more so if no definitive diagnosis has been made. When recovery is uncertain it is better to discuss this rather than giving false hope to the patient and family. This is generally perceived as a strength in the doctor–patient relationship and helps to build trust.
>
> (Ellershaw and Ward 2003: 30)

Ellershaw and Ward (2003) identify a range of barriers to the diagnosis of dying, including, among others: hope that the patient may get better, disagreements about the patient's condition, medico-legal issues and fears of foreshortening life.

The consequences that result from the problems that doctors have with defining dying and with prognostication are illuminated well by the findings from a well-known North American study: the Study to Understand Prognoses and Preferences for Outcomes and Risks of Treatment (SUPPORT Principal Investigators 1995). This study, which began in 1989, had the stated aim of achieving a clearer understanding of the character of dying in American hospitals.

Christakis, in his commentary on the SUPPORT study, notes that

> it is clear that discussion of prognosis occurred insufficiently frequently, since a majority of these seriously ill patients said they would have desired a discussion of the prognosis. Moreover, all had an objectively high risk of death within a few months, so *the prognosis was material to their care*, and there was ample opportunity for them to be provided with prognostic information, given that they were in hospital being seen daily by physicians . . . [as a result] patients generally had substantially unduly optimistic expectations about their prospects for recovery. These false prognostic impressions apparently influenced the choices that patients made, tilting patients in favour of active treatment of their illnesses rather than palliative care.
>
> (Christakis 1999: 188–9, our emphasis)

Box 10.1 Highlight on research: the Study to Understand Prognoses and Preferences for Outcomes and Risks of Treatment

SUPPORT enrolled a total of 9105 patients suffering from life-threatening illness in five hospitals over a 4-year period. Each patient's illness was judged to be such that they had a 50 per cent chance of death within the next 6 months. In the first phase of the study, the care and treatment that 4301 patients received was documented:

- 80 per cent of those who died during phase one had a 'Do-not-resuscitate' order, but almost half of these orders were written within 2 days of death.
- 31 per cent of patients in phase one expressed a preference (to researchers) not to be resuscitated, but this was understood by slightly less than half of their lead clinicians.
- Of those patients who died in phase one, 38 per cent spent 10 or more days in intensive care units.
- 50 per cent of all conscious patients who died in phase one were reported by their families as having moderate or severe pain.

The second phase of the study was the implementation and evaluation of an intervention aimed at resolving the problems highlighted in phase one. The remaining 4804 patients were involved in this phase. An intervention was designed that was aimed at improving communications between the relevant parties. First, researchers provided doctors with brief written reports on their patients' probability of surviving up to 6 months, likelihood of being functionally impaired at 2 months and probability of surviving cardiopulmonary resuscitation. Second, doctors were provided with brief written reports regarding patients' views on life-sustaining treatment, presence of pain and desire for information. Third, specially trained nurse facilitators were given responsibility for initiating and maintaining communication between patients, their carers and their health care team. Patients were randomized to receive either the intervention or to continue with the usual medical care. Data pertaining to the key issues highlighted in phase one were then gathered from the two groups and the results compared. The results indicate that there were no significant differences between the two groups regarding the four key issues: the timing of do-not-resuscitate orders remained the same; patient–physician communication did not improve; reported pain levels remained static; and high levels of technology attended a significant proportion of deaths.

One of the problems associated with achieving a medical definition of dying, and how and when it occurs, is that there is still a myth that dying is essentially a 'natural' phenomenon that exists independently of the activities and beliefs of those caring for the dying person. However, an examination of how matters of team interaction determine the status of ill persons as 'dying' reveals that dying is a fluid state heavily dependent not only on the technical and clinical work that informs prognostication, but also the social interaction between clinicians and their colleagues at the bedside of patients.

Interactional issues in defining dying

Writing in 1996, Turner made the sharp observation that it is illusory to think that the problem of recognizing imminent death is merely a matter of the inaccuracy of our *technical* abilities to define or diagnose dying:

> the problem, however, is not simply technical since there is an essential difference between medical death and social death. Dying is a social process, involving changes in behaviour and a process of assessment which do not necessarily correspond to the physical process of bodily death. Death, like birth, has to be socially organized and, in the modern hospital, is an outcome of team activities.
>
> (Turner 1996: 198)

Turner is arguing here that clinical work transforms the body and invokes, or produces, dying as an identity through the activities of teamwork and team discussions. The PhD research of one of us (Seymour 2001), summarized in Box 10.2, applied this latter insight to interpret the interactional processes that precede the withdrawal or withholding of life-prolonging treatments from people dying in intensive care units. In this study, the largely unspoken

---

Box 10.2 A summary of Seymour's research (Seymour 2001)

Seymour's ethnographic research examines the way in which problems of defining dying are resolved during medical work within the adult intensive care unit. She argues that issues of non-treatment in intensive care are emotive and, at times, contentious matters which hinge upon the resolution of 'problem[s] of social definition' (Glaser and Strauss 1965: 16). She then explores the way in which such resolution occurs and examines the navigation of 'uncertain death at an unknown time' (Glaser and Strauss 1965: 16) for people who were patients in the intensive care units of two city hospitals in the UK during the mid-1990s. At the outset, the study was envisaged as an attempt to slow down and dwell upon fast-moving action in intensive care to better understand the social processes that culminate in a definition of dying and precipitate an application of human agency (in the form of withholding or withdrawing life support) such that death can follow dying. Seymour presents an analysis of observational case study data and suggests that the definition of 'dying' in intensive care hinges upon four strategies. These are presented as a frame-work with which to interpret social interaction between physicians during end-of-life decision making in intensive care. They are as follows: First, the establishment of a 'technical' definition of dying – informed by results of investigations and monitoring equipment – over and above 'bodily' dying informed by clinical experience. Second, the alignment of the trajectories of technical and bodily dying to ensure that the events of non-treatment have no perceived causative link to death. Third, the balancing of medical action with non-action, allowing a diffusion of responsibility for death to the patient's body. Last, the incorporation of the patient's companions and nursing staff into the decision-making process.

negotiation that occurs between medicine and nursing during interaction was explored, with a focus on how the seemingly contradictory 'whole person work' of nursing and 'medical-technical' work of medicine are balanced during the care of dying patients.

In Seymour's study, the recognition that there are two potentially divergent trajectories of dying in intensive care ('technical' and 'bodily' dying) and two opposing foci of work ('whole body' and 'medical-technical') allows for an examination of the consequences for the care of (probably) dying patients and their families. The study shows clearly the deleterious outcomes for nurses as they struggle to achieve the 'good death' for patients in circumstances in which, because it is difficult to align technical and bodily dying, death is either precipitate or delayed. We see also the problems that result in trying to advance and protect the rights of families to participate in the decision-making process, when much of the interactional work that leads to critical decisions about the withdrawal and withholding of treatment takes place 'behind the scenes' and thus is insulated from all but the most determined of family members (Seymour 2001).

It might be easy to think that intensive care is somehow a 'special case', in which death is indeed profoundly problematic but has little relevance for other settings of care, and can therefore be set aside. More recently published work in the anthropological tradition seems to suggest that this is not the case and that similar problems frequently attend the definition of dying in less technological environments of care, and even at home. For example, Kaufman's (2003) study of a long-term care facility in North America for people in near persistent vegetative states alerts us very movingly to some of the ethical complexities that attend dying in our developed world. She speaks of the suffering endured by the sister of a man who exists, by virtue of severe brain injury as a result of a failed suicide attempt and the indecision of those caring for him about continuation or cessation of life-prolonging treatments, in the twilight world between living and dying. The sister feels that he should be allowed to die and is deeply distressed about the possibility that he is suffering even more profoundly than at the time of his unsuccessful suicide attempt. The team, having failed to resolve questions of decision making through reference to ethical principles, decide to 'wait and see' for another few months. Kaufman argues that

> medicine ponders a cluster of questions, constructed through the frame of bioethics, whose very formulation minimizes or ignores location and context. For example, how can professionals promote 'quality of life' when the idea is itself debatable? What is in the patient's 'best interest'? Those questions, based on the primacy of patient autonomy, underlie every medical intervention and every interaction even though patients' identities are actually invoked through inter-subjective relations . . . those questions and the rationalist, utilitarian moral philosophy from which they derive cannot, by themselves, reveal medicine's complicated ethical role in transforming and fabricating persons through its examinations and treatments. Nor do those questions speak to the realm of

compassion and emotional connection felt toward very impaired persons. Those questions, as debated in the public sphere, ignore a powerful and essential dimension of human relations.

(Kaufman 2003: 2259–60)

The questions that Kaufman raises here about 'bioethics', 'autonomy', 'quality of life', 'best interests' and the potential schism between the medical interpretations of an ill person's identity and those of others with an emotional attachment to the person, underpin much ethical and moral debate in palliative care and beyond. We turn now to look at a few selected issues in more detail.

Ethical issues in clinical practice at the end of life

As the means have become available to support life and to defer death for prolonged periods, so the moral and ethical complexities surrounding clinical practice at the end of life have multiplied. In palliative care, ethics centre on 'decisions which will enable us to satisfy the criteria for a peaceful death, dignified and assisted by a helpful society' (Roy and MacDonald 1998: 97). Medical and clinical ethics are those values and obligations of a moral nature that govern the practice of medicine and are enshrined in professional codes and standards of practice. *Medical ethics* change over time, although medicine in the UK has been guided by the Jewish/Christian and Hippocratic traditions, in which doctors' obligations to the sick have been emphasized. *Clinical ethics* are of more relevance when thinking about the nature of interdisciplinary teamwork in palliative care, and the need to engage with ethical issues across disciplinary and professional boundaries in order to give good care to dying patients. The field of *bioethics*, in which the rights of the individual are emphasized, emerged following the Second World War. Bioethics is rooted in the reaction to the 'medical' experiments conducted in Germany by scientists during the war and exposed during the Nuremberg Trials. In its contemporary form, bioethics focuses on the consequences for people of new health technologies and other scientific developments (ten Have and Clark 2002; Dingwall 2003).

Here, we provide a brief review of two particularly contentious issues in palliative care: euthanasia and artificial feeding and hydration. This choice is necessarily highly selective and we refer readers to the texts referenced at the end of this chapter. To begin, we highlight four critical cases from the UK that capture some of the issues involved and with which we are familiar.

The case of Lillian Boyes presents us with the very worst scenario in which death portrays the characteristics often cited when people imagine what a bad death would be like. Nigel Cox was convicted of attempted murder and admonished by the General Medical Council. He was eventually reinstated to his former post on the condition that he underwent training in palliative care and was supervised. This case, and those of Diane Pretty and

Box 10.3   Ethical issues at the end of life: four critical cases

Lillian Boyes

Lillian Boyes had been suffering from rheumatoid arthritis for many years, and for thirteen years she had been under the care of Dr Nigel Cox, a consultant rheumatologist at the Royal Hampshire County Hospital in Winchester, UK. Mrs Boyes had developed ulcers and abscesses on her arms and legs, a rectal sore penetrating to the bone, fractured vertebrae, deformed hands and feet, swollen joints, and gangrene from steroid treatment. Her weight was down to below 42 kg, and it was agony for her to be touched. In hospital, five days before she actually died, she pleaded for her life to be ended. When this was refused she asked for her treatment to be stopped, and the steroids were discontinued. Her pain became worse and the diamorphine Dr Cox had prescribed – up to 50 mg per hour – failed to lessen her agony. A nurse said that Mrs Boyes 'howled and screamed' when she was touched. On 16 August 1991, 70-year-old Lillian Boyes was not expected to last the day, and Dr Cox gave her 100 mg of diamorphine to ease her continued suffering. Mrs Boyes continued to cry out in pain, and so Dr Cox injected her with two ampoules of potassium chloride, which he noted in her records, and Mrs Boyes died.

(Dyer 1992: 731)

Diane Pretty

Diane Pretty was a woman of 43 who had late-stage motor neurone disease and applied during 2002 to the European Court of Human Rights to allow her husband to help her to commit assisted suicide. The application, which was rejected, was surrounded by publicity. Mrs Pretty eventually died in a hospice. It was widely reported that, in the days before her death, she had suffered the very symptoms she had feared, although these had eventually been well controlled. The case was supported by the Voluntary Euthanasia Society and the civil rights group 'Liberty'.

(BBC News, Monday, 13 May 2002: http://news.bbc.co.uk/1/hi/health/1983941.stm)

Miss B

A quadriplegic woman who fought and won a legal battle for the right to come off the ventilator which kept her alive, has got her wish and died peacefully in her sleep. Miss B, a former senior social worker, was moved three weeks ago to a London hospital where doctors had agreed to carry out her wishes, after those caring for her at another hospital for more than a year refused to take a step they regarded as killing her. Last-ditch attempts were made to persuade her to try rehabilitation, which would not have improved her physical condition but might have increased her quality of life through the use of mechanical aids. But 43-year-old Miss B, who was unmarried, was adamant that she did not want to live, as she was paralysed from the neck down and reliant on others for all her personal care. She died last Wednesday, but the death was announced yesterday. Miss B, who was paralysed after a blood vessel burst in her neck, made UK history last month as the first non-terminally ill patient to ask to be withdrawn from a ventilator. The Department of Health announced yesterday: 'Miss B _ has died peacefully in her sleep after being taken off the ventilator at her request.' Dame Elizabeth Butler-Sloss, President of the High Court's family division, ruled in the high court in London last month that Miss B had the 'mental capacity to give consent or refuse consent to life-sustaining medical treatment'.

(Dyer 2002)

Anthony Bland*

Since April 15, 1989, Anthony Bland has been in persistent vegetative state. He lies in Airedale General Hospital in Keighley, fed liquid food by a pump through a tube passing through his nose and down the back of his throat into the stomach. His bladder is emptied through a catheter inserted through his penis, which from time to time has caused infections requiring dressing and antibiotic treatment. His stiffened joints have caused his limbs to be rigidly contracted so that his arms are tightly flexed across his chest and his legs unnaturally contorted. Reflex movements in the throat cause him to vomit and dribble. Of all this, and the presence of members of his family who take turns to visit him, Anthony Bland has no consciousness at all. The parts of his brain which provided him with consciousness have turned to fluid. The darkness and oblivion which descended at Hillsborough will never depart. His body is alive, but he has no life in the sense that even the most pitifully handicapped but conscious human being has a life. But the advances of modern medicine permit him to be kept in this state for years, even perhaps for decades.

(Extract from Airedale NHS Trust v. Bland (C.A.), 19 February 1993, 2 Weekly Law Reports, p. 350, of Hoffman's description of Bland. Cited in Singer 1994: 58)

* Anthony Bland was fatally injured in the Hillsborough football stadium disaster of 1989 causing a persistent vegetative state. His feeding tube was withdrawn after a prolonged legal battle (Airedale Trust v. Bland [1993] 1 All ER 821 (HL)), and he died 10 days afterwards.

Miss 'B', highlight the clinical and public dilemmas that can surround caring for people at the end of their life. In particular, questions of how refractory symptoms can be managed, what should be done when a person no longer wants to live, or the person's life appears to be so tortured with suffering that death could be in that person's best interest. Is there a right to death, and does it ever outweigh the right to life? When a life has become unbearable, is it ever permissible to choose a path of clinical action or non-action that ends that life? Should a doctor ever help a patient die? How are we to understand the relationship between the moral principles of sanctity of life, autonomy, mercy and justice (Cobb 2003)? The differential resolutions of the cases of Miss B (who was taken off a ventilator at her own request and died shortly afterwards) and of Diane Pretty (whose husband was not allowed to assist her to commit suicide) provoked a storm of controversy, with some saying that there was little between the cases and that the judgments showed how disadvantaged certain groups of terminally ill people are by the laws surrounding the withdrawal and withholding of treatment. The distinction between the two cases hung on the difference perceived in English law between *acts of commission* (i.e. killing) and *acts of demission* (i.e. 'pulling the plug' or withdrawing treatment) (Shaw 1995). Shaw also refers to *acts of omission*, which relate to situations where treatments judged to be able to confer no benefit to a person are withheld. A further distinction relates to the way in which the Courts used the principles of autonomy and sanctity of life in making their judgments. In Miss B's case, autonomy was prioritized, whereas in Diane Pretty's case, sanctity of life, and the need to be seen to protect this for the good of society, triumphed (Huxtable and Campbell 2003).

As the medical technology exists increasingly not only to relieve the suffering associated with dying, but to prolong life or to procure early death, the clarification of the distinction between 'killing' and 'letting die' is perhaps one of the most pressing concerns facing society today. In the UK, it is now recognized that where death is inevitable, then life-prolonging treatments such as resuscitation, artificial ventilation, dialysis, artificial nutrition and hydration can be withdrawn or withheld, and the goal of medicine redirected to the palliation of symptoms and the provision of 'basic care' and comfort, which are mandatory (British Medical Association 2001). The case of Anthony Bland, depicted above, fundamentally informed the current position in the UK. Public concern about this case pushed forward the establishment of a House of Lords Select Committee on Medical Ethics, which reported in 1994. This committee ruled that Bland's death was a case of 'double-effect',[1] in which death was an unintended, although not unforeseen, consequence of the removal of futile life-prolonging medical therapy (House of Lords 1993–94).

Euthanasia[2]

As far as humans are concerned, the protection of innocent human life is regarded as the central principle to morality asserted in the United Nations' Universal Declaration of Human Rights (1948) and, in the UK, in the Human Rights Act of 1998. If we accept that all persons have full and equal moral status, then we also have to accept our obligations to one another, specifically to do no harm. However we may regard euthanasia, it is an act that violates this fundamental human right to life, and for this reason alone it is a highly contested subject. Causing the death of someone is usually considered wrong, but not always – take, for example, self-defence or war. Killing is therefore sometimes permitted, but in health care it seems to contradict the very purpose of what we set out to do, to save lives and bring about healing. Some argue, however, that under certain conditions, ending the life of a terminally ill patient in extreme suffering is consistent with the ethic of beneficence in that it is a compassionate and merciful response that brings relief. In the UK, the broad definition of euthanasia adopted by the House of Lords says that euthanasia is 'a deliberate intervention undertaken with the express intention of ending a life to relieve intractable suffering' (House of Lords 1993–94: 10). When, as appears to be the case with Lillian Boyes, there is a request for euthanasia from the patient who is a mentally competent adult, who is fully informed and who has arrived at a reasoned decision without coercion, then the act of euthanasia in response to the patient may be termed 'voluntary'. The act is 'non-voluntary' when the patient does not have the capacity to express a reasoned preference to request, agree or refuse to be killed.

When considering euthanasia, we become aware of the conflicts that can exist between an individual's call to be released from suffering and society's efforts to protect and sustain life. Clinically, this tension becomes focused in the health professional's duty to provide beneficial care to those in need, to refrain from harming them, and to respect an individual's choices.

Arguments for euthanasia: appealing to 'mercy', 'autonomy' and 'justice'

Mercy

Those who prioritize the moral value of 'mercy' in arguing for euthanasia assert that allowing euthanasia would produce more good than harm, since it would relieve uncontrolled suffering and reassure others that death is not painful. Proponents of this position argue that while modern medicine can, in most cases, relieve pain and suffering, it still cannot do so in all cases. For example, while most patients dying of cancer have little or no pain, some have pain that is erratic and very difficult to control. Those taking this position often also argue that there is no substantive distinction between 'killing' and 'letting die', and that the maintenance of this distinction disadvantages some groups of dying people because it leads to all sorts of difficulties about what should be withdrawn, when and how. The published critiques of the legal judgment on the Diane Pretty case (summarized by Huxtable and Campbell 2003) use these sorts of arguments. It is arguably the case that ethical confusion over these issues means that clinical behaviour can lurch from 'the abrupt cessation of treatment, minimalist palliative care and treatment directed at bringing about a rapid dying process, to excessive caution about being seen to be instrumental in causing death' (Ashby 1998: 74, cited in Seymour 2001). Most commonly, many of those who support the legalization of euthanasia on the grounds of 'mercy' suggest that it is a necessary solution to the problem of containing the unintended effects of 'medical heroism', in which dying may be prolonged in a profoundly undignified way. Le Fanu (1999, cited in Seymour 2001), in commenting on the 'transforming power' of the technological innovation of artificial ventilation and oxygenation that heralded the development of intensive therapy in the early 1950s, notes that 50 years later those same life-saving therapies have also become a means of prolonging the 'pain and misery of terminal illness' for many.

Autonomy

The principle of mercy is tied conceptually to the principle of autonomy (Pabst-Battin 1994). To impose 'mercy' on someone who wishes to live regardless of their pain and suffering would clearly be a contradiction of the mercy principle. Autonomy – meaning informed consent to treatment and the respect of a person's competent wishes where those do not violate other moral obligations or cause harm to others – is also crucially important. The 'right to die' lobby in both the USA and the UK use this principle to underpin their argument that individual choice for euthanasia should be respected and the law changed to ensure that medical actions to help people to die are permissible.

Justice

A final key principle that has been used to support euthanasia is that of justice. Here it is argued that some people have a 'meaningless existence' – those in deep, irreversible comas, for example, or suffering from late-stage Alzheimer's disease – and that in the interests of the fair distribution of scarce resources, laws against euthanasia should be relaxed to embrace these groups. One famous argument that has been used to back up this position has been put forward by an American ethicist, Daniel Callahan (1987), who argues that when people have had 'their fair innings' it should be recognized that health resources are better spent on younger people who are more likely to benefit and contribute to the overall wealth of a society. It is perhaps a short jump from this argument for rationing based on age to an extension of the same argument as a justification for euthanasia.

Arguments against euthanasia: the 'slippery slope'

Those who argue against the legalization of euthanasia suggest that such legalization will mean that there will inevitably be abuses of the law, and that vulnerable people will be put at risk. These arguments are known collectively as 'slippery slope' arguments. Slippery slope arguments recognize that individual treatment decisions are always constrained to a greater or lesser extent by wider economic and social factors. Proponents of this position suggest that there is a possibility that wholesale discrimination on a societal level may be unleashed against those considered, possibly arbitrarily, as an economic or social burden. A particularly powerful argument against the legalization of voluntary euthanasia has come from those who point to the possibility of 'co-erced' altruism becoming a significant element in requests for euthanasia. This theme was a major consideration in the rejection of euthanasia by the House of Lords Select Committee on Medical Ethics (1993–94) in the UK:

> we do not think it possible to set secure limits on voluntary euthanasia ... we conclude that it would be virtually impossible to ensure that all acts of euthanasia were truly voluntary and that any liberalisation of the law was not abused ... We also feel concerned that vulnerable people – the elderly, lonely, sick or distressed – would feel pressure, whether real or imagined – to request early death.
>
> (extracts from paras 238–9)

Many in the hospice and palliative care movement also reject euthanasia for precisely these reasons. They argue that there is a risk that euthanasia may become an easy alternative to the difficult challenge of addressing care delivery and planning for people as they approach the end of their lives. The general stance of the hospice and palliative care movement in the UK is summarized by Robert Twycross (1995). He responds to the arguments for euthanasia based on 'mercy' by saying that good palliative care for patients and families will mean that suffering can be relieved and the fears of dying and death greatly lessened. He frames the problem of euthanasia in terms of inadequate provision of palliative care services together with a lack of knowledge about how to respond appropriately to requests for euthanasia.

Twycross's position is similar to that of Roy and Rapin (1994), who compiled the First Position Paper on Euthanasia at the behest of the European Association for Palliative Care. In this, they argued unequivocally that 'we should firmly and without qualification, oppose the legalisation of euthanasia as both unnecessary and dangerous' (Roy and Rapin 1994: 58). Roy and Rapin used a definition of euthanasia which was very close to the UK definition put forward by the House of Lord's Select Committee on Medical Ethics, and to which we referred above.

A task force set up by the European Association for Palliative Care in 2002 set out a revised position paper on euthanasia (Materstvedt *et al.* 2003). This was in response to rapid social and clinical changes since 1994 when the first statement was issued; in particular, the legalization of euthanasia in Belgium subject to strict constraints, its decriminalization in the Netherlands, brief legalization in the Northern Territories of Australia, and the legalization of physician-assisted suicide in Oregon, USA.[3] The statement perhaps overturns the traditional opposition between palliative care and euthanasia, since it suggests that the two can, in certain circumstances, co-exist. It adopts a much narrower definition of euthanasia: 'Euthanasia is killing on request and is defined as: a doctor intentionally killing a person by the administration of drugs at that person's voluntary and competent request' (Materstvedt *et al.* 2003: 98). Following this definition, the Position Paper sets out a number of key issues, and calls for dialogue between the opposed camps in this debate. This provoked a huge commentary from across the world (*Palliative Medicine* 2003: 17(2)), showing that the issue is set to continue to arouse debate and contention well into the twenty-first century.

Artificial feeding in palliative care

Nutritional support can be provided artificially in two ways to people who are unable to swallow, digest or absorb adequate amounts of food and fluids:

- Parenteral feeding procedures are primarily intravenous methods of administering nutrients and water. Total parenteral nutrition refers to an intravenous procedure that supplies enough nutrients to maintain a person's body weight indefinitely.
- Enteral or tube feeding procedures, by which nutrients and water are infused into the patient's stomach or intestines via tubes.

These techniques are widely applied in health care. In the context of a literature review conducted by one of us (Seymour 2002), it is clear that they are used extensively among older people, many of whom might otherwise be in their final days and weeks of life. Yet these techniques are among the most contested and poorly understood of all life-prolonging technologies, and applied in practices seemingly based on ritual and entrenched habits.

Advantages and disadvantages of artificial nutritional support for dying people

In a systematic review of the effects of fluid status and fluid therapy on the dying process, Viola *et al.* (1997) point to the existence of polarized views regarding the risks and benefits of artificial hydration and nutrition for dying older people. Some clinicians argue that any thirst or discomfort produced by a dry mouth can be relieved effectively by the use of ice chips, sips of fluid and good oral care and that additional fluid therapy may aggravate symptoms or produce troublesome symptoms where none existed before. These include increased respiratory tract secretions resulting in increased dyspnoea and coughing, increased saliva-inducing sensations of choking, increased urine production leading to feelings of discomfort and agitation, increased risk of nausea and vomiting, and increased oedema and ascites. However, as Viola *et al.* observe, these arguments have a poor evidence base. Studies that have been conducted reveal conflicting findings because of the use of different outcome measures and small samples.

More recently, studies conducted in non-palliative care settings have shown that, except for patients in coma (Borum *et al.* 2000), artificial hydration and feeding have no benefits in terms of length of survival over hand feeding (Mitchell *et al.* 1997; Meier *et al.* 2001). Furthermore, commentators have observed that the need for restraint in older people who are being artificially fed is a significant contributor to their suffering during the final period of their lives (Peck *et al.* 1990) and may lead to increased use of sedation, the 'chemical cosh' (Gillick 2000).

However, it has been argued that some common problems among the terminally ill, such as delirium, can be aggravated by dehydration (for a review, see Holmes 1998). Others have argued strongly that artificial nutrition should be provided on ethical, social and biographical grounds. Concerns voiced by the families of dying people may be particularly powerful. For example, Kedziera (2001: 156) provides an example of an older man dying from cancer who, with his wife, had been a victim of the Holocaust. His wife found the idea of discontinuing food and fluids inconceivable and therefore he was supported with artificial feeding until he died.

In the field of palliative care, guidelines have been produced to assist in decision making in artificial feeding and hydration in dying people. These acknowledge the difficulties surrounding prediction of life expectancy in dying people and of the clinical response to treatments of this kind (EAPC 1996; NCHSPCS 1997). These difficulties give rise to significant concerns and variable practices among clinicians in relation to treatment and non-treatment decisions in artificial feeding, perhaps as a result of feelings of walking 'a tightrope between over treatment and neglect' (Goodhall 1997: 218).

Box 10.4 summarizes some findings from a study of the views of older members of the public about artificial feeding at the end of life (Seymour 2002). This project explored the views of older people living in Sheffield, UK, about life-prolonging and basic care technologies in end-of- life care. Artificial feeding was one issue that was introduced. The concept of 'natural death' and, specifically, how ideas about technologies used in palliative and end-of-life care are used actively to construct this, was employed as a theoretical framework.

Box 10.4 Technology and natural death: a study of older people*

Seventy-seven older people from three age cohorts (65–74, 75–84 and 85 years and over) and from three socio-economically contrasting areas of Sheffield, UK took part in interviews, focus groups, and a discussion day at the end of the project. The research team was assisted by an advisory group which included research participants.

During focus groups, participants were invited to comment on a simple *aide-mémoire* in which key themes were presented in words and pictures in slides projected on a portable screen. A simple synopsis of the Anthony Bland case was used as a resource to 'open up' a discussion about the role of artificial feeding in dying people. All of the focus participants had heard of the case of Tony Bland, and some had strong negative feelings about the role of artificial feeding in his care. This was valuable in so far as lively debates were generated around a subject that might otherwise have been difficult to discuss. A disadvantage may have been that attitudes to his situation were heavily influenced by recollections of the media coverage of the polarized debates that occurred at that time.

Many participants drew on personal experiences to express complex and sometimes paradoxical understandings of the boundaries between 'body' and 'person', between 'life' and 'death', and between 'artificiality' and 'natural'. Much discussion focused on the 'proper' roles of, and relationships between, families and clinical staff in end-of-life decisions, and to the expression of expectations about how participants' families should act to represent them in the event of their serious illness. There was recognition that the application of technological innovations to the management of dying had transformed a social order of dying in which 'doctor knows best' to one in which patients, clinicians and their families were caught in a shared dilemma imposed by medicalization. Participants made clear their views that all parties had to work together to establish the best course of action in impossible circumstances. However, it was recognized that, in these new circumstances, families had to be ready to assume a degree of responsibility for representing their dying relative, and that new risks were associated with this. Most importantly, participants recognized the difficulties of establishing whether a particular course of action constituted euthanasia or 'letting go', and recognized significant threats to the 'proper' relationship between family members. Some participants made repeated references to the role of 'God' and 'prayer' in aiding difficult end-of-life decisions or in negating the need for human intervention in difficult situations, while others reflected on the meaning of 'quality of life' and how this could be assessed.

* Funded (2001–2003) by the Economic and Social Research Council, grant number L218252047.

Experiences of dying

The individual experience of dying is shaped, at least in part, by a myriad of complex factors, all of which interrelate. Depending on the cause of death, and the type of treatment being given to a person, the trajectory of the dying process may be slow, sudden or take the form of a series of relapses and recoveries. As we have discussed above, in contemporary society, death has particular features which makes 'dying' difficult to anticipate, diagnose and plan for. The lack of recognition of dying associated with some chronic illnesses, for example heart failure, is arguably a major factor in the death experience for many. The place of death varies, and different places tend to give rise to different care practices and interpersonal relationships: these can fundamentally influence what sort of death experience a person has. For example, in spite of rhetoric to the contrary (and as we have discussed elsewhere in this book), to be in receipt of specialist palliative care in an in-patient hospice or at home remains largely dependent on having a diagnosis of cancer. Those dying of other diseases tend to die in hospitals or, when dying is associated with advanced old age, in care homes. The structure and organization of formal health care systems, and aspects of the dying person's social networks and living arrangements, are thus critically important. Beyond these lie wider belief systems, attitudes to death and the complex, shifting tapestry of meanings, values and representations of death in modern society. Age, gender, ethnicity, social class and culture, these have all been shown to affect the experience of dying, both in the sense of the access a person has to the material and social resources that can support them during dying and, existentially, in terms of the meaning and sense that a person makes of their dying (Field *et al.* 1997). Most notably, dying is part of the biography of an individual and will be seen by them in that context: the sorrows, regrets, joys and achievements of life, whether or not the dying person has lived through war, the way in which they have seen others close to them die, how they have experienced bereavement, their experience of family life. These are but a few of the many biographical factors that are likely to have a powerful influence on the experience of dying. By way of pointing out that death falls into recognizable categories or types, such as the 'gradual' death, the 'catastrophic' death or the 'premature' death, Clark and Seymour (1999) analyse how 'the social' interweaves with 'the individual' in powerfully shaping the experience of death and dying.

The most common contemporary experience of dying is that associated with chronic disease, especially in older age. This type of dying process may create dependencies on others, which can be experienced at one and the same time (by the dying person as well as their carers) as a welcome intimacy and a burdensome trouble. It may involve an increasing struggle to do those things on which everyday life depends, and the dying person's carers will be drawn, inexorably, into gradually assuming more and more caring responsibilities whether or not this is welcomed. For many, a sense of 'social death' may be experienced (Mulkay 1993) as a result of feeling that one is of diminishing importance to the lives and concerns of other people and no longer an active participant in the affairs of daily life. This is not something that just affects older people: it has been shown to be of relevance to children and young adults suffering from cancer and for whom the lack of sustained contact with friends is a significant contributor to their experience of suffering (Hodgson and Eden 2003). Lawton (2000), in a powerful ethnography of patients' experiences of dying in a hospice, argues that bodily unboundedness (incontinence and other problems encountered during the late stages of terminal illness) is a particularly powerful determinant of 'social death'. She claims, controversially, that hospices could be seen as places of 'sequestration', taking in patients who, because of their lack of bodily control, are no longer regarded as people. Lawton thus theorizes that 'self' is determined by the ability to control one's body, rather than the ability to maintain social relationships.

As Clark and Seymour (1999) have observed, death may be 'experienced as sheer hard work – as the illness advances and as the burdens of caring grow; but it may also be experienced as an opportunity – for personal development or fulfilment in relationships with others' (p. 12).

Sociologists draw our attention to the social-symbolic nature of human interaction (Leming and Dickenson 2002). This means that how death and dying are experienced is shaped by the way in which others react to a person once they know, or suspect, that individual is dying. To this extent, dying is a shared event. Leming and Dickenson (2002) identify a number of issues that are raised by the interactions that dying people have with their family, their friends and others. They list these from the perspective of how the dying person perceives others' behaviour:

- What people are willing to talk about with me and what they avoid.
- Whether they are willing to touch me, and how they touch me when they do.
- Where I am, or maybe where others have located me – hospital, nursing home, intensive care unit, isolation unit, or my room at home.
- Tangible and verbal gifts that others give to me.
- What people will let me do, or expect me to do, or will not let me do.
- The tone of voice that people use when they talk to me.
- The frequency and length of visits from others.
- Excuses that people make for not visiting.
- The reactions of others to my prognosis.

Taking a broader perspective beyond the close interaction emphasized by Leming and Dickenson, Kellehear (1990) has argued, on the basis of interviews with 100 people dying of cancer, that the social experience of dying is marked by five features. He argues that these are likely to be universal across cultures:

- Awareness: whether or not a person knows that they are dying.

- Social adjustments and preparations: the making of a will or preparing one's funeral, for example.
- Public preparations.
- Relinquishing of roles: one person may have many different roles, and their dying may leave many 'gaps'.
- Formal and informal farewells.

Kellehear argues that these are:

> Central recurrent concerns of organising dying despite variations to the content of that organisation ... individual styles of dying are bounded by the shape of that person's social and cultural existence. Cultures provide behavioural possibilities. In other words they supply broad prescriptions for how to act. In turn, individuals provide unique variations.
>
> (Kellehear 1990: 34)

In addition to Kellehear's classic study, there have been a number of fascinating studies that allow us to gain a perspective on the experience of dying, and which have been written drawing on accounts from dying persons (as opposed to being an account proffered by the analyst, or constructed through the 'proxy' accounts of the dying person's carers). We intend to highlight one of these studies here (see Box 10.5). The objective of the study highlighted in Box 10.5 was to describe the experiences of illness and needs and use of services in two groups of patients with incurable cancer, one in a developed country (Scotland) and one in a developing country (Kenya) (Murray *et al.* 2003). In Scotland 20 patients with inoperable lung cancer and their carers were interviewed, while in Kenya 24 patients with various advanced cancers and their carers were interviewed. The study found that people dying in Scotland were primarily concerned with the emotional pain of facing death, whereas those in Kenya were much more concerned about physical pain and financial issues. The district in Kenya where the research took place was an area of abject poverty, and what few health care services there were could only be accessed on payment of a fee, with the cost of admission to hospital the equivalent of 7 months' wages for an unskilled worker. In contrast, in Scotland, people had access to primary and secondary care free at the point of delivery and a social security system. Running water and all other domestic facilities that we take for granted in the West were available in Scotland but lacking in Kenya. In their conclusion, Murray *et al.* note that:

> Though living in a resource rich country, Scottish patients described unmet psychosocial needs. Meeting physical needs did not alone ensure a good death. In developing countries, while physical needs often go unmet, the family and local religious community can and do meet many of the psychological, social and spiritual needs: 'higher order' needs can be met amid physical distress, everting Maslow's typology of need.
>
> (Murray *et al.* 2003: 367)

Box 10.5   Summary of the issues raised by respondents in the study of Murray *et al.* (2003)

Scotland	*Kenya*
• Main issue is the prospect of death	• Main issue is physical suffering, especially pain
• Pain is unusual	• Analgesia unaffordable
• Anger in the face of illness	• Acceptance rather than anger
• Just keep it to myself	• Acceptance of community support
• Spiritual needs evident	• Patients comforted by belief in God
• Diagnosis brought active treatment and then a period of watching and waiting . . .	• Diagnosis signalled waiting for death
• Patients concerned about how carer will cope in the future	• Patients concerned about being a physical and financial burden to their family
• Support from hospital and primary care teams	• Lack of medical support, treatment options, equipment and basic necessities
• Specialist palliative care available	• Specialist palliative care services not available in the community
• Cancer a national priority	• Cancer not a national priority

---

At the beginning of this section, we drew attention to the myriad of factors that shape the experience of death. Murray and co-workers' study demonstrates this powerfully through the comparison of patients' experiences in a developed and a developing country, where vividly contrasting social, economic, political, cultural and spiritual contexts led to very different concerns and priorities among two groups of people dying from the same disease.

The nurse's role in caring for dying people

Of all those involved with the care of dying persons, except for close companions and friends, nurses have the closest and sustained contact with them. Indeed, it has been claimed that care of the dying is the 'quintessential' expression of nursing care (Bradshaw 1996). However, as we have seen elsewhere in this book, caring has not traditionally been afforded a high priority in developed health systems and this poses fundamental problems for nurses as they care for the dying. The early work of Quint (1967) was particularly influential in revealing how the lack of education given to nurses about how to care for dying patients in hospitals demonstrates the low status afforded to 'caring' work, and the negative impact of this on the physical and psychological care of those people.

In the UK, Field's (1989) study of nurses' experiences of caring for dying patients demonstrated that attitudes to disclosure of terminal prognoses had changed by the 1980s, with open awareness regarded as a necessary component of humane care. However, Field showed that nurses had relatively little autonomy in their work. This was especially the case on general surgical and medical wards, where medical staff exerted considerable power. This constrained nurses' ability either to communicate openly to dying patients or to respond to their needs in an individualized way. The enduring relevance of Field's work has been confirmed by similar findings in other contexts (Kiger 1994; Beck 1997).

At about the same time as Field's work was published, Degner and Beaton (1987) published their 4-year study of life and death decisions in acute care settings in Canada. Like Field, they suggested that nurses' conceptualization of their work leads frequently to disagreements, which were often not verbalized, with medical staff over the continuation of treatment for patients. Drawing on a follow-up study, Degner went on to publish a paper with colleagues (Degner *et al.* 1991) in which they identified a list of seven critical nursing behaviours in care for the dying. This was based on interviews with nurse-educators and palliative care nurses. The behaviours identified were:

- *Responding to the death scene*: involving maintaining a sense of calm, involving the family.
- *Providing comfort*: reducing discomfort, especially pain.
- *Responding to anger*: showing respect and empathy even when anger is directed at the nurse.
- *Enhancing personal growth*: showing that the nurse has defined a personal role in caring for the dying.
- *Responding to colleagues*: providing emotional support and critical feedback to colleagues.
- *Enhancing quality of life*: helping patients to do those things which are important to them.
- *Responding to the family*: responding to the need for information; reducing the potential for future regret; including the family in care or relieving them of responsibility according to their needs.

While other studies have identified further dimensions of the nurses' role in palliative care (see, for example, Chapter 3), this list seems to capture very well the complex responsibilities of nurses at the critical time of a patient's death. What stands out is the way in which competing demands and high levels of emotional engagement must be managed for death to be well managed. This is 'work' that involves the nurse relating not only to patients, but also to the patient's family and close companions and to other professional colleagues. De Raeve (1996) argues that nursing the dying involves a degree of professional self-exposure that makes the nurse vulnerable to harm.

In an empirical study of nurses' responses to exposure to repeated death, Saunders and Valente (1994) examined the relationship between nurses' perceptions of 'good death' and the maintenance of nurses' 'professional integrity, personal wholeness and self esteem' (p. 321). In their study, nurses delineated certain key conditions that characterize a 'good death': all relate to a protection of their patient's physical, psychological safety, to the appropriate location of death in time and space, and to a maintenance of 'family' and professional relationships. In a similar way to Field (1989) and Degner and Beaton (1987), Saunders and Valente identified that those situations where deaths were perceived by nurses as 'difficult' were marked by unresolved conflicts between health care staff over issues such as continuation of treatment or resuscitation. This issue of team relationships has been highlighted elsewhere as a problem among nurses in acute settings caring for the dying (Copp and Dunn 1993).

Whatever problems nurses face in caring for dying people, they need to be able to bring some sense of meaning to the experience. Maeve (1998) has suggested that nurses 'weave a fabric of moral meaning' into their work with dying people; in this, nurses use the dilemmas of their patients' lives to inform their own personal and professional lives, and thus come to terms with their own mortality and with the universal experience of suffering. Reflection on experiences of caring for dying patients and their families, then, clearly has the potential to become a reservoir of personal development. It also can be one valuable way in which nurses learn to provide high-quality and sensitive care. Wong (2001) reports on work with student nurses in Hong Kong, in which the latter attended problem-based learning sessions focused on group discussion of some fictional scenarios involving death and dying. The students documented their learning in reflective journals focusing on the care they gave to dying patients. Within these journals, there was compelling evidence that the nurses experienced anxiety about death and felt inadequate in dealing with dying patients. However, the dual processes of engaging in problem-based learning and of writing about their clinical experiences emerged as an effective strategy to enhance their awareness and sensitivity to dying patients and to facilitate their formulation of appropriate care plans for the dying.

Overview of chapters in Part Two

It has been our intention to provide a broad overview of the issues with which the authors of the subsequent chapters in this part of the book are concerned. We turn now to introduce these.

From its earliest foundations, hospice and palliative care has been associated with matters of religious and spiritual care, and there have been debates about who is best placed to identify needs and deliver care in this area (Walter 1997; Clark and Seymour 1999). In Chapter 11, Michael Wright examines how, through facing the inevitability of one's own mortality, spiritual activity occurs. This *may* involve religious observance but can be best understood, according to Wright, as a kaleidoscope involving: 'personhood', in the sense of values, belief and achievements; relationships a person has with themselves, with others, with the universe and with a 'life force' or with God; religion, which may involve private prayer, vocation, commitment and worship; a search for meaning about the 'big' questions of life; and transcendence, in the sense of becoming aware of something above and beyond oneself. Wright shows that as dying patients begin to address their religious and spiritual needs across these dimensions, health professionals have an opportunity to play a supportive and important role. Wright draws on his doctoral study of spiritual care in the UK in which he examined how hospices and hospitals in England organize the delivery of spiritual care and how this is perceived by patients.

Jessica Corner's chapter is about the challenge of managing difficult symptoms from which dying patients may suffer. She takes a critical approach to symptom control and, rather than offering a 'tool kit', explores how symptom control has become a dominant construct in palliative care in which 'personal' knowledge is marginalized *vis-à-vis* 'scientific' knowledge. This means that other forms of intervention, such as spiritual care, have received limited consideration in spite of the highly prized rhetoric of 'holism' in palliative care. While biomedical science is clearly essential in achieving good symptom control, Corner argues that we should not forget that not all the problems of dying experienced by patients are related to disease processes and their associated physical consequences. For example, it may be that patients prioritize complete eradication of pain less highly than do clinicians: they may be more concerned with the *meaning* of the pain (does it indicate that death is imminent? Will it mean that I cannot go home today?) rather than its complete control. To not appreciate this is to miss an important opportunity to begin to address with patients some wider issues about their dying. Here we enter the realm of suffering, which can be related to physical pain and other symptoms, but *may also* exist independently of those. Corner goes on to examine in some detail the management of difficult problems such as breathlessness, fatigue, emaciation, odour and exudate. She shows that symptoms are a product of mind *and* body, and that their control takes place in a social and cultural context, which itself shapes the experience of the symptom and the way in which it is managed. She concludes by drawing attention to the importance of developing an understanding of *why* a symptom is perceived as difficult and of listening to patients' stories in developing, with them, a meaningful approach to control in which 'self-management' is enhanced.

Silvia Paz and Jane Seymour follow Corner by focusing on pain. They look at pain and its management drawing on theoretical and historical perspectives to show how pain management has evolved across the twentieth and early twenty-first centuries. They draw particular attention to changing understandings of pain as a constellation of biopsychosocial factors not necessarily connected in a linear fashion to a particular disease process. They explore the distinction between chronic and acute pain states, and review the evidence about controlling cancer pain. They explore the role of the nurse in pain control, drawing attention to the importance of pain assessment and measurement. Throughout they emphasize the experience of pain as a multidimensional phenomenon that requires the very best standards of multidisciplinary teamwork for its management.

In Chapter 14, Mari Lloyd-Williams continues the theme of the interconnectedness of body and mind through an examination of how we may help and support patients who are facing feelings of depression and sadness at the end of their lives. She draws our attention to the impact that poor communication practices can have on patients and how important it is to recognize that not all suffering is physical. She calls for all professionals in palliative care to develop excellent communication and interpersonal skills, saying that for many patients 'the presence of a caring, empathic professional who is able to give honest information sensitively' can make the difference between being able to find the resources within themselves to face the future and finding it impossible to cope. Lloyd-Williams examines 'psychological distress', particularly depression, arguing that this should not be accepted as an automatic sequelae of dying but should be treated actively to maximize patients' quality of life even as the final days and weeks of their life draw near.

The next two chapters focus on family care-givers, in recognition that most of the care that dying people receive in the last year of life takes place within their own home, and that family care-giving is absolutely essential in helping patients remain at home if this is what they wish to do. Paula Smith explores the rewarding and challenging process of working with family care-givers, and examines how they perceive and shape their role. She presents a review of some important policy issues, which, although described from a UK perspective, have relevance elsewhere in the developed world. Drawing on the work of Nolan *et al.* (1996), Smith examines the notion that family care-givers have a particular type of expertise that we ignore at our peril. She draws on her doctoral research to examine how family carers construct their role and what satisfactions and difficulties they meet during caring for someone who is seriously ill or dying. She follows this with an examination of evidence about how family care-givers can best be supported and how their needs as individuals, as opposed to appendages of the patient, can be met. Elizabeth Hanson follows Paula Smith by looking more closely at the support needs of families of dying people and the types of interventions that can be offered to them. Again, Hanson draws on the work of Nolan *et al.* (1996) to emphasize that caring is a dynamic process that changes across time. She explores how new information and communication technologies can be harnessed to help family care-givers access information and sources of support from within their own homes. Here she suggests that such technologies enhance nurses' abilities to work collaboratively with family care-givers to meet their core support needs.

We have already briefly introduced the notion of social death and how the behaviours and attitudes of those in contact with dying persons can powerfully impinge on their experience of dying. In Chapter 17, Gail Johnston explores this phenomenon in more depth, drawing together a range of classic analyses and highlighting their significance for a greater appreciation of the complexities faced by dying persons. She relates the concept of social death to matters of social exclusion showing how, drawing on the theories of Erving Goffman, places of care can engender forms of social exclusion that function to isolate the dying person and dehumanize them. Here she examines the classic study by Hockey (1990) of older people dying in a nursing home and a hospice, as well as work that examines the management of people dying from dementia and those dying in hospital. Johnston concludes that the 'situation of social death is largely imposed by strategies both staff and carers use to distance themselves from those for whom death is inevitable . . . behaviours which encourage others to be labelled as socially dead or their own self-labelling will only be addressed when we begin to view death as a normal part of living'.

Johnston's chapter is complemented by Jonathan Koffman's analysis, in Chapter 18, of social exclusion in end-of-life care. Echoing our argument at the beginning of this overview chapter, Koffman notes that there is 'no second chance' to improve the care of individuals who are dying, and argues that it remains the case that significant 'silent' sections of the community are inadequately served at the end of life. This is a timely reminder of the way in which ethical issues are integral to palliative care. While Koffman's concern is to highlight social issues of equity and justice, ethical issues associated with the treatment of individual patients become especially important during dying. Here questions of the harms and benefits of forms of treatment, both for the individual and the society, must be resolved. We have spent some considerable time mapping out some general issues in this area: Bert Broeckaert's chapter follows this by examining closely, from a largely philosophical perspective, issues surrounding what he terms 'life-shortening' treatments. Broeckaert reflects on the different meanings of euthanasia and describes clearly the stance towards euthanasia adopted by the Netherlands and Belgium. He places particular emphasis on outlining issues surrounding 'palliative sedation' – arguably a core technique used in palliative care but one that is surrounded by controversy as to its meaning and significance.

Ethical issues are to some extent culturally contingent, and we have already explored how culture can shape dying both materially and existentially for those it directly affects. In Chapter 20, Kay Mitchell focuses on the influence of socialization on the dying process, arguing that this can fundamentally influence not only how we react to dying, but also the definition of the 'dead' state itself. Thus she explores how the concept of 'brain death', which allows the harvesting of transplantable organs, was, until very recently, not shared across all developed societies where the technologies exist to ventilate persons with catastrophic brain injuries. Although concentrating on differences between cultures, Mitchell also shows that differences within cultures are significant and often ignored. Here she echoes the concerns of Jonathan Koffman, and raises our awareness that cultural sensitivity is a necessary attribute of developing services that minimize social exclusion for people facing death. Like Bert Broeckaert, Kay Mitchell explores the issues of physician-assisted suicide and the meanings of palliative care and euthanasia. She concludes by noting that, while it is possible to talk of a shared understanding of the goals of palliative care, there may be many different approaches and paths for reaching that end.

This part of the book concludes with a chapter from Jeanne Katz, who examines the organization and delivery of palliative care in different types of institution. Katz picks up many of the issues explored elsewhere and shows how these translate into particular care practices and experiences for the dying person. Katz compares and contrasts hospices, hospitals, prisons and care homes in terms of the services they can provide to the dying, the social relationships they engender, and the constraints on quality of care imposed by their particular cultures and wider missions. Her analysis and description of initiatives in the USA to introduce hospice concepts into prisons show how it is possible to radically transform the quality of the dying experience even in the most difficult of circumstances.

▌Notes

1 While the Report of the House of Lords Select Committee on Medical Ethics (1993–94) states that the doctrine of double effect has some validity for the problems associated with end-of-life decision making (see paras 22, 242–3), it should be noted that this stance is not shared across Europe.
2 We are grateful to Mark Cobb for allowing us to draw on his lecture notes on the historical, social and clinical aspects of euthanasia delivered to medical students at the University of Sheffield between 2002 and 2003.
3 See the Guidance from the Standards Committee of the General Medical Council (2002) *Withholding and Withdrawing Life-Prolonging Treatments: Good Practice in Decision-Making* (http://www.gmc.org.uk).

▌References

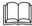

Ariès, P. (1981) *The Hour of Our Death*. London: Allen Lane.
Ashby, M. (1998) Palliative care, death causation, public policy and the law. *Progress in Palliative Care*, 6: 69–77.
Bauman, Z. (1992) *Mortality, Immortality and Other Life Strategies*. Oxford: Polity Press.
Beck, C.T. (1997) Nursing students' experiences caring for dying patients. *Journal of Nursing Education*, 36: 408–15.
Borum, M.L., Lynn, J., Zhong, Z. *et al.* (2000) The effect of nutritional supplementation on survival in seriously ill hospitalized adults: an evaluation of the SUPPORT data. Study to Understand Prognoses and Preferences for Outcomes and Risks of Treatments. *Journal of the American Geriatrics Society*, 48 (suppl. 5): S33–S38.

Bradshaw, A. (1996) The spiritual dimension of hospice: the secularisation of an ideal. *Social Science and Medicine*, 43(3): 409–20.

British Medical Association (2001) *Withholding and Withdrawing Life-Prolonging Medical Treatment*. London: BMA.

Callahan, D. (1987) *Setting Limits: Medical Goals in an Ageing Society*. New York: Simon & Schuster.

Christakis, N. (1999) *Death Foretold: Prophecy and Prognosis in Medical Care*. Chicago, IL: University of Chicago Press.

Clark, D. and Seymour, J. (1999) *Reflections on Palliative Care*. Buckingham: Open University Press.

Cobb, M. (2003) Euthanasia: historical, social and clinical issues. Lecture delivered to the School of Medicine, University of Sheffield, March.

Copp, G. and Dunn, V. (1993) Frequent and difficult problems perceived by nurses caring for the dying in community, hospice and acute care settings. *Palliative Medicine*, 7: 19–25.

Degner, L.F. and Beaton, J.I. (1987) *Life and Death Decisions in Health Care*. New York: Hemisphere.

Degner, L.F., Gow, C.M. and Thompson, L.A. (1991) Critical nursing behaviours in care of the dying. *Cancer Nursing*, 14(5): 246–53.

de Raeve, L. (1996) Dignity and integrity at the end of life. *International Journal of Palliative Care Nursing*, 2(2): 71–6.

Dingwall, R. (2003) Bioethics, in A. Pilnick (ed.) *Genetics and Society*. Buckingham: Open University Press.

Dyer, C. (2002) Miss B dies after winning fight to end care. *The Guardian*, Tuesday 30 April.

Dyer, C. (1992) Rheumatologist convicted of attempted murder. *British Medical Journal*, 305(26): 731.

Ellershaw, J. and Ward, C. (2003) Care of the dying patient: the last hours or days of life. *British Medical Journal*, 326: 30–4.

European Association for Palliative Care (EAPC) (1996) Guidelines on artificial nutrition versus hydration in terminal cancer patients. *Nutrition*, 12(3): 163–7.

Field, D. (1989) *Nursing the Dying*. London: Tavistock/Routledge.

Field, D. (1996) Awareness and modern dying. *Mortality*, 1(3): 255–65.

Field, D., Hockey, J. and Small, N. (1997) *Death, Gender and Ethnicity*. London: Routledge.

General Medical Council (2002) *Withholding and Withdrawing Life-Prolonging Treatments: Good Practice in Decision-Making*. Guidance from the Standards Committee of the General Medical Council. London: GMC.

Gillick, M.R. (2000) Rethinking the role of tube feeding in patients with advanced dementia. *New England Journal of Medicine*, 342: 206–9.

Glaser, B. and Strauss, A. (1965) *Awareness of Dying*. Chicago, IL: Aldine.

Goodhall, L. (1997) Tube feeding dilemmas: can artificial nutrition and hydration be legally or ethically withheld or withdrawn? *Journal of Advanced Nursing*, 25(2): 217–22.

Hockey, J. (1990) *Experiences of Death: An Anthropological Account*. Edinburgh: Edinburgh University Press.

Hodgson, A. and Eden, O.B. (2003) 'Everything has changed': experiences of young people with recurrent or metastatic cancer. Paper presented to the *Palliative Care Research Society Annual Scientific Meeting*, Royal College of Physicians, Edinburgh, 25 June.

Holmes, S. (1998) The challenge of providing nutritional support to the dying. *International Journal of Palliative Care Nursing*, 4(1): 26–31.

Hopkins, P.D. (1997) Why does removing machines count as 'passive' euthanasia? *Hastings Center Report*, 27: 29–37.

House of Lords (1993–94) *Report of the Select Committee on Medical Ethics* (HL Paper 21-I). London: HMSO.

Huxtable, R. and Campbell, A.V. (2003) The position statement and its commentators: consensus, compromise or confusion? *Palliative Medicine*, 17: 180–3.

Jennett, B. (1995) High technology therapies and older people. *Ageing and Society*, 15(2): 185–98.

Kaufman, S. (2003) Hidden places, uncommon persons. *Social Science and Medicine*, 56: 2249–61.

Kedziera, P. (2001) Hydration, thirst and nutrition, in B.R. Ferrell and N. Coyle (eds) *Textbook of Palliative Nursing*. Oxford: Oxford University Press.

Kellehear, A. (1990) *Dying of Cancer: The Final Year of Life*. Reading, PA: Harwood Academic.

Kiger, A.M. (1994) Student nurses' involvement with death: the image and the experience. *Journal of Advanced Nursing*, 20: 679–86.

Lawton, J (2000) *The Dying Process: Patients' Experiences of Palliative Care*. London: Routledge.

Le Fanu, J. (1999) *The Rise and Fall of Modern Medicine*. London: Little, Brown & Company.

Leming, M.R. and Dickenson, G.E. (2002) *Understanding Death, Dying and Bereavement*. Fort Worth, TX: Harcourt College Publishers.

Lofland, L. (1978) *The Craft of Dying*. Beverley Hills, CA: Sage.

Maeve, M.K. (1998) Weaving a fabric of moral meaning: how nurses live with suffering and death. *Journal of Advanced Nursing*, 27(2): 1136–42.

Materstvedt, L.J., Clark, D., Ellershaw, J. *et al.* (2003) Euthanasia and physician assisted suicide: a view from an EAPC Ethics Task Force. *Palliative Medicine*, 17(2): 97–101 (discussion 102–79).

McNamara, B. (1997) A good enough death? Paper presented to the *Third International Social Context of Death, Dying and Disposal. Conference*, Cardiff, April.

Meier, D.E., Ahronheim, J.C., Morris, J., Baskin-Lyons, S. and Morrison, R.S. (2001) High short-term mortality in hospitalised patients with advanced dementia: lack of benefit of tube feeding. *Archives of Internal Medicine*, 161(4): 594–9.

Mitchell, S.L., Kiely, D.K. and Lipsitz, L.A. (1997) The risk factors and impact on survival of feeding tube placement in nursing home residents with severe cognitive impairment. *Archives of Internal Medicine*, 157: 327–32.

Mulkay, M. (1993) Social death in Britain, in D. Clark (ed.) *The Sociology of Death*. Oxford: Blackwell/The Sociological Review.

Murray, S.A., Grant, E., Grant, A. and Kendall, M. (2003) Dying from cancer in developed and developing countries: lessons from two qualitative interview studies of patients and their carers. *British Medical Journal*, 7385: 326–68.

National Council for Hospice and Specialist Palliative Care Services and the Ethics Committee of the Association for Palliative Medicine of Great Britain and Ireland (1997) *Ethical Decision Making in Palliative Care: Artificial Hydration for People Who are Terminally Ill*. London: NCHSPCS.

Nolan, M., Grant, G. and Keady, J. (1996) *Understanding Family Care*. Buckingham: Open University Press.

Pabst-Battin, M. (1994) *The Least Worst Death: Essays in Bioethics on the End of Life*. Oxford: Oxford University Press.

Peck, A., Cohen, C.E. and Mulvihill, M.N. (1990) Long-term enteral feeding of aged demented nursing home patients. *Journal of the American Geriatric Society*, 38: 1195–8.

Quint, J.C. (1967) *The Nurse and the Dying Patient*. New York: Macmillan.

Roy, D.J. and MacDonald, N. (1998) Ethical issues in palliative care, in D. Doyle, G.W.C. Hanks and N. MacDonald (eds) *Oxford Textbook of Palliative Care*. Oxford: Oxford University Press.

Roy, D.J. and Rapin, C.-H. (1994) The EAPC Board of Directors: regarding euthanasia. *European Journal of Palliative Care*, 1: 57–9.

Saunders, J.M. and Valente, S.M. (1994) Nurses' grief. *Cancer Nursing*, 17: 318–25.

Seymour, J.E. (2001) *Critical Moments: Death and Dying in Intensive Care*. Buckingham: Open University Press.

Seymour, J.E. (2002) Artificial feeding at the end of life: older people's understandings, in C. Gastmans (ed.) *Between Technology and Humanity: The Impact of New Technologies on Health Care Ethics*. Brussels: Leuven University Press.

Shaw, A.B. (1995) Acts of commission, omission and demission or pulling the plug. *Journal of the Royal Society of Medicine*, 88: 18–19.

Singer, P. (1994) *Rethinking Life and Death: The Collapse of Our Traditional Ethics*. Oxford: Oxford University Press.

Singer, P. (2000) Recent advances in medical ethics. *British Medical Journal*, 321: 282–5.

SUPPORT Principal Investigators (1995) A controlled trial to improve care for seriously ill hospitalized patients: the study to understand prognoses and preferences for outcomes and risks of treatment (SUPPORT). *Journal of the American Medical Association*, 174: 1591–8.

ten Have, H. and Clark, D. (eds) (2002) *The Ethics of Palliative Care: European Perspectives*. Buckingham: Open University Press.

Turner, B.S. (1996) *The Body and Society*. London: Sage.

Twycross, R.G. (1995) Where there is hope, there is life: a view from the hospice, in J. Keown (ed.) *Euthanasia Examined: Ethical, Clinical and Legal Perspectives*. Cambridge: Cambridge University Press.

Viola, R.A., Wells, G.A. and Peterson, J. (1997) The effects of fluid status and fluid therapy on the dying: a systematic review. *Journal of Palliative Care*, 13(4): 41–52.

Walter, T. (1997) The ideology and organization of spiritual care: three approaches. *Palliative Medicine*, 11(1): 21–30.

Wong, F.K.Y. (2001) Educating nurses to care for the dying in Hong Kong: a problem based learning approach. *Cancer Nursing*, 24(2): 112–21.

11

Good for the soul?

The spiritual dimension of hospice and palliative care

Michael Wright

Confronting mortality in the face of approaching death may be a deeply disturbing experience (Ainsworth-Smith and Speck 1999; Lawton 2000). Yet amidst the imminence of separation and the disintegration of self, a well-spring of spiritual activity may frequently be found. In this chapter, I address such activity from three perspectives: the conceptual perspective, the patient and family perspective and the institutional perspective. I will show that as dying patients address their spiritual and religious needs, health professionals have an opportunity to play a vital and supportive role. Where appropriate, data will be presented from a doctoral study[1] undertaken by the author between 1998 and 2001 (Wright 2001a).

The conceptual perspective

Background

When Cicely Saunders founded St Christopher's Hospice (Sydenham) in 1967, she sought to recapture the spirit of the former Christian 'hospices', welcoming the sick and performing the works of mercy found in Matthew 25 verses 35 and 36[2] (Saunders 1986). At this time, her evangelical zeal was probably at its highest. In a letter to the Reverend Bruce Reed, she tellingly wrote: 'I long to bring patients to know the Lord' (Clark 1998: 50). Yet Dr Saunders did not establish a religious community, preferring instead to pioneer a new pattern of relationships exemplified by the multidisciplinary team.

As hospice philosophy developed, however, questions came to be asked about its religious foundations. Was the Christian perspective part of the essence of hospice, or did it merely provide a motivating force among like-minded pioneers? The debate surrounding these questions was influenced by three factors: the establishment of palliative care, a changing pattern of religious observance and the emergence of spirituality as a discrete phenomenon.

The introduction of palliative care was interpreted as a shift in emphasis away from the religious towards the secular (Maddocks 1997: 196). This shift caused misgivings among those who perceived 'a profound ideological rejection of the traditional understanding of the spiritual dimension of care, exemplified by Cicely Saunders' (Bradshaw 1996: 415). As the National Health Service opened its door to palliative medicine, so religiously based principles encapsulated within 'aim and basis' statements of hospices like St Christopher's[3] came to be regarded as institution-specific rather than generalizable. Alongside these changing perceptions, a universal register acknowledging 'human dignity' and 'quality of life' began to replace the religiously invested language of 'sympathy', 'love' and 'sanctity of life' (ten Have and Clark 2002: 6).

Currently, fewer people in Europe seem inclined to become religious. A survey (Gallup 1999) of 50,000 people across 60 countries found that only 20 per cent of respondents in Western Europe and 14 per cent in Eastern Europe worship on a weekly basis. In Britain, this figure has been estimated at 8 per cent (Brierley 1999), prompting concerns about the future of redundant churches (Churches Conservation Trust 2002).[4] Yet research undertaken by Davie (1994) indicates that beliefs have not been discarded. In her study of religion in Britain since 1945, seven out of ten adults claimed to believe in God, leading her to identify a contemporary population 'believing without belonging'.

Paradoxically, as religious observance has declined, interest in the spiritual has increased, producing a form of spirituality that has become dislocated from religion. The term 'spirituality' has its roots in seventeenth-century France, where it was used pejoratively to describe a form of contemplation (Wakefield 1993). Today's 'religion-free' spirituality is frequently associated with the New Age movement and its related ecological and feminist philosophies. Dictionary definitions relate 'spirituality' to its root, 'spirit', locating it within the non-physical aspects of humankind. Seen as a universal human attribute, spirituality has come to be regarded as somehow 'purer' than religion: further 'upstream', freer to access and more personally relevant.[5] As a result, formal religion waxes and wanes against a backdrop of a folk spirituality that intermittently emerges in the symbols and rituals formed around catastrophic events or personal tragedies[6] (Percy 2000).

This relational, ontologically based perception of spirituality has found a ready acceptance within health care (Stoll 1989; Stoter 1991; Department of Health 1992; Harrison 1993; Ross 1994; Elsdon 1995; NHS Executive 1995; NAHAT 1996; Harrison 1997; Ronaldson 1997; Speck 1998; Jewell 1999; Aldridge 2000). Nevertheless, it remains a contested area. Markham (1998) points to the strong association between spirituality and Christianity, and suggests that the term may not be recognized equally by other religious traditions. Pattison (2001) focuses upon a lack of conceptual clarity, causing him to liken spirituality to 'intellectual Polyfilla, changing shape and content conveniently to fill the space its users devise for it' (p. 37).

Meaning of spirituality

In the light of these divergent views, I conducted a phenomenological enquiry designed to identify the meaning of spirituality among a sample of spiritual care stakeholders.[1] Participants included representatives of major world faiths and those of no faith, who nonetheless regarded themselves as spiritual. Based on the philosophy of Husserl (1962) and later developed by Heidegger (1962) and Merleau-Ponty (1962), phenomenology seeks to describe the meaning of a phenomenon through the lived experience of human beings. Such approaches have been used both in health care research (Reiman 1986; Styles 1994; Hallorsdottir and Hamrin 1996) and in enquiries into the essence of religious experience (Otto [1902] 1968; Buber 1970). For these reasons, I considered the approach to be relevant to this study. A summary of interviewee perceptions is shown in Table 11.1.

An analysis of these perceptions produced the following taxonomy:

- *Personhood*: values, beliefs, achievements.
- *Relationships*: with self, others, the universe, a 'life force' or God.
- *Religion*: prayer, vocation, commitment and worship.

Table 11.1   Spiritual care stakeholders' perceptions of spirituality

1   All people are spiritual beings; spirituality recognizes each individual as a unique person
2   Spirituality is a life orientation shaped by culture and history, incorporating values and beliefs, practices, customs and ritual
3   Spirituality is about understanding suffering, preparing to die and letting go
4   Spirituality is like being on fire; all that's possible is flowing and quickening
5   Spirituality is being at one with the universe and in touch with nature and creation
6   Spirituality is concerned with something other than just the body; it is concerned with feelings, relationships, personal awareness and the mystery of our understanding of ourselves
7   Spirituality is concerned with the soul and its link with the spirit
8   Being spiritual is not the same as being religious
9   Spirituality can be expressed religiously or non-religiously
10   Spirituality is a submission to the commands of God
11   Spirituality is related to God's call and to the effects of that call
12   Christian spirituality orientates towards a life that is linked to the Holy Spirit and is patterned by Christ
13   Spirituality is expressed in worship, devotion and prayer
14   Spirituality is about questing and searching – that journey, that struggle – addressing the big questions of life, death, another life and the universe
15   Spirituality is an awakening to life and a focus upon the meaning, direction, purpose and achievements of individual lives
16   Spirituality is concerned with the intangibility of transcendence and the tuning in to something both beyond and within, something deeper, something wider
17   Spirituality is being aware of a life force – sometimes called 'God'

- *Search for meaning*: the 'big questions' of life and death, mortality.
- *Transcendence*: something beyond/something within.

A striking feature of this study is that 'spirituality' was meaningful to all of the participants, indicating an element of commonality. The conclusion may be drawn, therefore, that whatever the differences of faith (or lack of it), the term had assumed potency in the lived experience of this group of stakeholders.

Model of the spiritual domain

The above typology is emblematic of the range of perceptions summarized in the following model of the spiritual domain (Figure 11.1). This inclusive, overarching model recognizes that spirituality may be expressed *both* religiously *and* humanistically. It acknowledges dimensions of 'self', 'others' and the 'cosmos', the importance of the big questions of life and death, and the spiritually-related activities of becoming, connecting, finding meaning and transcending.

In some instances, religion and spirituality have become inseparable, providing the faithful with an all-encompassing vehicle to encounter the mysteries of their life, their relationships and their death (Butler and Butler 1996). The hospice ideal has come to interface with a broad spectrum of faiths prompting profound religious debate. Central to this debate is the recognition of shared values. In her study of the Koruna Hospice Service in Australia, McGrath (1998) notes how the Buddhist metaphysic resonates with the ethos of hospice, apparent in the concept of universal compassion. Within Judaism, a common purpose has been found between hospice philosophy and Jewish spirituality: to cherish each moment of a person's life

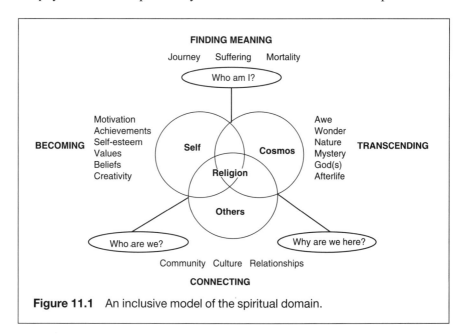

Figure 11.1   An inclusive model of the spiritual domain.

(Hegedus 2002); so too in Saudi Arabia with its strong Islamic culture and the submission of its people to the will of God (Gray *et al.* 1997); and in Hong Kong, with its diverse religious practices and differing approaches to death (Chung 1997). Christian spirituality is exemplified by the establishment of hospices with a Christian foundation,[7] and expressed through organizations such as St Columba's Fellowship (England),[8] the Sisterhood of St Elizabeth (Russia)[9] and the Sisters of Charity (global).[10] In its many forms, the religious articulation of hospice continues to feature prominently, both internationally and in Britain.

The spiritual activity of becoming centres on the unfolding life involving reflection, creativity and a sense of who one is (Ferrucci 1993). Within this activity are a number of discreet models, including:

- *Developmental models*: founded on the premise that as there are stages in physical growth, so there are stages in spiritual growth (Scott Peck 1987).
- *Needs-based models*: suggesting that human beings have a need for meaning, purpose and fulfilment in life (Renetzky 1979).
- *Values-based models*: associated with the 'ultimate' values of love, truth, forgiveness and reconciliation (Stoll 1989).
- *Personhood models*: relating to that which characterizes human beings – embodiment, cognition, the emotions and relationships (Wilson 1999).

Spirituality has become associated with connectedness, where meaning and fulfilment are found in loving relationships (Burkhardt 1994). In essence, the spiritual life is a community life (Erricker and Erricker 2001), a life with opportunities for belonging through the vehicles of language, ritual and art (Helman 1990). Within the activity of connecting, relationship and cultural models are especially relevant. Relationship models are exemplified by the notion of 'being there', an activity that involves sharing the patient's space, hopes and fears (Speck 1995). Cultural models occur at both macro and micro levels. Hervieu-Léger's (2000) notion of a chain of memory connecting past, present and future members of a community typifies the macro model. In this case, it has relevance to the care of the dying, and has parallels with the growing interest in patient-centred care shown during the last decade by countries of the former Soviet Union.[11] Rights of passage associated with hospice admission procedures exemplify the micro level. These procedures contextualize a ritual entry into a unique space – described as sacred and transitional – as people cross boundaries between one status and another (Froggatt 1997).

In the West, finding meaning has come to be regarded as a central feature of spirituality, due partly to the influence of Viktor Frankl (1959), a Holocaust survivor who formed the view that the purpose of human beings is not to avoid pain but to find a meaning in life. Metaphors of journey acknowledge the impact of illness upon the individual, likening the search for meaning to a sacred quest to discover the mysteries of life (Hawkins 1999). On this journey, suffering and mortality occupy a special place. The journey into death is considered by some to be the ultimate vehicle for spiritual discovery (Singh 1999).

Transcending the self has been described as 'going beyond', an action or state of being that exceeds the usual limits of human experience (Page 1995). It may be associated with a sense of awe and wonder in the presence of mystery and the beauty of nature, prompting questions about the existence of a creator and life after death. Within health care, writers frequently favour the 'vertical' idea of transcendent space: a dualist world-view in the Cartesian tradition that regards the natural and supernatural as essentially different from one another (Harrison 1993). Gill (1989: 3) argues for a re-thought, postmodern view of 'mediated transcendence' – a phenomenon whereby intangible reality can be encountered *in and through* the particulars of tangible reality. This fusion of the tangible and intangible suggests the possibility of fresh insights into patient transcendence and resonates with Kellehear's (2000) pragmatic view that transcendence may be achieved by searching for meanings in situations, in moral or biographical contexts and in religious beliefs.

A hospice nurse, drawn to the Buddhist tradition, explains how a broad view of spirituality has become integrated into his clinical practice:

> It's about caring for the person – whether it's going back after a while to ask whether the pain is less, or sitting with somebody whilst they cry or they laugh. It's about being able to engage in the big questions with people, things like: 'why is this happening to me?' – enabling them to talk about their fears and anxieties about the process of dying, and what will happen to them as well as to those who are left behind. For some people, it's about supporting them in trying to leave things, or say things, or do things, which they feel are important to leave or say or do before they die. It's trying to listen to people properly. Where possible, we try and let people tell us how they want things to be, and we try and make it be that way. I also think it's important that when a person can't communicate with us any more as themselves, that we continue to respect them as themselves up to the point at which they die.[12]

A postmodern description of the spiritual domain might liken it to a diamond, its multiple facets revealed or concealed depending on the viewer's angle of observation. At best, inclusive models resonate with concepts of holism and the values of acceptance and non-judgemental compassion. Such models recognize that among patients drawn from pluralistic societies, there is no single spiritual source but multiple explorations, multiple interpretations and multiple expressions.

Reflection

- How would you define spirituality?
- What influences shape your own spirituality?
- How do you become aware of the spiritual impact of the dying process on each individual patient?
- What barriers might be created by your own spiritual perceptions when dealing with the spiritual diversity of patients and their families?

Patient and family perspectives

Patient narratives

The spiritual needs of patients relate in no small part to their encounter with their illness. Within a whole-life context, these needs are grounded in the successes, failures, hopes and dreams of individual biographies. A feature of the late twentieth century has been the willingness of patients and relatives to reveal their experience of illness and what it has come to mean (Diamond 1998). In 1996, when journalist Ruth Picardie was diagnosed with breast cancer, she wrote a series of articles for *Observer Life* that gave the public insights into her deteriorating condition. What hurt most, she said, was losing the future: not being there to clap when her babies learnt to write or to kiss their knees when they fell off their bikes (Picardie 1998: 58).

The dimension of loss is an inescapable feature of illness, highlighted by admission to a health care institution that in itself bears witness to a loss of lifestyle and social status (Kleinman 1988; Ainsworth-Smith and Speck 1999). Vanstone (1982) notes how illness results in a change in outlook, increasing isolation and transition from activity to passivity. Such losses impact upon the dying patient (Nuland 1997), each loss bearing witness to the incremental dismantling of personhood (Rose 1996).[13]

Underpinning these losses is what may be termed woundedness. Arthur Frank (1995), a cancer survivor, notes how the wounded hip of Jacob authenticates the story of his biblical struggle with an angel (Genesis 32: 24–26). In essence, Frank regards the patient as a wounded storyteller, a raconteur whose wounds are emblematic of the story's potency. In this scenario, storytelling becomes a vehicle for recovering the voice which has been silenced by illness; a means of reclaiming power after diagnosis through the knowledge that an individual's story is both worth the telling and worthy of being heard.

Patient requirements

In the summer of 1999, I conducted a survey of hospices and hospital trusts in England and Wales to discover chaplains' perceptions of the most frequently expressed religious and non-religious requirements of patients.[1] Eighty-nine per cent of respondents in both groups indicated that patients most frequently require somebody to listen to them; someone to 'be there' followed closely behind. Hospital patients most frequently wish to discuss their concern for relatives, pain and death and dying; hospice patients wish to discuss their concern for relatives, suffering and death and dying. Of the activities of the Christian faith, patients within both hospice and hospital most frequently wish to receive communion, to pray and to worship (Table 11.2).

Interview data from a multiple case study in four health settings – analysed according to an adaptation of Kellehear's model of spiritual needs –

Table 11.2 Chaplains' perceptions of the most frequent spiritual requirements of patients

	Hospital		Hospice	
	n	*%*	*n*	*%*
Non-religious requirements				
Someone to listen	103	89	128	89
Someone to 'be there'	100	86	106	74
Spiritual issues				
Why me?	43	37	81	56
Pain	81	71	81	57
Meaning of life	36	32	51	36
Value of one's own life	51	45	53	37
Suffering	51	44	84	58
Forgiveness	13	11	16	11
Transcendence	5	5	6	4
The nature of God	15	13	26	18
Concern for relatives	102	88	116	81
Death and dying	79	69	83	58
Afterlife	22	19	24	17
Religious requirements				
Prayer	49	43	88	61
Texts	3	3	16	11
Worship	25	22	51	36
Special rituals	9	8	39	28
Baptism	0	0	11	8
Confession/absolution	7	6	6	4
Communion	51	44	94	65
Anointing	10	9	19	13
Last rites	15	14	42	30

provide insights into the individual requirements of patients.[1] Within the category of 'situational transcendence', indicators of hope and connectedness were found among all ten patients. Some hopes relate to the patient's condition or for a return to normality by going home. Amanda voiced her hope for a painless death. She felt neglected by the medical profession and, as her symptoms remained uncontrolled, both she and her family had pressed for treatment. 'I don't have to fight anymore. I hope it's not painful, that's the only thing I'm worried about, but apart from that – just a painless death.'

Connectedness focused mainly upon friends and family. Social presence featured prominently for seven patients, with nurses playing a key role. The opportunity to talk was seen to be advantageous. Christine has cancer of the rectum. Reflecting upon her life, she found many regrets: leaving her husband, entering an unfulfilling relationship and losing all contact with her children. Yet as her illness progressed, Christine's relationship with her daughter improved, to her great joy. 'I could never show [my daughter] me feelings, but this last fortnight when she's 'phoned I've told her I love her, and I've come to accept what a wonderful daughter I've got.'

Within the moral and biographical category, nine patients believed in God or a 'larger being', although all of them strongly claimed to be 'not religious'. Seven patients sought transcendence through prayer, three patients admitting to daily prayer and one patient to 'praying all the time'. Christine says, 'I just pray to God. I don't go to church, but I pray to God every morning and every evening. Just because I don't go to Church it doesn't mean to say I don't believe in him, because I would say he giveth and he taketh.'

Despite nine patients describing themselves as 'not religious', eight displayed evidence of religious needs and three gave indications of divine support. Religious leaders played a significant role for three patients and two patients focused upon an afterlife. Hettie is a widow whose daughters live abroad, causing her to feel isolated and lonely. To her surprise, she found unexpected strength when she was moved to the ward where her husband had died. She felt close to him and looked forward to joining him in an afterlife. 'I believe there's something there, somewhere. My husband died in this hospital and I've said to him many times, "ne'er mind lad, I'll be there with you before long, I've just this and that to see to". Then, sometimes, a day like today, I've thought: Oh I wish it were today!'

Only one patient, Jasmine – a Jehovah's Witness – considered herself to be religious. Although she was shocked by her cancer diagnosis, Jasmine received constant support from members of her family and congregation who visited frequently to pray with her. Jasmine professed a deep, personal faith and recounted an unusual experience of God: 'when I were praying to him, I put my hand over the trolley when I were going to theatre, and in my mind, because my faith was so strong, he was holding my hand'.

Relative narratives

In their ground-breaking article,[14] Rosemary and Victor Zorza (1978) tell how their daughter, Jane, developed a painful melanoma and was admitted to an Oxford hospice where she died 8 days later. She was 25 years old. Surprised by the change in Jane's demeanour after admission and charged with the task of making her last days happy, the Zorzas write as follows:

> As things worked out, the time of greatest suffering was when the doctors were refusing to tell her what her chances of survival were. Once she was told . . . there was no great anguished sobbing, but a sad, resigned little sigh, almost of relief, and just a few tears. 'Now that I know, she said, I want to enjoy every day I have left and I want to be happy, and I want you to help me to be happy.'
>
> (Zorza and Zorza 1978)

Against the backdrop of cancer, a source of happiness for both Jane and her parents was her new-found ability to transcend the disease and rediscover the presence of beauty: in music, in the sunset, in the flowers she wore in her hair. Victor recalls a poignant moment. 'One morning, I had put on a Mozart tape for her, just as she was waking up. She slowly opened her eyes, listened with obvious enjoyment for a few minutes and glanced at me . . . "How beautiful you are making it for me to die" she said slowly' (Zorza and Zorza 1978).

More recently, Grinyer (2002) has provided a telling account of 28 young adults seen from their parents' perspectives as they encounter illness and, in some cases, death. Serious issues emerge, such as the tension between dependence and independence and the loss of a child on the threshold of adulthood. Spiritual issues figure prominently. George is a case in point. As his physical strength decreased, his spirituality increased, becoming a source of strength not only for himself but also for his mother. Finding meaning in the spiritual domain is important for both patients and relatives. Referring to George and her own son, Alexander, Denise C ascribes a greater meaning to their deaths – and lives – when she says, 'I do believe that our respective sons must have been so very special in God's eyes that he handpicked them for greater works' (Grinyer 2002: 158).

For those with a religious faith, having beliefs and belonging to a Church can provide powerful support. Anne says: 'another lifeline for me has been my local church who have all been very supportive. I think my belief in an afterlife has got me through some very dark days' (Grinyer 2002: 158).

Yet religious beliefs may also be problematic. Turning to data from my doctoral study,[1] Karen comes from a Roman Catholic family and has lived with her partner, Arthur, for 14 years. Arthur has cancer of the bladder and has been admitted to a hospice. In the following extract, Karen indicates some pressures arising from her religious background:

> I met Arthur just about 15 years ago, and I was – yes, I was divorced by that time. We never really wanted to get married because we felt that, I suppose, our relationship was OK as it was, and I'd been married, and – I'm steeped in Catholicism, that's the first thing, steeped in it – I don't practise now, although I do – well, we've just had a family party, and our family parties always start with mass – so it's still very much part of my family. How did I get on to that? So there was quite a lot of pressure to marry, and I suppose me mum still thinks that I committed adultery or something. There are loads of things I don't like about religion, but, if you say 'am I religious?', I'm not sure really, 'cos it's quite a comfort to think of God.

David is 92 years old and has prostate cancer. His daughter, Annette, says that having experienced the death of her grandmother, she is able to cope with her father and accept him as he is on any one day. She finds it helpful to 'just get on with life'. A non-churchgoer, she resorts to prayer in a crisis: 'I pray if father's not so good, or if there's – my younger daughter unfortunately got married and the marriage was over within a fortnight of the honeymoon; so something like that, but otherwise, not particularly.'

June is anxious about her mother, who has cancer. Having seen her father die from the same disease, she worries constantly and succumbs to sudden changes of mood. An ambivalent attitude towards her mother's prognosis prompts a sense of guilt: 'Part of me wants her to get on with her life and the other part of me wants it to be over. Yeah. I then think "stop being so selfish", you know, and then I start feeling guilty for wanting it to be over.'

In the context of woundedness and loss, the narrative of illness places mortality centre stage, prompting an increase in spiritual activity for both patients and relatives. Despite the risk of a lost faith, there is also the possibility that faith may be strengthened. Remarkably, many patients who describe themselves as 'not religious' believe in God and pray daily. Not churchgoers, they have nevertheless rediscovered the language and imagery of the Church, in some cases learnt during childhood. In effect, a familiar landscape has emerged as patients move towards the end of their lives. This pentimento (Denzin 1989), or re-appearance, has been likened to that within a painting, where shadows of previously drawn lines gradually come to the surface to provide an insight into a once obscured domain.

Reflection

- What do you consider to be the most frequently required religious and non-religious spiritual requirements of patients?

- How would you respond to a patient who claimed to be 'not religious' but wanted to talk about God, prayer or an afterlife?

- What would you say to a patient who asked you what it is like to die?

- How would you respond to a relative who felt guilty for 'wanting it to be over'?

| Institutional perspectives

Historical links between caring for the sick and the work of religious orders were incorporated into the British National Health Service (NHS) in 1948 when the Ministry of Health advised hospital authorities to provide spiritual care by appointing paid chaplains from different traditions. Further guidance (NHS 1948) advised authorities to establish a chapel and arrange schedules so that nurses and others could attend services of their denomination. By the close of the twentieth century, the religious climate had changed. Reflecting the multicultural nature of contemporary society, the *Patient's Charter* (Department of Health 1991) set a national standard regarding respect for religious and cultural beliefs. New guidance (Department of Health 1992) advised the NHS to recognize the needs of both

Christians and non-Christians. Managers now face the complex task of providing spiritual care across a range of religious traditions and none (Cobb 2001).

Responses from a survey conducted in 1999 show that 56 (40 per cent) hospitals and 62 (57 per cent) hospices had published a policy statement on spiritual care. Multifaith guidelines were in place in 124 (86 per cent) hospitals and 64 (60 per cent) hospices. Within the hospitals, 73 (29 per cent) chapels and 86 (91 per cent) multifaith rooms opened during the 1990s. During the same period, 41 (44 per cent) chapels and 16 (55 per cent) multifaith rooms opened in hospices. Within hospitals, all chaplaincies were funded within a range of 30 to 368 hours per week; 98 per cent of these hours were allocated to Christians. Within hospices, 72 per cent of chaplaincies were funded within a range of 3 to 88 hours per week; 99.5 per cent of these hours were allocated to Christians. These figures suggest that in England and Wales:

- spiritual care is not fully integrated at the policy level of hospitals and hospices;

- although multifaith guidelines were in place in most hospitals, they were lacking in 40 per cent of hospices;

- a changing religious landscape was reflected in the establishment of multifaith rooms within both types of institution;

- funded chaplaincy is almost exclusively Christian.[15]

At the unit level, both hospitals and hospices attempt to inform patients of their spiritual care provision. Methods range from the publication of newsletters and information packs to the use of videotape played on strategically placed monitors. In a bedside leaflet, a chaplaincy department was introduced as follows:

> The name 'chaplaincy' derives from the Latin word *cappella*, which means 'cloak'. As human beings we are called to serve one another, to bring a touch of comfort, healing and strength. The symbol of chaplaincy in this Hospital Trust is of one person holding another by the hand, while both are enfolded, or cloaked, within the love and protection of God.

Identification of spiritual needs

Survey responses from 97 (71 per cent) trusts and 102 (88 per cent) hospices indicate that an assessment was made of spiritual needs. Around three-quarters of hospices include items about worship, sacraments and preferences for a minister; fewer than half of the hospitals include these items. Spiritual assessments are complex, however, illustrated perhaps by their absence in 29 per cent of hospitals and 12 per cent of hospices. The National Health Service Executive Northern and Yorkshire Chaplains and

Pastoral Care Committee (1995) suggests that a patient's spiritual needs should be assessed during an interview conducted shortly after admission. Attention would focus on the interface between religion and health care; information would be collected on the patient's religious and cultural requirements and, if appropriate, there may be an exploration of the patient's wishes in the event of death.

Questions arise about what is being assessed. A record of patient wishes surrounding worship, diet or ritual washing may be seen as a note of spiritual *behaviours* rather than an assessment of spiritual *needs*. Cobb (1998) suggests that Bradshaw's taxonomy of social need – normative need, felt need, expressed need and comparative need – helps to illuminate the issues for both patients and health professionals. Difficult to assess, however, are the elusive 'felt needs': the need for meaning, purpose and fulfilment in life.

A variety of measures are currently used within the spiritual domain. Stoll (1979) set the scene when she published her spiritual history guide. Using in-depth interviews, data were gathered concerning the patient's concept of God, sources of strength, and perceptions regarding the relationship between spiritual beliefs and health status. Other measures have come to rely heavily on interview techniques, together with the skills of discernment when being with, observing or listening to a patient (Hay 1989; Emblem and Halstead 1993; King *et al.* 1995; NAHAT 1996). The relationship between spirituality and well-being has received increasing attention since Paloutzian and Ellison (1982) developed their Spiritual Well Being Scale in the early 1980s. Similar measures include the JAREL Spiritual Well Being Scale (Hungelmann *et al.* 1996) and the Spiritual Perspective Scale (Reed 1987). In the quality of life arena, existential issues have been included in the McGill Quality of Life Questionnaire (Cohen *et al.* 1996) and in Wyatt and Friedman's (1996) quality of life model for long-term survivors of breast cancer. At present, a spiritual well-being module is currently being developed in Europe under the auspices of the European Organization for Research and Treatment of Cancer Quality of Life Study Group (Vivat and Young 2002).

The case study discovered that institutions were using both formal and informal means to identify spiritual needs. All units encouraged patients to make their own needs known, which was very important in the case of the acute hospital with 1000 beds. Common to all institutions was a formal checklist, used to gather information around admission. Supplementary assessments and patient reviews figured prominently in both settings. Informal means encompassed a receptiveness to patient questions, observing the patient's demeanour and obtaining the perceptions of relatives.

Spiritual care

Institutions deliver spiritual care in various ways. Physical resources such as chapels, quiet rooms and prayer rooms, together with facilities for viewing and handling the dead, have a part to play. Alongside these physical resources is the need for human resources: chaplains, chaplaincy volunteers and local faith leaders. In some institutions, opportunities for worship and the celebration of world-faith festivals form part of a religious calendar; so, too, do broadcast services, guided reflection, meditation and prayer, accompanied by opportunities for the occasional baptism, marriage and funeral service.

A key factor within spiritual care provision is the expertise of staff and the creation of a spiritual ethos. Attempts to meet a diverse range of spiritual needs contribute to this ethos. In addition, good communication and notions of 'being there', 'sharing the patient's journey' and 'helping a person to find meaning' have the capacity to engage on a spiritual level. Ultimately, the activities of giving time and listening are crucial.

Spiritual care-givers

Traditionally, chaplains have assumed a special responsibility for spiritual care-giving. A comparison, however, of the chaplain's duties reported by the first Commission of the Hospital Chaplaincies Council (1951) and findings of the study reported in this chapter shows how the role has changed. While chaplains retain a core responsibility for conducting services and administering the sacraments, gone are any assumptions that every patient will receive a visit on their day of admission. Increasingly, chaplains are being asked to manage a broadly based spiritual care service, monitor activity, contribute to education, liaise with leaders of other faiths and manage – rather than become involved with – a bereavement service.

Historically, certain groups who care for the sick have acknowledged the place of spirituality. Nursing is a case in point. Florence Nightingale was a committed Unitarian with a strong faith that caused her to regard nursing as a religious calling. Today, evidence remains of this tradition (Carson 1989; Fry 1997). Theorists such as Watson (1974) advise nurses to create a supportive spiritual environment and Abdella seeks to facilitate progress towards the patient's spiritual goals (Abdella *et al.* 1960). Among the grand nursing theories, the Roy's (1976) Adaptation Model and the Neuman's (1995) Systems Model both identify the place of the spiritual self. Significantly, Travelbee (1971) regards suffering as a spiritual encounter.

In 1984, the UK Central Council for Nursing, Midwifery and Health Visiting (UKCC) considered it a nurse's duty to take account of the customs, values and spiritual beliefs of patients. This view became incorporated into Project 2000, a new basic training programme designed to produce a different type of nurse – a 'knowledgeable doer' more actively involved in the delivery of care. One element of this course was the provision of student opportunities to identify the spiritual needs of patients and devise a plan of care (UKCC 1986).

Despite suggestions that nurses find the concept of spirituality less than meaningful and experience discomfort within the spiritual domain (Narayanasamy 1993; Golberg 1998); the burgeoning literature on spirituality and nursing suggests a growing interest (Bollwinkel 1994; Elsdon 1995; Ross

1995; Halstead and Mickley 1997; Mickley *et al.* 1998). Within the case studies I undertook, spiritually aware nurses were found in all institutions. Typical of nurses' responses is the following: 'I always did equate spirituality with religion, you know, religious beliefs and that, until I came here [hospice]. Now my sort of thing is "What has my life been about? What is the meaning of life? Has it been worthwhile?" Those kind of questions'.

An analysis of patient contacts showed that all patients in all units had encounters with spiritually aware personnel (Table 11.3). In this instance, 'spiritually aware personnel' is taken to mean those members of staff or volunteers who have undertaken some form of professional training, either in-depth or at a basic level. This latter form is amplified by the following comment from a spiritual care director:

> Part of my role with staff in the non-clinical areas is around helping people to understand that they actually do contribute to the wellbeing of patients by how they receive them in reception, by how they present the food – the spiritual aspects of all that – and people need to be helped sometimes to see the connections.

In all cases, encounters with spiritually aware personnel included a Christian chaplain or chaplaincy volunteer whether or not patients professed the

Table 11.3   Patient encounters with spiritually aware personnel

	Patients									
	Hospice 1		Hospice 2				Hospital 1		Hospital 2	
	A	B	C	D	E	F	G	H	I	J
Recorded religion:	C/E	None	C/E	C/E	J	C/E	C/E	C/E	RC	JW
Practising/non-practising:	NP	NP	NP	NP	NP	NP	NP	NP	NP	P
Chaplain (Free Church)	•	•						•		
Chaplain (Roman Catholic)			•	•	•	•			•	
Chaplain (Church of England)							•		•	•
Chaplain (student)		•								
Chaplaincy volunteer			•	•	•	•	•	•	•	•
Visiting minister/elder					•				•	•
Visiting believers					•					•
Palliative care physician	•	•	•	•	•	•	•	•		
Nurse (palliative care specialist)	•	•	•	•	•	•	•	•		
Nurse (trained care of dying)	•	•	•	•	•	•	•	•	•	•
Nurse (unit trained)	•	•	•	•	•	•		•		
Health care assistant (unit trained)	•	•	•	•	•	•	•			
Social worker	•	•	•	•	•	•				
Support staff (receptionists, domestics)	•	•	•	•	•	•				
Care staff (personal faith)	•	•	•	•	•	•	•	•		

Abbreviations: C/E = Church of England, J = Jewish, RC = Roman Catholic, JW = Jehovah's Witness, NP = non-practising, P = practising.

Christian faith or regarded themselves as religious. In addition, Patient E received visits from the Rabbi, Patient J from the congregation of Jehovah's Witnesses, and Patient I from her Roman Catholic parish priest.

The separation of religion from spirituality has become a marked feature of current thought. Consequently, although the care-giving of chaplains may include a unique denominational role, a broader role that relates to the spiritual activities of transcending, finding meaning and connecting has come to attract a wider ownership: an ownership that includes the psychologist, the physician, the complementary therapist and the nurse. A consequence of this wider ownership has led to a patchwork of spiritually aware personnel. Some, such as chaplaincy volunteers, have a strong religious faith. Others have no faith, yet relate easily to the spiritual personhood of the confused – or routinely create privacy and accompaniment for the dying. They include staff whose spiritual awareness has been raised through in-depth education alongside those who have spent just a little time reflecting upon how their role contributes to the spiritual ethos of the institution; all in addition to chaplains and all found in the field. The contemporary challenge for those charged with spiritual care delivery is how to blend a cohesive team of spiritually aware personnel, drawn from disparate spiritual perspectives, which owns an inclusive vision and gently meets the patient with affirmation and compassion at the point of need.

Reflection

- Who are the spiritual care-givers in your institution?
- In what areas of spiritual care do you feel comfortable/uncomfortable?
- What are your training needs?
- How could spiritual assessment be further developed?

Conclusions

- The separation of religion from spirituality has become a marked feature of current thought.
- The narrative of illness places mortality centre stage, prompting an increase in spiritual activity for both patients and relatives.
- Many patients who describe themselves as 'not religious' believe in God and pray daily.
- A key factor of spiritual care provision is the expertise of staff and the creation of a spiritual ethos.
- Within the case studies I undertook, spiritually aware nurses were found in all institutions.
- An analysis of patient contacts showed that all patients in all units had encounters with spiritually aware personnel.

- Although the care-giving of chaplains may include a unique denominational role, a broader role that relates to the spiritual activities of transcending, finding meaning and connecting has come to attract a wider ownership: an ownership that includes the psychologist, the physician, the complementary therapist and the nurse.

- The contemporary challenge for those charged with spiritual care delivery is how to blend a cohesive team of spiritually aware personnel, drawn from disparate spiritual perspectives, which owns an inclusive vision and gently meets the patient with affirmation and compassion at the point of need.

Notes

1 The objectives of this study were to identify: the nature of spirituality; the means whereby spiritual needs are assessed and met; and the perceptions of spiritual care stakeholders, patients and relatives. A multi-method, three-phase design was used, incorporating:

(i) A survey by postal questionnaire of the views of chaplains in 151 hospices and 195 trusts in England and Wales. The survey's purpose was to discover chaplains' perceptions of the most frequently expressed religious and non-religious requirements of patients. Chaplains were selected as questionnaire recipients in view of their institutional responsibility for both religious and non-religious spiritual care. The response rate was 76 per cent (Wright 2001b).

(ii) A phenomenological enquiry into the spiritual care perceptions of palliative care stakeholders (defined here as people with experience of spiritual care-giving who had opportunities to influence praxis). Data were collected by means of semi-structured, recorded interviews with 16 participants who represented the Jewish, Christian, Hindu, Muslim and Buddhist traditions. Some held high office: as a rabbi, a bishop or an imam. Also included were individuals of no faith, who nonetheless regarded themselves as 'spiritual'. To ensure disparity, participants were selected using purposive sampling techniques. Backgrounds and length of service varied. Roles included: chief executive, manager, nurse, medical director, therapist, artist, chaplain and volunteer. Not everyone was born in Britain. The data were analysed using NUD*IST software (Wright 2002).

(iii) A multiple case study in four health settings. Purposive sampling techniques identified two hospices and their neighbouring acute hospitals. Data were collected from multiple sources by a variety of means. On each site, recorded interviews were conducted with the senior chaplain, a focus group of nurses, patients and, where possible, a matched relative. Approval to interview patients and their relatives was obtained from two local research ethics committees. Where transcripts have been used in this chapter, patients and relatives have been anonymized by the use of false names. Most of the patients were coming towards the end of their lives. In these circumstances, they were asked about their fears, their beliefs and their hopes. Both patient and relative interviews were treated as oral history and analysed according to what Denzin (1989) calls the biographical method. In addition, Kellehear's (2000) theoretical model of spiritual needs provided a framework within which the spiritual needs of patients could be articulated and analysed. Based on the premise that human beings have a desire to transcend their suffering and find meaning, Kellehear suggests that spiritual needs such as hope and connectedness may lead to 'situational transcendence'; the need for peace and prayer may lead to 'moral and biographical transcendence'; and the need for divine support, religious rites, and discussion about eternal life may lead to 'religious transcendence'. An adaptation of this framework saw the added dimension of belief in God – without any religious implications or membership of a faith community [Davie's (1994) 'believing without belonging'] – allocated to the moral and biographical category. Individual narratives displayed evidence of movement between theoretical categories.

2 'I was hungry and you gave me food, I was thirsty and you gave me drink, I was a stranger and you welcomed me, I was naked and you clothed me, I was sick and you visited me' (*The Bible*, Revised Standard Version 1952).

3 For example, 'St Christopher's was established and has grown as a Christian foundation, not simply in terms of its care, but from a belief that the God revealed in Christ shares the darkness of suffering and dying and has transformed the reality of death' (Saunders 1997: 7).

4 The Trust was previously known as the 'Redundant Churches Fund' and has in its care over 325 churches no longer needed for regular worship, all of which are of historic interest. The current report expresses concern that if the disengagement from institutional religion continues, the number of redundant churches will fall outside of the resources of the Trust.

5 Exemplified by the following statement: 'the first lesson that we should learn is that religion is a man-made institution, but Spirituality is given to us by the Creator' (Renault and Freake 1996: ix).

6 Consider, for example, the ritual and symbolism that developed after the Hillsbrough disaster or the death of Princess Diana.

7 Such as: Bethesda (Lutheran) Children's Hospice, Budapest (Hungary); Southwest Christian Hospice, Georgia (USA); Our Lady's Hospice, Lusaka (Zambia); Mary Potter (Little Company of Mary) Hospices in Wellington (New Zealand) and Korce (Albania); Haven of Hope (Hong Kong) and Caritas Christi ('Love of Christ') hospice in Kew (Australia).

8 Founded in 1986 and based in Windsor with Prue Clench as Director. Motto: 'A Christian presence in the Hospice Movement'. The Fellowship provides education and retreats for palliative care staff.

9 Based at Lakhta Hospice, St Petersburg, under the leadership of Elena Kabakova. Volunteers in the Russian Orthodox tradition provide a programme of educational, religious and material support for orphans whose parents have died in the hospice.

10 The Sisters of Charity were founded in Ireland by Mother Mary Aikenhead in 1815. They played a role in the care of the dying during the nineteenth century in England and Australia and during the twentieth century became established in Africa, North and South America and East Timor.

11 This represents a cultural change from Soviet ideology that regarded medicine as a means of maintaining the workforce (Field 2002).

12 From an interview with John Hunt, undertaken as part of the author's doctoral study.

13 Personhood has been described as a unique human dimension that is 'coherent,

bounded, individualised, intentional, the locus of thought, action and belief, the origin of its own actions, the beneficiary of a unique biography' (Rose 1996: 3).

14   This article was syndicated worldwide and received a reported mailbag of 10,000 letters. It was followed by a book, published in Britain 2 years later (Zorza and Zorza 1980).

15   It is also dominated by the Church of England. Within hospitals, 60 per cent of funded chaplaincy hours were allocated to Anglicans; within hospices, the figure was 70 per cent.

References

Abdella, F.G., Beland, I.L., Martin, A. and Matherny, R. (1960) *Patient-Centred Approaches to Nursing*. New York: Macmillan.

Ainsworth-Smith, I. and Speck, P. (1999) *Letting Go*. London: SPCK.

Aldridge, D. (2000) *Spirituality, Healing and Medicine: Return to the Silence*. London: Jessica Kingsley.

Bollwinkel, E.M. (1994) Role of spirituality in hospice care. *Annals of the Academy of Medicine, Singapore*, 23(2): 261–3.

Bradshaw, A. (1996) The spiritual dimension of hospice: the secularization of an ideal. *Social Science and Medicine*, 43(3): 409–19.

Brierley, P. (1999) *Religious Trends*. London: Marshall Pickering.

Buber, M. (1970) *I and Thou*. Edinburgh: T. & T. Clark.

Burkhardt, M.A. (1994) Becoming and connecting: elements of spirituality for women. *Holistic Nursing Practice*, 8(4): 12–21.

Butler, B. and Butler, T. (1996) *Just Spirituality in a World of Faiths*. London: Mowbray.

Carson, V.B. (1989) Spiritual development across the life span, in V.B. Carson (ed.) *Spiritual Dimensions of Nursing Practice*. Philadelphia, PA: W.B. Saunders.

Chung, L.S.T. (1997) The hospice movement in a Chinese society – a Hong Kong experience, in C. Saunders and R. Kastenbaum (eds) *Hospice Care on the International Scene*. New York: Springer.

Churches Conservation Trust (2002) *Heart and Identity: Report 2001–2002*. London: Churches Conservation Trust.

Clark, D. (1998) Originating a movement: Cicely Saunders and the development of St Christopher's Hospice, 1957–1967. *Mortality*, 3(1): 43–63.

Cobb, M. (1998) Assessing spiritual need: an examination of practice, in M. Cobb and V. Robshaw (eds) *The Spiritual Challenge of Health Care*. London: Churchill Livingstone.

Cobb, M. (2001) *The Dying Soul: Spiritual Care at the End of Life*. Buckingham: Open University Press.

Cohen, S.R., Mount, B.M., Tomas, J.J.N. and Mount, L.F. (1996) Existential wellbeing is an important determinant of quality of life. *Cancer*, 77: 576–86.

Davie, G. (1994) *Religion in Britain since 1945*. London: Blackwell.

Denzin, N.K. (1989) *Interpretive Biography*. London: Sage.

Department of Health (1991) *The Patient's Charter*. London: HMSO.

Department of Health (1992) *Meeting the Spiritual Needs of Patients and Staff*. HSG (92)2. London: HMSO.

Diamond, J. (1998) *C: Because Cowards get Cancer Too*. London: Vermillion.

Elsdon, R. (1995) Spiritual pain in dying people: the nurse's role. *Professional Nurse*, 10(10): 641–3.

Emblem, J.D. and Halstead, L. (1993) Spiritual needs and interventions: comparing the views of patients, nurses and chaplains. *Clinical Nurse Specialist*, 7(4): 175–82.

Erricker, C. and Erricker, J. (2001) *Contemporary Spiritualities: Social and Religious Contexts*. London: Continuum.

Field, M.G. (2002) Soviet medicine, in R. Cooter and J. Pickstone (eds) *Medicine in the Twentieth Century*. Amsterdam: Harwood Academic.

Frank, A. (1995) *The Wounded Storyteller*. London: University of Chicago Press.

Frankl, V.E. (1959) *Man's Search for Meaning*. London: Touchstone Press.

Froggatt, K. (1997) Rites of passage and the hospice culture. *Mortality*, 2(2): 123–35.

Ferrucci, P. (1993) *What We May Be: The Vision and Techniques of Psycho-synthesis*. New York: Harper Collins.

Fry, A.J. (1997) Spirituality: connectedness through being and doing, in S. Ronaldson (ed.) *Spirituality: The Heart of Nursing*. Melbourne, VIC: Ausmed Publications.

Gallup (1999) International Millennium Survey, in G. Sturdy (ed.) Europe 'leads world in godlessness', *Church Times*, 17 December.

Gill, J.H. (1989) *Mediated Transcendence: A Postmodern Reflection*. Macon, GA: Mercer University Press.

Golberg, B. (1998) Connection: an exploration of spirituality in nursing care. *Journal of Advanced Nursing*, 7(4): 836–42.

Gray, A., Ezzart, A. and Boyer, A. (1997) Palliative care for the terminally ill in Saudi Arabia, in C. Saunders and R. Kastenbaum (eds) *Hospice Care on the International Scene*. New York: Springer.

Grinyer, A. (2002) *Cancer in Young Adults through Parents' Eyes*. Buckingham: Open University Press.

Hallorsdottir, S. and Hamrin, E. (1996) Experiencing existential changes: the lived experience of having cancer. *Cancer Nurse*, 19: 29–36.

Halstead, M.T. and Mickley, J.R. (1997) Attempting to fathom the unfathomable: descriptive views of spirituality. *Seminars in Oncology Nursing*, 13(4): 225–30.

Harrison, J. (1993) Spirituality and nursing practice. *Journal of Clinical Nursing*, 2: 211–17.

Harrison, R.L. (1997) Spirituality and hope: nursing implications for people with HIV disease. *Holistic Nursing Practice*, 12(1): 9–16.

Have, H. and Clark, D. (2002) *The Ethics of Palliative Care: European Perspectives*. Buckingham: Open University Press.

Hawkins, A.H. (1999) *Reconstructing Illness: Studies in Pathography*. West Lafayette, IN: Purdue University Press.

Hay, M. (1989) Principles in building spiritual assessment tools. *American Journal of Hospice Care*, September/October, pp. 25–31.

Hegedus, K. (2002) Interview in the Palliative Care in Eastern Europe project: Jewish Charity Hospital, Budapest, 26 July 2001, in D. Clark and M. Wright (eds) *Transitions in End of Life Care: Hospice and Related Developments in Eastern Europe and Central Asia*. Buckingham: Open University Press.

Heidegger, M. (1962) *Being and Time*. Oxford: Blackwell.

Helman, C. (1990) *Culture, Health and Illness*. London: Butterworth Heinemann.

Hervieu-Léger, D. (2000) *Religion as a Chain of Memory* (translated by S. Lee). New Brunswick, NJ: Rutgers University Press. First published in 1993 as *La Religion pour Mémoire*. Paris: Éditions du Cerf.

Hospital Chaplaincies Commission of the Church Assembly (1951) *CA 1003: Final Report*. London: SPCK.

Hungelmann, J.A., Kenkel-Rossi, E., Klassen, L. and Stollenwerk, R. (1996) Focus on spiritual wellbeing: harmonious interconnectedness of mind–body–spirit – use of the JAREL Spiritual Wellbeing Scale. *Geriatric Nursing*, 17: 262–6.

Husserl, E. (1962) *Ideas: General Introduction to Pure Phenomenology*. New York: Collier.

Jewell, A. (ed.) (1999) *Spirituality and Ageing*. London: Jessica Kingsley.

Kellehear, A. (2000) Spirituality and palliative care: a model of needs. *Palliative Medicine*, 14: 149–55.

King, M., Speck, P. and Tomas, A. (1995) The Royal Free interview for religious and spiritual beliefs: development and standardization. *Psychological Medicine*, 25(6): 1125–34.

Kleinman, A. (1988) *The Illness Narratives: Suffering, Healing and the Human Condition*. New York: Basic Books.

Lawton, J. (2000) *The Dying Process: Patients' Experience of Palliative Care*. London: Routledge.

Maddocks, I. (1997) Is hospice a western concept? A personal view of palliative care in Asia, in D. Clark, J. Hockley and S. Ahmedzai (eds) *New Themes in Palliative Care*. Buckingham: Open University Press.

Markham, I. (1998) Spirituality and the world of faiths, in M. Cobb and V. Robshaw (eds) *The Spiritual Challenge of Health Care*. London: Churchill Livingstone.

McGrath, P. (1998) Buddhist spirituality – a compassionate perspective on hospice care. *Mortality*, 3(3): 251–63.

Merleau-Ponty, M. (1962) *Phenomenology of Perception* (translated by C. Smith). London: Routledge & Kegan Paul.

Mickley, R.J., Pargament, K.I., Brant, C.R. and Hipp, K.M. (1998) God and the search for meaning among hospice caregivers. *The Hospice Journal*, 13(4): 1–17.

Narayanasamy, A.M. (1993) Nurses' awareness and educational preparation in meeting their patients' spiritual needs. *Nurse Education Today*, 13: 196–201.

National Association of Health Authorities and Trusts (1996) *Spiritual Care in the NHS: A Guide for Purchasers and Providers*. Birmingham: NAHAT.

National Health Service (1948) *Appointment of Chaplains*. HMC (48) 62. London: HMSO.

National Health Service Executive Northern and Yorkshire Chaplains and Pastoral Care Committee (1995) *Framework for Spiritual Faith and Related Pastoral Care*. Leeds: The Institute of Nursing, University of Leeds.

Neuman, B. (1995) *The Neuman Systems Model*. Norwalk, CT: Appleton & Lange.

Nuland, S.B. (1997) *How We Die*. London: Vintage.

Otto, R. ([1902] 1968) *The Idea of the Holy* (translated by J.W. Harvey). London: Oxford University Press.

Page, R. (1995) Transcendence and immanence, in A.V. Campbell (ed.) *A Dictionary of Pastoral Care*. London: SPCK.

Paloutzian, R.D. and Ellison, C.W. (1982) Loneliness, spiritual wellbeing and the quality of life, in L.A. Peplau and D. Perlman (eds) *Loneliness: A Sourcebook of Current Theory, Research and Therapy*. New York: Wiley.

Pattison, R. (2001) Dumbing down the spirit, in H. Orchard (ed.) *Spirituality in Health Care Contexts*. London: Jessica Kingsley.

Percy, M. (2000) A knowledge of Angles: how spiritual are the English? *The Eric Symes Abbott Memorial Lecture* delivered at Westminster Abbey, 4 May 2000. London: The Dean's Office, King's College.

Picardie, S. (1998) *Before I Say Goodbye*. London: Penguin.

Reed, P.G. (1987) Spirituality and wellbeing in terminally ill hospitalised adults. *Research in Nursing and Health*, 10: 335–44.

Reiman, D.J. (1986) The essential structure of a caring interaction, in P.L. Munhall and C.J. Oiler (eds) *Nursing Research: A Qualitative Perspective*. Norwalk, NJ: Appleton-Century-Crofts.

Renault, D. and Freake, T. (1996) *Native American Spirituality*. London: Thorsons.

Renetzky, L. (1979) The fourth dimension: applications to the social services, in D.O. Moberg (ed.) *Spiritual Wellbeing: Sociological Perspectives*. Washington, DC: University Press of America.

Ronaldson, S. (ed.) (1997) *Spirituality: The Heart of Nursing*. Melbourne, VIC: Ausmed Publications.

Rose, N. (1996) *Inventing Ourselves: Psychology, Power and Personhood*. Cambridge: Cambridge University Press.

Ross, L. (1994) Spiritual care: the nurse's role. *Nursing Standard*, 8(29): 35–7.

Ross, L. (1995) The spiritual dimension: its importance to patients' health, wellbeing and quality of life and its implications for nursing practice. *International Journal of Nursing Studies*, 32(5): 451–68.

Roy, C. (1976) *Introduction to Nursing: An Adaptation Model*. Englewood Cliffs, NJ: Prentice-Hall.

Saunders, C. (1986) The modern hospice, in F. Wald (ed.) *In Quest of the Spiritual Component of Care for the Terminally Ill*. New Haven, CT: Yale School of Nursing.

Saunders, C. (1997) Hospices worldwide: a mission statement, in C. Saunders and R. Kastenbaum (eds) *Hospice Care on the International Scene*. New York: Springer.

Scott Peck, M. (1987) *The Different Drum*. London: Arrow Books.

Singh, K.D. (1999) *The Grace in Dying: How We are Transformed Spiritually as We Die*. Dublin: Newleaf.

Speck, P. (1995) *Being There: Pastoral Care in Time of Illness*. London: SPCK.

Speck, P. (1998) Spiritual issues in palliative care, in D. Doyle, G.W. Hanks and N. MacDonald (eds) *Oxford Textbook of Palliative Medicine*. Oxford: Oxford Medical Publications.

Stoll, R.I. (1979) Guidelines for spiritual assessment. *American Journal of Nursing*, September, pp. 1574–7.

Stoll, R.I. (1989) The essence of spirituality, in V.B. Carson (ed.) *Spiritual Dimensions of Nursing Practice*. Philadelphia, PA: W.B. Saunders.

Stoter, D. (1991) Spiritual care, in J. Penson and R. Fisher (eds) *Palliative Care for People with Cancer*. London: Arnold.

Styles, M.K. (1994) The shining stranger: application of the phenomenological method in the investigation of the nurse–family spiritual relationship. *Cancer Nurse*, 17(1): 18–26.

The Bible (Revised Standard Version) (1952) W.M. Collins & Sons & Co Ltd for The British and Foreign Bible Society.

Travelbee, J. (1971) *Interpersonal Aspects of Nursing*. Philadelphia, PA: F.A. Davis.

UK Central Council for Nursing, Midwifery and Health Visiting (1984) *Code of Professional Conduct for the Nurse, Midwife and Health Visitor*. London: UKCC.

UK Central Council for Nursing, Midwifery and Health Visiting (1986) *Project 2000: A New Preparation for Practice*. London: UKCC.

Vanstone, W.H. (1982) *The Stature of Waiting*. London: Darton, Longman & Todd.

Vivat, B. and Young, T. (2002) *The Construction of a Spiritual Wellbeing Module: Preliminary Report, Phases 1 and 2*. Internal document. Report for the EORTC Quality of Life Study Group.

Wakefield, G.S. (1993) Spirituality, in A.E. McGrath (ed.) *The Blackwell Encyclopaedia of Modern Christian Thought*. London: Blackwell.

Watson, J. (1974). *Nursing: The Philosophy and Science of Caring*. Boston, MA: Little, Brown & Company.

Wilson, P.H. (1999) Memory, personhood and faith, in A. Jewell (ed.) *Spirituality and Ageing*. London: Jessica Kingsley.

Wright, M.C. (2001a) Spiritual health care: an enquiry into the spiritual care of patients with cancer within the acute hospital and specialist inpatient palliative care unit in England and Wales. Unpublished PhD thesis, University of Sheffield.

Wright, M.C. (2001b) Chaplaincy in hospice and hospital: findings from a survey in England and Wales. *Palliative Medicine*, 15: 229–42.

Wright, M.C. (2002) The essence of spiritual care: a phenomenological enquiry. *Palliative Medicine*, 16: 125–32.

Wyatt, G.K.H. and Friedman, L.L. (1996) Developing and testing of a quality of life model for long-term female cancer survivors. *Quality of Life Research*, 5: 387–94.

Zorza, V. and Zorza, R. (1978) Death of a daughter. *Washington Post Outlook*, 22 January.

Zorza, R. and Zorza, V. (1980) *A Way to Die*. London: André Deutsch.

12

Working with difficult symptoms

Jessica Corner

Rather than providing a toolkit for working with difficult symptoms as in many other palliative care texts, a critical view of symptom management is offered here, as well as some different ideas about approaches that may be adopted while working with people facing physical, emotional or practical problems as a result of life-limiting illness. I have chosen to adopt a critical and reflective stance, since this seems to be a more fruitful avenue to finding ways of working with some of the most challenging problems faced in caring practice. I have chosen not to offer a set of solutions or guidance on the management of difficult symptoms, since these are unlikely to be addressed through this kind of approach; the problems are both complex and bound up in the particular contexts in which people with life-limiting illness live. I do, however, draw out some ideas that might be used to guide the development of caring practice.

Cribb (2001), in writing about knowledge and caring, identifies two worlds, the world of science and the 'human world'; that is, there is scientific knowledge and there are 'lay beliefs'. He argues that the human world is being displaced and colonized by the natural and human sciences, so that personal and common sense knowledge is being displaced by 'expert' knowledge. Cribb argues that alongside this knowledge there is also what he calls 'real knowledge'; that is, knowledge about how to do things that cannot be gained through textbooks – how to ride a bike, conduct a conversation, be a good listener, for example. It is this real knowledge that is primary, as it provides the frame of reference on which all other knowledge rests or is made use of. Other authors have outlined ways of knowing in the context of nursing practice (see, for example, Carper 1978; Johns 1995; Nolan and Lundh 1998). Like the 'real' knowledge of Cribbs, these authors argue that there is knowledge that comes from direct involvement with situations or experiences.

Cribb (2001) argues that 'the stories that weave our domestic lives indicate a reality just as substantial as the stories which tell us about the material of which they are made' (p. 17). Cribb suggests that a different relationship between expert and lay 'knower' may be needed; that instead of falling short of knowledge, the lay person, with their 'every day knowing', has knowledge that is continuous with more specialized forms of knowledge. It is understanding the relationship between expert knowledge and 'lay', or what might also be called 'embodied' knowledge (Benner and Wrubel 1989), that seems to be at the heart of how we should consider the approach to managing difficult symptoms. Valuing different kinds of knowledge, particularly the knowledge that people have about the problems of their own limiting illness, has influenced the way I set out my thoughts here.

Symptom management as a dominant construct in palliative care

A powerful impetus for palliative care has been the goal to relieve the symptoms and problems that accompany life-limiting illness and are part of the process of dying. From the outset, hospice and palliative care services were established to tackle the particular needs of people dying from cancer. Symptom management, a core function in palliative care, has largely focused on a set of symptoms and problems commonly associated with advanced or metastatic stages of cancer, the most prevalent symptom being pain. The early success of the hospice and palliative care movement in developing effective approaches to the management of cancer pain using opioid drugs was an important driving force behind how palliative care as a speciality subsequently evolved, and has been instrumental in its success. As Robbins (1998) states: 'a large part of the impetus of setting up hospices and palliative care teams was the belief that the pain of terminal illness, especially the pain of progressive cancer, can be controlled effectively . . . relief of symptoms is largely the foundation upon which all other aspects of palliative care rest' (p. 20). Thus, 'symptom management' is now seen as an essential part of the skills required in providing palliative care and, although not the exclusive form of help or intervention offered to patients and families, it is often the focus for the intervention of specialist palliative care teams.

While offering symptom management to people who are dying has become a major part of the *raison d'être* of palliative care, the way in which symptom management has become the primary focus has implications for the way care is organized and experienced. Palliative care, originating in the work of Cicely Saunders and others in the 1950s and 1960s, set out to offer a radical and alternative model of care to the prevailing model of increasingly institutionalized and medically managed care for people who were dying. Although the palliative care approach was devised as an alternative model, it has over time increasingly become embedded within the traditions, or discourses, of health care, particularly that of biomedicine. This has been a natural consequence of the professionalization of hospice services, but also means that approaches to managing the problems associated with dying have become defined and addressed in particular ways.

Palliative care as it exists in contemporary health care, defined by a dominant culture orientated to the 'management' or 'control' of symptoms, places heavy emphasis on the biomedical model of disease management, and is one aspect of the so-called 'medicalization' of death described by Field (1994). Field suggests that while the hospice movement was founded on a desire to reject the trend whereby dying was increasingly becoming the province of health workers and managed within highly technical health care institutions, palliative care is perhaps unintentionally perpetuating some aspects of the medicalization of dying. There is, for example, a trend towards the heavy use of technical procedures and medical technology. Also, palliative care becoming the overarching speciality for care in life-limiting illness has moved the emphasis away from dying and death to an unspecified time earlier in the course of illness, thereby focusing attention away from dying and death.

The point here is not to revisit a rather well-trodden path in relation to the critique of medicalization of society [see, for example, Ivan Illich's ([1976] 1990) now seminal critique *Limits to Medicine, Medical Nemesis: The Expropriation of Health*], whereby medicine is revealed and denigrated for having acquired extraordinary power and control over people's lives, or over people in medical encounters. Rather, it is to understand that the biomedical paradigm has provided a system of knowledge and practices that can, because they are dominant, define our very experience of ourselves; they become part of the way we understand and live our lives (Lupton 1997). This has not been intentional; rather, it is an effect of the very success of biomedicine. It does, however, have some consequences and in the context of palliative care and in the management of difficult symptoms these are apparent. Clark (1999), for example, traces the origins of the concept of 'total pain' in the work of Cicely Saunders. Clark notes a paradox in the concept resulting from the radical intention to move the relief of pain arising from terminal cancer into territory where wider dimensions of suffering are acknowledged, and beyond the biomedical paradigm whereby pain is seen as simply a sensation arising from largely physical causes. It nevertheless can also be seen to be an extension of medical dominion where 'pain relief' is also an instrument of power. Clark argues that the principle of giving regular analgesia and thereby constant control of pain, can be seen to extend to the 'constant control of the patient' – that is, patients offered pain control regimes in palliative care are no longer expected to articulate their needs, since these will be anticipated in advance by someone else. Thus pain relief is achieved, but at the cost of loss of personal autonomy. The concept of 'total pain' that incorporates psychological, spiritual and social aspects of the pain experience can also be seen as extending the range of medical 'gaze', which Clark argues has an imperialist feel about it. From this perspective, then, holism 'is revealed as something other than we might suppose. Paradoxically and contrary to its own claims, this is a strategy of power, one which in subjecting human suffering to a new nosology, at the same objectifies it and prescribes strategies for its relief. In this sense "total pain" becomes a nomenclature of inscription, albeit unintended by its author' (Clark 1999: 734).

The foundation for palliative care within the discourse of biomedicine has led to the belief that the problems of dying should be understood as manifestations of disease, rather than more generally how one dies. Since symptoms are considered to be disease-related problems, it is assumed that they are properly managed by health professionals within the formal structures of health care. These assumptions tend to generate a particular set of responses to problems and excludes others. One assumption, for example, is that for individuals to have a peaceful death they must, as far as is possible, be symptom-free. While this is a laudable goal for care, it also focuses the activity of those involved in providing ever more effective symptom management, even when the goal to be 'symptom-free' while dying may be unrealistic. Another consequence is that there is little room for acknowledging social, professional or individual constraints that may operate as part of the dying process and that may contribute to the experience of difficult symptoms, or that may prevent the development of supportive but also more liberating regimes of care, for example those that prioritize preservation of personal autonomy.

The consequences of a biomedical construction for symptom management in palliative care

It is worth exploring for a moment the ways in which symptom management has become defined and practised within palliative care. The ability to manage cancer pain through a biomedical approach using morphine was a very significant discovery for the hospice movement. The approach of using powerful drugs, or combinations of drugs, for cancer pain led to the search for new and better drugs and other treatments, first for pain and then for other symptoms common in cancer. A consequence of the success in using drugs to manage symptoms is that, in many instances, not only is 'symptom management' the primary endeavour, but drug treatments have become the primary approach used in tackling problems. Frequently, drug treatment for problems reported by a patient is the first approach or perhaps the only solution considered. While this may be entirely appropriate, it also has had certain consequences for the way palliative care has developed and become organized. Care constructed around the use of drug treatments for symptoms emphasizes 'relief', 'control' or 'management' of the symptoms, the object being the removal, obliteration or disguise of symptoms as manifestations of the disease patients are dying from. The goal of care is 'relief' or 'control', reducing the symptom to a level such that it is in the background or absent entirely. It is arguable that in pursuing this strategy to 'relieve' or 'control' symptoms, other aspects of the experience of symptoms, such as suffering, distress, the ability to function and even personal autonomy, independently have been relegated to secondary importance. Also, the assumption that the perception of a symptom such as pain, once removed or reduced using powerful pharmacology, ceases to be of concern to the person who experienced it, overlooks the possibility that suffering or the ability to function may not be addressed by the treatment.

The dominance of symptom management as the central goal of palliative care has had other ramifications. As a pharmacological approach became dominant, the doctor as the person who prescribes treatment aimed at symptom management also became the natural leader of services, reinforcing the trend towards biomedical or pharmacological solutions to the problems patients bring to the attention of palliative care services. An illustration of the dominance of this approach can be seen in the palliative care research literature; there has been a preoccupation within palliative care research to chart or map the prevalence of symptoms among people who are dying. This has been motivated no doubt by a need to record demand for palliative care and to provide information on which to make decisions in determining where to target limited resources. For example, in a historical review of palliative care research, studies of symptoms – especially symptom prevalence studies among patients admitted to hospices and palliative care services – were found to be the most common form of research published in the palliative care literature (Corner 1996). These studies have commonly used retrospective case note reviews, or groups of patients were asked to indicate which of a list of symptoms they were experiencing.

Symptom prevalence studies provide an indication of the common and most difficult symptoms for patients and yield insights into the problems that palliative care services are most commonly attempting to alleviate. However, the symptoms identified in these studies are largely defined by palliative care clinicians or the researcher undertaking the research and, as a result, reflect biomedical categories of different manifestations of disease, rather than problems identified and defined by people with life-limiting illness themselves. It is difficult to know whether or not 'common symptoms' identified through this process would be broadly similar if there had been more room for patients or family members to define for themselves the nature of their problems. If the emphasis for palliative care services is on managing symptoms as constructed through these various studies, there is a risk that palliative care is not currently addressing need more broadly. Also important is that less attention has been paid to the extent to which palliative care services have achieved 'symptom relief' for individuals who are dying. There has been relatively little work into the effectiveness of symptom control, as constructed through this model of care. We know little about the extent to which the symptoms of people with cancer are indeed 'relieved' or 'managed'; indeed, there is evidence that in many circumstances this is not the case (see, for example, Higginson and McCarthy 1989; Hinton 1994; Addington-Hall and McCarthy 1995).

Our understanding of what it is like to live with particular symptoms is benefiting from research, although there is still much that is unknown. Studies have been conducted of the frequency with which symptoms and problems occur among patients receiving palliative care and a few have reported detailed work into how these develop over time, or are manifested in the last weeks of life. The orientation of research has been to examine a particular set of clinical problems that are deemed amenable to intervention by palliative care services. Little work has been undertaken from a more insider or user/consumer oriented perspective. It is surprising that no concerted effort has been made to determine which symptoms or problems individuals may wish to be 'managed' on their behalf by health professionals, an issue I shall return to later. Importantly, since the very word 'managing' implies a certain stance when working with people who are ill or dying, this also warrants critical exploration.

Among the various limitations of the biomedical model identified is the biomedical construction of the body. Critical accounts of biomedicine identify the term 'symptom' as a biomedical construction; that is, it has developed as part of the way in which medicine has developed systems of knowledge and understanding of the body and of illness, but that is only one way of understanding one's body and the way one feels. It belongs firmly to the territory of 'expert' or scientific knowledge identified by Cribb. Armstrong (1995), for example, drawing on the work of Michel Foucault ([1973] 1986), identifies the biomedical 'spatialization of illness', where the relationship of symptoms and illness are configured in a three-dimensional framework: symptom, sign and pathology. The symptom is understood to be a marker of illness experienced by the patient, a sign is the intimation of disease elicited by the doctor, for example through physical examination, and together these are used to infer pathology. However, this spatialization or ordering of how illness is determined is not seen to be entirely benign. To align the three elements, the body of the patient is submitted to the 'gaze' – medical investigations which the patient must submit to. The patient is only required to answer questions that are deemed relevant to the identification of biomedically defined pathology and its treatment; other issues that may be deemed important by the person who is ill are not explored.

According to Lyon and Barbalet (1994), the model whereby biomedicine regards the body as an external object assumes that the practitioner is in control of the body of the patient; the patient is subordinate to the practitioner. Biomedicine deals with malfunctioning organs or other subsystems of the body, and with symptoms, but not the 'body' that is the person:

> The medical body is passive; any active capacities it may display are regarded as internal to its physiology, and these can be revealed to external observers as external knowledge. The body is readily subordinated to the authority of medical practice. It is disciplined and made, or at least made better, through the social institution of medicine. The medical body is a partial body. It is partial in a dual sense: it is the internal body, and it is the body patients have, but not the body patients *are* in the full sense.
>
> (Lyon and Barbalet 1994: 53)

Lyon and Barbalet (1994) argue that 'the medical body' is but one among a number of different constructions of the body that can be identified and have been variously described in scholarly writing. For example, 'the consumerist body' – that is, the body in consumerist society as manifested in magazines or in relation to our beliefs about the health products we buy. Another construction could be described as the 'social body' – that is, the body that is subject to social and cultural norms and practices. An alternative to the biomedical view of the body, where mind or self and physical body are considered separate entities, is the notion of 'embodiment'; that is, the idea that the body is experienced and is where and how 'self' is located. From this perspective, it is argued that the body, being one with self, acts to construct its own world; it is not a discrete physical entity external to the self. It is inter-communicative and active. Within health care and more particularly palliative care, these different ways of understanding the body are largely unacknowledged. There is, however, a developing interest in exploring the implications of acknowledging these different 'bodies', as well as the potential value of incorporating such understanding into approaches to offering health care.

The notion of a 'social body' recognizes that individuals are subject to power relations at large within society, such as the influence of doctors in medical encounters, and that how the body is understood is socially determined rather than 'real'. For example, how one should 'manage' one's bodily processes to be socially acceptable is generated and passed on through history and culture; it is socially determined and not simply the province of individuals. As Taussig (1980) states: 'things such as the signs and symptoms of disease . . . are not only biological and physical, but are also signs of social relations disguised as natural things, concealing their roots in human reciprocity' (p. 3).

The notion of an 'embodied body' proposes that the 'lived body' is experienced as a fluid, a combination of physicality and emotionality. It is 'a pre-objective structure of lived experience; one in which mind and body, reason and emotion, pleasure and pain are thoroughly interfused' (Williams and Bendelow 1998: 133). Williams and Bendelow (1998) explain how, in chronic illness, the taken-for-granted normal state of embodiment, experienced as a kind of bodily disappearance in which one is not conscious of one's body as distinct from oneself, can be radically disrupted. In these circumstances, one becomes suddenly very aware of one's bodily failings and one's bodily identity is undermined. As a consequence, loss of self becomes a fundamental form of suffering in illness. This process can be reinforced and exacerbated by biomedical approaches to managing and treating disease, since these tend to disregard the importance of 'self'. Where symptoms are treated as physical manifestations of disease that need to be controlled or managed, we may fail to acknowledge emotional, social or individual processes that create the very experience of the symptom.

McNamara (2001) notes that symptom relief is a medicalized, technical and pharmacologically driven response to the dying process that 'masks' the physical process of dying, and has been prioritized above psychological, spiritual or other forms of care. McNamara does not elaborate on precisely what she believes to be 'masked' through this; however, this highly technical and externally 'managed' system of symptom control may well remove the possibility of self-management, or what Williams (1996) describes as achieving a 'negotiated settlement' with illness or dying. In relation to living with chronic illness, Williams notes that over time individuals reach for themselves a kind of resolution, a realignment of body, self and society.

While the relief of physical symptoms among people who are dying is an important and legitimate goal, it is worth considering why it has become a priority and what other aspects of caring may have been excluded or neglected as a result. While in many instances pharmacological interventions and other technical treatments are of value, all too often problems are only partially alleviated or are viewed as 'intractable', since they are not readily amenable to pharmacological intervention. Once labelled as 'intractable', symptoms may be overlooked as other avenues for assisting people experiencing the problem are not pursued. Moreover, those who are thought to have 'intractable' or difficult to manage symptoms, because they do not respond to symptom control strategies as expected or who have socially unacceptable problems, may themselves be identified as 'difficult'. Intractable symptoms challenge staff members in hospice and palliative care settings, since they confront widely held beliefs about what is a 'good' death and raise questions as to whether this is being provided (McNamara 2001).

Thought needs to be given to how one might start to work with some of the themes already outlined with people experiencing difficult symptoms at the end of their lives, and some principles for working with the various problems highlighted need to be established. However, it is also important to acknowledge that the mere act of identifying a particular symptom as 'difficult' could also mean that individuals risk being designated as outsiders, beyond help, and when this occurs it may challenge the very ability of staff to care.

What are difficult symptoms?

The term 'difficult' suggests symptoms or problems in illness that are difficult to manage, that are perhaps difficult to bear or that cannot be controlled. What becomes defined as 'difficult' in practice is interesting, since there is often a discrepancy between symptoms that one might anticipate would be understood to be 'difficult' and those that in reality are labelled as such. The term could denote illness problems that cause an individual suffering, in which case all symptoms are potentially difficult, even those that may be possible to control in physical terms. However, many problems are defined as 'difficult' because health professionals or carers may feel that they do not know what to offer or that they have failed to provide 'relief'. Symptoms may be difficult to watch; for example, extreme breathlessness can be very distressing to observe, especially if it appears that there is little effective intervention available and can leave health professionals and family members feeling extremely helpless. Problems such as loss of appetite may not be perceived as a problem for the person concerned but can be deeply distressing to family members, since eating is life sustaining and not eating is a clear manifestation of the dying process. Other problems remain unrecognized as symptoms and therefore are left unresolved, perhaps because they have not been defined within a logical symptom 'category' in biomedical terms or because the person experiencing them finds it difficult to express the nature of the problem, yet these may cause considerable distress and suffering. Finally, there may be instances where patients have difficult symptoms or problems resulting from their illness that challenge social taboos, or result in them exhibiting demanding or highly emotional behaviour, or that are simply beyond relief; in these situations, patients themselves may become defined as 'difficult'. This suggests that there is a close relationship between symptoms and a person's self and identity (as described in Chapter 1).

Difficult symptoms: some exemplars

The many complex problems that arise for people while living with life-limiting illness and while dying cannot be defined using a neat list of symptoms or strategies for dealing with each listed, although this is typically how many textbooks on palliative care present symptom management. I have argued elsewhere that symptoms are often a constellation of states of mind and body where problems such as pain, breathlessness, fatigue, anxiety or depression are often experienced simultaneously, each problem related to and often difficult to distinguish from all the others (Corner and Dunlop 1997). They are problems that take on significant meanings when someone is knowingly facing death and although they are a result of physiological decline due to illness, they are experienced as part of that person's own social and cultural world. The person's own reactions and ways of understanding and living with problems directly influence the particular constellation of problems and needs that arise, as does the response of others. I now describe some common problems of life-limiting illness. These are used as examples of the issues already identified and also to illustrate some themes around which nurses and other health professionals might approach offering support to people who experience them.

Fatigue

Fatigue is acknowledged to be a very common problem in life-limiting illness and considerable research has been undertaken into fatigue associated with cancer and cancer treatment, although relatively little work has been undertaken in the context of palliative care. Richardson and Ream (1996) define fatigue as 'a total body feeling ranging from tiredness to exhaustion creating an unrelenting overall condition which interferes with an individual's ability to function to their normal capacity' (p. 527). While tiredness is a normal and everyday experience, fatigue experienced during chronic or life-limiting illness is of a different order and strategies such as resting or sleeping are often of little help. In these circumstances, fatigue can be extremely incapacitating and distressing and yet it is often difficult to convey the extent of fatigue as a problem to others because it is such a normal and everyday experience; perhaps this is also because the language available to people when describing their fatigue draws on the same language used to express the everyday and normal experience of tiredness.

In a study of 15 patients with advanced cancer suffering from fatigue who were being cared for in a palliative care unit, Krishnasamy (2000) reveals a complex condition that patients found difficult to put into words and a limited dialogue between patients and professional carers about the condition. Medical and nursing records made very little specific reference to the problem of fatigue even when the patients reported being severely disabled by it; the patients experienced it to be of an entirely different quality and order than day-to-day tiredness. There was also no reference to intervention or help being offered. The severity of fatigue reported was not related in any way to physiological indicators such as anaemia or hypercalcaemia, but it was described as having a profound emotional impact on those who were suffering from it. The study used several standardized measures of fatigue, anxiety and depression and of functional status. What was interesting was that scores recorded using the measures did not appear to reflect the depth of distress and difficulty that patients described during interviews. Somehow the research measures seemed to miss the point. Only three of the 15 patients' scores on the Hospital Anxiety and Depression Scale, for example, indicated evidence of 'clinical depression'; when asked about this, one of the three patients who was 'apparently' depressed rejected the suggestion that the score might indicate this because he felt that low mood was a normal response to his situation. The measurement of functional status was also rejected as a useful means of assessing the impact of fatigue, as the measure tended to assume that a problem is fixed, so that scores relating to severity or impairment can be recorded as a reflection of the problem at a given point in time. Patients described their fatigue as an unpredictable and patternless problem and thus could not be neatly 'captured' in this way. Fatigue for these patients was a diffuse, inexpressible experience with no obvious cause. Yet it was also the very means by which they understood that they were deteriorating; the symptom 'told' them that they were dying. For family members and friends, watching someone become so incapacitated by fatigue was deeply distressing.

The mismatch between the experience of fatigue and it 'falling below the line of detection' for physiological parameters or quality-of-life measures partly explains why it seemed not to be recognized or addressed by health professionals. Somehow it does not fit into standard assumptions about symptoms and problems in palliative care. This was expressed by a woman who participated in Krishnasamy's study: 'He [a doctor] has no idea . . . he doesn't listen to what it's like, really like to feel like this all the time, you see, they don't take it seriously, this is taking it seriously, talking about . . . it, and listening, really listening, to me tell you this is awful.'

This important study reveals a recurrent theme in relation to how health professionals might respond to and work with people experiencing difficult symptoms. That is, listening to and making it possible for people to talk about and express their experiences of difficult symptoms and of their illness is important. Acknowledging the problem is in itself experienced as supportive and helpful.

Eating and emaciation

Loss of appetite is commonly reported in life-limiting illness and may be associated with weight loss. Equally, weight loss may occur as a consequence of loss of appetite or as a result of disease processes. Eating has social meanings that go much further than simply being a means of obtaining sustenance; it is associated with the most deeply felt human experiences and has many symbolic meanings (Lupton 1994). The significance of not being able to participate in the rituals and social processes surrounding food preparation and consumption are profound, yet have received little attention in palliative care.

A recent review of studies on the weight loss and loss of appetite of patients with advanced cancer and their carers identified only 50 studies covering such issues as measurement, incidence and prevalence, the experiences of patients and carers, and interventions (Poole and Froggatt 2002). Few of these studies attempted to assess the distress associated with anorexia or weight loss. Problems with eating were found to be rather different from fatigue, where the symptoms appear to be uniquely experienced by individuals, since this is also profoundly difficult for those closest to the person who is ill, especially if they are responsible for preparation of meals. Weight loss in contrast to eating difficulties is a highly visible manifestation of life-limiting illness. Tate and George (2001) explored the impact of weight loss among HIV-positive gay men. Weight loss that occurred as part of illness for these men had a dramatic effect on their lives and led them to avoid social activities because they were conscious of their emaciated appearance. Emaciation in this context was an indisguisable manifestation of their disease and their sexuality.

What is revealed by the little work that has been undertaken into what is difficult about weight loss or eating difficulties is not simply that they are inevitable and often irreversible manifestations of the process of dying, but that they are inextricably bound up with deeply held cultural beliefs and practices, and therefore they disrupt intimate and more public social relationships. The 'managing' of the problems associated with difficulties in eating or with emaciation, then, may more fruitfully lie in working with the interplay between self and an individual's social world rather than more direct nutritional interventions.

Odour and exudate

In her important observational study, Lawton (2000) observes that many symptoms requiring 'control' in hospice settings appear to share the distinctive feature that they are associated with or a cause of the body's surfaces rupturing or breaking down. Lawton describes people as having 'unbounded bodies', meaning the literal erosion of the body's physical boundaries. Here, symptom control was observed to be directed at a range of bodily ailments such as incontinence of urine and faeces, uncontrolled vomiting including faecal vomit, fungating tumours and weeping limbs from skin breaking down in lymphoedema. Symptom 'control' was aimed at controlling the body's boundaries to minimize the effects of 'unboundedness'.

Lawton presents the case of Annie, a woman dying of cervical cancer with a recto-vaginal fistula; faecal leakage from the fistula was completely unmanageable and resulted in a severe stench that filled the hospice. Annie's problem was the profound effect this had on her sense of self, and resulted in her desire to withdraw from family life and remain in the hospice rather than return home. Her situation deteriorated and her diarrhoea became so bad that Annie, feeling such a profound fear and loss of self-esteem, asked to be sedated. Her request was granted and she was sedated until she died 2 weeks later. Lawton describes the use of sedation in Annie's case as a kind of imposed and orchestrated social death by hospice staff – she was, following sedation, removed to a side room and visits from her family ceased soon after. Annie's symptoms were profoundly difficult – practically unmanageable (her severe diarrhoea and odour) but also socially difficult because of the profoundly unacceptable nature of her problem. 'Control' in these circumstances meant removing Annie's consciousness of her predicament.

It seemed to Lawton that symptom 'control' in cases such as that of Annie was about imposing control on what was becoming uncontrollable, those things in normal situations that would be considered to be socially unacceptable. For patients whose bodies were becoming 'unbounded', symptom control – when it was successful – provided the function of restoring the body's 'boundedness' and enabled a return to normal life. When it fails, the consequence for patients could be a profound loss of self. Lawton theorizes that hospices have become places where people with unbounded bodies and who are undergoing 'dirty' dying may be sequestered or shut away, and symptoms are only 'managed' in the sense that the hospice permits and provides for their removal from society.

Lawton's account is shocking not because palliative care staff struggle with dealing with these enormously challenging problems, but because symptom control as a form of social control and yet relief of profound suffering in Annie's case could not have been said to have been achieved. Annie's problems were 'unmanageable', but her case challenges us to find ways of more effectively supporting people in a similar predicament.

Breathlessness

Breathlessness is a very common problem among patients needing palliative care. Since the physical causes of breathing difficulties are irreversible, bio-medical intervention often at best only offers partial relief. Breathlessness can be disabling and terrifying at the same time, so that simply addressing it as a physical problem does not assist people to deal with the intense fear of dying that the symptom often engenders or the practical problems of managing everyday activities when these trigger breathlessness. Several carefully researched accounts have been published of the experience of breathlessness in different illness contexts; see, for example, Williams (1993) and Skilbeck *et al.* (1998) in relation to chronic respiratory illnesses, and Roberts *et al.* (1993) and O'Driscoll *et al.* (1999) in relation to advanced lung cancer. These accounts reveal the complex interplay of mind and body in the experience of breathlessness in life-limiting illness.

Breathlessness is an example of a symptom where some attempts have been made to address the issues and difficulties outlined. In trying to respond to the particular circumstances of people with lung cancer who develop difficulties with breathing, together with colleagues I have developed and evaluated an approach to working with breathlessness, describing this as a parallel model of management (Corner 2001a; see Figure 12.1). The model has been developed and formally evaluated over a series of studies. These indicate that patients appear to derive benefit from the approach when compared with patients not offered it (Corner *et al.* 1996; Bredin *et al.* 1999).

An integrative model of breathlessness was adopted, in which the emotional experience of breathlessness is considered inseparable from the sensory experience and from the pathophysical mechanisms. The approach to managing breathlessness is rehabilitative in its orientation even though

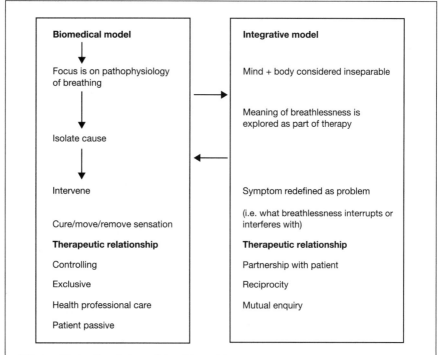

Figure 12.1   Parallel models of breathlessness management. Reprinted with permission from Corner (2001a).

patients may be at the very end of their lives. Care is directed at assisting individuals to manage the problem of breathlessness themselves, rather than to find ways of eliminating it or taking charge of it as a health professional.

The relationship with the person with breathlessness is considered a reciprocal one; breathlessness is viewed as a problem about which both patient and nurse have a mutual interest. Ways of managing breathlessness are therefore discovered together. The nurse is therapist, but the object of therapy (i.e. breathlessness) is the subject of mutual enquiry by both patient and nurse. The relationship is therefore one of equality. Care is focused on agreed goals to reduce the duration and frequency of episodes of breathlessness and to improve function.

The importance of encouraging and listening to the patient's story of their illness and how breathlessness is experienced as part of this is recognized and is a central part of intervention. Intervention begins with assessment in the form of facilitating storytelling, or narration, about illness and breathlessness; this becomes an ongoing part of care. In developing this approach, we were influenced by Kleinman's (1988) notion of 'illness narratives' and the importance of working with such narratives with patients who have chronic health problems. Fundamental is the recognition that much of what is therapeutic in listening to patients' stories of their breathlessness is hearing and 'holding' fear and distress associated with the symptom. In describing the approach as 'therapy', Bailey (1995) draws on Bion (1977) and Fabricius (1991) to explain the process of therapeutic work. The nurse as 'therapist' makes herself available, psychically, as a container for anxieties that are intolerable. This is a maternal function whereby, like a mother with an infant, intolerable stress is contained and processed and, in time, fed back in a more tolerable form. The primal link between breathing and life, ceasing to breathe and dying, is frequently central to fear of breathlessness and may itself evoke or exacerbate attacks of the symptom. Often patients fear they will die during the next attack of breathlessness, yet often have never voiced this fear. In exploring experiences of breathlessness, the aim is to assist patients to understand how and why such associations and fears arise and that these are in themselves not real. Hearing about sadness, anger or frustration may also be therapeutic.

Intervention employs a number of techniques from respiratory rehabilitation, including breathing re-training, energy conservation, life adaptation, and relaxation and distraction techniques. These are strategies that can be used by patients, often supported by close family members or carers, to manage episodes of breathlessness or situations that have become difficult or unmanageable because of breathlessness. The integrative model is realized in practice through a complex balancing of practical assistance and facilitation of adjustment to the limitations of breathlessness, with explicit and implicit recognition of the distress and fear that accompanies the symptom. What has been important to me over the years when working with people experiencing breathlessness is what I have learnt about talking with them and using their experiences within the supportive framework that I could offer as a nurse. 'Managing' symptoms using this approach is about helping people to manage the problem for themselves; this may also mean learning to live with the problem, and 'control' is about handing back 'control'. As Bailey states:

> There is scope for developing nursing roles within a framework that makes it possible to be more accepting of patients' 'conscious and unconscious demands', to employ nursing as therapy. The order of nursing situations; the routine; the way in which 'symptoms' are dealt with at a high level of abstraction; the prevalence of models or algorithms that 'stand for' human entities without expressing them; the splitting of human experience into neatly bound categories, setting aside the undisciplined whole; all of this stands in the way, provides a means to become detached, to leave painful things untouched. If nursing can change these things, the opportunities are unlimited.
>
> (Bailey 1995: 189)

Working with difficult symptoms: some ideas

It is not possible to draw up a set of definitive guiding principles for working with difficult symptoms; indeed, it would be unwise to try, especially as the intention of this chapter has been to reveal the impossibility of finding 'neat' solutions for the hugely challenging problems identified. However, it is possible to identify some themes that might at least offer a starting point for developing thinking and work with people in this area. The first and possibly most important is to adopt the kind of critical and reflective stance used here to develop understanding about why particular problems are 'difficult' and what might need to change so that care addresses the issues identified. Also, to consider whether 'symptom management' should continue to occupy the primary place it does currently.

The second is the potential importance of people's narratives in developing therapeutic approaches for difficult symptoms. The possibility of using a person's particular story as the starting point for intervention or support has been revisited throughout this chapter. Bury (2001) reminds us that it is no accident that there is an increasing interest in patients' narratives, since this reflects wider social trends, in particular the increasing emphasis on self in modern identity, the rise of chronic illness where everyday living with illness becomes paramount, and the various challenges to a single medical authority over illness. Bury also points out that illness narratives are themselves a constructed form of 'storytelling' in which the teller makes choices about the form in which the story is told and is influenced by the listener. As such, these are not 'truer' pictures of illness; they are, however, rich sources of insight into the problems of life-limiting illness that are as yet largely unexplored. Kleinman (1988), however, does promote the active facilitation of 'storytelling' as a therapeutic approach to the problems of chronic illness and this warrants further examination for its potential value in the context of palliative care.

Third, the idea of nurse or health professional as facilitator of the person's own journey in learning to live with, manage or find relief from the particular problems they are facing seems more fruitful than presenting oneself as the agent of 'control' for symptoms. Thus the principle of fostering 'self-management' brings a fresh perspective that might usefully be explored further (Corner 2001a). Self-management or 'self-care' does not necessarily mean remaining entirely self-maintaining or fully functional. It does, however, mean maintaining one's usual practices of self-care; those things that are important and unique to oneself in maintaining one's sense of self. Self-management also implies being given the means to master or deal with problems, rather than relinquishing them to others. This could be in relation to managing attacks of breathlessness for oneself or it could mean reaching some level of comfort with oneself while facing death. The important thing is that these are active strategies owned and used by people who are ill.

Finally, more work is needed into the variety of problems faced by people with life-limiting illness to provide a more detailed understanding of the nature of what it is that is 'difficult' about the symptoms or problems experienced.

Ideas for working with difficult symptoms

- Adopt a critical and reflective stance to understanding why particular problems are 'difficult' and to trying to understand what might need to change so that problems are addressed from a broader perspective.

- Use the person's story as the starting point for intervention or support. Hearing about the problem can in itself be therapeutic and may offer insights into how the problem may be tackled.

- Facilitating the person's own journey in learning to live with, manage or find relief from problems may be more fruitful than presenting oneself as the agent of 'control' for symptoms.

- Enabling self-management; that is, maintain activities and practices that are unique to oneself in maintaining one's sense of 'self'. Learning to master or deal with problems rather than relinquishing them to health professionals may be an important new direction for what has to date been know as 'symptom management'.

Figure 12.2

Conclusions

It may appear that more criticism than guidance has been offered here; this has not been the intention. However, I wanted to avoid glib or facile solutions to the most challenging aspects of working with people with life-limiting illness. I have chosen to explore why certain problems are difficult and why the way we construct our responses to them may also be part of the problem. I have tried to make reference to key texts that support the arguments and issues set out so that these may be used as sources for further reading. I have also tried to adopt a critical and reflective stance, as I believe this is the route to learning about more supportive and ultimately more effective health care. As Nikolas Rose (1994) states: 'in revealing the complex contingencies that have made up the territory we inhabit and the horizons of our experience, in showing that things could have been different, such analyses encourage us to weigh up the costs as well as the benefits of the present we inhabit. They thus allow us to dream of a time in which our times could be different again' (p. 71).

References

Addington-Hall, J. and McCarthy, M. (1995) Dying from cancer: results of a national population-based investigation. *Palliative Medicine*, 9: 295–305.

Armstrong, D. (1995) The rise of surveillance medicine. *Sociology of Health and Illness*, 17(3): 393–404.

Bailey, C. (1995) Nursing as therapy in the management of breathlessness in lung cancer. *European Journal of Cancer Care*, 4: 184–90.

Benner, P. and Wrubel, J. (1989) *The Privacy of Care: Stress and Coping in Health and Illness*. Menlo Park, CA: Addison-Wesley.

Bion, W. (1977) Learning from experience. *Seven Servants: Four Works*. New York: Jason Aronson.

Bredin, M., Corner, J., Krishnasamy, M. *et al.* (1999) Multicentre randomized controlled trial of nursing intervention for breathlessness in patients with lung cancer. *British Medical Journal*, 318: 901–4.

Bury, M. (2001) Illness narratives: fact or fiction? *Sociology of Health and Illness*, 23(3): 263–85.

Carper, B.A. (1978) Fundamental patterns of knowing in nursing. *Advances in Nursing Science*, 1: 13–23.

Clark, D. (1999) 'Total pain', disciplinary power and the body in the work of Cicely Saunders, 1958–1967. *Social Science and Medicine*, 49(6): 727–36.

Corner, J. (1996) Is there a research paradigm for palliative care? *Palliative Medicine*, 10: 201–8.

Corner, J. (2001a) Management of breathlessness in lung cancer: new scientific evidence of developing multidisciplinary care, in M. Muers, F. Macbeth, F.C. Wells and A. Miles (eds) *The Effective Management of Lung Cancer*. London: Aesculapius Medical Press.

Corner, J. (2001b) *Between You and Me: Closing the Gap Between People and Health Care*. London: The Nuffield Trust/The Stationery Office.

Corner, J. and Dunlop, R. (1997) New approaches to care, in D. Clark, J. Hockley and S. Ahmedzai (eds) *New Themes in Palliative Care*. Buckingham: Open University Press.

Corner, J., Plant, H., A'Hern, R. and Bailey, C. (1996) Non-pharmacological intervention for breathlessness in lung cancer. *Palliative Medicine*, 13: 375–84.

Cribb, A. (2001) Knowledge and caring: a philosophical and personal perspective, in J. Corner and C. Bailey (eds) *Cancer Nursing: Care in Context*. Oxford: Blackwell Science.

Fabricius, J. (1991) Running on the spot or can nursing really change. *Psychoanalytic Psychotherapy*, 5: 97–108.

Field, D. (1994) Palliative medicine and the medicalization of death. *European Journal of Cancer Care*, 3: 58–62.

Foucault, M. ([1973] 1986) *The Birth of the Clinic*. London: Routledge.

Higginson, I. and McCarthy, M. (1989) Measuring symptoms in terminal cancer: are pain and breathlessness controlled? *Journal of the Royal Society of Medicine*, 82: 264–7.

Hinton, J. (1994) Can home care maintain an acceptable quality of life for patients with terminal cancer and their relatives? *Palliative Medicine*, 8: 183–96.

Illich, I. ([1976] 1990) *Limits to Medicine, Medical Nemesis: The Expropriation of Health*. London: Penguin.

Johns, C. (1995) Framing learning through reflection within Carper's fundamental ways of knowing nursing. *Journal of Advanced Nursing*, 22: 226–34.

Kleinman, A. (1988) *The Illness Narratives: Suffering, Healing and the Human Condition*. New York: Basic Books.

Krishnasamy, M. (2000) Fatigue in advanced cancer: meaning before measurement. *International Journal of Nursing Studies*, 5: 401–14.

Lawton, J. (2000) *The Dying Process: Patients' Experiences of Palliative Care*. London: Routledge.

Lupton, D. (1994) Food, memory and meaning: the symbolic and social nature of food events. *Sociological Review*, 42: 664–85.

Lupton, D. (1997) *Medicine as Culture: Illness, Disease and the Body in Western Societies*. London: Sage.

Lyon, M.L. and Barbalet, J.M. (1994) Society's body: emotion and the 'somatization' of social theory in T.J. Czordas (ed.) *Embodiment and Experience*. Cambridge: Cambridge University Press.

McNamara, B. (2001) *Fragile Lives: Death, Dying and Care*. Buckingham: Open University Press.

Nolan, M. and Lundh, U. (1998) Ways of knowing in nursing and healthcare practice, in P. Crookes and C. Davies (eds) *Research into Practice*. Edinburgh: Ballière Tindall.

O'Driscoll, M., Corner, J. and Bailey, C. (1999) The experience of breathlessness in lung cancer. *European Journal of Cancer Care*, 8: 37–43.

Poole, K. and Froggatt, K. (2002) Loss of weight and loss of appetite in advanced cancer: a problem for the patient, the carer, or the health professional. *Palliative Medicine*, 16: 499–506.

Richardson, A. and Ream, E. (1996) Fatigue: a concept analysis. *International Journal of Nursing Studies*, 33(5): 519–25.

Robbins, M. (1998) *Evaluating Palliative Care*. Oxford: Oxford Medical Publications.

Roberts, D.K., Thorne, S.E. and Pearson, C. (1993) The experience of dyspnoea in late stage cancer. *Cancer Nursing*, 16: 234–6.

Rose, N. (1994) Medicine, history and the present, in C. Jones and R. Porter (eds) *Reassessing Foucault: Power, Medicine and the Body*. London: Routledge.

Skilbeck, J., Mott, L., Page, H. *et al.* (1998) Palliative care in chronic obstructive airways disease: a needs assessment. *Palliative Medicine*, 12: 245–54.

Tate, H. and George, R. (2001) The effect of weight loss on body image in HIV-positive gay men. *AIDS Care*, 13: 163–9.

Taussig, M.T. (1980) Reification and the consciousness of the patient. *Social Science and Medicine*, 14: 3–13.

Williams, S. (1993) *Chronic Respiratory Illness*. London: Routledge.

Williams, S. (1996) The vicissitudes of embodiment across the chronic illness trajectory. *Body and Society*, 2(2): 23–47.

Williams, S. and Bendelow, G. (1998) In search of the 'missing body': pain suffering and the (post) modern condition, in G. Scrambler and P. Higgs (eds) *Modernity, Medicine and Health*. London: Routledge.

13

Pain

Theories, evaluation and management

Silvia Paz and Jane Seymour

It is only during the last 50 years that pain has been recognized as a condition that requires specialized treatment and dedicated research. Before the availability of analgesics and anaesthetics, pain was regarded as a natural and an expected part of life, and was explained primarily in terms of a religious belief system within which medicine had little part to play. During the nineteenth century, with the emergence of 'modern' medical and scientific ideas, advances in anatomy, physiology, chemistry and pharmacy heralded the discovery of analgesics and anaesthetics, together with techniques for their application. As a result, medical and research interest in the subject was generated, and by the beginning of the twentieth century physicians engaged not only in controlling pain but also in finding a scientific explanation for it. Until the 1960s, pain was considered by most clinicians as an inevitable sensory and physiological response to tissue damage: there was little recognition or understanding of the effects on pain perception of individual expectations, anxiety, past experience or genetic differences. Moreover, no distinction was made between 'acute' and 'chronic' pain states. It is only in more recent years that the physiological, psychological and socio-cultural factors that contribute to the perception of pain have begun to be understood, and the necessary differentiation made in treatments of acute and chronic pain. The aims of this chapter are to: provide a framework for understanding theories of pain and pain mechanisms, and how these have developed over time; describe basic principles for the management of chronic and cancer pain; and examine the role of the nurse in the assessment and measurement of pain, and in the administration of analgesics.

What does 'pain' mean: contemporary definitions

Pain is difficult to define because of the complexity of its anatomical and physiological foundations, the individuality of its experience, and its social and cultural meanings. Pain has had different significances and meanings throughout the ages and in various societies existing at the same time. In spite of this, definitions have been developed that are widely accepted as both clinically useful and phenomenologically valid. Thus, the International Association for the Study of Pain (IASP) defines pain as 'an unpleasant sensory and emotional experience associated with actual or potential tissue damage, or described in terms of such damage' (Merskey and Bogduk 1994: 210). In other widely accepted definitions, pain is described as being 'whatever the experiencing person says it is, existing whenever he says it does' (McCaffery 1968, cited by Fink and Gates 2001: 95) or as 'what the patient says hurts' (Twycross and Wilcock 2002: 17). These three 'classic' definitions present pain as:

- being an individual experience;
- comprising emotional and sensorial components;
- having temporal characteristics;
- having undefined boundaries.

In the next section, we review how pain has been understood across the course of the last century and we outline current concepts of acute, chronic and cancer pain. We present recognized methods for pain assessment and pharmacological and non-pharmacological approaches for adequate pain control, emphasizing the role of the nurse in chronic and cancer pain relief.

Theories of pain and pain mechanisms

For centuries, medical physicians and scientists have been engaged in establishing a theoretical explanation for questions about how the human body perceives pain, why the experience of pain is different from other sensations, and why individuals perceive pain differently in objectively similar conditions. A *theory* is primarily an attempted solution to a problem. The theory is usually formulated on the basis of a collection of several clues that may lead to a guess about the nature of the solution. It is made up of a mix of facts and assumptions that need to be tested. After the theory has been formulated, new facts are tested against it to see whether they fit. If they support the theory, all the clues may fit together to make a coherent picture (Melzack and Wall 1996). Here we intend to review the following theories of pain: specificity theory, patterning theory, gate control theory and the neuromatrix theory. A variety of key concepts have been used within these (see Box 13.1).

Specificity theory

During the first half of the twentieth century, the most enduring theory of pain was 'specificity theory' (Melzack and Wall 1996). This proposes that a

---

Box 13.1   Pain concepts

- *Receptor* is a three-dimensional structure localized in the cell membrane with special architectural features that enables it to bind different molecules, such as drugs, to form a 'drug–receptor' complex. By binding their specific receptors, drugs and other molecular mediators have their effect in the body
- *Nociceptor* is a receptor preferentially sensitive to a noxious stimulus or to a stimulus that would become noxious if prolonged
- *Noxious stimulus* is one which is damaging to normal tissues
- *Nociception* is the physiological process necessary for pain to occur. It is a sensory process that involves three steps:

  (a)   nociceptor activation in the periphery (transduction)
  (b)   relay of the information from the periphery to the central nervous system (transmission)
  (c)   neural activity that leads to control of the pain transmission pathway (modulation)

- *Pain perception* is the awareness of pain frequently initiated by a noxious stimulus, such as an injury or a disease, or by lesions in the peripheral or central nervous system, such as diabetic neuropathy, spinal cord compression and stroke. Pain is a perceptual phenomenon that involves higher central nervous system mechanisms
- *Pain behaviours* are the things somebody does or does not do that can be described as a result of the presence of pain and the menace of tissue damage or disease that it represents. Examples of pain behaviours are grimacing, anger, lying down, stopping working, crying, recourse to medical advice

---

specific 'pain pathway' in the spinal cord carries messages from pain receptors in the skin to a pain centre in the brain, and pain is evidenced by the withdrawal of the relevant body part from the noxious stimulus as a result of the action of nerves (Horn and Munafo 1997: 2). This principle was first formulated by Descartes in 1664 (Melzack and Wall 1996: 150). It emphasized the mechanistic nature of pain and implied a 'linear causality', with no modulating factors acting between the stimulus, the receptor and the response (Horn and Munafo 1997: 1–2). The psychological and affective dimensions of pain, together with social factors, were ignored. This concept underwent little change through the next three centuries and, during the nineteenth century, further findings in anatomy and physiology supported its basic principles.

By the middle of the nineteenth century it was first stated, by Johannes Müller, that sensory nerves carried information about external objects to the brain: the doctrine of 'specific nerve energies' (Melzack and Wall 1982: 151). Müller's theory posited a linear system from the sensory organ to the brain centre, which was responsible for the sensation (Melzack and Wall 1982: 151).

The four modalities of skin sensation, touch, warmth, cold and pain were differentiated by von Frey in 1894 in a 'theory of cutaeneous senses' (Melzack and Wall 1982: 152). Von Frey assumed that the human skin comprises a multitude of unique sensory 'spots' for touch, warmth, cold and pain, and identified two types of structures in the skin: (1) *free nerve endings*, in the upper layers of the skin; and (2) *nerve fibres*, wrapped around hair follicles. Von Frey associated free nerve endings with the detection of pain in the periphery and assumed these to be the *pain receptors* (Melzack and Wall 1982: 151–2). Von Frey's theory encouraged others to seek for specific pathways from the receptors to the spinal cord and then the brain (Horn and Munafo 1997: 4). Subsequent studies and operations in humans and animals suggested that the anterolateral quadrant of the spinal cord was critically important for relaying pain sensation to the brain, and the spinothalamic tract that ascends in the anterolateral aspect of the spinal cord came to be known as 'the pain pathway'. To this day, the location of the pain centre in the brain is still a source of controversy and extensive research (Melzack and Wall 1982: 154).

The greatest weakness of the specificity theory of pain is its assumption that there is a rigid and direct relationship between the physical stimulus and a sensation felt by the individual. The idea of the existence of specific pain receptors implies that stimulation of these receptors will result invariably in the sensation of pain (Horn and Munafo 1997: 5), but clinical evidence of phantom limb pains, neuralgias and causalgias constitute a strong challenge to the idea of a fixed, direct-line nervous system and thus to the simplicity of the specificity theory of pain. In all these latter syndromes, the central nervous system has been damaged and gentle-touch, vibration and any other type of non-noxious stimuli can trigger excruciating pain (Melzack and Wall 1982: 156).

Patterning theory

In an early critique of specificity theory, Goldscheider hypothesized in 1894 that pain was due to excessive peripheral stimulation that produces a pattern of nerve impulses interpreted centrally as pain (Horn and Munafo 1997: 5). He based this hypothesis on observations of patients with unusual pain perceptions due to late-stage syphilis who sometimes reported bizarre pain as a result of a mild stimulus, such as burning pain when repeatedly touched by a warm stimulus (Horn and Munafo 1997: 5). Goldscheider proposed that all fibre endings were alike, that intense stimulation of non-specific receptors produced different patterns for pain, and that the transmission of peripheral sensory information was 'summated' at the dorsal horn. Pain information would be transmitted to higher levels (the brain) and perceived only if the level of output at the dorsal horn exceeded a threshold (Horn and Munafo 1997: 5). He formulated the theory of pattern generation of pain, popularly known as the 'patterning theory of pain'. The important contribution made by this theory to the understanding of pain was the idea of the summation phenomenon in the spinal cord implying that 'something else' needs to happen at the transmission level before the pain sensation would be perceived.

An emergent critique of specificity and pattern theories: the impact of the First and Second World Wars

It could be said that the advances made in the understanding of pain during the first half of the twentieth century resulted from (1) the work undertaken by Rene Leriche during the First World War, which introduced the concept of visceral pain and its components, and (2) the invaluable observations made in battlefields by Henry Beecher during the Second World War, which highlighted that pain was a multidimensional and individual experience.

In the post-war periods, the idea of a 'specific pain pathway' led to the development of numerous surgical techniques to control pain. It was believed that by sectioning the pain pathway the perception of pain would be avoided. These surgical sections could be done at different levels of the pain path, such as a 'neurotomy' to section a nerve branch, a 'radicotomy' to section posterior spinal nerve roots, or a 'cordotomy' to section the spino-thalamic tract of the spinal cord (Rey 1995: 307). This emerging neuro-surgical field seemed to proffer tempting solutions when other available therapeutic options were insufficient. It was also a time when addiction to morphine, or 'morphinomania', was becoming a major medical and social concern. In comparison, surgery was seen as an opportunity to attack and potentially eradicate pain directly, without resorting to morphine use (Rey 1995: 308).

The French surgeon Rene Leriche was, arguably, a pioneer of the 'surgery of pain'. His work covered two types of surgical operations: one performed on the sensibility tracts of the central nervous system as previously mentioned, and the other performed on the sympathetic nervous system. The latter was the area in which Leriche made his most significant contribution (Rey 1995). During the First World War, Leriche saw many soldiers with injuries that compromise both motor and visceral structures. By performing different interventions to the sympathetic nervous system, he was able to define the two elements of 'visceral pain': the 'true' and the 'referred' pain, concepts hotly debated at the time (Rey 1995: 312–15).

Later, an anaesthetist, Henry Beecher, had a considerable influence based on his observations of wounded soldiers during the Second World War, when he reported that many rarely complained of pain (Beecher 1946, cited in Meldrum 1998). He hypothesized that this was because of their culture of stoicism, their relief that they survived, or their expectation that they would now be able to return home. From these observations and his subsequent clinical work, Beecher theorized that the perception of pain was largely dependent upon a 'reaction component' that depended on such variables as age, gender, ethnicity, experience, culture and distraction. The main thrust of Beecher's critique of laboratory-based pain was that *experimentally induced* and *clinically relevant* pain were not comparable because:

> the reaction or processing of sensations that travel over the peripheral pain apparatus and emerge in consciousness is determined by past experience, by conditioning, by memory, by judgement, by present meaning . . . This reaction is never alike for any two individuals and, indeed, with the passing of time and accumulation of life experience, is never exactly the same for the same individual from one time to another.
>
> (Beecher 1956: 12)

Another American anesthetist, John Bonica, built on Beecher's work, putting forward the radical view that pain was a *composite* of neurophysiologic and psychological factors that should be 'apprehended clinically as a whole' (Baszanger 1998: 27). Most notably, Bonica argued that the mental and physical effects of pain needed to be understood as catalysts of each other. This overturned a position in which the approach to pain was confined to diagnosis and cause, and in which any emotional or 'subjective' element was excluded (Baszanger 1998: 29).

In the decades after the Second World War, the study of pain gained momentum primarily for two reasons. First, the search for strong and non-addictive analgesics as alternatives to morphine and aspirin led to the study of pain under laboratory-controlled conditions with the aim of detecting and measuring changes in pain perception in order to document the efficacy of the analgesics (Meldrum 1998). Until then, morphine and aspirin were the only painkillers widely used and easily accessible. While morphine and other opium derivatives had many medical uses, aspirin was the first drug purely marketed as an analgesic. Second, published observations made by physicians of their clinical practice began to provide a richer understanding of pain as a multidimensional and individual experience.

The emergence of 'gate control' theory

By the 1960s, pain was defined by unconnected concepts of patterning, possible modulation in the dorsal horn of the spinal cord, ascending pain pathways from the periphery to the brain, and the multidimensional qualities of the *pain experience*. Although it became apparent that the spinal cord might have an active role in the mechanism of pain, much emphasis was still concentrated on the periphery and the pain receptors. The spinal cord was conceived as a passive transmission station, and the brain as a final receptive station.

In 1965, Ronald Melzack and Patrick Wall presented a new theory – the 'gate control theory of pain' – which effectively provided a comprehensive model that was, for the first time, able to account for both neurophysiological and psychological factors. They suggested that input signals from primary sensory neurons were actively modulated in the spinal cord by a neural mechanism, the 'gate'. A balance between inhibitory and facilitatory influences arising both locally and descending from the brain determined which signals were let through and relayed to the brain. These signals would then be perceived as a painful stimulus. The balance between peripheral (ascending and facilitatory) and central (descending and inhibitory) inputs would open or close the 'gate'. As a result, both the spinal cord and the brain were actively involved in the pain process. The spinal cord was presented as a controlling centre where activations, inhibitions and modulation occurred, and the brain as an active system that filters, selects and also modulates sensory inputs. The gate control theory pointed to the dorsal horn of the spinal cord as the crucial place that determines whether an individual would be in pain (Melzack and Wall 1965). In this way, it allows us to explain: (a) the cultural, affective and emotive dimensions of pain that make severely wounded patients feel less pain than expected (Beecher 1946); (b) pain without evident tissue damage, such as migraine or chronic low back pain.

After the publication of the gate control theory, an explosion in research on the physiology and pharmacology of the dorsal horn of the spinal cord and the descending control systems from the brain occurred. Psychological factors started to be seen as an integral part of the pain process and new approaches for pain control were opened, such as the transcutaneous electrical nerve stimulation (TENS) technique that later became an important modality for the treatment of chronic and acute pain (Tulder *et al.* 2000).

The neuromatrix theory

In 1999, Ronald Melzack proposed a model to explain how the human body perceives pain in relation to itself and the outside world. He called his model the 'neuromatrix theory of pain'. When we are in pain, several events occur simultaneously. For instance, we become aware of our current pain state by being able to define its severity, its duration, what makes it worse or better. We tend to look for reasons that might be causing the pain and for ways to control it. But what the pain means to us and how we react to it and behave depend upon several factors, such as our previous experiences of similar circumstances, our ability to cope with stressful situations, our genetic disposition to perceive and tolerate pain, and our expectations of the immediate and near future in relation to the painful condition. To explain how all these aspects come together to build up our individual experience of pain, Melzack proposed that the whole body is represented in a neural network in the brain, the *neuromatrix*. He suggested that its structure is determined genetically and modified by experience over time. The perception of pain by the neuromatrix in the brain results from the summary of sensory inputs that arrive from the site of injury, current concentrations of endocrine products of stress release in response to the pain, such as cortisol, adrenaline and glucose, and emotive inputs derived from past individual experiences. In this way, Melzack emphasizes the importance of incorporating other disciplines, such as endocrinology and genetics, in the multidisciplinary approach of pain management (Dickenson 2002).

Neuroplasticity

Today, it is acknowledged that when tissue is damaged many different chemical inflammatory messengers form locally an 'inflammatory soup' and sensitize a network of neural structures (Dickenson 2002). These peripheral changes then alter the activity in central systems and drive central compensations and adaptations, so that the mechanisms involved in the pain are likely to be multiple and located at a number of sites. As a result of these observations, potential new targets for analgesic therapy are currently being researched and a rationale on which to base the use of opioids and other analgesics has emerged. On the other hand, it has also been suggested that sensory neurons share the ability to use information previously acquired to respond to current demands following a neuronal 'learning' process. This capacity of sensory neurons to change the pattern of transmission according to previous experience and the surrounding environment is recognized as the plasticity of the nervous system or 'neuroplasticity' (Dickenson 1995).

Pain and the brain: contemporary understandings

During recent decades, the major challenge in the study of pain mechanisms has been to understand how the brain works (Melzack and Wall 1996: 154). Reasons for lack of appropriate evidence have included ethical concerns and limitations, lack of interest in the subject compared with other medical fields and lack of suitable examination techniques (Berman 1995). However, the development of relatively non-invasive imaging techniques has made possible the study of functional brain activity during the process of pain. There are three relevant imaging techniques currently available for the study of pain:

- single photon emission computed tomography (SPECT);
- positron emission tomography (PET); and
- functional magnetic resonance imaging (fMRI).

These imaging techniques have been applied to the problem of localizing brain areas associated with a variety of experimental and clinical pain conditions. They can also be used in human beings to study the distribution of brain receptors. For instance, positron emission tomography has been widely used to map opioid receptors. However, these techniques have several limitations: they rely on the experience of the operator and on the integrity of anatomical structures, and they only provide information at a 'macro' level with no precision on the cells involved in the process of pain and their functions (Berman 1995).

We now provide a brief summary of the variety of understandings of pain and their evolution (see Box 13.2).

Box 13.2   Summary of pain understandings

Before the nineteenth century	People expected to suffer pain as a life natural event. It had magical and religious connotations. Raw opium was the only medicine available with analgesic properties, although alcohol was also used to dull the senses. Principles of anesthesia were unknown

Nineteenth century

- Morphine was first isolated from opium in 1804 and subsequently other opioids were found
- Anaesthetic techniques started to be developed and the principles for anaesthesia became to be understood
- The study of pain gained more interest alongside developments in surgical procedures
- Acetylsalicylic acid (aspirin) was first discovered in 1873 and was the first medicine marketed as a painkiller or analgesic
- The *specificity theory of pain* was formulated following a mechanistic understanding of the pain process as rigid, unidirectional and structured. Pain receptor (skin) → pain pathway (spinal cord) → pain centre (brain)

First half of the twentieth century

- The specificity theory of pain further developed and dominated understandings of pain mechanisms
- Surgical techniques to 'cut' the 'pain pathway' were developed and used to control severe chronic pains
- Patients who suffered from pain of uncertain origin with no evidence of tissue damage (e.g. migraine, low back pain) were sent to psychiatrists, as it was not possible to explain their painful conditions with the knowledge at the time
- Visceral pain was described and recognized as a possible variety of pain
- The need for further alternative analgesics led to the study of pain in experimental and clinical settings
- Earliest observations and documentations of the emotive, affective and cultural aspects of pain gained recognition

Second half of the twentieth century

- Cancer and chronic pain started to gain medical recognition as a relevant public health problem
- In 1960, the *gate control theory of pain* incorporated the physical and psychological components of pain, changing the way in which the pain process was understood and researched

> - The hospice movement and the development of pain clinics emphasized the need for a multi-professional approach to pain relief
> - Pain became to be seen as a multidimensional phenomenon with physical, social, psychological, emotional and cultural components
> - A significant development in analgesic interventions and methods for the administration of painkillers developed
> - Imaging techniques helped to study the brain behaviour of human beings during painful events

Different types of pain: classifications

Two main types of pain can be identified according to the reaction they generate: (1) functional or physiological pain and (2) clinical pain. *Functional* or *physiological pain* has a primary protective role: it warns us of imminent or actual tissue damage and elicits coordinated reflex and behavioural responses to keep such damage to a minimum. It does not require medical intervention. Examples of physiological pain are present in everyday life, such as the way we quickly remove our hand when touching a hot plate. By contrast, *clinical pains* comprise persistent pain syndromes that offer no biological advantage and cause suffering and distress. Clinical pains are summarized in Box 13.3. People presenting with any type of clinical pain seek medical advice and frequently need regular assessment and supervision.

As Box 13.3 indicates, clinical pains can be described in a temporal sense as being *transient*, *acute* or *chronic*. They can also be described in terms of the type of tissue damage with which they are associated. *Inflammatory pain* is associated with visceral or somatic tissue damage or inflammation; *neuropathic pain* results from damage to the peripheral or central nervous systems.

Box 13.3   Clinical pain

	Inflammatory		Neuropathic
	Visceral	*Somatic*	*Neuropathic*
Transient	Painful endoscopy	Intramuscular injection	Shooting pain elicited by knocking the elbow
Acute	Inflamed appendix	Broken bone	Trigeminal neuralgia
Chronic	Metastatic enlargement of the liver	Low back pain	Diabetic neuropathy

Transient pain

This can appear in the absence of any tissue damage and is elicited by the activation of sensitive receptors in the skin or other tissues. It has been suggested that this type of pain probably develops to protect people from physical damage due to an adverse surrounding or due to over-stress of the body tissues (Loeser and Melzack 2001). In the clinical setting, transient pain is seen in procedural manoeuvres, such as during an endoscopy or an intramuscular injection.

Acute pain

This has been defined as 'the normal, predicted physiological response to an adverse chemical, thermal or mechanical stimulus associated with surgery, trauma and acute illness' (Federation of State Medical Boards of the United States 1998). It typically results from tissue injury or inflammation, and it can be considered to have a biologically reparative function. Because tissue damage has already occurred and cannot be prevented, the presence of acute pain enables healing and repairs to occur undisturbed, making the injured or inflamed area and surrounding tissue hypersensitive to all stimuli so that contact with any external stimulus is avoided. Usually, the local injury does not overwhelm the body's reparative mechanisms and 'healing' occurs without medical intervention (Carr and Goudas 2001). However, medical interventions may be useful in preventing or reducing pain and speeding up the healing process by shortening the duration of the injury (Loeser and Melzack 2001). Clinical observations indicate that the biological and psychological foundation for chronic pain is in place within hours of an acute injury. Early control of acute pain can shape its subsequent evolution and prevent it from transforming to persistent and long-term pain. For many patients minimization of pain can improve clinical outcomes (Carr 1998). Patients' attitudes, personalities and previous experiences will strongly influence their immediate reaction to acute pain, a typical example of which is post-operative pain.

Chronic pain

Chronic pain persists long after the tissue damage that initially triggered its onset has resolved, and in some people chronic pain presents without any identified ongoing tissue damage or antecedent injury, such as chronic low back pain or migraine (Bonica 1990, cited by Ashburn and Staats 2001). The inability of the body to restore its physiological functions to normal homeostatic levels distinguishes acute from chronic pain (Niv and Devor 1998). In some cases, chronic pain exists because the injury exceeds the body's capability for healing. This occurs in cases of extensive trauma and subsequent scarring, loss of a body part, or when the nervous system is affected by the injury itself (Loeser and Melzack 2001). For other chronic pain syndromes, such as chronic low back pain, headache, neuropathic pain and phantom limb pain, the available knowledge about their underlying pathophysiology is limited. These chronic pain syndromes are usually diagnosed and treated on the basis of clinical criteria alone, without existing definitive scientific evidence or confirmatory studies (Ashburn and Staats 2001). The traditional classification, based on the duration of pain, that describes acute pain as pain of recent onset and short duration and chronic pain as persistent pain after an injury has healed, is increasingly questionable (Carr and Goudas 2001). A 1994 report of the International Association for the Study of Pain Task Force on Taxonomy (Merskey and Begduk 1994) acknowledged that acute pain associated with new tissue injury might last for less than 1 month, but at times for longer than 6 months. However, since the healing process usually takes a few days or a few weeks, pain that persists for several months or years tends not to be classified as acute. Chronic pain tends to have a more profound impact on patients' general state than acute pain: it often affects the patient's mood, personality and social relationships. People with chronic pain usually experience concomitant depression, sleep disturbance, fatigue and decreased overall physical and mental functioning (Ashburn and Staats 2001).

Approaches to managing chronic pain

In the 1950s, John Bonica developed an interdisciplinary approach designed to integrate the efforts of health care providers from several disciplines, each of whom specializes in different features of the pain experience (Baszanger 1998). Bonica's legacy has been the concept of the 'pain clinic': a model for managing chronic pain that has been adopted across the world. Bonica's work in the USA was mirrored in many respects by the pioneering work on cancer pain of Cicely Saunders in the UK during the 1960s (Clark 1998).

It is now widely understood that the management of chronic pain should be an interdisciplinary endeavour, with a core team typically comprising a pain management physician, a psychologist, a nurse specialist, a physical therapist and a pharmacist. The team tailors the care plan according to the individual needs of the patient, with a focus on achieving measurable treatment goals in reasonable periods of time established with the patient. Cognitive and behavioural therapies are used in the management of chronic pain to alter the effect of the pain on the individual's life (see Box 13.4).

Nociceptive and neuropathic pain

The term 'nociceptive' is applied to pains that are presumed to be maintained by continual tissue injury (Twycross and Wilcock 2002). *Nociceptive pain* is called 'somatic' when it is produced by damage of structural tissues, such as skin, bone, muscle or joint (Woolf 1995). Pain of somatic origin is usually focal and well localized, dull or stabbing. It usually responds well to conventional analgesics, such as non-steroidal anti-inflammatory and opioid drugs. Nociceptive pain is known as *visceral pain* when it is produced by an injury of internal organs, such as lung, heart or gut. Visceral pain has five important clinical characteristics (Cervero and Laird 2001):

Box 13.4   Roles of members of an interdisciplinary pain management team (adapted from Ashburn and Staats 2001: 4)

Physician	Nurse	Psychologist	Physical and occupational therapist	Pharmacist
• Regular assessment and neurological and musculo-skeletal examination • Review of preview interventions • New therapy considerations • Specialist referral • Education	• Coordination of care • Education to medical and non-medical staff • Regular assessment of patient's and relatives' needs • Continuous support • Consideration and provision of non-pharmaco-logical interventions	• Comprehensive psychological support • Regular psychological assessment • Coping skills reinforcement • Cognitive behaviour therapies • Education on the use of self-management techniques	• Regular assessment of physical endurance • Regular assessment of the work site and home • Management of physical rehabilitation techniques	• Regular review of past and current pharmaco-logical interventions. • Education with regard to adequate use of pharmaco-logical interventions. • Regular update on available alternative pharmaco-logical interventions

- It is not evoked from all viscera (organs such as liver, kidney, most solid viscera and lung parenchyma are not sensitive to pain). Pain in the area of these organs is usually due to inflammation, distention or irritation of the surrounding tissues (e.g. pain due to distention of the liver capsule due to hepatic malignant infiltration).
- It is not always linked to visceral injury (cutting the intestine causes no pain, whereas stretching the bladder is painful).
- It is diffuse and poorly localized.
- It is referred to other locations.
- It is accompanied by motor and autonomic reflexes, such as nausea, vomiting and local muscle tension, such as the lower back muscle tension that occurs in renal colic.

There are two distinct types of localization of visceral pain: deep, 'true' visceral pain, and superficial, 'referred' visceral pain. The pain that is perceived as being deep within the body is often called 'true' visceral pain. It is usually perceived as arising in the midline, and perceived as anterior or posterior. 'True' visceral pain is usually extensive rather than focal and with diffuse boundaries. It is frequently associated with a sense of nausea and being ill. Autonomic and motor reflexes are often extreme and prolonged.

'Referred' visceral pain appears in distant structures from the affected organ. The area of referral is often superficial and segmental, that is to muscle, skin or both, innervated by the same spinal nerves as the affected viscus. The site of referral may additionally show hyperalgesia and it might be tender to the touch. 'True' and 'referred' visceral pain may be present at the same or different times (Cervero and Laird 2001).

Tissue damage provokes a local inflammatory response that alters the sensitivity of sensory fibres in the periphery. The inflammatory response is characterized by the local release of many different chemical messengers, such as growth factors – histamine, bradykinin, cytokines, substance 'P' – which are responsible for the sensitization of the peripheral sensory fibres. They tend to act synergistically together rather than individually, by producing a 'soup' or 'cocktail', usually called the 'inflammatory soup' (Loeser and Melzack 2001). Non-steroidal anti-inflammatory drugs, such as aspirin and ibuprofen, act by modifying this inflammatory soup. For this reason, they are of particular benefit for pains in which inflammation is a major component, such as bone metastasis and tissue infiltration (Twycross and Wilcock 2002). Figure 13.1 depicts this process.

The term *neuropathic pain* is used when the pain results from damage to the nervous system, such a peripheral nerve, the dorsal root ganglion or dorsal root, or the central nervous system (Woolf and Mannion 2001). It is sustained by an aberrant somatosensory processing in either the peripheral or the central nervous system. In cancer patients, for instance, neuropathic pain appears when a peripheral nerve is trapped by the growth of the tumour. Other more complex syndromes are also labelled as neuropathic pains, namely central pain, neuropathies (either mononeuropathies or polyneuropathies) and complex regional pain syndromes (see Box 13.5).

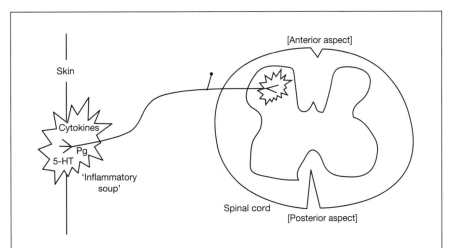

Figure 13.1 Inflammatory messengers are released at the site of the injury. They sensitize sensory peripheral fibres and also induce changes at the central processing of the pain message (adapted from Twycross and Wilcock 2002: 33).

Box 13.5   Neuropathic pain syndromes associated with an injury of a nervous system structure

- *Central pain* is the pain initiated or caused by a primary lesion or dysfunction in the central nervous system, such as post-stroke pain and spinal cord compression pain
- *Neuropathies* represent a disturbance of function or pathological change in a peripheral nerve:
  - in one nerve, *mononeuropathy*
  - if diffuse and bilateral affecting several nerves, *polyneuropathy*
- *Complex regional pain syndromes*, such as:
  - *causalgia* is a syndrome of sustained burning pain and allodynia after a traumatic nerve lesion, often combined with vasomotor and sudomotor dysfunction and later trophic changes

---

Many patients with neuropathic pain exhibit persistent or paroxysmal pain that is independent of a stimulus (Woolf and Mannion 2001). This pain appears without any identified stimulus and it can be shooting, stabbing or burning. It may depend on activity in the sympathetic nervous system. Stimulus-evoked pain is a common component of peripheral nerve injury and has two key features: hyperalgesia and allodynia. Although neuropathic pain can respond well to conventional analgesics, in many patients it does not respond to non-steroidal anti-inflammatory drugs and it is resistant or insensible to opioid drugs. Patients are usually treated with combinations of drugs that may include: opioid analgesics, such as morphine; non-steroidal anti-inflammatory drugs, such as diclofenac; tricyclic antidepressants, such as amitriptiline; serotonin uptake inhibitors, such as sertraline; and anticonvulsants, such as carbamazepine or gabapentin. Local anaesthetic blocks targeted at trigger points, peripheral nerves, plexi, dorsal roots and the sympathetic nervous system have useful but short-lived effects. Chronic epidural administration of drugs such as clonidine, steroids, opioids or midazolam has also been used with variable results (Woolf and Mannion 2001). Overall, the diagnosis of neuropathic pain indicates the need for a combination of therapies and the aim of the treatment is often to help the patient to cope by means of psychological, complementary or occupational therapies, rather than to eliminate the pain completely (see Figure 13.2).

The ability to clinically differentiate inflammatory – either visceral or somatic – from neuropathic pain has relevant therapeutic implications, since different analgesics are better at controlling different types of clinical pains. Box 13.6 presents a summary of this section of the chapter.

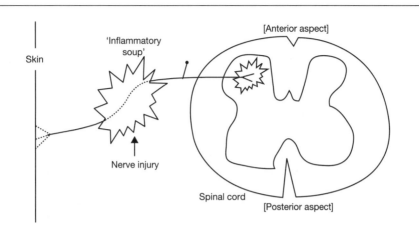

Figure 13.2   Neuropathic pain appears when there is an injury that affects any structure of the nervous system. Inflammatory messengers are also released at the site of the injury and play an important role in the development of neuropathic pain (adapted from Twycross and Wilcock 2002: 33).

Box 13.6   A summary of types of pain

- *Somatic pain* is the pain elicited when the body's structural elements, such as bone or muscle, are damaged
- *Visceral pain* is the pain caused by the injury of internal organs or their surrounding tissues, such as liver, heart and appendix
- *Neuropathic pain* is the pain initiated or caused by a primary lesion or dysfunction in the nervous system
- *Referred pain* is a feature of visceral pain. The area of referral is generally localized to distant structures, segmental and superficial, that are muscle, skin or both, innervated by the same spinal nerves as the affected internal organ
- *Breakthrough* (*unpredictable*) *pain* is an intermittent exacerbation of pain that can occur spontaneously, usually not related to a specific activity or weight-bearing
- *Incident* (*predictable*) *pain* is a type of intermittent pain that is related to a specific activity, such as eating, defecation, weight-bearing or walking. Also referred to as 'movement-related pain'
- *End of dose failure pain* occurs shortly before the next dose of regular analgesics is due. It is usually controlled with an increase in the regular dose of analgesics
- *Hyperalgesia* is an increased response to a stimulus, which is normally painful. It appears when a noxious stimulus applied on the skin causes more pain than that expected in a normal tissue
- *Allodinya* is the pain caused by a stimulus that would not normally produce pain
- *Dysesthesia* is an abnormal painful sensation, such as burning, caused by a non-noxious stimulus

Cancer pain

The prevalence of chronic pain in cancer patients has been estimated to be 30–50 per cent among patients with cancer who are undergoing active treatment for a solid tumour and 70–90 per cent among those patients with advanced disease (Portenoy and Lesage 2001). Box 13.7 summarizes data from the World Health Organization (Pan-American Health Organization 1999).

Prospective surveys indicate that as many as 90 per cent of patients could attain adequate relief with simple drug therapies, but this success rate is not achieved in routine practice (Pargeon and Hailey 1999). Inadequate management of pain is the result of various factors, including a deficiency in proper education of physicians and other health professionals on pain control and palliative care; fear among health professionals of drug dependence and addiction that results in under-prescription and under-use of analgesics; lack of general awareness that pain can be adequately controlled; misguided drug legislation and inappropriate availability of suitable drugs (WHO Expert Committee Report 1990). The World Health Organization advocates a strategy to respond to these issues (WHO 1996). It relies on three key components:

- *Government policies* emphasizing the need to alleviate chronic cancer pain.
- *Drug availability*, improving the prescription, distribution, dispensation and administration of drugs (especially opioids).
- *Education* of the public, health care professionals, drug regulators and policy makers.

Cancer pain management has had several implications for public health initiatives and policies and has recently been suggested as a possible indicator of adequate health service provision (Breivik 2002).

Box 13.7   Palliative care and adequate cancer pain relief needs: the World Health Organization figures (Pan-American Health Organization 1999)

- Nine million people a year worldwide develop cancer and 6 million others die from the disease
- Twenty-five per cent of all cancer patients throughout the world die without relief from severe pain
- Cancer pain occurs in about one-third of patients receiving anti-cancer therapy and more than two-thirds of patients with advanced disease experience pain
- Eighty per cent of patients in developing countries are incurable at diagnosis
- Terminal patients are inadequately managed in a significant number of cases in both developed and in developing countries

Pain syndromes in cancer

A cancer patient might present acute and chronic pain syndromes that are associated with the tumour or other painful condition unrelated to the neoplasm (Pargeon and Hailey 1999). Chronic pain syndromes in cancer patients may result from a direct effect of the neoplasm, may be related to therapies administered to manage the disease or to disorders unrelated to the disease or its treatment (Portenoy and Lesage 2001). Although most acute pain syndromes are caused by common diagnostic or therapeutic interventions, acute flare-ups of pain are common among patients with chronic pain (see Box 13.8). Many patients with well-controlled chronic pain have transitory 'breakthrough' pains. Recognition of cancer pain syndromes helps to identify the specific aetiology responsible for the pain, guide the need for additional evaluation, suggest specific therapies or assist in assessment of patients' outcome.

Tumour-related somatic pain syndromes might be due to neoplastic invasion of bone, joint, muscle or connective tissue causing persistent somatic pain. The spine is the most common site of bone metastases and many patients with cancer have back pain. Extension of a malignant tumour from the vertebra has the potential to damage the spinal cord, causing devastating neurological disorders. With early diagnosis and treatment, the neurological complication can be prevented. For this reason, a high level of suspicion of this complication is extremely important to prevent it and to ask for immediate medical assessment is mandatory. Different visceral and somatic pain syndromes can be caused by obstruction, infiltration or compression of visceral structures and connective supporting tissues. Tumour infiltration or compression of nerve, plexus or dorsal roots ganglion can be the reason for neuropathic pain syndromes. These can also be a consequence of the remote effect of malignant disease on peripheral nerves. The syndromes are highly variable. Patients react differently to each situation and they may refer aching pains or dysesthesias (abnormal pain sensations, such as burning) anywhere innervated by the damaged neural structure (Portenoy and Lesage 2001).

Iatrogenic pain syndromes may emerge after chemotherapy or radiotherapy or a combination of both. However, in general, specific somatic pain syndromes related to chemotherapy, radiation therapy or surgery are rare (e.g. radiation-induced or corticosteroid-induced necrosis of femoral or humeral head). More frequently, patients may complain of general malaise and aching, a flu-like syndrome, after these interventions have been preformed. Visceral pain can follow intraperitoneal chemotherapy or abdominal radiation therapy. These syndromes can mimic tumour-related pains and in the assessment it is important to exclude recurrence. Most pain syndromes that appear some time after the treatment has been completed are neuropathic. Radiation-induced fibrosis can damage a peripheral nerve or nerves and cause neuropathic pain; symptoms usually occur months to years after treatment. The neuropathic pain can be associated with slowly progressive weakness, sensory

Box 13.8   Acute pain syndromes in cancer patients (adapted from Portenoy and Lesage 2001: 3–4)

Acute pain may be associated with:
1   Diagnostic procedures:

- lumbar puncture headache
- bone marrow biopsy
- venepuncture
- paracentesis
- thoracentesis

2   Analgesic techniques:

- acute pain after strontium therapy of metastatic bone pain

3   Therapeutic procedures:

- pleurodesis
- tumour embolization
- nephrostomy insertion

4   Chemotherapy:

- intravenous or intraperitoneal infusions
- painful peripheral neuropathy (platins and taxanes)
- diffuse bone or muscle pain from colony-stimulating factors
- oral pain due to chemotherapy-induced mucositis

5   Hormonal therapy:

- painful gynaecomastia

6   Immunotherapy:

- arthralgia and myalgia from interferon and interleukin (flu-like syndrome)

7   Radiation therapy:

- headache after brain metastasis irradiation
- acute post-radiation proctocolitis or enteritis

Acute pain can be due to:
1   Tumour-related pathology:

- vertebral collapse
- pathological fracture
- headache from intracranial hypertension

2   Intercurrent infection:

- pain associated with wound infection or abscesses

3   Intercurrent pathology:

- cardiac angina
- ureteral colic pain

disturbances, radiation changes of the skin and lymphoedema (Portenoy and Lesage 2001).

The patient with pain due to cancer: the nurse's role in pain assessment and pain measurement

Patients with cancer are likely to experience a range of psychological, social and spiritual problems that extend far beyond the experience of physical pain. The concept of 'total pain' first coined by Cicely Saunders (Clark 1998), and subsequently developed by Twycross (see for example Twycross 1997), captures the range of issues with which nurses and other members of the multidisciplinary team need to be concerned when caring for patients suffering from pain due to cancer (see Figure 13.3).

The concept of 'total pain' alerts us to the fact that pain is a deeply personal experience that cannot be understood as merely a biological phenomenon. One of the nurse's greatest challenges and contributions to pain management is to facilitate the expression of each individual's encounter with pain (Krishnasamy 2001), and to begin to understand what factors, beyond the purely physical and physiological, impinge upon this. Although exploring what pain means to the person experiencing it can be very difficult, Krishnasamy identifies a range of questions that can be used to begin to evaluate and assess the experience of pain for a person with cancer and thus inform an effective care strategy (see Box 13.9).

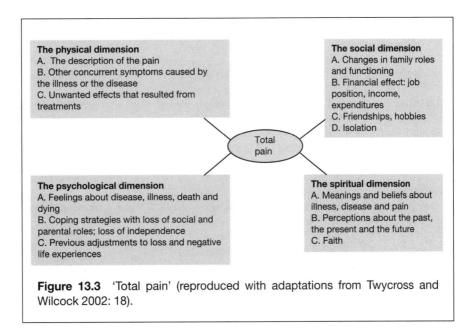

Figure 13.3 'Total pain' (reproduced with adaptations from Twycross and Wilcock 2002: 18).

While these questions are invaluable for understanding the personal experience of pain and the impact that pain has on the lives of patients and their family carers, nurses will also be responsible for contributing to *measuring* the severity of pain such that the effectiveness of therapeutic interventions can be evaluated. Pain measurement refers to a quantified measure of one aspect of the pain experience – its severity. The measurement of pain relies on a patient's self-reports, or the inferences that health professionals make on the basis of the patient's behaviour. Several methods are used to measure pain severity: numeric scales, descriptive rating scales, visual analogue scales and box scales.

One of the most frequently used instruments to measure pain is the McGill Pain Questionnaire (Turk and Okifuji 2001). It has three parts:

1 The first part includes a descriptive scale that rates the intensity of the present pain. Numbers are assigned to each of five adjectives: 1 (mild), 2 (discomforting), 3 (distressing), 4 (horrible), 5 (excruciating).

2 In the second part, patients can mark the location of their pain on ventral and dorsal views of a human figure.

3 The third part explores the sensory, affective and cognitive components of pain. It comprises 20 categories grouped in a pain-rating index.

Although this questionnaire provides a great deal of information, it requires a long time to complete. A shorter version has been produced.

Categorical verbal rating scales have been used to assess how effective a given analgesic is. The patient is asked to rate the pain and the analgesic effect and the observer documents the patient's ratings. They are one of the most reliable, sensitive and reproducible tools, although the information they provide about other pain characteristics is very limited (Carroll and Bowsher 1993). The Oxford Pain Chart (McQuay 1990) incorporates cat-

---

Box 13.9 Evaluate and assess the experience of pain for a person with cancer to inform an effective care strategy (from Krishnasamy 2001: 341)

- When did you first notice you were ill?
- How have things been with your family and friends?
- What was happening in your life when the cancer was diagnosed?
- Did you experience any pain when you were first ill?
- What makes it better?
- Is the pain the same now or has it changed?
- What are your fears for the future?

- How have things been since you were told about the cancer?
- How have things been for your family and friends?
- What plans in your life has it disrupted or stopped?
- When did you first experience any pain?
- What makes it worse?
- What are your expectations and hopes for the future?
- What does the pain mean to you?

egorical scales into a pain diary. For 7 days, the patient is asked to fill in a pain diary before going to bed. Each day, the patient should rate the intensity of the pain and the relief obtained with the treatment and tick a box (Carroll and Bowsher 1993: 24):

How bad has your pain been today?

severe   ☐

moderate   ☐

mild   ☐

none   ☐

How much pain relief have the tablets given today?

complete   ☐

good   ☐

moderate   ☐

slight   ☐

none   ☐

There is also a space for the patient to describe side-effects: *Has the treatment upset you in any way?* Finally, the patient is asked to estimate the effectiveness of the treatment over the week by circling a choice:

How effective was the treatment this week?

poor   fair   good   very good   excellent

☐   ☐   ☐   ☐   ☐

There are many other tools for pain measurement. There are no rules as to which pain measurement tool should be used or which is the best one. It may be useful to find out what tools are used by colleagues and what their perceptions about available tools are. Functional scales are useful in measuring patients' ability to engage in functional activities, such as walking up stairs, sitting or resting for a specific time, and performing activities of daily living. They are self-report measures that require no more than 5–10 minutes to complete. Another approach would be to ask the patient to keep a diary of the activities performed during the day, the pain related to them and the actions taken to control it. In patients who are unable to communicate, autonomic reactions to pain and distress can be measured, such as high heart rate, perspiration and nausea. Similarly, 'pain behaviours' (such as grimacing, restlessness or protection of a painful limb) can be observed and quantified (Turk and Okifuji 2001).

Pain 'assessment' is distinguished from pain 'measurement' by denoting a combination of an attempt to understand the experience, quality and duration of pain, to quantify its severity through measurement and to contribute to a clinical diagnosis of its cause. As such, pain assessment requires that nurses consider the interrelationship between pain and the experience of suffering in terms of the degree of spiritual or existential distress that someone may be experiencing (Brant 2003), and that they are aware of issues that relate to the particular characteristics of the patient for whose care they are responsible (Aranda 1999). For example, nurses should be aware that pain and clinical depression are frequently found together in patients with chronic pain, and that therefore it is extremely important to assess depression in this group of patients (see Chapter 14).

Pain assessment should be carried out at regular intervals and be well documented so that all members of the multidisciplinary team have access to an understanding of the patient's pain problem (Fink and Gates 2001: 55) and so that a comprehensive pain management strategy can be developed.

Pain management: pharmacological and non-pharmacological interventions

In 1982, a panel of experts were invited by the World Health Organization to create an easily applicable approach for the management of pain: this is known as the *WHO three-step analgesic ladder* (see Box 13.10). The three-step ladder is the method most widely accepted and recognized as the basis for adequate pain control. Its methodology involves a stepwise approach to the use of analgesic drugs, going from the first to the third step in analgesic strength. It recommends that analgesics should be used:

- *By the mouth*: the mouth is the standard route for the administration of opioids, including morphine.

- *By the clock*: emphasizing the importance of a preventive attitude towards pain control. Analgesics should be given regularly and prophylactically.

- *By the ladder*: using the three-step analgesic ladder, moving always up the ladder and not sideways in the same efficacy group (Twycross and Wilcock 2002: 30–1).

- *Review:* on a regular basis to assess response to analgesics, to adjust doses and to identify different sources of pain and possible aggravating factors.

The emphasis on the use of oral opioids for moderate to severe pain has been recognized as the most important reason for the success of the three-step ladder. Moreover, it constitutes a framework of conceptual principles, which are easy to teach and to remember, and practical to implement. It is not a rigid protocol and allows considerable flexibility in the choice of

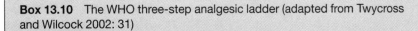

Box 13.10   The WHO three-step analgesic ladder (adapted from Twycross and Wilcock 2002: 31)

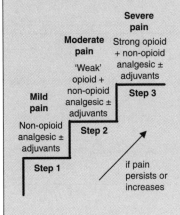

- The *first step* is the use of acetaminophen, aspirin or another non-steroidal anti-inflammatory drug (NSAID) for mild to moderate pain
- When pain increases or persists, a 'weak' opioid such as codeine should be added to the NSAID (*second step*)
- When higher doses of 'weak' opioids are needed and the maximum therapeutic dose has been reached, or the pain has not been well controlled, they should be replaced with strong opioids such as morphine (*third step*)
- Adjuvant drugs are used at any time to enhance analgesic efficacy (*broad-spectrum analgesia*)
- Opioids and non-opioid analgesics are used systematically by the clock, and by the mouth whenever possible
- The right dose is the one which relieves the pain in that particular patient (*individualized treatment*)

REVIEW, REVIEW, REVIEW . . .
The division of opioids into 'weak' and 'strong' is arguable and arbitrary. Pharmacologically, there is no logic to use weak opioids, as small doses of strong opioids can be used instead. Step 2 of the WHO analgesic ladder would either represent full doses of 'weak' opioids or small doses of 'strong' opioids. However, due to reasons of non-availability or restricted supplies of morphine and other strong opioids in many countries worldwide, Step 2 has been placed for practical reasons within an international perspective (Twycross *et al.* 2002: 159).

specific drugs. Pain treatment can be started at the first, second or third step in the ladder according to the pain intensity and, in many circumstances, the second step may need to be ignored. The mainstay approach for the management of cancer pain is opioid-based pharmacotherapy, using opioids (such as morphine, methadone, fentanyl), usually in combination with non-opioid analgesics, such as acetaminophen (paracetamol), NSAIDS (non-selective COX-2 inhibitors, such as aspirin and selective COX-2 inhibitors, such as celecoxib), and analgesic adjuvants, such as corticosteroids (e.g. dexamethasone), tricyclic antidepressants (e.g. amitryptiline) and anti-convulsants (e.g. gabapentin) (see Box 13.11).

In 2001, an expert working group of the research network of the European Association for Palliative Care (EAPC) published a series of 20

Box 13.11   Commonly used analgesics

Acetaminophen (paracetamol)	*NSAIDS*	*'Weak' opioids*	*'Strong' opioids*	*Adjuvants*
	Acetyl salicylic acid (aspirin)	Codeine	Morphine	Corticosteroids
	Diclofenac Ibuprofen	Hydrocodone Tramadol	Hydromorphone Fentanyl	Anticonvulsants Tricyclic antidepressants
	Selective COX-2 inhibitors	Buprenorphine	Diacetylmorphine	Biphosphonates
		Propoxyphene	Oxycodone Methadone	

recommendations for the use of morphine and alternative opioids in cancer pain control (Hanks *et al.* 2001). Each of these recommendations has been based on the best available evidence at the time of the publication. Box 13.12 reproduces these.

The World Health Organization and the European Association for Palliative Care thus recommend morphine as the opioid of first choice to be considered for cancer pain relief. The oral route is the preferred one and it should always be considered in the first instance. If morphine is given orally, it should be titrated upward in gradually increasing doses until a dose is found that maintains continuous pain relief. The goal is to make the patient pain-free at all times (Melzack and Wall 1996: 277). The attitude towards cancer pain control should be preventive and proactive without waiting until the patient is in pain to administer the required dose of opioid. Doses of painkillers and adjuvant medications need to be given regularly and extra doses should be advised and available to be taken 'as required' by the patient to relieve episodes of 'breakthrough' and 'incidental' pain.

Adjuvant analgesics are a miscellaneous group of drugs; their primary indication is not for pain control but they can relieve pain in specific circumstances. They include:

- *Corticosteroids*, such as dexamethasone and prednisolone are specially helpful for the reduction of pain associated with nerve root or spinal cord compression. Their general anti-inflammatory effect reduces the oedema surrounding the tumoral mass.

- *Antidepressants*, such as amitriptiline.

- *Anticonvulsants*, such as sodium valproate and gabapentin

Antidepressants and anticonvulsants can act both at the level of the peripheral nerve and at the dorsal horn of the spinal cord. They are used

Box 13.12   The European Association for Palliative Care (EAPC) recommendations for the use of morphine and alternative opioids in cancer pain management (Hanks *et al.* 2001)

1   Morphine is the opioid of first choice for moderate to severe cancer pain
2   The optimal route of administration of morphine is by mouth. Ideally, two types of formulations are required: normal release (for titration) and modified release (for maintenance treatment)
3   The simplest method of dose titration is with a dose of normal release morphine given every 4 hours and the same dose for breakthrough pain. This 'rescue' dose may be given as often as required (up to hourly) and the total daily dose of morphine should be reviewed daily. The regular dose can then be adjusted to take into account the total amount of rescue morphine
4   If pain returns consistently before the next regular dose is due, the regular dose should be increased. In general, normal release morphine does not need to be given more often than every 4 hours and modified release morphine more often than every 12 or 24 hours (according to the intended duration of the formulation). Patients stabilized on regular oral morphine require continued access to the rescue dose to treat 'breakthrough' pain
5   Several countries do not have a normal release formulation of morphine, although such a formulation is needed for adequate pain management. A different strategy is needed if treatment is started with modified release morphine. Changes to the regular dose should not be made more frequently than every 48 hours. The dose titration phase will be prolonged
6   For patients receiving normal release morphine every 4 hours, a double dose at bedtime is a simple and effective way of avoiding being woken by pain
7   Several modified release formulations are available. There is no evidence that the 12-hourly formulations (tablets, capsules, liquids) are different in their duration of effect and relative analgesic potency
8   If patients are unable to take morphine orally, the preferred alternative route is subcutaneous. There is generally no indication for giving morphine intramuscularly for chronic cancer pain because subcutaneous administration is simpler and less painful
9   The average relative potency ratio of oral morphine to subcutaneous morphine is between 1 : 2 and 1 : 3
10   In patients requiring continuous parenteral morphine, the preferred method of administration is by subcutaneous infusion
11   Intravenous infusion of morphine may be preferred in patients:

   • who already have an indwelling intravenous line
   • with generalized oedema
   • who develop erythema, soreness or sterile abscesses with subcutaneous administration
   • with coagulation disorders
   • with poor peripheral circulation

12   The average relative potency ratio of oral to intravenous morphine is between 1 : 2 and 1 : 3
13   The buccal, sublingual and nebulized routes of administration of morphine are not recommended because there is no evidence of clinical advantage over the conventional routes at the present time
14   Oral transmucosal fentanyl citrate (OTFC) is an effective treatment for 'breakthrough pain' in patients stabilized on regular morphine or any other alternative Step 3 opioid
15   Successful pain management with opioids requires that adequate analgesia be achieved without excessive adverse effects. The application of the WHO and the EAPC guidelines permit effective control of chronic cancer pain in the majority of patients
16   A small proportion of patients develop intolerable adverse effects with oral morphine (in conjunction with a non-opioid and adjuvant analgesic as appropriate) before achieving adequate

pain relief. In such patients, a change to an alternative opioid or a change to the route of administration should be considered

17   Hydromorphone or oxycodone, if available in both normal release and modified release formulations for oral administration, are effective alternatives to oral morphine

18   Methadone is an effective alternative but may be more complicated to use than other opioids because of pronounced inter-individual differences in its plasma half-life, relative analgesic potency and duration of action. Its use by non-experienced practitioners is not recommended

19   Transdermal fentanyl is an effective alternative to oral morphine but is best reserved for patients whose opioids requirements are stable

especially in the case of nerve compression due to malignant invasion or compression.

- *NMDA-receptor-channel blockers* are usually used when neuropathic pain does not respond well to standard analgesics together with an antidepressant and an anti-epileptic. Ketamine, which is the NMDA-receptor-channel blocker most widely used, is an anaesthetic induction agent. Methadone, a synthetic opioid, also seems to act in the NMDA-receptor-channel. It represents a very good opioid alternative in these circumstances. It has a comparatively lower cost. However, due to its long half-life, it may remain in the bloodstream for a long time leading to higher risk for accumulation and side-effects.

- *Antispasmodics*, such as hyoscine butylbromide and glycopyrronium, are used to relieve visceral distension pain and colic pain.

- *Muscle relaxants*, such as diazepam (which is a benzodiazepine), are used in cases of painful muscle spasm (cramps). Relaxation therapies are recommended as complementary therapies in these situations.

Generally, adjuvant analgesics should be given in combination with morphine, or another opioid, and a NSAID. The relief of pain would be obtained gradually. The first step is to help the patient obtain a good night's sleep; the second step is to reduce the intensity of pain during the day to a bearable level, and the third step is to obtain sustainable and adequate pain control round the clock. The patient needs to be informed that a week or so might be necessary to obtain major benefits (Twycross and Wilcock 2002: 51–8).

A range of potential strategies can also be considered for each patient that complement the pharmacological treatment, such as palliative radiation therapy and chemotherapy for pain relief, behavioural therapies, lifestyle therapies, complementary therapies and local anaesthetic techniques. Symptomatic drug treatment is used in an integrated way with disease-modifying therapies and non-drug measures. The main aim remains always to provide adequate pain control to help patients to improve their functioning despite the pain and, at more advanced stages, to guarantee comfort and the best possible quality of life when nearing the end of their life (see Box 13.13).

> **Box 13.13** The principles of cancer pain management (based on Krishnasamy 2001: 339)
>
> - Recognize and promptly assess pain in cancer patients
> - Identify psychological and spiritual influences on pain perception and management
> - First aim to alleviate pain at night, then at rest and, finally, on movement
> - Maximize independence and best possible quality of life
> - Address and relieve current fears about pain
> - Anticipate and discuss possible concerns about future painful episodes and therapeutic options
> - Provide support and encouragement for family members, friends and professional care-givers
> - Invite participation of the patient, family and other informal carers
> - Adopt a collaborative, multidisciplinary approach
> - Design analgesic regimens tailored to each patient's needs and tolerance
> - Regular outcome follow-up
> - Refer early to pain specialist services if pain control is not achieved.

Routes of analgesic administration

Many options are available for the delivery of analgesics in the management of acute, chronic and cancer pain. It is essential to consider that the relieving of chronic and cancer pain requires a long-term therapeutic strategy that is dynamic and individually tailored. The decision to use one preparation or delivery system over another should take into consideration the ability of the patient to manage a specific type of delivery system, the efficacy of that system to deliver acceptable analgesia, the ease of use by the patient and his or her carers, the potential complications associated with that system and the costs attached to its use (Stevens and Ghazi 2000). For nursing practice, it is particularly important to be familiar with different routes for the administration of analgesics, especially opioids, and with the formulations available in each individual place of work. This knowledge allows the confident use of several options for appropriate pain control when it is necessary.

The oral route

The oral route is the easiest, least invasive, cheapest and most common route used for the administration of analgesics in patients with chronic and cancer pain. There are no major complications associated with its use. There are usually two types of formulations: 'normal release' and 'slow (or modified) release' formulations. Slow release formulations have been designed to provide long-lasting analgesia. Morphine, oxycodone and hydromorphone are the opioids currently available in slow release formulations. They are usually given twice a day. Normal release formulations are used to titrate opioid requirements against pain and should always be available for breakthrough pain relief.

Some patients may find it difficult or impossible to take oral medications. For instance, in patients with head and neck cancer or oesophageal or gastric cancer, the malignant growth might obstruct the anatomical passages and make it impossible to swallow. In the case of severely ill, debilitated or very confused patients, the oral route might be better avoided. In all these circumstances, other routes for the administration of analgesics need to be considered.

The intravenous route

The intravenous route for the administration of analgesics should only be considered when the use of other less invasive routes does not control a patient's pain. This route has several disadvantages: it requires an indwelling intravenous central or peripheral catheter; the preparation of the opioid solution by a pharmacist; the use of an external infusion pump; and outpatient and inpatient skilled nursing support. All these aspects increase costs significantly. On the other hand, any indwelling intravenous catheter can serve as an entry port for infection and for this reason it requires regular and skilled nursing attention. Intravenous infusions of opioids can be given as continuous infusions, or they can be used in conjunction with a patient-controlled analgesia (PCA) device, which provides continuous infusion plus on-demand boluses that the patient self-administers. PCA devices are not recommended in confused patients (Stevens and Ghazi 2000).

The subcutaneous route

When use of the oral route is not appropriate, the subcutaneous route is a simple method of parental administration of analgesics (Stevens and Ghazi 2000). There is no need for vascular access and problems associated with indwelling intravenous catheters are avoided. The subcutaneous route can be used to give medications by bolus or for continuous infusions. An area on the chest, abdomen, upper arms or thighs is shaved and cleaned with antiseptic and a 25- or 27-gauge butterfly needle is inserted. When continuous infusion of analgesics is considered, the tubing is attached to an infusion pump or a syringe driver. If not, a loop of tubing is secured with adhesive tape and used to give subcutaneous bolus injections. A clear plastic occlusive dressing is applied to cover the needle. The injection site should be changed weekly or as needed, and allergies to metal needles should always be assessed. The volume of fluid that can be injected per hour represents the main limiting factor. It has been suggested that infusion rates of 2–4 ml per hour can be administered safely without causing pain at the site of injection (Bruera *et al.* 1987). Taking adequate precautions, such as cleaning and rotating sites for injection, the rate of skin infection is very low (1 in 117 patients in one study) (Swanson *et al.* 1989, cited by Stevens and Ghazi 2000).

The transdermal route

The transdermal route is a non-invasive option for continuous administration of opioids for patients unable, or unwilling, to take oral medications (Stevens and Ghazi 2000). Fentanyl has been available to be given through the skin for several years. The delivery system consists of a reservoir of fentanyl and alcohol that holds a 3-day supply of fentanyl in the form of a patch, similar to the better known nitroglycerine or oestrogen patches. A permeable membrane separates the drug reservoir from the skin and controls the release of fentanyl from the reservoir. An adhesive layer saturated with fentanyl holds the system in place. After the patch is applied, a bolus of fentanyl is delivered to the bloodstream through the skin. Fentanyl saturates the subcutaneous fat beneath the patch to form a subcutaneous 'depot'. Steady-state plasma fentanyl concentrations are reached after approximately 12 hours and these concentrations are maintained for about 72 hours. Once it has been placed, the patch releases fentanyl at a constant rate until the reservoir is depleted. Multiple patches may be placed if higher doses than that in one patch are needed. In case of opioid toxicity, the patch should be removed. It takes many hours to resolve opioids' side-effects after the removal of a patch due to a prolonged elimination of the drug from the body. However, adverse effects of the fentanyl patch, such as dermatological reactions, are rare and are usually easily treated. The transdermal route is best suited for patients with stable pain in whom the 24-hour opioid requirement has already been determined. It is not suitable for rapid titration of opioid requirements in patients with uncontrolled pain. Some sort of breakthrough pain coverage is usually needed (e.g. immediate-release oral morphine). In patients unable to take oral medications, the transmucosal (e.g. fentanyl lozenge), rectal (e.g. morphine suppository) and subcutaneous (e.g. subcutaneous diamorphine) routes are available for 'breakthrough' administration of fast-acting opioids (Stevens and Ghazi 2000). Recently, buprenorphine patches were introduced to the market.

The transmucosal and the sublingual routes

These routes for analgesic administration are useful as an alternative in patients who cannot tolerate the oral route because of nausea, vomiting or dysphagia and in those that cannot receive parental opioids due to emaciation, coagulation defects or lack of venous access (Stevens and Ghazi 2000).

Compared with the oral route, the sublingual region guarantees rapid absorption and entry of medications to the system and a quicker onset of action due to its rich venous drainage. It is very simple; it requires little expertise, preparation or supervision. More lipophilic drugs, such as methadone, fentanyl or buprenorphine, are better absorbed sublingually than hydrophilic ones. The transmucosal route is similar to the sublingual route. It differs from the sublingual route in that the absorption of the medication takes place mainly through the oral mucosa of the cheek. A fentanyl lozenge has been specially formulated for transmucosal absorption for the treatment of 'breakthrough' pain. The lozenge needs to be rubbed against the mucosa of the cheek, rather than sucked. Side-effects associated with the use of the sublingual and the transmucosal routes are a bitter taste and a burning sensation when the formulation first comes is in contact with the mouth (Stevens and Ghazi 2000). Sublingual formulations are much cheaper options than the fentanyl lozenge.

The rectal route

This route constitutes an alternative to the oral route, especially in an emergency when the oral route is not suitable due to altered consciousness, severe nausea or vomiting, or gastrointestinal tract obstruction. It is also useful when the motility of the gastrointestinal tract is compromised or gastric emptying is severely compromised. The most suitable form for the rectal route is the suppository, although, if necessary, any tablet or capsule of any opioid that is used for oral administration can be used rectally (Stevens and Ghazi 2000). The disadvantage of the rectal route is the wide anatomical variations among individuals, which requires titration and individualization of doses. Due to the small surface area of the rectum, the absorption of drugs may be delayed or limited. It can also be interrupted by defecation and the small amount of fluid available in the rectum may slow down the dissolution of tablets or capsules. When constipated, medications may be absorbed into faeces. The rectal route should not be used if the patient finds it unpleasant or if the patient has painful anal conditions, such as fissures, anal tumour or inflamed haemorrhoids.

'Interventional' approaches to pain control

Although the vast majority of patients with chronic and cancer pain can be appropriately relieved by the administration of analgesics via the oral, subcutaneous, rectal or transmucosal routes, a small proportion of patients may fail to obtain adequate analgesia despite the use of large systemic doses of analgesics, or they may suffer from uncontrollable side-effects, such as nausea, vomiting, constipation, confusion or over-sedation while still in pain. These patients may benefit from the administration of opioids, local anaesthetics and other medications via the perispinal route and from the use of nerve blockade procedures and surgical interventions. The latter procedures are indicated only in patients with severe, intractable pain in whom less aggressive manoeuvres are ineffective or intolerable because of either poor physical condition or the development of intolerable side-effects (Stevens and Ghazi 2000).

The perispinal (epidural or intrathecal) route

The goal of perispinal opioid therapy is to place a small dose of an opioid and/or local anaesthetic close to the spinal opioid receptors situated in the dorsal horn of the spinal cord to enhance analgesia and reduce systemic side-effects by decreasing the total daily opioid dose. An indwelling catheter is placed into the epidural or intrathecal space and the medications are delivered using an external or implantable pump. Smaller doses of opioids can be effectively administered to act locally and directly at the opioid receptor level, and only small amounts of drugs reach the systemic circulation causing fewer side-effects. The various perispinal approaches for opioid delivery include epidural bolus, continuous epidural infusion, intrathecal injection and continuous intrathecal infusion. Deciding between epidural and intrathecal placement or external and implantable pumps to deliver the opioid is based on multiple factors, including duration of therapy, type and location of the pain, disease extent, central nervous system involvement, opioid requirement and individual preference and expertise. The complications and side-effects associated with the use of this route can be divided into three categories:

- *Procedural and surgical complications*: infection, bleeding at various sites, postdural puncture headache.
- *Complications related to a system malfunction*: kinking, obstruction, disconnection, tearing or migration of the catheter.
- *Pharmacological complications*: including possible overdoses and pump filling errors.

In general, with the exception of constipation, side-effects of perispinal opioids in patients already tolerant to opioids are rare (Stevens and Ghazi 2000).

Sympathetic blockade

The sympathetic chain exists along the vertebral column and carries nociceptive information mainly of visceral origin (Miguel 2000). It is suitable for intervention at various levels (see Figure 13.4) for respective pain complaints and the blockade of sympathetic ganglia may improve visceral pain. It can also be considered an option for the diagnosis of pain and possible long-term pain relief. For instance, this procedure has been most commonly used for the control of abdominal pain due to pancreatic cancer and pelvic pain resulting from cervical cancer (Leon-Casasola 2000).

Neurolysis

Neurolysis implies the use of neurolytic agents or techniques to destroy nerves and interrupt the conduction of pain. It can be: (a) *chemical*, with concentrations of 50 or 100 per cent alcohol, or 7 to 12 per cent phenol; (b) *thermal*, applying cryoanalgesia or radiofrequency lesioning; or (c) *surgical*,

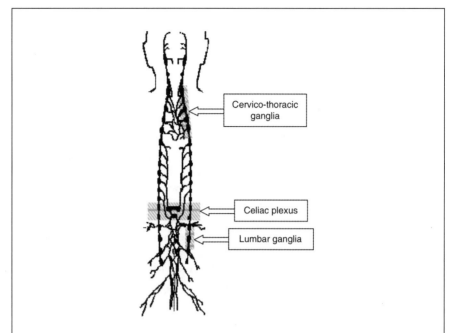

Figure 13.4 The three levels of sympathetic blockade (reproduced with adaptations from Carroll and Bowsher 1993: 226).

by surgically interrupting the nerve pathway. Chemical neurolysis is the most common modality. The results of the injection of alcohol or phenol are similar to those obtained by sectioning the nerve, although the effect is usually seen for only 3–6 months. An example in which a trial injection is useful is in areas where pain is limited to a very circumscribed section, such as a tumoral rib invasion, or rib metastases treated with intercostals neurolysis. Its effect is not permanent, and pain returns either from a re-growth of neural structures or by progression of the underlying disease beyond the treated area. A risk–benefit ratio should be made before implementing any invasive analgesic method.

The nurse's role and responsibility in analgesic administration

The nurse spends more time with the patient than any other health professional and is thus in an ideal position to constantly assess and evaluate the effectiveness of their pain treatments (McCaffrey and Beebe 1994). For these reasons, nurses play a very active role in ensuring good pain control in patients suffering from unrelieved pain. McCaffrey and Beebe (1994: 54–8) identify that nurses should:

- Determine whether the analgesic is to be given and, if so, when.
- Choose the appropriate analgesic(s) when more than one is prescribed.
- Be alert to the possibility of certain side-effects as a result of the analgesic.

- Evaluate effectiveness of the analgesic at regular frequent intervals following each administration, but especially the initial doses.
- Report promptly and accurately to the doctor when a change is needed.
- Make suggestions for specific changes, such as route of administration, interval, formulations.
- Advise the patient about the use of analgesics.
- Inform the patient about non-pharmacological interventions for pain relief.
- Develop a preventive approach with analgesics by teaching the patient to request painkillers as soon as pain occurs or before it increases, and by regularly assessing the patient and enquiring about the pain. A preventive attitude towards pain relief has several benefits:
  - the patient spends less time in pain;
  - doses of analgesics can be lower than if pain is allowed to increase or become severe;
  - fewer side-effects due to lower doses;
  - decreased concerns about obtaining relief when needed;
  - overall increase in activities;
  - decreased anxiety about the return of pain.

Non-pharmacological interventions

Although drug therapy is one of the major modalities used in managing chronic and cancer pain, it represents only one of many methods available. Pharmacological interventions are most effective when used in combination with other non-pharmacological approaches and psychosocial support.

Cognitive-behavioural therapy

Cognitive-behavioural therapy (CBT) involves changing people's thoughts and behaviour and enhancing their coping skills. In the context of chronic pain, CBT aims to teach patients the skills they need to cope better with the pain to reduce their suffering and enhance their overall quality of life. The therapeutic work is structured and planned according to the patient's own set of relevant and achievable goals. Activity is increased in small, steady steps at a rate set jointly by the therapist and patient towards the long-term goal. Instead of a reduction in pain, goals achieved and improvements in quality of life and mood represent the successful outcomes of an adequate treatment (Carroll and Bowsher 1993: 60–2).

Relaxation techniques

These have been used as therapeutic tools for the treatment of pain because pain is frequently associated with muscular tension, and stress and anxiety are usually associated with the onset and maintenance of pain (Horn and Mufano 1997). Techniques involve the progressive relaxation of skeletal muscle groups over a period of 20–40 minutes. Relaxation needs to take place in a quiet environment and in a comfortable posture on a bed or a couch. Some schedules include some sort of calming mental exercise or a period of controlled breathing after the muscular relaxation. It has been reported that successful relaxation is associated with decreased autonomic stimulation and decreased skeletal muscle tension (Horn and Mufano 1997). It may also act as a distracter because it involves focused attention to instructions, and it can also have a positive impact on the management of pain because it is an essentially self-management technique that may enforce a sense of self-control and self-efficacy (Horn and Mufano 1997).

Biofeedback

This comprises the use of instruments to enhance and transform information from the body, such as temperature of the skin or the amount of tension in skeletal muscles, into a vivid form like a flashing light or oscilloscope readout, a tone or a series of clicks (Horn and Mufano 1997). In this way, physiological responses associated with stress or tension and not normally under voluntary control are measured and displayed to the patient (Carroll and Bowsher 1993). Operant conditioning is the learning paradigm, and knowledge of results acts as reinforcement as it signals success. In the treatment of pain, physiological parameters subjected to biofeedback conditioning include muscle tone, finger temperature, temporal pulse and alpha EEG activity (Horn and Mufano 1997). It is often used with a relaxation procedure, and the measurement provides the person with an objective appreciation of the extent to which relaxation has been achieved.

Physiotherapy may be applied to help cure or alleviate the tissue source of pain, or to reduce the severity of the pain the patient is experiencing. Physical therapies can be grouped into four categories: electrical therapy; massage and manipulative procedures; exercise therapy, including hydrotherapy; and relaxation procedures. In the four categories, the patient subjectively assesses the degree of pain relief. They differ on the amount of patient cooperation they require. While electrical therapy, massage and other manipulative procedures are applied to patients who passively receive them, the last two categories require active cooperation from the patient (Carroll and Bowsher 1993).

Transcutaneous electrical nerve stimulation

This is an example of electrical therapy. Sensory cutaneous nerve endings in the skin are stimulated by an electrical current generated by the TENS unit. These electrical impulses feel like a buzzing, vibratory sensation on the skin under the electrodes. It has been suggested that as the brain selectively concentrates upon skin sensation rather on deeper sensations, TENS helps to reduce the conscious experience of pain (Carroll and Bowsher 1993). TENS has been used to relieve the pain of rheumatoid arthritis, neck and back pain, labour pain, metastatic pain and acute unpleasant pain due to peripheral nerve injuries.

Complementary therapies

Several complementary therapies have gained popularity in the treatment of chronic and cancer pain, such as massage, aromatherapy, reflexology, hypnosis, guided imagery, visualization and shiatsu. Their aim is usually to add another source of comfort and relief to pharmacological approaches.

Conclusions

Pain is a complex subject. Interventions for its relief have become established over the last 50 years and, for cancer pain, promoted under the auspices of the World Health Organization. The rationale for, and popularity of, particular interventions over time can be related to changing understandings of the relationship between the perception of pain and the reaction to pain: gate control theory and the development of techniques for the use and administration of opioids are perhaps the most notable scientific advances that influence contemporary understandings of pain, cancer pain and pain control. Less well charted is the role of charismatic figures such as John Bonica in the pain field, and Cicely Saunders in the hospice and palliative care field. Their attempts resulted, arguably, in a movement away from a narrow biomedical focus in the management and assessment of pain towards a broader frame of reference, in which understanding the individual experience of pain and suffering and valuing the collaborative contributions of the multidisciplinary team in measuring, assessing and relieving pain are understood to be crucially important. Pain is now understood as the 'fifth vital sign' (Heller 2000). This chapter has elucidated the historical developments that have led to this reformulation and has attempted to distil from contemporary sources the information necessary to underpin evidence-based care for persons in pain. We provide a range of sources below which we hope can aid further enquiry into this fascinating subject.

References

Aranda, S. (1999) A pain assessment approach to nursing the person with complex pain, in M. O'Connor and S. Aranda (eds) *Palliative Care Nursing: A Guide to Practice*. Melbourne, VIC: Ausmed Publications.

Ashburn, M.A. and Staats, P.S. (2001) Management of chronic pain. *The Pain Series* (available at: www.thelancet.com/journal/vol357/isss1/full/llan.357.s1.pain_series.15831.1), accessed September 2002.

Baszanger, I. (1998) *Inventing Pain Medicine: From the Laboratory to the Clinic*. New Brunswick, NJ: Rutgers University Press.

Beecher, H.K. (1946) Pain in men wounded in battle. *Annals of Surgery*, 123(1): 96–105.

Beecher, H.K. (1956) Limiting factors in experimental pain. *Journal of Chronic Disability*, July, pp. 11–21.

Berman, J. (1995) Imaging pain in humans. *British Journal of Anaesthesia*, 75: 209–16.

Bonica, J. (1990) Definition and taxonomy of pain, in J. Bonica (ed.) *The Management of Pain*, 2nd edn. Philadelphia, PA: Lea & Febiger.

Brant, J. (2003) Pain management, in M. O'Connor and S. Aranda (eds) *Palliative Care Nursing: A Guide to Practice*, 2nd edn. Melbourne, VIC: Ausmed Publications.

Breivik, H. (2002) International Association for the Study of Pain: update on WHO-IASP activities. *Journal of Pain and Symptom Management*, 24(2): 97–101.

Bruera, E., Brenneis, C. and MacDonald, R.N. (1987) Continuous sc infusion of narcotics for the treatment of cancer pain: an update. *Cancer Treatment Reports*, 71: 953–58.

Carr, D.B. (1998) Preempting the memory of pain. *Journal of the American Medical Association*, 279: 1114–15.

Carr, D.B. and Goudas, L.C. (2001) Acute pain. *The Pain Series* (available at: www.thelancet.com/journal/vol357/isss1/full/llan.357.s1.pain_series.15828.1), accessed September 2002.

Carroll, D. and Bowsher, D. (1993) *Pain Management and Nursing Care*. Oxford: Butterworth-Heinemann.

Cervero, F. and Laird, J.M.A. (2001) Visceral pain. *The Pain Series* (available at: www.thelancet.com/journal/vol357/isss1/full/llan.357.s1.pain_series.15834.1), accessed September 2002.

Clark, D. (1998) An annotated bibliography of the publications of Cicely Saunders 1: 1958–67. *Palliative Medicine*, 112(3): 181–93.

Descartes, R. ([1664] 1901) L'Homme (translated by M. Foster), in *Lectures on the History of Physiology During the 16th, 17th and 18th Centuries*. Cambridge: Cambridge University Press.

Dickenson, A.H. (1995) Spinal cord pharmacology of pain. *British Journal of Anaesthesia*, (75): 193–200.

Dickenson, A.H. (2002) Editorial I. Gate Control Theory of pain stands the test of time. *British Journal of Anaesthesia*, 6(88): 755–7.

Federation of State Medical Boards of the United States (1998). *Model Guidelines for the Use of Controlled Substances for the Treatment of Pain*. Euless, TX: The Federation. Cited in Carr, D.B. and Goudas, L.C. (2001) Acute pain. *The Pain Series* (available at: www.thelancet.com/journal/vol357/isss1/full/llan.357.s1.pain_series.15828.1), accessed September 2002.

Fink, R. and Gates, R. (2001) Pain assessment, in B.R. Ferrell and N. Coyle (eds) *Textbook of Palliative Nursing*. Oxford: Oxford University Press.

Hanks, G.W., Conno, F., Cherny, N. *et al.* (2001) Expert Working Group of the Research Network of the European Association for Palliative Care – morphine and alternative opioids in cancer pain: the EAPC recommendations. *British Journal of Cancer*, 84(5): 587–93.

Heller, K.S. (2000) Implementing pain management guidelines (editorial). *Innovations in End of Life Care: Practical Strategies and International Perspectives*, 1: 107–10.

Horn, S. and Munafo, M. (1997) *Pain: Theory, Research and Intervention*. Buckingham: Open University Press.

Krishnasamy, M. (2001) Pain, in J. Corner and C. Bailey (eds) *Cancer Nursing Care in Context*. Oxford: Blackwell Science.

Leon-Casasola, O.A. (2000) Critical evaluation of chemical neurolysis of the sympathetic axis for cancer pain. *Cancer Control*, 7(2): 142–8.

Loeser, J.D. and Melzack, R. (2001) Pain: an overview. *The Pain Series* (available at: www.thelancet.com/journal/vol357/isss1/full/llan.357.s1.pain_series.15830.1), accessed September 2002.

McCaffery, M. and Beebe, A. (1994) *Pain* (adapted from the US edition by J. Latham with D. Ball). London: C.V. Mosby.

McQuay, H.J. (1990) Assessment of pain and effectiveness of treatment, in A. Hopkins and D. Costain (eds) *Measuring the Outcomes of Medical Care*. Cited in Carroll, D. and Bowsher, D. (1993) *Pain Management and Nursing Care*. Oxford: Butterworth-Heinemann.

Meldrum, M.L. (1998) 'Tell me if this hurts': the problem of pain and analgesic measurement, 1940–1960. Paper presented to the *History of Pain Symposium: Pain and Suffering in History. Narratives of Science, Medicine and Culture*, University of California, Los Angeles, CA, 13–14 March.

Melzack, R. (1999) From the gate to the neuromatrix. *Pain* (suppl. 6): S121–S126.

Melzack, R. and Wall, P.D. (1965) Pain mechanisms: a new theory. *Science*, 3669(150): 971–9.

Melzack, R. and Wall, P.D. (1982) *The Challenge of Pain*. Harmondsworth: Penguin Books.

Melzack, R. and Wall, P.D. (1996) *The Challenge of Pain*, 2nd edn. Harmondsworth: Penguin Books

Merskey, H. and Bogduk, N. (eds) (1994) *Classification of Chronic Pain: Descriptions of Chronic Pain Syndromes and Definitions of Pain Terms*. Report by the International Association for the Study of Pain Task Force on Taxonomy, 2nd edn. Seattle, WA: IASP Press.

Miguel, R. (2000) Interventional treatment of cancer pain: the fourth step in the World Health Organization analgesic ladder? *Cancer Control*, 7(2): 149–56.

Niv, D. and Devor, M. (1998) Transition from acute to chronic pain. Cited in Carr, D.B. and Goudas, L.C. (2001) Acute pain. *The Pain Series* (available at: www.thelancet.com/journal/vol357/isss1/full/llan.357.s1.pain_series.15828.1), accessed September 2002.

Pan-American Health Organization (1999) Non-Communicable Diseases Program. *HCN Palliative Care* (available at: http://165.158.1.110/english/hcn/hcnpain_1.htm), accessed November 2002.

Pargeon, K.L. and Hailey, B.J. (1999) Barriers to effective cancer pain management: a review of the literature. *Journal of Pain and Symptom Management*, 18(5): 358–68.

Portenoy, R.K. and Lesage, P. (2001) Management of cancer pain. *The Pain Series* (available at: www.thelancet.com/journal/vol357/isss1/full/llan.357.s1.pain_series.15835.1), accessed September 2002.

Rey, R. (1995) *Historie de la Douleur* [*The History of Pain*] (translated by L.E. Wallace, J.A. Cadden and S.W. Cadden). London: Harvard University Press.

Stevens, R.A. and Ghazi, S.M. (2000) Routes of opioid analgesic therapy in the management of cancer pain. *Cancer Control*, 7(2): 131–41.

Swanson, G., Smith, J., Bulich, R. *et al.* (1989) Patient controlled analgesia for chronic cancer pain in the ambulatory setting: a report of 117 patients. *Journal of Clinical Oncology*, 7: 1903–8.

Tulder, M.W., Cherkin, D.C., Berman, B., Lao, L. and Koes, B.W. (2000) Acupuncture for low back pain (systematic review). *Cochrane Database of Systematic Reviews*, 2: CD001351.

Turk, D.C. and Okifuji, A. (2001) Assessment of patients' reporting of pain: an integrated perspective. *The Pain Series* (available at: www.thelancet.com/journal/vol357/isss1/full/llan.357.s1.pain_series.15829.1), accessed September 2002.

Twycross, R. (1997) *Oral Morphine in Advanced Cancer*, 3rd edn. Beaconsfield: Beaconsfield Publishers.

Twycross, R. and Wilcock, A. (2002) *Symptom Management in Advanced Cancer*, 3rd edn. Oxford: Radcliffe Medical Press.

Twycross, R., Wilcock, A., Charlesworth, S. and Dickman, A. (2002) *Palliative Care Formulary*, 2nd edn. Oxford: Radcliffe Medical Press.

Woolf, C.F. (1995) Somatic pain: pathogenesis and prevention. *British Journal of Anaesthesia*, 75: 169–76.

Woolf, C.J. and Mannion, R.J. (2001) Neuropathic pain: aetiology, symptoms, mechanisms, and management. *The Pain Series* (available at: www.thelancet.com/journal/vol357/isss1/full/llan.357.s1.pain_series.15833.1), accessed September 2002.

World Health Organization (1990) *Cancer Pain Relief and Palliative Care*. Technical Report Series 804. Geneva: WHO.

World Health Organization (1996) *Cancer Pain Relief*, 2nd edn, *With a Guide to Opioid Availability*. Geneva: WHO.

14

Emotions and cognitions

Psychological aspects of care

Mari Lloyd-Williams

The presence of psychiatric morbidity in terminally ill patients and the fact that it is often not diagnosed is well recognized (Rodin and Voshart 1986; Kathol *et al.* 1990; Pirl and Roth 1999; Murray *et al.* 2002). Nursing staff have an important role in identifying patients who may have psychiatric symptoms (Valentine and Saunders 1989; McVey 1998). Nurses spend more time in direct patient contact, enabling them to observe behaviour more closely, and the nature of intimate nursing tasks may provide an opportunity for patients to express any psychological distress. Sadness and depression exist along a continuum. In this chapter, I explore how patients can be supported in coping with their feelings when confronted with a terminal illness, focusing in particular on depression and anxiety and the difficulties involved in diagnosis. Brief case histories will be used to illustrate the issues discussed; all names and details have been changed to protect anonymity.

Case history

Andrew was 46 years old, worked in an office and was the proud father of three small children. He noticed he was passing some blood mixed with the stool and after presenting to the GP was referred for barium enema and colonoscopy that revealed a cancer of the rectum. Andrew was told his diagnosis at the outpatient clinic with, as he recounted later, 'the world and his wife also there'. He was told that the surgery would probably mean a stoma and was admitted a week later for surgery. This was followed by 20 fractions of radiotherapy and chemotherapy. He found the stoma difficult to accept, but returned to work after finishing his treatment. Eighteen months later he developed a series of chest infections, which were resistant to antibiotic treatment. An X-ray revealed that he had multiple pulmonary metastases and an abdominal ultrasound revealed liver metastases. This was devastating to Andrew who believed he had 'beaten' the cancer. He withdrew from family and friends and said he was no longer any use to them and they had better get used to life without him. He stayed in bed for most of the day and could not tolerate the chatter of his small sons when they returned from school. His wife found his withdrawn behaviour difficult to handle and they were now having frequent rows during which Andrew would often say, 'If I had a gun I would just end it all.' Andrew was referred to the palliative care outpatient clinic and asked to talk about how he felt. 'What's the point of you talking to me? I'm no use to anybody' was his response.

The support of patients

All of us will have met patients like Andrew and the case reflects how patients perceive and remember how bad news is communicated. When a patient is told that their disease is incurable, they tend to show a characteristic emotional response. There is a period of shock and disbelief followed by a period of turmoil with anxiety, irritability and disturbance in appetite and sleep pattern. Concentration on daily tasks is impaired and thoughts regarding the diagnosis and fears for the future may intrude. There is also the grief that life will be shortened and the loss of future hopes and dreams. These symptoms usually resolve within 7–10 days with support from family and friends (Massie and Holland 1992). There is wide acknowledgement that all patients with a terminal illness should be given honest information and patients with terminal cancer are usually given such information; in the case of other diseases, this may not be the case and there is considerable cultural variation (Higginson and Costantini 2002). Research has shown, for example, that although the majority of relatives wished to be told if they themselves developed dementia, they did not wish this information to be conveyed to the patient (Maguire *et al.* 1996). This can be compared with the communication of a cancer diagnosis and the similar reasons given 30 years ago for withholding information – that being truthful with patients would precipitate anxiety and depression. In reality, many patients in the early stages of dementia are fully aware of their cognitive impairment and withholding such information is likely to do more harm. Sensitive communication of the diagnosis can have benefits, as patients may be able to participate in decisions regarding their future health care and also decisions regarding life-sustaining treatment before their condition deteriorates and they are rendered incapable of making such decisions themselves (Barnett and Meyers 1997). The emergence of new therapies for patients with dementia although palliative (Mechatie 1997), further supports the need for patients to be told their diagnosis so they may opt for treatment.

When conveying a diagnosis, medical and nursing staff can help by providing information and more importantly reassuring the patient that they will not be abandoned or die in pain or distress. For a significant number of patients, however good and appropriate this support is, their distress escalates; these are the patients who present with anxiety or develop a depressive illness. It is thought that patients with little social support are more likely to go on to develop psychiatric morbidity (Goldberg and Cullen 1986) than those who have more supportive family and friends, but the existence of excellent family and social support by no means precludes patients from developing anxiety or a depressive illness, which is illustrated by Andrew's case history.

To provide patients with terminal illness with optimum psychological care as well as palliation of physical symptoms, health care professionals should have excellent communication and interpersonal skills. For many patients, the presence of a caring, empathic professional who is able to provide honest information sensitively will be adequate. Such a professional may, for example, be a member of the primary care team or nurse specialist. The need for professionals with specific skills in psychosocial care, in addition to those members of nursing and medical staff with generic skills, has been identified in the area of cancer. In an effort to improve the provision of psychosocial care, the National Council for Hospice and Specialist Palliative Care Services (NCHSPCS; an umbrella organization of palliative care representing professionals from different disciplines involved with care of the patient with advanced cancer) set up a working party to look more closely at the issues of psychosocial care and its provision.

An occasional paper on psychosocial care (NCHSPCS 1997) has been published that specifies skills at three levels:

- *Level 1*: skills that are general communication skills desirable for all care-giving staff and volunteers.
- *Level 2*: skills, including excellent interpersonal and communication skills, that are appropriate to staff members with an extensive first-line role in palliative care (e.g. clinical nurse specialists in palliative care).
- *Level 3*: skills that are required by a specialist in psychosocial care.

The occasional paper defines as central to the application of these skills the ability of all staff to recognize when they have reached the ceiling of their skills, or the situation has become too complex and staff are unable to refer appropriately. Specialists in psychosocial care are specified as chaplain or spiritual adviser, psychologist, psychiatrist, and social worker or family therapist. To summarize, all nursing and medical staff require excellent communication skills but also need to be aware of the patients who may benefit from referral to another professional, either from within or from outside the team (e.g. psychologist or liaison psychiatrist). The remainder of this chapter will focus on those patients who develop anxiety or depression and the strategies that can be employed to support these patients and their families.

Aetiology of psychological distress

The exact aetiology of psychological morbidity in cancer and other terminal illness is unknown, but theories have been put forward. Goldberg and Cullen (1986) believed that the five psychosocial factors leading to significant psychological symptoms are disruption of key relationships, dependence, disability, disfigurement and approaching death. Patients referred to palliative care, for example, will normally have undergone a considerable part of their 'cancer journey' and already have experienced a range of emotions. The shock and disbelief of diagnosis, the acceptance of treatment and the fact that something can be done, is followed by the uncertainty of radiotherapy and chemotherapy. The detection of metastases, the hope that further treatment may help and final referral to a palliative care team is the 'emotional cancer journey' for the majority of patients referred for palliative care. Some of the earliest work looking at the physical and mental distress of dying patients was undertaken by Hinton (1963). He studied 102 patients who were dying in hospital and used hospital inpatients that were not terminally ill as controls in a study looking at psychological distress. Informal structured interviews of 30 minutes duration were conducted with the respondents and Hinton found that terminally ill patients had higher physical and emotional distress, with 24 per cent being depressed and 37 per cent suffering from anxiety. He concluded that both depression and anxiety had significant associations with the degree and duration of the terminal illness, with patients under 50 years of age having greater physical and mental distress. Addington-Hall and McCarthy (1995) explored care-givers' perceptions of patients' symptoms in the last year and week of life and found that perceptions of feeling low and miserable were reported by 69 per cent during the last year and 52 per cent during the last week of life.

Age appears to be an important factor in adjustment to cancer – younger patients react more acutely and dramatically than older patients, but have a greater capacity to adapt and develop new interests than older patients (Novotony *et al.* 1984). Younger patients with cancer are at a greater risk of developing depression and other psychiatric morbidity; Harrison *et al.* (1995) found in their study that cases of anxiety and depression were found in a significantly younger population.

A sense of hope is vital to all patients and even in the terminal stages of illness hope can still be fostered, ensuring that patients feel supported and cared for. There is a need for psychosocial interventions to be an integral part of every palliative care patient's management plan (Fallowfield *et al.* 1995). In cancer, where the majority of research has been carried out, it is recognized that psychiatric disorders occur more frequently in cancer patients than in the general population. It is estimated that 50 per cent of patients will have no significant psychiatric symptoms, 30 per cent will have what is defined as an adjustment reaction and 20 per cent will have a formal psychiatric diagnosis, the most common being depression. It is estimated that for a quarter of all patients admitted to a palliative care unit, depression will be a significant symptom (Barraclough 1994). In a review paper, Bergevin and Bergevin (1995) highlight the following facts: the prevalence of depression in the general population is 6–10 per cent, a number of patients with advanced cancer may have a pre-existing psychiatric disorder and the advancing cancer will place these patients at greater risk of developing further episodes. Research in renal disease (Kimmel 2002) and end-stage pulmonary disease (Singer *et al.* 2001) has also identified that many patients have unidentified psychological morbidity and that nursing, medical and paramedical staff have a role in identifying patients who may have psychiatric symptoms (Valentine and Saunders 1989; Fincannon 1995; McVey 1998).

In a questionnaire study of 100 oncology nurses caring for 475 patients in the USA on one particular day, Pasacreta and Massie (1990) found that nurses perceived that 55 per cent of patients had symptoms requiring further psychiatric evaluation – a higher figure than would be expected – which included 13 per cent already under psychiatric care. They concluded that although nurses may not be able to identify specific psychiatric disorders, they are skilful in recognizing significant psychological distress.

Anxiety

Anxiety is a normal emotion experienced by everybody at some time in their lives. Patients with any form of terminal illness will almost universally experience some anxiety, especially at the time of diagnosis and at times when their disease status changes. This 'normal' anxiety often dispels when patients adjust to their new situation, but in a proportion of patients anxiety can become severe and disabling. Patients with severe anxiety complain of both physical and psychological symptoms. The physical symptoms can be explained by increased autonomic activity and include palpitations, sweating, headaches, breathlessness, gastrointestinal symptoms and feelings of an inability to swallow (i.e. 'lump in the throat'). Anxiety can be present most of the time – the so-called free-floating anxiety present in certain situations (e.g. anticipatory anxiety during chemotherapy). A generalized anxiety disorder can be defined as an unrealistic or exaggerated anxiety with regard to life events and has a duration of more than 6 months (Steifel and Razavi 1994). Anxiety and depression are often present in the same patient (Cassileth *et al.* 1986). Risk factors include previous anxious predisposition, poor social support and social isolation. Often the anxiety is related to fear of illness and death, but anxiety itself causes physical symptoms, thus leading to a vicious circle of thought processes. Anxious patients tend to selectively remember the more 'threatening' information given to them and often the process of explanation of their diagnosis or treatment plan by a knowledgeable professional can be therapeutic in itself.

When caring for a patient for whom anxiety is a major problem, the patient may be reluctant to provide a true history of how they feel and the history may need to be obtained from a friend or relatives. The history often reveals that the patient has been tearful, completely preoccupied and unable to think of anything other than their illness. Their sleep patterns and eating habits will invariably have been disturbed, leading to autonomic disturbance (e.g. bowel disturbance).

Prevention of some anxiety is possible – much anxiety could be prevented by better organization of services for patients. Informing patients of the results of investigations as soon as possible, ensuring that all information is communicated between primary and secondary care, and that those caring for patients possess good communication skills can all minimize morbidity. Often patients may require medication to remove the feelings of anxiety and a short-acting benzodiazepine (e.g. Lorazepm or Diazepam) is helpful. It is important that fears are addressed and that they are discussed with the patient and his or her main carer if appropriate. Anxiety management groups or individual anxiety management can also be therapeutic and are often offered under the supervision of a liaison psychiatry or psychology service. Complementary therapies (e.g. aromatherpy and massage) and specific interventions (e.g. hypnosis, relaxation and imagery) are all beneficial. Referral to a palliative care day centre can similarly reduce the sense of isolation for a patient and also offer support for their family (Goodwin *et al.* 2002).

Depression

Depression can present in a variety of ways, including agitation, retardation and withdrawal. Patients are often reluctant to disclose their feelings of being low for fear of being thought a 'bad' or 'difficult' patient or because they may fear troubling or upsetting their doctor. It is important, therefore, that depression is acknowledged and thought about in palliative care as much as the assessment of pain or nausea. One of the main difficulties is distinguishing between depression and sadness – all patients can be expected to be sad at the end of life, but how can we distinguish between what can be called 'appropriate sadness' from a treatable depressive illness? What are useful indicators that a patient is depressed? Feelings of overwhelming hopelessness and helplessness, guilt and thoughts of self-harm are all thought to be useful indicators of depression (Casey 1994).

A very wise psychiatrist when asked how he was able to distinguish sadness from depression in patients with advanced cancer stated that patients who are depressed blame themselves for how they feel, whereas patients who are sad blame their illness for how they feel; from clinical experience this is invariably the case. Patients who are depressed frequently look more unwell than they really are. There may also be difficulties with symptom management; depression should be considered in the patient for whom no analgesia appears to work and whose symptoms are never fully resolved. Recent research with patients with end-stage renal disease has suggested that psychological distress can contribute to greater morbidity and earlier mortality in this population (Christensen and Ehlers 2002), and research of the need for palliative care for non-cancer patients has reported that the need for psychological care is as great as in those dying of malignant disease (Luddington *et al.* 2001).

How much of a problem is depression for palliative care patients?

The prevalence of depression differs widely from 3 per cent to 50 per cent depending on the criteria used and the way in which they are applied (Buckberg *et al.* 1984; Grassi *et al.* 1996; Minagawa *et al.* 1996; Hoptof *et al.* 2002). As the prevalence of depression in the general population is 6–10 per cent, a number of patients who present with advanced disease may have a pre-existing psychiatric disorder and the advancing disease will place these patients at greater risk of developing further episodes (Bergevin and Bergevin 1995). Grassi *et al.* (1996), studying 86 terminally ill patients being cared for at home and using the HAD scale and quality of life tool EORTC QLQ-C30, found that 45 per cent of patients were depressed and reported correlations between quality of life and depression. Buckberg *et al.* (1984) interviewed 62 oncology patients according to the criteria of the *Diagnostic and Statistical Manual of Mental Disorders-III* (American Psychiatric Association 1980) and found that 42 per cent met the criteria for major non-bipolar depression and 14 per cent had symptoms of depression that did not meet the criteria for major depression. In Hughes's (1985) prospective study, of 50 patients with advanced inoperable lung cancer, 16 per cent had a major depressive illness. Ramsay (1992) evaluated all referrals to a liaison psychiatry service during one year; there were 26 such referrals or 10 per cent of the patients admitted to the unit during the year. Of these 26 patients, 50 per cent had a diagnosis of depression. More recent work comparing patients with lung cancer and end-stage chronic pulmonary obstructive disease (COPD) has suggested that 90 per cent of patients with COPD suffered clinically relevant anxiety and depression, compared with 52 per cent of patients with terminal lung cancer (Gore *et al.* 2000). Up to 80 per cent of the psychological and psychiatric morbidity that develops in cancer patients goes unrecognized and untreated (Maguire 1985).

One reason for this low rate of detection is thought to be non-disclosure by patients, who may either feel they are wasting the doctor's time or that they are in some way to blame for their distress and therefore choose to hide it (Maguire and Howell 1995). There are no universally accepted criteria for diagnosing depression in the medically ill. In the physically healthy population, depression is diagnosed if patients have a persistent low mood and at least four of the following symptoms were present most of the day in the preceding 2 weeks:

- diminished interest or pleasure in all or almost all activities;
- psychomotor retardation or agitation;
- feelings of worthlessness or excessive and inappropriate guilt;
- diminished ability to concentrate and think;
- recurrent thoughts of death and suicide;
- fatigue and loss of energy;
- significant weight loss or gain;
- insomnia or hypersomnia.

In patients with advanced cancer, the last three symptoms in this list are almost universal and there has been considerable controversy as to whether physical symptoms should be included when diagnosing depression in the terminally ill. Buckberg *et al.* (1984) believed that anorexia, loss of appetite and low energy are such common symptoms in the medically ill that he proposed eliminating these somatic symptoms as criteria for the diagnosis of depression. They also found that the point prevalence of major depression dropped from 42 to 24 per cent when all somatic symptoms were eliminated as criteria. Such criteria therefore need to be used with caution in palliative care.

Assessment for depression is difficult when a patient has a terminal illness – asking patients about their mood or their spirits over the last week, or a general 'How are you feeling in yourself', may just be the opening required. Asking about previous history of depression and also establishing the patient's fears should also be part of the examination. Rating scales are widely used, with the Hospital Anxiety and Depression Scale (Zigmond and Snaith 1983) being the most common. This scale, however, has poor validity in terminally ill patients and can be difficult to use (Urch *et al.* 1999; Lloyd-Williams *et al.* 2001). The Edinburgh Depression Scale (Cox *et al.* 1987) has been found in recent work to have a sensitivity and specificity of over 80 per cent at a cut-off threshold of 13 and may be worth considering as an appropriate screening tool for palliative care (Lloyd-Williams *et al.* 2000). Although developed for the use with mothers in the post-natal period, it contains symptoms such as hopelessness, worthlessness, guilt and thoughts of self-harm, which are thought to be particularly discriminating symptoms in the palliative care population (Casey 1994). It must be stressed, however, that screening is not a solution in itself and that patients who are screened and score above a pre-determined and validated cut-off threshold require further assessment.

Research has suggested that asking patients if they are depressed is a useful indicator of whether they are or not; Chochinov *et al.* (1997) reported a sensitivity and specificity of 100 per cent for this item, making it almost a diagnostic tool. Further research in the UK population using the single question 'Are you depressed?' has found that this item does not perform so well (Lloyd-Williams *et al.* 2003). Additionally, patients under-report their psychological and psychiatric symptoms and may be reluctant to respond truthfully to such questions if asked in isolation (Maguire

1985). Visual analogue scales have been used in patients with cancer (Coates *et al.* 1983; Lees and Lloyd-Williams 1999), but the subjective experience of the patient may lead to either under- or over-scoring and many patients experience difficulty in understanding the concept of a visual analogue scale.

Management of depression

The management of depression in palliative care patients is similar for all other patients, but time is frequently shorter. Explaining to the patients and their relatives that depression is common in cancer can itself be part of the healing process, as many patients believe they are somehow not coping as they should. Trying to uncover what is really bothering the patient (i.e. in terms of their families, their disease or mode of death) can also help to lessen the feelings of isolation associated with depression. While psychological support is of course vital, there is no evidence to suggest that counselling alone is effective for these patients; indeed, a recent study suggested that in patients for whom time is limited, counselling alone should not be recommended (Chilvers *et al.* 2001).

Antidepressants are not prescribed as frequently as they should be (Lloyd-Williams *et al.* 1998; Maguire 2000). There is considerable debate as to which antidepressant to choose. Most doctors favour the selective serotonin reuptake inhibitors (SSRI) (e.g. Fluoxetine, Sertraline and the newer Mirtazapine) rather than the older tricyclic antidepressants (e.g. Dothiepin, Amitryptilene). Clinical evidence suggests that the SSRIs cause fewer side-effects in the terminally ill and are also safer in overdose. The main reason why antidepressant therapy is ineffective is that it is started too late in the patient's illness or there are difficulties with compliance; considerable encouragement may be required to enable a patient to persevere with medication while waiting for a therapeutic benefit. It is suggested that, if possible, treatment should be maintained for at least 3 months. Patients may benefit from support from community nurses or palliative care specialist nurses. Complementary therapies (e.g. aromatherapy, relaxation) can also enhance a feeling of well-being and may be of benefit to the patient. Seventy per cent of cancer patients treated with antidepressants had a full therapeutic response in one prospective study (Chaturvedi *et al.* 1994), but some patients may be very resistant to taking medication. A trial of one antidepressant for 4–5 weeks with no therapeutic benefit and proven compliance may require the intervention of a psychiatrist to assess the patient and suggest further strategies for management. For patients with long-standing mental health problems who also develop life-threatening illness, there may be particular issues surrounding medication, which may require specialist intervention from a psychiatrist.

Friends and relatives may require considerable support in knowing how to help the depressed patient, who may have withdrawn from them.

When things go wrong

Suicide is anecdotally thought to be a rare event in terminally ill patients, but a recent survey of palliative care units found 21 suicides and 37 attempted suicides within a 5-year period in the UK (Grzybowska and Finlay 1997). Female cancer patients are nearly twice as likely and male cancer patients 1.3 times more likely to die of suicide than the general population (Louhivori and Hakama 1979) and a far higher than expected number of suicides occur in patients with malignant disease (Whitlock 1978). When this happens, support may be required not only for the family but also for other members of the team, who may feel they have failed the patient.

Supporting the staff

Some patients are very depressed at the end of life when little can be done therapeutically and occasionally all measures fail. Penny was 42 years old and the mother of two children aged 5 and 3 when she presented with suicidal ideas and was admitted to the hospice with metastatic melanoma at her general practitioner's request. She was withdrawn, agreed she was depressed and refused to get out of bed. Over 5 weeks, staff spent a large amount of time encouraging her; she was offered several interventions, including relaxation and aromatherapy, all of which she declined. She was seen by a psychiatrist and agreed to take antidepressant medication but declined it 2 days later and remained withdrawn and uncommunicative until her death 4 weeks later.

After her death, members of staff from all disciplines were left with feelings of despondency that they had done nothing to help her. During a discussion of the case, it was realized that Penny had always remained in control during her life and by her actions remained in control during her dying – true holistic palliative care is all about acceptance and the knowledge that despite combined best efforts, we won't always in our own view 'get it right'; it is staying alongside the patient whatever they are going through that is most important.

Conclusions

A role for palliative care in non-cancer patients is increasingly being recognized. While the appropriate palliation of physical symptoms is important, the recognition of psychological distress and the assessment and treatment of anxiety and depression are vital to ensure that patients are able to use effectively and enjoy what remaining time they have left.

References

Addington-Hall, J. and McCarthy, M. (1995) Dying from cancer: results of a national population-based investigation. *Palliative Medicine*, 9(4): 295–305.

American Psychiatric Association (1980) *Diagnostic and Statistical Manual of Mental Disorders-III*. Washington, DC: APA.

Barnett, S. and Meyers, B. (1997) Telling patients they have Alzheimer's disease. *British Medical Journal*, 314: 321.

Barraclough, J. (1994) *Cancer and Emotion*. Chichester: Wiley.

Bergevin, P. and Bergevin, R. (1995) Recognising depression. *American Journal of Hospice and Palliative Care*, 12(5): 22–3.

Buckberg, J., Penman, D. and Holland, J. (1984) Depression in hospitalised cancer patients. *Psychosomatic Medicine*, 46(3): 199–211.

Casey, P. (1994) Depression in the dying – disorder or distress? *Progress in Palliative Care*, 2(1): 1–3.

Cassileth, B., Lusk, E. and Walsh, W. (1986) Anxiety levels in patients with malignant disease. *The Hospice Journal*, 2(2): 57–69.

Chaturvedi, S., Maguire, P. and Hopwood, P. (1994) Antidepressant medications in cancer patients. *Psycho-Oncology*, 3(1): 57–60.

Chilvers, C., Dewey, M., Fielding, K. *et al.* (2001) Antidepressant drugs and generic counselling for treatment of major depression in primary care: randomised trial with patient preference arms. *British Medical Journal*, 322: 772–5.

Chochinov, H., Wilson, K., Enns, M. and Lander, S. (1997) Are you depressed? Screening for depression in the terminally ill. *American Journal of Psychiatry*, 154(5): 674–6.

Christensen, A. and Ehlers, S. (2002) Psychological factors in end-stage renal disease: an emerging context for behavioural medicine research. *Journal of Consulting Clinical Psychology*, 70(3): 712–24.

Coates, A., Dillenbeck, C.F., McNeil, D.R. *et al.* (1983) On the receiving end. II. Linear analogue self-assessment (LASA) in evaluation of aspects of the quality of life of cancer patients receiving therapy. *European Journal of Cancer and Clinical Oncology*, 19(11): 1633–7.

Cox, J., Holden, J. and Sagovsky, R. (1987) Detection of postnatal depression: development of the 10 item Edinburgh Postnatal Depression Scale. *British Journal of Psychiatry*, 150: 782–6.

Fallowfield, L., Ford, S. and Lewis, S. (1995) No news is not good news: information preferences of patients with cancer. *Psycho-Oncology*, 4(3): 197–202.

Fincannon, J. (1995) Analysis of psychiatric referrals and interventions in an oncology population. *Oncology Nurses Forum*, 22(1): 87–92.

Goldberg, R. and Cullen, L. (1986) Depression in geriatric cancer patients: guide to assessment and treatment. *The Hospice Journal*, 2(2): 79–98.

Goodwin, D., Higginson, I., Myers, K., Douglas, H. and Normand, C. (2002) What is palliative day care? A patient perspective of five UK services. *Supportive Care Cancer*, 10(10): 556–62.

Gore, J., Brophy, C. and Greenstone, M. (2000) How well do we care for patients with end stage chronic pulmonary disease (COPD)? A comparison of palliative care and quality of life in COPD and lung cancer. *Thorax*, 55(12): 1000–6.

Grassi, L., Indelli, M., Marzalo, M. *et al.* (1996) Depressive symptoms and quality of life in home-care assisted cancer patients. *Journal of Pain and Symptom Management*, 12(5): 300–7.

Grzybowska, P. and Finlay, I. (1997) The incidence of suicide in palliative care patients. *Palliative Medicine*, 11(4): 313–16.

Harrison, J., Maguire, P. and Pitceathly, C. (1995) Confiding in crisis: gender differences in patterns of confiding among cancer patients. *Social Science and Medicine*, 41(9): 1255–60.

Higginson, I. and Costantini, M. (2002) Communication in end of life cancer care: a comparison of team assessments in three European countries. *Journal of Clinical Oncology*, 20(17): 3674–82.

Hinton, J. (1963) The physical and mental distress of the dying. *Quarterly Journal of Medicine*, 32(1): 1–21.

Hotopf, M., Chidgey, J., Addington-Hall, J. and Lan, L.K. (2002) Depression in advanced disease: a systematic review. Part 1: Prevalence and case finding. *Palliative Medicine*, 16(2): 81–97.

Hughes, J. (1985) Depressive illness and lung cancer. II: Follow-up of inoperable patients. *European Journal of Surgical Oncology*, 11(1): 21–4.

Kathol, R., Noyes, R., Williams, J. *et al.* (1990) Diagnosing depression in patients with medical illness. *Psychosomatics*, 31(4): 434–40.

Kimmel, P. (2002) Depression in patients with chronic renal disease: what we know and what we need to know. *Journal of Psychosomatic Research*, 53(4): 951–6.

Lees, N. and Lloyd-Williams, M. (1999) Assessing depression in palliative care patients using the Visual Analogue Scale: a pilot study. *European Journal of Cancer Care*, 8(4): 220–3.

Lloyd-Williams, M., Friedman, T. and Rudd, N. (1998) A survey of antidepressant prescribing in hospices. *Palliative Medicine*, 13(3): 293–8.

Lloyd-Williams, M., Friedman, T. and Rudd, N. (2000) The validation of the Edinburgh Postnatal Depression Scale in the terminally ill population. *Journal of Pain and Symptom Management*, 20(4): 259–65.

Lloyd-Williams, M., Friedman, T. and Rudd, N. (2001) The validation of the Hospital Anxiety and Depression scale in terminally ill patients. *Journal of Pain and Symptom Management*, 22(6): 990–6.

Lloyd-Williams, M., Dennis, M., Taylor, F. and Baker, I. (2003) A prospective study to determine whether it is appropriate to ask palliative care patients 'are you depressed?'. *British Medical Journal*, 327: 372–3.

Louhivori, K. and Hakama, M. (1979) Risk of suicide among cancer patients. *American Journal of Epidemiology*, 109(1): 59–65.

Luddington, L., Cox, S., Higginson, I. and Livesley, B. (2001) The need for palliative care for patients with non-cancer diseases: a review of the evidence. *International Journal of Palliative Nursing*, 7(5): 221–6.

Maguire, C., Kirby, M. and Cohen, R. (1996) Family members' attitudes toward telling the patient with Alzheimer's disease their diagnosis. *British Medical Journal*, 313: 529–30.

Maguire, P. (1985) Improving the detection of psychiatric problems in cancer patients. *Social Science and Medicine*, 20(8): 819–23.

Maguire, P. (2000) The use of antidepressants in patients with advanced cancer. *Supportive Care and Cancer*, 8(4): 265–7.

Maguire, P. and Howell, A. (1995) Improving the psychological care of cancer patients, in A. Houses, R. Mayou and C. Mallinson (eds) *Psychiatric Aspects of Physical Disease*. London: Royal College of Physicians and Royal College of Psychiatrists.

Massie, M. and Holland, J. (1992) The cancer patient with pain: psychiatric complications and their management. *Journal of Pain and Symptom Management*, 7(2): 99–109.

McVey, P. (1998) Depression among the palliative care oncology population. *International Journal of Palliative Nursing*, 4(2): 86–93.

Mechatie, E. (1997) New Alzheimer's drug delays sentence. *Clinical Psychiatry News*, 25(1): 28.

Minagawa, H., Uchitomi, Y., Yamawaki, S. and Ishitani, K. (1996) Psychiatric morbidity in terminally ill cancer patients: a prospective study. *Cancer*, 78(5): 1131–7.

Murray, S.A., Boyd, K., Kendall, M. *et al.* (2002) Dying of lung cancer or cardiac failure: prospective qualitative interview study of patients and their carers in the community. *British Medical Journal*, 325: 929–32.

National Council for Hospice and Specialist Palliative Care Services (1997) *Feeling Better: Psychosocial Care in Specialist Palliative Care*. Occasional Paper No. 13. London: NCHSPCS.

Novotony, E., Hyland, J., Coyne, L., Travis, J. and Pruyser, H. (1984) Factors affecting adjustment to cancer. *Bulletin of the Menninger Clinic*, 48(4): 318–28.

Pasacreta, J. and Massie, M. (1990) Nurses' reports of psychiatric complications in patients with cancer. *Oncology Nurses Forum*, 17(3): 347–53.

Pirl, W. and Roth, A. (1999) Diagnosis and treatment of depression in cancer patients. *Oncology*, 13(9): 1293–302.

Ramsay, N. (1992) Referral to a liaison psychiatrist from a palliative care unit. *Palliative Medicine*, 6(1): 54–60.

Rodin, G. and Voshart, K. (1986) Depression in the medically ill: an overview. *American Journal of Psychiatry*, 143(6): 696–705.

Singer, H., Ruchinskas, R., Riley, K., Broshek, D. and Barth, J. (2001) The psychological impact of end-stage lung disease. *Chest*, 120(4): 1246–52.

Steifel, F. and Razavi, D. (1994) Common psychiatric disorders in cancer patients: anxiety and acute confusional states. *Supportive Care in Cancer*, 2(4): 233–7.

Urch, C., Chamberlain, J. and Field, G. (1999) The drawback of the Hospital Anxiety and Depression Scale in the assessment of depression in hospice inpatients. *Palliative Medicine*, 12(5): 395–6.

Valentine, S. and Saunders, J. (1989) Dealing with serious depression in cancer patients. *Nursing*, 12: 44–7.

Whitlock, F. (1978) Suicide and cancer. *British Journal of Psychiatry*, 132: 477.

15

Working with family care-givers in a palliative care setting

Paula Smith

Working with family care-givers can be a rewarding and challenging process, particularly within the field of palliative care. Despite a rapid increase in the general care-giving literature based in the gerontological field over the last 20 years, there remains much we do not know or understand about the perceived needs and support for this group of people (George 1994). In this chapter, I will begin to address some of the issues that are emerging in the literature as being particularly relevant to the family care-giver in palliative or end-of-life care. By reflecting on individual family care-givers' perception of their role, it is anticipated that health and social care professionals will be able to consider their own interactions and support of this group of people in a more systematic way.

The chapter is divided into three sections. First, I focus on the current UK context and social policy relating to family care-givers. Next, I consider the development and understanding of the family care-giver role, relating this to a research study conducted with family care-givers in a palliative care setting. Finally, I consider the implications of this research for practice.

Definitions used within the chapter

One of the difficulties of having some clarity about working with family care-givers is the myriad of terms and definitions that are used within the literature to define this group and the activities they undertake. In this chapter, I will use the term 'family care-givers' to refer to the person or persons who have primary responsibility for the day-to-day care of the person with incurable disease or who is nearing the end of life. They may or may not recognize themselves as a carer or family care-giver, but nevertheless will often be involved in providing emotional, physical, social and/or spiritual support to the ill person. Care-givers will generally be participating in caring for familial, friendship or kinship reasons, and will usually be co-resident with the cared for person. They will generally be providing care in an unpaid capacity, although in some countries may be in receipt of financial benefits. They may or may not have formal training and qualifications in caring in general, although many will develop expertise in caring for the ill person.

One other source of confusion, which may affect the working relationship between family care-givers and health and social care professionals within a palliative care setting, is the term 'specialist palliative care'. Specialist palliative care in this chapter will refer to care provided by individuals who have additional training and expertise. General palliative care will refer to the palliative care provided by all health professionals across a range of settings. It is important to note that specialist palliative care in the UK has largely developed in relation to cancer patients and their families. Although provision of this service is not always exclusive to this particular group of patients, those with a chronic non-cancer diagnosis may have difficulty accessing the additional services and expertise provided by specialist palliative care providers. This, in turn, can result in a variable amount of support being offered to the family care-giver in developing and maintaining their caring role.

Family care-giving and current UK social policy

An ageing population, improving treatment regimes and changes within the National Health Service (NHS) within the UK have resulted in an increasing expectation of family participation in care-giving, particularly within a palliative care setting. Family care-givers are increasingly being relied on to provide most daily care, including the management of the physical, emotional and psychological consequences of advanced malignant disease (Kennedy *et al.* 1999; Weitzner and McMillan 1999). The impact on family care-givers of policy changes such as those in the UK, which have resulted in an emphasis on community care and a movement away from care delivered in institutions, remains unclear. It is important, therefore, that professional service providers are aware and understand the complex nature of the caring role assumed by family care-givers so that they can meet their information and support needs both adequately and appropriately (Kennedy *et al.* 1999).

Despite the increasing use of the term 'carer' within the general gerontological literature over the last few years (Heaton 1999), understanding and conceptualizing the role remains ambiguous (Smith 2000). This may be due in part to the origin of the term, which stemmed from a professional service orientation and related to individuals whose paid occupation was within a caring profession or organization (Twigg *et al.* 1990). Increasingly however, the term has been adopted to represent care that is provided by close family and friends and is based on pre-existing relationships such as familial or kinship obligations and responsibilities. Various terminologies have been applied to the family and friends who undertake such a caring role, including family care-givers, informal carers, lay carers, home carers, and unpaid or untrained carers. The use of these terms in relation to individuals who have generally not received training or payment for their work has led to an implication that professional care is somehow more desirable than informal or unpaid care. Within this position family carers may be viewed as the 'given' or 'taken-for-granted' background to professional service care, and may be relied on by professional service providers to form the basis underpinning additional professional support (Twigg and Atkin 1994). Heaton (1999) argues that this has resulted in a polarization of informal and formal carer roles in social policy that has conceptualized informal carers as the primary providers of care in the community and formal care as a sustainer of the informal network providers.

Such a view, however, is not cognisant of the acquired experience and expertise that family care-givers develop over time (Nolan *et al.* 1996a). An alternative typology proposed by Nolan *et al.* (1996a), based on their work with family carers in the gerontological field, views informal carers as 'experts' in caring. Within this framework, the informal carers' expertise may be supplemented or enhanced by that of professional carers. Services in this scenario work with the informal carer to provide optimum care and support to the cared for person, while acknowledging the developing expertise that these individuals acquire. Traditionally, family care-givers' expertise may have developed over a prolonged period, particularly in the case of chronic diseases other than cancer. However, the development of such expertise is also increasingly true for family care-givers who are caring for a family member with cancer. For some, the duration of symptoms may extend over a number of years and phases throughout the disease trajectory, including periods of recurrence, active treatment and remission (Thomas *et al.* 2002). This may result in some family care-givers adopting the role of representative of the ill person (Friedrichsen *et al.* 2001), or becoming the coordinator of care between the visiting health and social care professionals and the patient (Smith 2000).

Thus, being sensitive to the individual needs of each person and being able to provide an all-encompassing policy in relation to family care-givers may be difficult. Rather, there is a need to be aware of the differences each family care-giver may bring to a situation in order to work most effectively with them to ensure the safety and well-being of both the family care-giver and the person they are caring for.

Understanding the family care-giver role

The question, then, is who is the family care-giver in palliative care and how can health and social care professionals (a) recognize them and (b) provide appropriate information and support? In discussing these issues, I will refer to my own research (see 'The research study' on page 316) and illustrate the issues with summaries, quotes and case studies from some of the family care-givers who participated in this research.

How is caring constructed?

Definitions of informal caring often revolve around the overt, instrumental or tangible aspects of care. This view is reflected in the literature and in social policy in the UK. The Carers (Recognition and Services) Act 1995 sought to raise the profile of family care-givers and their support needs. However, it has been only partially effective, as it emphasized the physical burden of caring (Nolan *et al.* 1996b) and the implicit assumptions underlying the role. The Carers (Recognition and Services) Act 1995 did result in the launch of the Carers National Strategy (Department of Health 1999), which highlighted some of the key issues in being a carer. These include a desire to maintain the well-being of the cared for person, having a life of their own outside of caring, maintaining their own health, having confidence in the services they receive, and having a say in service provision. Furthermore, the Carers National Strategy emphasized the importance of shared responsibility for care and included in this a respect and acknowledgement of the family care-giver's knowledge. Although this strategy recognizes certain features relating to caring, it does still assume that the individual will identify with the term 'carer' and is able and willing to undertake these roles and activities.

For health and social care professionals, then, family care-giving may be constructed as negative, unwelcome and burdensome. Perhaps for this reason much of the care-giving literature views overt care-giving as having a negative impact on family care-givers' quality of life. Indeed, family caregivers within palliative care have been found to suffer from more anxiety than the ill person (Hinton 1994a). The negative impact on quality of life that may be found as a result of adopting the role of carer is often referred to in the general care-giving literature as a sense of burden. Some studies have attempted to explore what factors might constitute identification of caregivers who might be 'at risk' of a sense of burden. For example, Meyers and Gray (2001) found that the care-giving role negatively affected care-givers' quality of life and this was particularly noticeable among long-term caregivers who lived in a rural locality. They suggested that care-givers falling into this category would benefit from additional support from hospice or palliative care services.

That is not to say that all family care-givers find their role burdensome. Indeed, many family care-givers describe mixed emotions regarding their role and highlight both positive and negative aspects. Often family caregivers recall a sense of satisfaction to feelings of reciprocity and being able to return care received in the past, or as a way of demonstrating their love for the ill person (Grbich *et al.* 2001). For others, there may be social or moral obligations to participate in care-giving that negates the difficulties encountered. Recognizing the potential positive outcome of family care-giving is now being acknowledged in the literature and studies are beginning to emerge that suggest satisfaction with the care-giving role despite the difficulties this might cause (Nolan *et al.* 1996a; Grbich *et al.* 2001).

Who is the family care-giver?

Within palliative care, there has always been a strong emphasis on supporting the family of the terminally ill person (Seale 1989), although there is little guidance as to what such support involves or indeed how to achieve it. It is clear, however, that should the family care-giver's ability to maintain the care required by the ill person be compromised, there may be additional and sometimes distressing admissions to hospital or hospice (Addington-Hall *et al.* 1991; Hinton 1994a). This, in turn, can result in dissatisfaction for both the cared-for person and the family care-giver, as well as a sense of frustration and failure on the part of the health or social care professional.

The general care-giving literature, and that of the gerontological and dementia fields in particular, suggests that this role may be fulfilled by a number of the ill person's friends and relations working together to provide individual and holistic care (Linkewich *et al.* 1999). In practice, what usually happens is that one person, usually co-resident with the ill person, takes the predominant care-giving role and is supported in this by more extended family and friend networks (Smith 2000; Thomas *et al.* 2002). Keating *et al.* (1994) argue that the view of one family care-giver providing all care fails to explore or take account of the wider social dynamics involved in this type of caring. In addition, it is traditionally assumed in many cultures that care-giving is part of a woman's role (Neale and Clark 1992). Despite this, large numbers of men participate in caring, particularly if they are the spouse of the cared-for person (Arber and Gilbert 1989), and in the older generation will engage in equal amounts of co-resident care (Arber and Ginn 1990).

▌The research study

The case study examples provided in this chapter are from my own research, which explored the dynamic and changing nature of caring for a family member in a palliative care setting. I first became interested in exploring the needs and support of this group as a result of my clinical experience as a district nurse. The study was based on a case study approach similar to that described by Yin (1994), who acknowledged important background and situational information should be considered as part of the data collection and analysis within the research. One of the study's aims was to identify how the family care-giver's circumstances might change over time. To accomplish this, I used a longitudinal design. Sixteen family care-givers (eight husbands, six wives and two adult daughters) from two areas in the south of England were interviewed over 4 months. The age range of the family care-givers was 33–73 years with a mean age of 56.8 years. All were recruited through the visiting specialist palliative care professionals with whom they had contact, and all were caring for someone with cancer with a prognosis of 6 months or less.

Each family care-giver was visited up to four times over the 4-month period. Detailed interviews were conducted with the family care-givers alone if possible, although seven chose to be interviewed with the person they were caring for. The interviews focused on their role and relationship with visiting health professionals and other sources of support. All interviews took place in the care-giver's own home and lasted between one and two and a half hours.

Each interview was tape-recorded and later fully transcribed. Each transcript was then subjected to a continuous reading and re-reading to elicit themes and issues that were relevant to the family care-givers.

Identification with the family care-giver 'role'

Identification with the role of 'carer' is sometimes unclear, particularly when the role has been adopted for kinship and obligation reasons in a gradual and progressive way. The caring activities undertaken as a result are not, therefore, identified as being part of a particular role or job as the term 'carer' might imply. In the research highlighted in 'The research study', it was found that family care-givers who had been involved in caring for a prolonged period of time would often identify strongly with the term 'carer'. However, those that had only recently undertaken such role changes strongly resisted being called a carer (see Case study 1).

Case study 1

Mrs Vaughan was a lady in her mid-fifties who had a life-long history of caring and strongly identified with this role. She was an active member of her local carers' support group and was currently caring for both her husband, who had cancer, and her mother, who had Parkinson's disease: 'I've been a carer all my life. I've always done something for somebody. I've never had nursing training, but it's a natural instinct, it's born in me.' In part due to her strong allegiance to the carer role, Mrs Vaughan's greatest concern was what she would do if both her husband and mother should die at the same time. She posed the question: 'What do the carers do when the caring ends?'

Mr Lloyd, on the other hand, did not identify with the term carer and saw his involvement as being much more related to marital obligations and reciprocity for care received by his wife in the past. Mr Lloyd was in his late thirties and had never been involved in caring before.

'Cos when you're actually married to someone you're there through thick and thin any way aren't you? If I was ill she'd look after me, and if she was ill I'd look after her. Um, I remember when I was in hospital, I had two bad injuries playing rugby where I was put in hospital and I had an operation. When I came out I couldn't, I was on crutches. She always looked after me then. I mean it's just this is, I don't know, a bit longer that's all.

Mr Lloyd admitted that he had found the caring role, which included looking after their three young children and taking on additional household responsibilities, a shock: 'I do everything around the house. Do the cleaning, cooking, looking after the kids, washing. Just got used to it now [laughs] . . . when she was well I just used to come home and have my dinner ready made for me. Big shock this!'

While family care-givers are often happy to undertake additional roles and responsibilities in support of the cared for person, they may face a number of restrictions and losses to their own valued activities and interests (Duke 1998). If this is perceived to be for a limited period of time, such as is often assumed on being given a cancer diagnosis, family care-givers may be happy to put their own needs and activities on hold. Expectations of potential time-frames from diagnosis to death are particularly common with certain diseases such as cancer. However, while this may be true in some cases – for example, lung cancer generally has a poor prognosis – this is not the case for other cancers, particularly if they are diagnosed and treated at an early stage. If caring continues beyond the anticipated time-frame, the level and intensity of support may become unsustainable (see Case study 2). Similarly with other chronic diseases, the potential time-frame for which caring will be required may not be realistically considered at the beginning of the caring journey, as this is often unpredictable.

Case study 2

Some people who had become involved in family care-giving at the point of diagnosis with cancer found it increasingly difficult to maintain their involvement at the original level when the caring was extended over a prolonged period. This was especially noticeable for the younger and middle-aged care-givers who were juggling other roles, such as being a partner, parent, adult child and worker.

Mrs Page was in her late fifties and worked full-time. She had been 'keeping an eye' on her mother since the death of her father 4 years earlier. This involved daily visits to her mother either before or after going to work to check that her mother was well and had no immediate needs. Although her mother had a number of paid carers who heated a meal at lunchtime and assisted with dressing, it was Mrs Page who took on responsibility for ensuring that the shopping was done, finances organized, bills paid, tablets sorted and numerous other jobs around the house attended to. Mrs Page also anticipated her mother's current and future needs by instigating and organizing appropriate services as required. She would sometimes do things herself and sometimes call in professional services to deliver this care. After her mother was diagnosed with cancer, Mrs Page increased the time and attention she gave to visiting and supporting her mother. However, one year later she was torn between spending time looking after her mother and looking after her husband, who had also retired early due to ill health at about the same time as her mother was diagnosed with cancer: 'You can't split yourself in two, you know. You can't be over the road there and over here as well . . . If you please one, you upset the other. And I know lately I have more often than not upset my husband rather than upset my mother.'

Mrs Foster was also in her mid fifties and worked full-time. She and her husband had limited contact with their children as they lived a long way away, and so had to rely on friends and neighbours for support. Although her employers were sympathetic to her circumstances, Mrs Foster was finding it increasingly difficult to juggle her work and provide support for her husband, particularly through his treatment regime: 'You sort of run out of momentum sometimes . . . Because you begin to wonder yourself sometimes, which is only, you know, understandable is there going to be an end?'

What is family care-giving?

The amount and type of care given by family care-givers is not generally static and may change and develop throughout the disease trajectory. Nolan *et al.* (1995) suggest that throughout the care-giving experience, family care-givers are likely to engage in 'anticipatory care'. This involves anticipating what they will do should the ill person suffer from a real or imagined deterioration. Anticipatory care does not necessarily involve direct or instrumental care-giving, although it may well be as time-consuming and worrying for the family care-giver as more direct involvement in supporting the ill person. Furthermore, Nolan *et al.* (1995) suggest that the level of information and knowledge the family care-giver has in relation to the disease trajectory can become important in reducing what they term 'speculative anticipation', which is characterized by a lack of information or knowledge about the situation. This can result in over- or under-anticipation of future needs, which may have a detrimental effect on the family care-giver. Informed anticipation, on the other hand, can result in greater shared care and planning. By recognizing and acknowledging anticipatory care, health and social care professionals can reduce the invisibility of speculative anticipation.

The difficulty arises within palliative care when the very uncertainty of the disease trajectory and potential deterioration in the cared-for person's condition make anticipating future needs difficult. Increasingly within cancer care, family care-givers are faced with responding to the cyclical nature of the disease trajectory, including periods of remission, recurrence and active treatment that can have a negative impact on their ability to cope (see Case study 3).

Case study 3

Mr Lloyd found that the oscillation in his wife's condition between treatments for cancer resulted in him taking on the full responsibility for the domestic and child care chores at selected points and then relinquishing these to his wife as she recovered and wished to resume her normal role. Mr Lloyd struggled to adapt to this constant change in roles: 'On the one hand I'm glad she feels better the way she does. On the other side it's like she's just taking over what I'm doing all the time. I've got used to doing it now she's taking over sort of thing . . . It causes a few ructions actually. But then it's just getting used to it I suppose. Feel redundant.'

Family care-giving activities

Often becoming involved in family care-giving can result in a number of role changes and routines (Denham 1999). This can range from simply providing companionship and undertaking household tasks, to assisting with personal care, transport and, for some, quite complex nursing care (Payne *et al.* 1999; Aranda and Hayman-White 2001; Thomas *et al.* 2002). In a large-scale study following bereavement, Wyatt *et al.* (1999) found that family care-givers had been highly involved in assisting the cared-for person with activities of daily living, often averaging 10.8 hours a day of direct care-giving and 8.9 hours of providing companionship. The level of involvement that the family care-giver has in these activities will depend on several factors, such as the ill person's condition, their previous relationship with the ill person, their own health and ability to undertake such care, the level and type of support they receive from professional and social networks.

For many family care-givers, the most significant aspect of the care-giving role is to provide emotional support to the cared-for person, as observed in their desire to maintain a positive outlook and a sense of normality (Thomas *et al.* 2002). This creates a particular difficulty for family care-givers within palliative care when it is known and openly acknowledged that the cared-for person is going to deteriorate and will not recover to their pre-illness status. Juggling both of these positions at the same time can result in a state of tension for the family care-giver between wanting to remain positive on the one hand and yet having to acknowledge that the situation is not going to improve on the other. For some, one way of dealing with this conflict is to ignore it and focus only on the present, especially when with the cared-for person. Often significant family events or outings will be planned as something to look forward to (see Case study 4).

Case study 4

Mrs Gardner was in her mid-eighties and had been caring for her disabled husband for a number of years before he was diagnosed with cancer. They had both been looking forward to enjoying her birthday meal with all the family, including their 6-year-old grandson: 'On Saturday they were here for my birthday so we all went out for a meal . . . And er, we had a lovely meal and it was very nice, you know, it was very nice to have the little family together. The little boy was very good he sat and had his meal.'

Sometimes activities that are undertaken become increasingly complex, particularly during the terminal phase of the illness (Cameron *et al.* 2002). For example, Aranda and Hayman-White (2001) found that family care-givers were significantly involved in the symptom management of the ill person and undertook assessment, monitoring and delivery of complex therapeutic interventions such as pain and symptom control. In addition, they took on almost total responsibility for routine household tasks. Aranda and Hayman-White concluded that there is a need, therefore, to move towards the development of care-giver-focused nursing interventions. Providing practical, emotional and informational support to enable family care-givers to undertake this role may be particularly important at this time if they are to be able to participate fully in this activity (Rose 1999; Bakas *et al.* 2001), if that is the wish of both the family care-giver and the cared-for person. While it is commendable to provide adequate and appropriate support to family care-givers who wish to undertake additional caring roles and responsibilities, it is important to acknowledge that there may well be certain caring tasks that both the family care-giver and the cared-for person feel uncomfortable participating in; for example, the provision of intimate personal care or specific nursing roles such as catheter care. This may be particularly important if there are gender differences and or generational issues (such as a daughter caring for her father) that the health professional should be aware of and take into account when negotiating and providing information and support in undertaking these roles and responsibilities.

Implications for practice

What, then, are the implications for practice given the increasing awareness of the family care-giver role and perception of their needs?

Understanding the family care-giver role

Although family care-givers are acknowledged within palliative care, and are generally considered integral to the care of the ill person, a clear understanding of the nature of their role and relationship with health and social care professionals remains elusive. The difficulty lies in determining how joint care with family care-givers may be organized so that equity of support can be delivered to both the ill person and their associated family care-givers. If health professionals are unclear about the extent of their responsibility to the family, there is likely to be a privileging of the patient's needs and wishes over those of the family care-giver, despite the rhetoric of concern for the whole family. Privileging the patient's needs and concerns in this way fails to take account of the rights of the family care-giver, even though some decisions may have a direct consequence on their health and well-being. For example, if the patient wishes to die at home and the family care-giver feels unable to provide this level of care, to what extent should services be provided so that the patient's wishes are met? If the time before death is fraught with anxiety and worry about how the situation can be managed, the family care-giver may feel let down and could remember the cared-for person's death in a negative light, which may have implications for their own well-being during their bereavement.

By developing a clearer definition of what the role of family care-giver within palliative care involves, there is less likelihood of family care-givers being unexpectedly placed in the position of accepting a role or level of responsibility that they may feel uncomfortable with. In addition, understanding the role that the family care-givers themselves associate with their involvement may be important in tailoring the appropriate level and type of information and support required by the individual (Friedrichsen *et al.* 2001). Explicit recognition of the role would also result in an open acknowledgement of the family care-giver position, which, in turn, would have the benefit of highlighting the rights and needs of these carers. This would help health and social care professionals to identify clear areas of responsibility and priority in relation to the family care-giver.

Supporting the family care-giver

Within the palliative care literature, family care-givers' perception, experience and identification of needs has recently begun to receive more attention (Andershed and Ternestedt 2001; Smith 2001; McKay *et al.* 2002; Thomas *et al.* 2002). Understanding these factors could be one way of preventing unplanned admissions to hospital or hospice due to a breakdown in family care-giving arrangements.

Where there is a known disease trajectory of limited duration, specialist palliative care services are often introduced at an early stage. However, where there is a less clear disease progression and a potentially long illness, it is often difficult to determine when specialist palliative care services should be introduced. This can potentially result in family care-givers being the only ones involved in caring for a long period of time. For example, the cared-for person may experience a number of distressing symptoms and adaptations to various losses during the course of their illness. This may also impact on the family care-giver in a negative way. Such symptoms and adaptations have been linked to a sense of burden and anxiety in the family care-giver (Andrews 2001). Doyle-Brown (2000) found that the transitional phase of a person's illness between active participation in daily activities and being bed-bound was a time of increased anxiety for family care-givers. Being able to identify factors associated with this time and educate the family regarding this process could potentially help the family care-giver to continue with end-of-life care without the need for admission to hospice or hospital (Doyle-Brown 2000).

Another issue that may be a particular difficulty for family care-givers in a palliative care setting is the inevitability of the impending death. This creates a tension for the family care-giver whereby they want to prolong the life of the cared-for person and enjoy their company and shared experiences for as long as possible on the one hand, but they do not wish them to suffer or become distressed on the other. The tension, therefore, is one of conflict between attempting to prolong the life and quality of the cared-for person and at the same time preparing for their death and mourning the anticipated loss of shared experiences (Smith 2000).

For some family care-givers there may be particular times throughout the disease trajectory when additional support or information needs may be required (McKay *et al.* 2002). The point of diagnosis can often have a significant and profound effect on the family care-giver. If this time is addressed sensitively and information is given at an appropriate level, the family care-giver may be assisted to cope. Alternatively, if the communication between the family care-giver and health profession is poor at the start of an illness, this may well impact on the family care-giver's ability to negotiate and interact with other health professionals later in the disease trajectory. Also, as the family care-giver becomes increasingly involved in instrumental or 'doing for' caring, they may have specific practical and information needs related to providing such care that the health and social care practitioner may be able to provide.

Adequate assessment of need

Family care-giving is a complex and dynamic process, often involving a substantial amount of effort and commitment by the care-giver. Over a prolonged period of time, such an investment may not be viable for several reasons. First, the emotional roller-coaster that this type of uncertainty produces may be one reason that family care-givers exhibit increased anxiety and negative psychological consequences (Hinton 1994b). Second, if the family care-giver is able and willing to give up, or reduce, other social contacts, there is a possibility that the very mechanisms that may support them during the care-giving experience and following the death of the cared-for person will be unavailable when they are most needed. This is particularly important if the care-giving experience is conducted over a prolonged period. For example, both of the daughters in the research (see 'The research study') commented on the negative effect the period of care-giving had on their own interactions with their spouses and children. Similarly, those family care-givers who were still in employment had experienced a variety of reactions from their employers to their need to take time off work to care for the ill person. This ranged from full and active support of the family care-giver in undertaking this role, to open hostility and sanctions regarding the necessity of this course of action. If the supportive social relationships with extended family members or active employment roles are damaged during the care-giving experience, this may result in difficulties for the family care-giver following bereavement when there is an expectation that people will reintegrate into society. In this situation, an ongoing assessment of the family care-giver's perceived level of responsibility and resources to support the ill person may highlight the need for additional information, educational or counselling needs for the carer.

Information and education for family care-givers

Importance continues to be attached to the practical and burdensome aspects of caring within the literature, which fails to acknowledge the positive aspects that many family care-givers in palliative care report. However, while it is important to recognize that not everyone involved in family care-giving will be burdened by this role, some may. For those that are burdened by their role, there is an implicit assumption that there will be consequences for the individual's own health and well-being either during or after bereavement. Although there is little evidence available in the literature to link inadequate support for family care-givers with bereavement difficulties, a study by Kurtz *et al.* (1997) found that care-giver optimism, pre-bereavement depressive symptomatology and level of social support were critical in determining depressive symptomatology during bereavement. They concluded that understanding these factors could help health professionals to identify those family care-givers who may be at increased risk of exhibiting depressive symptoms following bereavement.

Adequate preparation for care-giving may be one way of preventing the family care-giver becoming overburdened with their role. In a UK study, Scott (2001) found that insufficient preparation for care-giving contributed significantly to the negative effects on the mental health of the family care-giver. A lack of information and acknowledgement by staff may increase the sense of isolation and difficulty that family care-givers experience. Andershed and Ternestedt (2001) describe this situation as 'involvement in the dark', whereby relatives report 'groping around in the dark' in their attempts to support the patient. Alternatively, when relatives are well informed and develop a sound working relationship with staff based on trust, then a more meaningful experience of caring may result (Andershed and Ternestedt 2001; Mok *et al.* 2002). Clearly, early intervention and informational support to new family care-givers is important in this process (Scott 2001). In the longer term, regular respite and opportunities to maintain social contacts may be important in supporting the family care-giver in palliative care (Scott 2001).

Families of those with cancer frequently report that their information and support needs are not being met satisfactorily (Lewis *et al.* 1997; Rose 1999; Flanagan 2001). Some studies have explored the effectiveness of educational training for family care-givers and the health professionals who are supporting them (Pickett *et al.* 2001). However, the evidence supporting these interventions as being effective is less clear. In a US study, Robinson *et al.* (1998) described a combined educational programme for both care-givers and health and social care workers. At the end of the programme, care-givers reported feeling less overwhelmed and better able to cope with the care-giver experience. However, McCorkle and Pasacreta (2001) found that data supporting the effectiveness of care-giver interventions is limited.

Conclusions

In this chapter, I have explored some of the issues faced by family care-givers within a palliative care setting, focusing particularly on the role of the family care-giver and the nature of their support needs. This has highlighted the need for acknowledgment and appropriate support of the family care-giver, which is an explicit part of the palliative care philosophy. However, implementing such support remains difficult due to the complex and individual nature of the situations arising in this setting. Despite this, there are clearly some areas that are worthy of consideration by health and social care practitioners (see 'Key issues for consideration'). These include being aware of the type of support needs of the family care-giver at various points along the disease trajectory. There need to be developments in educational programmes for both professionals and family care-givers to support both the practical and emotional aspects of managing a caring role in a palliative care situation. Finally, it is clear that any such initiative should be adequately researched to determine the effectiveness of such interventions and, if possible, the effect they might have on subsequent bereavement outcomes for family care-givers.

Key issues for consideration

- Understanding the role and perspective of the family care-giver to enable health and social care practitioners to liaise with and negotiate caring responsibilities in a more systematic way.

- Assessment and reassessment of family care-givers' needs to ensure that they are provided with adequate and appropriate information and support at appropriate points in the disease trajectory. This will help to reduce speculative anticipation in the caring role and enable family care-givers to focus on real problems and needs rather than imagined needs.

- Further work needs to be considered to explore the effectiveness and usefulness of any interventions with family care-givers from their perspective, particularly in relation to any educational programmes introduced.

References

Addington-Hall, J., MacDonald, L., Anderson, H. and Freeling, P. (1991) Dying from cancer: the views of bereaved family and friends about the experiences of terminally ill patients. *Palliative Medicine*, 5: 207–14.

Andershed, B. and Ternestedt, B.M. (2001) Development of a theoretical framework describing relatives' involvement in palliative care. *Journal of Advanced Nursing*, 34(4): 544–62.

Andrews, S.C. (2001) Caregiver burden and symptom distress in people with cancer receiving hospice care. *Oncology Nursing Forum*, 28(9): 1469–74.

Aranda, S.K. and Hayman-White, K. (2001) Home caregivers of the person with advanced cancer: an Australian perspective. *Cancer Nursing*, 24(4): 300–7.

Arber, S. and Gilbert, N. (1989) Men: the forgotten carers. *Sociology*, 23: 111–18.

Arber, S. and Ginn, J. (1990) The meaning of informal care: gender and the contribution of elderly people. *Aging and Society*, 10: 429–54.

Bakas, T., Lewis, R.R. and Parsons, J.E. (2001) Caregiving tasks among family caregivers of patients with lung cancer. *Oncology Nursing Forum*, 28(5): 847–54.

Cameron, J.I., Franche, R.L., Cheung, A.M. and Stewart, D.E. (2002) Lifestyle interference and emotional distress in family caregivers of advanced cancer patients. *Cancer*, 94(2): 521–7.

Denham, S.A. (1999) Part 2: family health during and after death of a family member. *Journal of Family Nursing*, 5(2): 160–83.

Department of Health (1999) *Caring about carers: a National Strategy for Carers.* London: Department of Health.

Doyle-Brown, M. (2000) The transitional phase: the closing journey for patients and family caregivers. *American Journal of Hospice and Palliative Care*, 17(5): 354–7.

Duke, S. (1998) An exploration of anticipatory grief: the lived experience of people during their spouses' terminal illness and in bereavement. *Journal of Advanced Nursing*, 28(4): 829–39.

Flanagan, J. (2001) Clinically effective cancer care: working with families. *European Journal of Oncology Nursing*, 5(3): 174–9.

Friedrichsen, M.J., Strang, P.M. and Carlsson, M.E. (2001) Receiving bad news: experiences of family members. *Journal of Palliative Care*, 17(4): 241–7.

George, L.K. (1994) Caregiver burden and well being: an elusive distinction. *The Gerontologist*, 34(1): 6–7.

Grbich, C., Parker, D. and Maddocks, I. (2001) The emotions and coping strategies of caregivers of family members with a terminal cancer. *Journal of Palliative Care*, 17(1): 30–6.

Heaton, J. (1999) The gaze and visibility of the carer: a Foucauldian analysis of the discourse of informal care. *Sociology of Health and Illness*, 21(6): 759–77.

Hinton, J. (1994a) Which patients with terminal cancer are admitted from home care? *Palliative Medicine*, 8: 197–210.

Hinton, J. (1994b) Can home care maintain an acceptable quality of life for patients with terminal cancer and their relatives? *Palliative Medicine*, 8: 183–96.

Keating, N., Kerr, K., Warren, S., Grace, M. and Wertenberger, D. (1994) Who's the family in family caregiving? *Canadian Journal on Aging*, 13(2): 268–87.

Kennedy, C., Lockhart-Wood, K. and Fielding, H. (1999) Pain management: use of the syringe driver in the community setting. *British Journal of Community Nursing*, 4(5): 250–7.

Kurtz, M.E., Kurtz, J.C., Given, C.W. and Given, B. (1997) Predictors of post-bereavement depressive symptomatology among family caregivers of cancer patients. *Supportive Care in Cancer: Official Journal of the Multinational Association of Supportive Care in Cancer*, 5(1): 53–60.

Lewis, M., Pearson, V., Corcoran-Perry, S. and Narayan, S. (1997) Decision making by elderly patients with cancer and their caregivers. *Cancer*, 20(6): 389–97.

Linkewich, B., Setliff, A.E., Poling, M. *et al.* (1999) Communicating at life's end. *The Canadian Nurse*, 95(5): 41–4.

McCorkle, R. and Pasacreta, J.V. (2001) Enhancing caregiver outcomes in palliative care. *Cancer Control: Journal of the Moffitt Cancer Centre*, 8(1): 36–45.

McKay, P., Rajacich, D. and Rosenbaum, J. (2002) Enhancing palliative care through Watson's carative factors. *Canadian Oncology Nursing Journal*, 12(1): 34–8.

Meyers, J.L. and Gray, L.N. (2001) The relationships between family primary caregiver characteristics and satisfaction with hospice care, quality of life, and burden. *Oncology Nursing Forum*, 28(1): 73–82.

Mok, E., Chan, F., Chan, V. and Yeung, E. (2002) Perception of empowerment by family caregivers of patients with a terminal illness in Hong Kong. *International Journal of Palliative Nursing*, 8(3): 137–45.

Neale, B. and Clark, D. (1992) Informal palliative care. *Journal of Cancer Care*, 3: 85–9.

Nolan, M., Keady, J. and Grant, G. (1995) Developing a typology of family care: implications for nurses and other service providers. *Journal of Advanced Nursing*, 21: 256–65.

Nolan, M., Grant, G. and Keady, J. (1996a) *Understanding Family Care: A Multidimensional Model of Caring and Coping*. Buckingham: Open University Press.

Nolan, M., Grant, G. and Keady, J. (1996b) The Carers Act: realising the potential. *British Journal of Community Health Nursing*, 1(6): 317–22.

Payne, S., Smith, P. and Dean, S. (1999) Identifying the concerns of family carers in palliative care. *Palliative Medicine*, 13(1): 37–44.

Pickett, M., Barg, F.K. and Lynch, M.P. (2001) Development of a home-based family caregiver cancer education program. *Hospice Journal*, 15(4): 19–40.

Robinson, K.D., Angeletti, K.A., Barg, F.K. *et al.* (1998) The development of a family caregiver cancer education program. *Journal of Cancer Education*, 13(2): 116–21.

Rose, K.E. (1999) A qualitative analysis of the information needs of informal carers of terminally ill cancer patients. *Journal of Clinical Nursing*, 8(1): 81–8.

Scott, G. (2001) A study of family carers of people with a life-threatening illness. 2: Implications of the needs assessment. *International Journal of Palliative Nursing*, 7(7): 323–30.

Seale, C. (1989) What happens in hospices: a review of research evidence. *Social Science and Medicine*, 28(6): 551–9.

Smith, P.C. (2000) Family caregivers in palliative care: perception of their role and sources of support. Unpublished PhD thesis, University of Southampton.

Smith, P.C. (2001) Who is a carer? Experiences of family caregivers in palliative care, in S. Payne and C. Ellis-Hill (eds) *Chronic and Terminal Illness*. Oxford: Oxford University Press.

Thomas, C., Morris, S.M. and Harman, J.C. (2002) Companions through cancer: the care given by informal carers in cancer contexts. *Social Science and Medicine*, 54(4): 529–44.

Twigg, J. and Atkin, K. (1994) *Carers Perceived: Policy and Practice in Informal Care*. Buckingham: Open University Press.

Twigg, J., Atkin, K. and Perring, C. (1990) *Carers and Services: A Review of Research*. London: Social Policy Research Unit.

Weitzner, M.A. and McMillan, S.C. (1999) The Caregiver Quality of Life Index-Cancer (CQOLC) Scale: revalidation in a home hospice setting. *Journal of Palliative Care*, 15(2): 13–20.

Wyatt, G.K., Friedman, L., Given, C.W. and Given, B.A. (1999) A profile of bereaved caregivers following provision of terminal care. *Journal of Palliative Care*, 15(1): 13–25.

Yin, R.B. (1994) *Case Study Research: Design and Methods*, 2nd edn. London: Sage.

16

Supporting families of terminally ill persons

Elizabeth Hanson

This chapter provides an empirical overview of the support needs of families of terminally ill persons and the types of interventions that can be employed by nurses to offer support, based on Nolan and co-workers' (1996) temporal model of family caring. The focus, wherever possible, is on the support needs of families caring for seriously ill older people at home. A Swedish information and communication technology (ICT) project will be drawn upon to illustrate the benefits and limitations of using technology to support families. The chapter concludes with a summary of nurses' support work with families of terminally ill persons.

Overall support needs for families caring for terminal ill people

Within the empirical literature on family care-giving of terminally ill persons, it is clear that the focus remains to a large extent on cancer patients approaching the end of life. Andershed's (1999) literature review of the role of the family carer at the end of life highlighted that the majority of the 229 chosen articles published in peer-reviewed academic journals from the early 1980s through to 1998 were largely concerned with cancer patients. However, from this review and her own empirical studies (Andershed 1999; Andershed and Ternestedt 2001), three key themes of knowing, being and doing were identified in relation to the principal support needs of families of terminally ill persons. I have used Andershed's themes as a framework to explore the empirical literature from 1999 through to 2002 regarding the support needs of families caring for terminally ill relatives. More specifically, I have prioritized literature addressing the support needs of family carers of older people at the end of life wherever possible. An overview of the literature review findings is presented in Table 16.1.

Table 16.1 Support needs for families caring for terminally ill persons based on Andershed's (1999) core themes of knowing, being and doing

Knowing		Being		Doing	
Aimed at	Individualized information, advice and support regarding	Aimed at	Individualized information, advice and support regarding	Aimed at	Individualized information, advice and support regarding
Planning for the remaining length of time	• the relative's disease, diagnosis, accompanying symptoms, treatment, care, prognosis, survival estimates and ongoing health status	Being with one's relative	• spending time together • 'sharing the illness and struggle together' • taking time off work and accompanying one's relative on hospital visits • making the best of the time one has together • trying to achieve a sense of normality	Practical caring acts or 'care work'	• dealing with personal care • dealing with regular household chores • securing appropriate practical support services, such as good transport, assistance with filling in forms and help with daily caring activities and housework • taking on new roles, including intimate aspects of care and learning new skills • getting extra help round the clock as necessary during the final phase • asking for informal support: practical, emotional as well as social from family, friends and/or voluntary organizations
To prepare for the impending death	• what the death will be like • discussion of personal fears to reduce anxiety about the future	'Emotional work'	• managing the emotions of their relative as well as their own • talking openly about the impending death as well as their fears for the future and being left alone • balancing emotions • experiencing and gathering memories • sensing changes in their own identity		
Being fully aware of the nature of the caring role	• knowing what to expect and what to do in particular situations				
Maintaining an income for the carer	• financial benefits available	Time for himself or herself	• securing rest, relaxation and sleep • to have time for oneself as well as spending time with others • regular respite services to enable carer to get a regular break from caring		
Knowing what services are available and the help to secure them	• the range of specialist services available • the role and responsibilities of different professionals involved				

Knowing

Knowing is a central theme within the empirical palliative care-giving literature and centres upon family members as well as terminally ill persons themselves being informed about a range of issues. Given that this chapter is
concerned with supporting families, relatives' needs form the focus of the
discussion and it is assumed that the terminally ill person himself or herself
is also in a state of 'knowing'.

First, Andershed and Ternestedt (2001) point out that it is extremely
important for carers to know about the relative's disease, diagnosis, prognosis, accompanying symptoms, treatment and care as well as ongoing
health status. Lamont and Christakis (2001) highlight the complexity surrounding issues of prognostication, including the difficulties surrounding
communication of survival estimates, as well as the need for physicians to
improve their skills regarding prognostication. However, it is increasingly
acknowledged that it is important for family members who directly request
it to be given honest information so that they are able to plan for the remaining length of time with their relative (Steinhouser *et al.* 2000a,b). An
accompanying theme is allowing families to have an opportunity to prepare
for the impending death. In particular, to be able to know what the death will
be like, to make preparations for death and to discuss personal fears to
reduce anxiety about the future (Payne *et al.* 1999).

The palliative care-giving literature emphasizes the importance of family members being fully aware of the nature of the caring role, such as what
to expect and knowing what to do in particular circumstances (Rose 1999;
Scott *et al.* 2001). Sheldon (1997) argues that it is crucial for carers to be
informed of the financial benefits available to them due to the challenges of
maintaining an income for the carer as well as the extra costs incurred when
caring for a seriously ill person at home. Knowing what services are available
and the help to secure them is also important for family carers. Jarrett *et al.*
(1999) highlighted that families are often unaware of the range of specialist
services available. Similarly, there is often confusion regarding the role and
responsibilities of the different professionals involved (Wiles *et al.* 1999).

Andershed (1999) argued that if family carers of terminally ill persons
are informed about relevant issues that are of concern to them, then they are
more likely to be enabled 'to be' and 'to do'.

Being

'Being' is another central theme within the palliative care-giving literature
and can be summarized as togetherness and partnership (Duke 1998; Kellett
and Mannion 1999; Wennman-Larsen and Tishelman 2002). This principally means being with one's relative, to spend time together and to be close
to one another. As Kellett and Mannion (1999) explain, it involves 'sharing
the illness and struggle together'. It also includes the ability, for example,
to take time off work and to accompany one's relative for hospital visits
(Andershed 1999).

At first glance, it would appear to be a rather idealistic and optimistic concept. However, 'being' is also described within the literature as trying to make the best of the time one has together and attempting to achieve a sense of ordinariness and normality (Rose *et al.* 1997). Efraimsson *et al.* (2001) explained how remaining at home was viewed by all family carers in their interview study as a prerequisite for preserving a sense of normality.

Several empirical studies have also acknowledged the stressful nature of the 'emotional work' that carers have to manage – that is, managing the emotions of their relative as well as their own feelings, such as guilt, anger, sadness and uncertainty (Kellett and Manion 1999; Scott *et al.* 2001; Soothill *et al.* 2001; Thomas *et al.* 2002; Wennman-Larsen and Tishelman 2002).

A central element of 'being' is the ability for the family and relative to be able to talk openly about their feelings together. However, it is readily acknowledged that, for many families, it is often difficult to share feelings about their relative's impending death as well as feelings related to being left alone and associated fears for the future (Rose *et al.* 1997; Thomas *et al.* 2002). Wennman-Larsen and Tishelman (2002) referred to bereavement studies in which a number of family carers reported their regrets for not being able to express their feelings openly with their dying partner.

Duke (1998) also notes how some family carers in her interview study reported feelings of being in suspense, of holding their feelings in a precarious emotional balance, such as enjoying time with one's loved one but knowing it would not last and would change. Carers also referred to experiencing and gathering memories, such as treasuring events as they happened, knowing that this might be their last experience of such an event.

Soothill *et al.* (2001) revealed complex issues surrounding carers sensing changes in their identity and appearance. This leads to the final element within the concept of being, which is the ability of the carer to be able to have time for himself or herself as well as to be able to spend time with others so as to reduce their feelings of isolation. A central theme within the palliative care-giving literature is the importance of a range of ongoing respite services to promote the well-being of carers and reduce their burden. Respite services enable carers to get a regular break from caring and gives them an opportunity to participate in activities and interests (Herlitz and Dahlberg 1999; Wiles *et al.* 1999; Cameron *et al.* 2002). Scott's (2001) study of palliative family care-givers highlighted their feelings of fatigue and, in some cases, exhaustion as a result of caring for a dying relative at home in the last months of life. She referred to Maslow's hierarchy of needs to argue the importance of securing basic requirements for rest, relaxation and sleep before then being able to deal with one's emotions such as anxiety, fear and uncertainty and one's higher-order needs of self-esteem and self-actualization.

Doing

Doing is the final theme within the empirical literature and refers to practical caring acts or 'care work'. This involves a range of tasks and activities from personal care, dealing with symptoms and assistance with medications, through to regular household chores of shopping, cleaning, cooking, gardening and home maintenance. The UK literature in particular highlights the practical needs of palliative family carers and the problems with securing appropriate practical support services, such as the prompt installation of aids and adaptations at the point of need to make care-giving feasible at home (Sheldon 1997; Jarrett *et al.* 1999), access to good transport (Thomas *et al.* 2002) and assistance with filling in forms (Soothill *et al.* 2001). In a study of 30 palliative family care-givers, Grande *et al.* (1997) found that just under half admitted that more help should be provided with daily caring activities and housework.

Wennman-Larsen and Tishelman's (2002) Swedish study revealed that 'doing' for female spousal palliative family care-givers often also meant taking on new roles and learning new skills, such as financial management skills and simple household repair and maintenance skills. In relation to taking on new roles, Rhodes and Shaw's (1999) interview study of bereaved palliative family care-givers emphasized the additional problems experienced by male carers when carrying out intimate care for their dying relative, as it encroached on the boundaries of their previous relationship.

It is also recognized within the empirical literature that practical tasks and activities are often significantly onerous within the last weeks of life and extra help is often required, such as at night and over the weekend (Axelsson and Sjöden 1998; Beaver *et al.* 1999). Problems are also highlighted with regard to securing extra help from family and friends, as family carers are often reluctant to ask for extra help, preferring instead to be as independent and self-reliant as possible (Payne *et al.* 1999) Difficulties regarding reciprocity were mentioned by family carers in the study of Steele and Fitch (1996). Thus, informal support is more likely to be of a social nature rather than in the form of practical or emotional support (Cohen *et al.* 1994). Yet, bereaved palliative family care-givers in Wennman-Larsen and Tishelman's (2002) study admitted, in retrospect, that they wished they had asked for more help with routine tasks from family and friends.

It would appear that family carers are also reluctant to seek support from professional carers, viewing them as primarily being concerned with the patient and thus lacking the resources, including the time, to help them (Grande *et al.* 1997; Soothill *et al.* 2001). Where formal support is available, drawbacks are reported by carers in terms of the numbers of health professionals involved and a lack of continuity of care (Jarrett *et al.* 1999). Several palliative family carers in the study of Efraimsson *et al.* (2001) described how this made them feel that their home was no longer their own and became, instead, 'a public room'.

Andershed's (1999) themes provide a useful framework to explore the empirical evidence regarding the overall support needs of families caring for a dying relative at home. However, given the continued predominance of cancer care-givers within the palliative care-giving literature to date, I now turn to highlight the specific support needs of families caring for a seriously ill older relative with advanced chronic illness.

Specific support needs of families caring for seriously ill older people

Seale (1999) concluded from his retrospective survey of bereaved relatives, friends and neighbours of older people in the last year of life, that there needs to be a much broader perspective on death and dying that emphasizes the needs of older people. Seymour and Hanson (2001) noted the emerging body of empirical literature highlighting the inverse care needs of seriously ill older people and their families. With regard to family care-giving of older people at the end of life, additional challenges are noted to those identified in the cancer care-giving literature. Seale (1999) and Mezey *et al.* (1999) note the complexities surrounding prognosis and accompanying preparation for death. This is due to the likelihood of multiple existing diseases and the associated range of long-term symptoms, as well as the nature of the dying process for older people living with advanced chronic illness, which is, typically, a gradual decline and a lengthy trajectory. This often leads to an additional burden for older family carers who may also have chronic health problems themselves. As an older spousal carer participant explained to Meyers and Gray (2001), 'I knew I could do anything for a few months, but this has gone on forever. I don't know how long I can go on like this.'

In addition to physical strain, there are often additional emotional demands surrounding the delivery of long-term highly personal care to a loved spouse or parent who is often unable to recognize anyone, or no longer resembles the person they once were and is often unable to provide reciprocity. Mezey *et al.* (1999) conclude that there is a need for educational models to support families and professional carers in providing end-of-life care for older people. Mike Nolan (personal communication) has argued that while the knowing, being and doing needs of families are all important considerations, most research and practice to date has focused on the 'doing' and, to a lesser extent, 'knowing', to the neglect of 'being', which is likely to require a change of orientation for staff.

I now turn to consider the types of interventions that can be used by nurses to offer support, with particular consideration to the support needs of families caring for seriously ill older people at home.

Working in partnership with families: nursing interventions in relation to the temporal model of family care-giving

Nolan and co-workers' (1996) temporal model of family caring has had a considerable influence on researchers, policy makers and practitioners in the field of gerontology with regard to providing an appropriate framework to understand the dynamics of family care-giving and to work in partnership with families. More specifically, the temporal model of family care-giving acts as a useful educational model for nurses to help them in their support work with families caring for a terminally ill relative at home (see Table 16.2).

Table 16.2 Nursing interventions in relation to the temporal model of family caring (Nolan *et al.* 1996)

Phases	Concerned with	Nursing interventions
Building on the past	Recognition of the nature of the caring relationship with the relative and its influence on the current and future situation	• being aware that a carer's past relationship with their relative influences their decision to take on board the role of carer, and shapes the nature of their caring situation
Recognizing the need	Being aware of the changing relationship with their relative	• enabling the family member to recognize their changing relationship with their relative as a result of his or her illness or confirming the suspicions as appropriate of family members that suspect their relative is ill
Taking it on	The family carer making a decision if he or she should take on board the role as carer	• providing informed anticipatory care about the nature of family caring and the services available
Working through it	Learning to carry out a range of care-giving tasks and managing the emotional aspects of caring	• providing individualized information, advice and support • facilitating skill development in novice carers • recognizing experienced family carers as the experts regarding their caring situation • encouraging family carers to use a broad range of coping strategies to enhance their coping abilities, including exploring with family carers the satisfying aspects of caring • ensuring carers have access to regular respite services • being aware of, and advising carers of, the role of informal sources of support and the range of informal respite services • referring carers to pastoral support as appropriate
Reaching the end and a 'new beginning'	The carer reaching the end of instrumental care-giving and the transition into widowhood, the bereavement period and entering a new life situation	• proactively working with families to reduce the potential for future regret • giving permission as appropriate regarding entry to nursing home • enabling carers to negotiate roles with care staff at home, nursing home or hospital • working together with carers to ensure a 'good' death • facilitating carers to re-negotiate roles with family and friends • assessing carer's bereavement needs and referring them as appropriate to sources of support

A core element of the temporal model of family caring is working in partnership with families to provide optimal support by recognizing the different needs for support at different stages of, or transitions within, the caring trajectory. It can be seen that the core needs of knowing, being and doing outlined above within the palliative care-giving literature are clearly interwoven within many of the phases of the caring process.

Building on the past

Nolan *et al.* (1996) describe how the caring process begins by 'building on the past', which is a stage before caring in its formal sense and includes recognition of the nature of the caring relationship with the relative and its influence on the current and future situation.

Recognizing the need

The second stage, 'recognizing the need', involves the family member being aware of their changing relationship with their relative. This is particularly pertinent to family members when a relative has a chronic illness with a gradual onset such as dementia. At this stage, family members may consult with professionals to confirm their suspicions regarding the changed behaviour of their relative.

Taking it on

'Taking it on' is the next phase and is often a brief phase involving decision making about the formal caring role – namely, 'Can I do it?' and 'Should I take it on board?' A crucial element within the model of Nolan *et al.* is the recognition that support work is as much about helping family members to decide if caring is for them as it is about helping them to continue caring. They acknowledge that in many circumstances, such as the rapid onset of stroke, families have very little time to make informed decisions about taking on the role of family carer. As Ward-Griffin (2001) highlighted in her study of family care-givers of older people, the lack of options led many spousal carers to believe that they had no choice but to provide the bulk of the care. For many spousal carers, filial obligation is also an important factor, as an older family carer expressed to Wennman-Larsen and Tishelman (2002): 'This is his home, of course he should be here.'

In contrast, Nolan and colleagues argue it is important to work proactively with families. For nurses, this means carrying out what Nolan *et al.* (1996) call 'informed anticipatory care', which means providing carers with the necessary information and advice to make informed choices about their situation. This reflects the knowing need outlined earlier within the palliative care literature.

Working through it

'Working through it' is concerned with the day-to-day aspects of the caring role and involves 'hands-on care' as well as emotional aspects of care. Nolan *et al*. (1996) note the importance of appropriate information, education and advice to enable novice family carers to be optimally involved in daily care-giving. The palliative care-giving literature highlights the problems experienced by family carers when their relative is first discharged home and their subsequently having to learn by 'trial and error' to carry out a range of care-giving tasks (such as the 'doing' tasks). This is often recognized as being an onerous and time-consuming process (Rose 1998; Efraimsson *et al*. 2001; Wennman-Larsen and Tishelman 2002). In keeping with the temporal model of family caring, the palliative care-giving literature emphasizes the need to ensure that information-giving by nurses is individualized and that checks are frequently made about the assimilation of information over time (Rose 1999; Carter 2001; Cameron *et al*. 2002).

Nolan *et al*. (1996) explain that as family carers 'work through it', over a period of time they often become experts in their care-giving activities. Mezey *et al*. (1999) refer to the special knowledge about their older relative which makes family carers experts in care. Nolan *et al*. argue that such an approach requires nurses to work in partnership with families by acting as facilitators and enablers as opposed to 'doers or providers'. They also explain that this involves nurses sharing their knowledge and learning from family carers. In this way, nurses can increase carers' competence and enable them to move quickly from novice to expert and help to sustain them in the expert role over the course of the caring process.

However, as acknowledged earlier within the 'being' needs of palliative family care-givers, Nolan *et al*. (1996) also recognize that 'working through it' involves dealing with the emotional aspects of caring. They argue that nurses can enable family carers to cope more effectively by exploring with them the satisfying aspects of care, so that these can be enhanced. For example, in their longitudinal study, Nijboer *et al*. (1999) found that a number of family carers gained an increased sense of self-esteem from being able to care for their partner to the best of their ability at home.

Nolan *et al*. (1996) also explain the importance of encouraging family carers to use a broad range of coping strategies to help them manage. Within the palliative family care-giving literature, recommended strategies include: taking each day as it comes; maintaining hope; managing time effectively, such as developing a routine and having a window of time for oneself; normalizing; using humour; finding meaning and a sense of control in care-giving activities; and engaging in relaxation activities (Steele and Fitch 1996; Rose *et al*. 1997; Rose 1998; Kellett and Mannion 1999; Scott *et al*. 2001; Wennman-Larsen and Tishelman 2002). Cohen (1994), Steele and Fitch (1996) and Seale (1999) also highlight in their respective studies of palliative family care-givers the importance of faith in a higher power for many carers.

As highlighted earlier within the 'being' needs of family carers, Nolan *et al.* (1996) emphasize the importance of nurses helping family carers to manage their situation by ensuring that they have access to respite services that match their particular problems and are flexible to changes over time. This includes nurses recognizing the invaluable role of informal sources of support from other family carers. Scott (2001) highlights that talking and meeting other carers helps new carers to realize that they are not alone. Informal respite services can take the form of carer support groups, study circles, voluntary telephone help-lines, home visiting and sitting services (Almberg 2002).

Reaching the end and a new beginning

The final phase within the temporal model of family caring is 'reaching the end' and a 'new beginning' and relates to the phase when the carer reaches the end of instrumental care-giving. Nolan *et al.* (1996) highlight the difficulties involved for family carers when an older relative is admitted to a nursing home, describing the 'legacy of guilt' that often ensues as a result of a lack of support by care staff to enable them to create 'a new beginning'. Nolan and Dellasega (1999) note that nurses need to engage proactively with families to reduce the potential for future regret so that a 'new beginning' is made possible. This can be accommodated by nurses creating opportunities for family carers to engage with them in an open and honest appraisal of their individual caring situation. It may also involve the professional carer supporting the family carer by directly 'giving permission' to the family carer for their relative to enter a nursing home (Winslow 1998). Once a decision has been reached about institutional placement, creating a new beginning can also be achieved by carers negotiating roles with care staff in the home (Sandberg *et al.* 2002).

I would argue that this final phase within palliative family care-giving refers to the last weeks of life of the relative, the death of the relative and the subsequent preparation of the body and funeral arrangements, after which the family carer reaches the end of instrumental caring. However, this final phase is recognized as the most challenging within the palliative care-giving literature. This is because the family carer requires active and sustained support to manage the burden of caring for a dying relative at home as well as the emotions surrounding the impending death of their loved one (Duke 1988). It is important that the nurse works together with the family to ensure as good a death as possible. Rhodes and Shaw (1999) highlight that lack of good pain and symptom control often necessitate hospital admission within the last weeks of life. Similarly, they acknowledge that dying at home may be rather idealized and some family carers fear the prospect of witnessing a death at home and living in a house in which a relative has died.

I would also argue that a 'new beginning' for palliative family carers includes the transition to widowhood and the bereavement period, in which the family member adjusts to being alone and enters a new life situation, which includes renegotiating roles with family and friends (Duke 1998; Wennman-Larsen and Tishelman 2002). Nurses can play a valuable role in assessing family carers' bereavement needs and referring them to appropriate sources of support (Sheldon 1997).

Thus, it can be seen that Nolan and co-workers' (1996) temporal model of family care-giving acts as a useful conceptual framework for nurses to use in their support work with palliative family care-givers – namely, by working in partnership with families to meet their core needs of knowing, being and doing over time. In this way, nurses are able to empower families by enabling them to be better informed in relation to their caring situation.

I now turn to explore how the temporal model of family caring can be used as a basis for considering innovative ways of delivering support. In particular, I consider the use of information and communication technology (ICT) and provide an example of an innovative support intervention in Sweden.

Example of an innovative information and communication technology support intervention in Sweden

In her study of hospice family care-givers, Scott (2001) acknowledges that ICT will increasingly have a role to play in the future in terms of opening up avenues of advice, support and companionship for family carers. She refers directly to the ACTION Project (Assisting Carers using Telematic Interventions to meet Older Persons' Needs) as an innovative example of providing information, advice, skill development and support via the medium of ICT.

I provide an overview of the ACTION concept and give examples of how it is supportive by referring to data from the initial testing of an interactive multimedia programme on end-of-life care that has been developed in Sweden.

The ACTION concept

The ACTION concept arose out of the EU-funded ACTION Project, which made use of ICT to provide older people and their family carers with education, information and support in relation to their caring situation. A key feature of the ACTION services is that they were developed in close collaboration with older people and their family carers and were subsequently tested by a number of families in their own homes across the partner countries of Sweden, England, Northern Ireland, the Republic of Ireland and Portugal (Magnusson *et al.* 2002).

The conceptual framework of ACTION is based on Nolan and co-workers' (1996) temporal model of family care-giving, as it was acknowledged that it is important to work in partnership with family carers by providing education, information and support as necessary to help them initially to decide whether to take on board the role of family carer and, if so, to support them through the entire caring trajectory. A central theme is the recognition that an experienced family carer is the expert regarding their relative's care.

The ICT initially consisted of the family's television set, a personal computer and a remote control through which they could access a range of multimedia caring programmes on the TV screen. Each partner country set up a local family carers' user group, which met regularly to help develop the scope and content of the programmes. Family carers requested that the programmes should be focused on practical as well as emotional aspects of caring, such as moving and handling, incontinence, emergency situations, respite care, planning ahead, coping, and claims and benefits.

The ACTION concept also used a video-phone by which families could get in touch with other participating families as well as care professionals at the research sites. In Sweden, families were given the option to use the computer to access the caring programmes as well as the Internet and e-mail facilities; nearly all families chose to do so. Many families had no experience of using a computer and thus group educational sessions were provided as well as the possibility to have individual training at home.

An End-of-Life Caring programme was developed in the Swedish ACTION Project (consisting of further research and development work in Sweden funded by the Ministry of Health and Social Affairs, 2000– 2002) in response to requests from several Swedish family carers who had direct experience of their spouse dying during the term of the project. They considered that the existing programmes were too broad and were unable to focus specifically on care for a seriously ill older person at home.

The request of the Swedish ACTION family carers was a timely one, as it clearly resonated with recent Swedish policy initiatives that acknowledged the work that needed to be done concerning the palliative care needs of Swedish citizens and, in particular, recognition of the vital role of family carers (Andershed 1999; Sundström *et al.* 2002). I now provide a snapshot of the Swedish policy context so that the reader can gain an awareness of the contextual backdrop to the palliative programme development work in Sweden.

The Swedish policy context of palliative care and the role of family carers

As in the UK, health and social care services in Sweden are delivered separately. Health care is delivered at a regional level and district nurses operate at this level providing home health care. Social care is delivered by the municipalities, mainly by assistant nurses who provide personal care and home help to older citizens. Specific palliative care services centre on hospital-based home care teams, which were pioneered by Beck-Friis in the 1970s.

The teams consist largely of physicians and nurses delivering 24-hour care, mainly to cancer patients, who are linked to a hospital unit (Fürst *et al.* 1999).

Again like in the UK, the current trend is towards reduced hospital care and increased home care services for frail older people. Andersson *et al.* (1999) highlighted that end-of-life care dominates advanced home health care services. Nearly three-quarters of patients receiving home care services were over 65 years of age and just over half were women. However, most seriously ill older people, as in the UK, are cared for in nursing homes run by municipalities. In contrast to the UK, however, there are far fewer hospices and fewer palliative care physicians (Fürst *et al.* 1999). Yet Sandman (2001), in his concept analysis work of palliative care in Sweden, noted the extension of the concept of palliative care beyond the end-stage of an illness and to incorporate illnesses other than cancer. This shift in focus has also been mirrored in recent government policy.[1]

Traditionally in Sweden, unlike in the UK, there has been much less reliance on voluntary support services for seriously ill people and their families. More recently, however, there has been a national initiative, 'Family Carer 300',[2] to support family carers and to encourage active partnerships between statutory and voluntary services, as in the UK. This initiative reflects a growing trend of informal care for older people in Sweden, largely delivered by spouses and adult children (Wimo *et al.* 2002; Johansson *et al.* 2003).

The ACTION End-of-Life Caring programme

Against this backdrop, the ACTION End-of-Life Caring programme was primarily designed to provide user-friendly education, information and support to family carers of terminally ill older persons living at home. An outline of the programme was based on an analysis of interview data with several family carers who had experienced the death of their relative during the period of the ACTION Project, as well as key findings from a review of relevant empirical literature in the field of palliative family care-giving.

The interview data revealed that needs centred on both practical as well as emotional aspects of family care-giving, in keeping with Andershed's (1999) core themes. Practical aspects centred on the need for information about medicines, aids and adaptations for safe movement at home, pressure sore prevention in bed, advice about food and the range of support services available. Emotional aspects focused on the nature and role of the family carer, as well as information and support about the advancement of the cared for person's illness and the risk of unexpected death and support after death. The initial structure of the programme is shown in Table 16.3.

This initial working prototype of the programme was reviewed by eight family carers who had direct experience of caring for a seriously ill relative in the last year of life at home (see Box 16.1). Two carers were participants in

Table 16.3 End-of-Life Care Programme: initial version

Chapters/headings	Parts/subheading
1 Read this first (an introduction)	• About death and dying • A good death • Palliative care
2 Living with dying	• Loss • Emotions and experiences • Suffering • Physical problems
3 Being a family carer	• When death is near • When death has occurred • The funeral • Mourning • Re-investing in life

4 Personal care	• Hygiene
	  ○ personal hygiene
	  ○ clothes and laundry
	• Food and drink
	  ○ difficulties with eating and drinking
	  ○ food and drink with different consistencies
	  ○ help with food and medicine
	• Moving and handling
	  ○ transfer in bed
	  ○ transfer out of bed
	  ○ prevention of pressure sores

5 Support services	• Support in and outside the home • Claims and benefits
6 Poems and relaxation exercises	
7 Links to other parts of the general ACTION service	

the Swedish ACTION Project and the remaining family carers were recruited with the help of a local pastoral care worker. Local ethical approval was secured before carrying out the research and development work with the programme. Two research nurses, who were experienced in care for older people, carried out the reviews. They provided support as appropriate during and after the reviews. Box 16.1 provides a brief description of the family carer participants and a selection of their comments about the ways in which the programme was supportive.

Key benefits and limitations

Contrary to the stereotypes surrounding older people and the use of new technology, this first phase of testing with family carers revealed the potential benefits of ICT to provide information, education and support to families caring for seriously ill relatives at home. Family carer participants with no previous experience of using a computer, after some initial training (of approximately 20 minutes duration), were able to effectively manage the multimedia programme.

Several family carer participants considered that the End-of-Life Caring programme would have helped to make their everyday role as a family carer for a terminally ill relative much easier. This was related to the inclusion of practical care-giving information and advice that centred upon 'doing', such as tips in the programme about food and drink when a family member is seriously ill and does not feel like eating. Elements of 'knowing' found to be important in the programme by participants included information on the range of services available, such as home help services, technical aids to help family carers in their daily caring activities and also financial aspects, such as the benefits available to family members taking care of a dying relative at home.

However, in addition to practical aspects of caring, 'being' needs were frequently raised by participants in relation to their individual caring situation as they reviewed the programme. In many cases, particular parts of the programme triggered participants to recall their own caring situations, including the range of emotions they experienced. For example, guilt was expressed by a carer regarding the death of her spouse in a nursing home, by a spouse when he spent time away from his wife to engage in a leisure activity and by a daughter who felt she could have done more to help her mother prior to her death. This resonates with the 'legacy of guilt', identified by Nolan *et al.* (1996), that is frequently experienced by carers in the final stages of caring.

One male participant acknowledged that the desire for a terminally ill relative to die at home is not so clear-cut, as noted by Rhodes and Shaw (1999), and described the fear surrounding death at home as opposed to feelings of security attached to the hospice. Another participant openly acknowledged his feelings of grief following the death of his wife, as well as feelings of loss regarding his role as carer, as highlighted by Duke (1998). And in line with the findings of Rose *et al.* (1997) and Thomas *et al.* (2002), both these male carers admitted experiencing difficulty in engaging in an open and honest conversation about death with their dying spouses.

Thus, it can be argued that the End-of-Life Caring programme has the potential to help carers by enabling them to recognize that emotions such as guilt are normal and understandable reactions when caring for a seriously ill relative. Also, other experiences, such as difficulty talking about death and dying, are commonly encountered by other family carers as they take care of their dying relative at home. In this way, as recommended by Soothill *et al.* (2001), Thomas *et al.* (2002) and Sheldon (1997), the carer is informed that

Box 16.1 Family carer participants: End-of-Life Caring programme review and their summary comments

Comments regarding the programme	*Family carer participants*
Overall comments: I'd have found this programme very useful if I'd had it while I was a family carer. I think to be honest that I'd have been able to care for my husband longer at home. It's important to think of timing – of when the programme can be most useful for families (Anna).	**Inga, ACTION family carer, 68 years,** cared for her husband, Barbro, at home for 3 years. They had ACTION immediately before her husband's discharge home from hospital following his stroke. Barbro later became seriously ill and was admitted to hospital for heart surgery. Barbro entered a nursing home and he died several weeks later
I'd have found it very useful at the beginning when my wife became very ill – I'd have got advice and tips about my situation and the different kinds of help available (Hans).	
Food and drink: The practical things like the tips about food and drink are very useful because my sister worried about being able to manage things without being sick (Helena).	**Anna, ACTION family carer, 75 years,** cared for her husband at home for 15 years. He had a severe stroke. They had ACTION a year before her husband's death. Anna cared for her husband at home until 5 days before his death when he was transferred to the local hospital due to heart failure
Depression: The information about depression is very good as my sister was very down when she knew she was going to die (Helena).	
Support services: My husband needed a lot of help with things at home and I didn't know that I could have family care support while I cared for my husband – I didn't have any home help or technical aids either – it's good to see about those things in the programme (Gun).	**Helena, sibling family carer, 77 years,** cared for her sister who was 80 years old and had metastatic sarcoma of her left leg. Helena helped her sister everyday. She stayed at home until the last 3 weeks before her death, when she decided to enter the nursing home because of severe pain and dyspnoea
I cared for my wife round the clock and I didn't want help from anyone – she was able to put up with me and support me for all those years so it goes without saying that I'd be there for her (Emil).	
I had home care services in the last 3 weeks before my wife's death – had I known that it would work so well, I'd have gladly accepted that help sooner (Hans).	**Katrina, family carer and professional carer, 57 years,** helped care for her mother at home up until the last month of her life when she was transferred to the local hospice. Her mother had metastatic breast cancer. Katrina was a paediatric nurse and she explained that she had not got over the death of her father when her mother became very ill
Technical aids: I didn't know about all these – I went out and bought incontinence pads myself (Gustav).	
When he saw a vertically adjustable bed and a glide mat he commented, 'just think if I'd have had them!' (Hans).	

Gun, experienced family carer, 68 years, cared for her husband at home for 10 years. He had heart disease and diabetes. She had worked at a day nursery and a youth recreation centre before her husband's illness. She had also cared for her mother who had been ill for a longer period and died a year before her husband

Birgitta, spousal family carer and professional carer, 57 years, was a district nurse and cared for her husband who had been seriously ill for about a year with a brain tumour. He had been ill for a long time before this and they did not receive a diagnosis until after his death

Emil, spousal family carer, 86 years, cared for his wife for 10 years. She had Parkinson's disease and later developed dementia. They had travelled a lot together. He explained they had had a good life together even during the last 10 years

Hans, spousal family carer, 79 years, cared for his wife who had cancer and diabetes without any help until the last 3 weeks of her life when they received home care services. His wife was transferred in the last week of life to an oncology ward at the local hospital. He had worked as a travel agent and they had gone on many trips abroad together, which they had enjoyed

Claims and benefits: I only became aware of the benefits I was entitled to the week just before my wife died (Hans).

Emotions and experiences: I wonder if I could have done more to help my mum – it would have been good to have talked with the doctor after her death (Gun).

Our family and friends didn't understand my wife's illness so they stopped coming . . . we never talked about dying to one another (Emil).

I used to feel guilty leaving my wife at home sometimes to watch the local football match – I worried all the time I was away – now when I know how little time she had left I could have stayed at home instead (Hans).

I found it so difficult to talk with my wife about dying – she wanted to talk about it, but I couldn't manage it – it didn't feel natural for me to do that (Hans).

When death is near: I wonder if people really do want to die at home, it can be rather frightening and, some people, as in my mum's case, may feel more secure to die in a hospital or hospice (Katrina).

When death has occurred: After my husband's death, my family and I chose a special outfit we'd bought when he was well and we buried my husband in it – this was important for us (Birgitta).

After my wife's death, I felt awful, I felt my task in life was over – I didn't feel needed as much as before (Emil).

The funeral: Inga told her story of her husband's funeral and about his death in the nursing home. She explained, 'I killed him you know by him going there.'

their needs are valid in their own right. The programme also goes one step further by informing the family carer about the different kinds of support available to them and how to secure it.

A second version of the programme is currently underway that builds on the initial testing phase and it is intended that the whole ACTION service, of which the End-of-Life Caring programme is a part, will be tested by ten consenting families who are caring for a terminally ill older relative in their own home.

To summarize, the main benefit of ACTION is that it empowers families because it provides them with the choice to decide if, when and for how long to access the information, advice and support that is available to them via the computer, from the comfort of their own home. However, it is important to acknowledge that the use of new technology to support families of terminally ill persons is not without some limitations and it is to these that I now turn.

Information and communication technology support services, such as ACTION, are intended to complement existing statutory and voluntary services for older people and their families. They are not intended, nor are they able to replace, core services, such as home help and home health care. Thus, it can only help to inform families of the range of services that provide 'hands-on' care. It cannot provide practical care directly, which is an essential element of support at the end of life.

One family carer raised the issue of optimal timing of the introduction of the End-of-Life Caring programme to families. Results thus far highlight the importance of introducing ACTION as early as possible within the caring trajectory to optimize its supportive effects. Problems arise when it is introduced much later, such as towards the end of the 'working through it' phase, as it can be viewed as 'too little, too late'. In such cases, core services such as home help and district nursing services are often required to help relieve the burden of caring (Hanson and Clarke 2000).

Yet, could ACTION replace the nurse's advisory and educative role? It is argued that ACTION gives nurses the opportunity to work in partnership with families, as advocated by Nolan *et al.* (1996), by enabling them to provide individualized advice and support at the point of need. This could be carried out by a more traditional home visit or, where time is limited and travelling times are long, it can be carried out via the video-phone. Where appropriate, nurses can also direct families to specific ACTION programmes, or particular sections of a programme that will help families to be more informed about their specific caring situation and the types of services that are available to them.

A key issue relates to Nolan and co-workers' (1996) original premise that support services should, wherever possible, enable family members to make an informed choice as to whether to take on board the role of family carer. Does ACTION subtly coerce family carers to continue caring? How can family carers withdraw from the service once ACTION is in their own home? These questions relate more to the way in which the service is introduced to families and, I would argue that the problems can be minimized if the nurse openly discusses with individual families the support options available to them. Wherever possible, this should take place at the beginning of the 'taking it on' phase. Nurses working with ACTION at a local call centre for family carers in a municipality in Sjuhärad, West Sweden, acknowledge that ACTION is not suitable for all families and is not a 'panacea for all ills'; rather, it requires careful assessment on the part of the nurse together with the individual family concerned (Magnusson 2003).

One ethical consideration also concerns the difficulties faced by the local municipalities involved to withdraw the ACTION service from families such as after the death of their relative or when a relative enters a nursing home. Case study data from the Swedish ACTION Project have highlighted the benefits of ACTION for several family carers in the initial bereavement period, in terms of providing informal and formal support via the video-phone. Similarly, several family carers and their relatives have been able to maintain regular face-to-face contact with each other more easily using the video-phone which is linked from the local nursing home to the family carer's own home (Magnusson 2003).

Conclusions

- Nolan and co-workers' (1996) temporal model of family care-giving enables nurses to work in partnership with families of terminally ill persons to meet their core support needs of knowing, being and doing over the course of the caring trajectory.

- To actively work in partnership with families, nurses must be prepared to share their knowledge with family carers as well as being open to learn from family carers themselves.

- To help empower family carers, nurses need to acknowledge experienced family carers as experts on their individual caring situation.

- Nurses can help family carers to manage the emotional aspects of caring by enabling them to explore the satisfactions of caring.

- ICT services such as ACTION can be used to complement existing services to provide nurses with new ways of working with families, which will enhance their educative and support role.

Acknowledgements

The Swedish ACTION Project was funded by the Ministry of Health and Social affairs in cooperation with University College of Borås, School of Health Sciences, the West Sweden region, the municipalities of Borås and

Mark and ÄldreVäst Sjuhärad. I would like to express my thanks to all the participating families in the project as well as to the members of the project team that worked together to develop and test ACTION. Finally, I would like to thank Mike Nolan for his thoughtful comments on an earlier draft of the manuscript.

Notes

1   See Statens Offentliga Utredningar (SOU) (2001) *Döden angår oss alla, värdig vård vid livets slut* [*Death Concerns Us All: Dignified Care at the End of Life*], p. 6. Government White Paper, Final Report of the Commission for Care at the End of Life. Stockholm: SOU.
2   Family Carer 300 (2000–2002) was so-called because the Swedish Board of Health and Welfare provided fundings to a total of 300 million Swedish crowns, approximately €35 million, to a variety of care-giver research and development initiatives in all interested municipalities in Sweden.

References

Almberg, B. (2002) *Family Carer 300: Final Report*. Stockholm: Swedish Board of Health and Welfare.
Andersson, A., Beck-Friis, B., Britton, M. *et al.* (1999) *Advanced Home Health Care and Home Rehabilitation: Reviewing the Scientific Evidence on Costs and Effects.* Stockholm: Swedish Council of Technology Assessment in Health Care.
Andershed, B. (1999) *The Role of the Family Carer at the End of Life: An Evidence-Based Literature Review*. Stockholm: Swedish Board of Health and Welfare.
Andershed, B. and Ternestedt, B.M. (2001) Development of a theoretical framework describing relatives' involvement in palliative care. *Journal of Advanced Nursing*, 34(4): 554–62.
Axelsson, B. and Sjöden, P.O. (1998) Quality of life of cancer patients and their spouses in palliative home care. *Palliative Medicine*, 12: 29–39.
Beaver, K., Luker, K. and Woods, S. (1999) The views of terminally ill people and lay carers on primary care services. *International Journal of Palliative Nursing*, 5(6): 266–74.
Cameron, J., Franche, R.L., Cheung, A. and Stewart, D. (2002) Lifestyle interference and emotional distress in family caregivers of advanced cancer patients. *Cancer*, 94(2): 521–7.
Carter, P. (2001) A not-so-silent cry for help. *Journal of Holistic Nursing*, 19(3): 271–84.
Cohen, C., Teresi, J. and Blum, C. (1994) The role of caregivers' social networks in Alzheimer's disease. *Social Science and Medicine*, 38(11): 1483–90.
Duke, S. (1998) An exploration of anticipatory grief: the lived experience of people during their spouse's terminal illness and in bereavement. *Journal of Advanced Nursing*, 28(4): 829–39.
Efraimsson, E., Höglund, I. and Sandman, P.O. (2001) 'The everlasting trial of strength and patience': transitions in home care nursing as narrated by patients and family members. *Journal of Clinical Nursing*, 10: 813–19.

Fürst, C.J., Valverius, E. and Hjelmerus, L. (1999) Palliative care in Sweden. *European Journal of Palliative Care*, 6(5): 161–4.

Grande, G.E., Todd, C.J. and Barclay, S.I.G. (1997) Support needs in the last year of life: patient and carer dilemmas. *Palliative Medicine*, 11: 202–8.

Hanson, E.J. and Clarke, E. (2000) The role of telematics in assisting family carers and frail older people at home. *Health and Social Care in the Community*, 8(2): 232–41.

Herlitz, C. and Dahlberg, L. (1999) Causes of strain affecting relatives of Swedish oldest elderly. *Scandinavian Journal of Caring Sciences*, 13: 109–15.

Jarrett, N., Payne, S., Turner, P. and Hillier, R. (1999) 'Someone to talk to' and 'pain control': what people expect from a specialist palliative care team. *Palliative Medicine*, 13: 139–44.

Johansson, L., Sundström, G. and Hassing, L. (2003) State provision down, offspring's up: the reverse substitution of old-age care in Sweden. *Ageing and Society*, 22: 1–12.

Kellett, U. and Mannion, J. (1999) Meaning in caring: reconceptualizing the nurse–family carer relationship in community practice. *Journal of Advanced Nursing*, 29(3): 697–703.

Lamont, E. and Christakis, A. (2001) Prognostic disclosure to patients with cancer near the end of life. *Annals of Internal Medicine*, 134: 1096–105.

Magnusson, L. (2003) *The Swedish ACTION Project: Final Report*. Stockholm: Ministry of Health and Social Affairs.

Magnusson, L., Hanson, E., Brito, L. *et al.* (2002) Supporting family carers through the use of information technology – the EU project ACTION. *International Journal of Nursing Studies*, 39(4): 369–81.

Meyers, J. and Gray, L. (2001) The relationship between family primary caregiver characteristics and the satisfaction with hospice care, quality of life and burden. *Oncology Nursing Forum*, 28(1): 73–82.

Mezey, M., Miller, L. and Linton-Nelson, L. (1999) Caring for caregivers of frail elders at the end of life. *Generations*, 23(1): 44–51.

Nijboer, C., Triemsta, M., Tempelaar, R., Sanderman, R. and van den Bos, G. (1999) Determinants of caregiving experiences and mental health of partners of cancer. *Cancer*, 86(4): 577–88.

Nolan, M. and Dellasega, C. (1999) 'It's not the same as him being at home': creating caring partnerships following nursing home placement. *Journal of Clinical Nursing*, 8: 723–30.

Nolan, M., Grant, G. and Keady, J. (1996) *Understanding Family Care*. Buckingham: Open University Press.

Payne, S., Smith, P. and Dean, S. (1999) Identifying the concerns of informal carers in palliative care. *Palliative Medicine*, 13: 37–44.

Rhodes, P. and Shaw, S. (1999) Informal care and terminal illness. *Health and Social Care in the Community*, 7(1): 39–50.

Rose, K. (1998) Perceptions related to time in a qualitative study of informal carers of terminally ill cancer patients. *Journal of Clinical Nursing*, 7: 343–50.

Rose, K. (1999) A qualitative analysis of the information needs of informal carers of terminally ill cancer patients. *Journal of Clinical Nursing*, 8: 81–8.

Rose, K., Webb, C. and Waters, K. (1997) Coping strategies employed by informal carers of terminally ill cancer patients. *Journal of Cancer Nursing*, 1(3): 126–33.

Sandberg, J., Nolan, M.R. and Lundh, U. (2002) 'Entering a new world': emphatic awareness as the key to positive family/staff relationships in care homes. *International Journal of Nursing Studies*, 39(5): 507–15.

Sandman, L. (2001) Palliative care in Sweden, in H. ten Have and R. Janssens (eds) *Palliative Care in Europe: Concepts and Policies*. Amsterdam: IOS Press.

Scott, G. (2001) A study of family carers of people with a life-threatening illness. 2: Implications of the needs assessment. *International Journal of Palliative Nursing*, 7(7): 323–30.

Scott, G., Whyler, N. and Grant, G. (2001) A study of family carers of people with a life-threatening illness. 1: The carers' needs analysis. *International Journal of Palliative Nursing*, 7(6): 290–7.

Seale, C. (1999) Caring for people who die: the experiences of family and friends. *Ageing and Society*, 10: 412–28.

Seymour, J. and Hanson, E. (2001) Palliative care and older people, in M. Nolan, S. Davies and G. Grant (eds) *Working with Older People and their Families: Key Issues in Policy and Practice*. Buckingham: Open University Press.

Sheldon, F. (1997) *Psychosocial Palliative Care*. Cheltenham: STP.

Soothill, K., Morris, S., Harman, J. *et al.* (2001) Informal carers of cancer patients: what are their unmet psychosocial needs? *Health and Social Care in the Community*, 9(6): 464–75.

Steele, R. and Fitch, M. (1996) Coping strategies of family caregivers of home hospice patients with cancer. *Oncology Nursing Forum*, 23(6): 955–60.

Steinhouser, K., Clipp, E., McNeilly, M. *et al.* (2000a) In search of a good death: observations of patients, families and providers. *Annals of Internal Medicine*, 132: 825–32.

Steinhouser, K., Christakis, N., Clipp, E. *et al.* (2000b) Factors considered important at the end of life by patients, family, physicians and other care providers. *Journal of the American Medical Association*, 284(19): 2476–82.

Sundström, G., Johansson, L. and Hassing, L. (2002) The shifting balance of long term care in Sweden. *The Gerontologist*, 42(3): 350–5.

Thomas, C., Morris, S. and Harman, J. (2002) Companions through cancer: the care given by informal carers in cancer contexts. *Social Science and Medicine*, 54: 529–44.

Ward-Griffin, C. (2001) Negotiating care of frail elders: relationships between community nurses and family caregivers. *Canadian Journal of Nursing Research*, 33(2): 63–81.

Wennman-Larsen, A. and Tishelman, C. (2002) Advanced home care for cancer patients at the end of life: a qualitative study of hopes and expectations of family caregivers. *Scandinavian Journal of Caring Sciences*, 16: 240–7.

Wiles, R., Payne, S. and Jarrett, N. (1999) Improving palliative care services: a pragmatic model for evaluating services and assessing unmet need. *Palliative Medicine*, 13: 131–7.

Wimo, A., von Strauss, E., Nordberg, G., Sassi, F. and Johansson, L. (2002) Time spent on informal and formal care giving for persons with dementia in Sweden. *Health Policy*, 61: 255–68.

Winslow, B. (1998) Family caregiving and the use of formal community support services: a qualitative case study. *Issues in Mental Health Nursing*, 19: 11–27.

17

Social death
The impact of protracted dying

Gail Johnston

In this chapter, I examine the notion of social death, the factors which predispose someone to be defined as socially dead and the impact of such a definition for patients and families. In so doing, I examine the theoretical origins of the concept, its behavioural enforcement by health professionals and the psychological and social consequences of such behaviour. In particular, I draw attention to the way in which a diagnosis of cancer can impose a state of social deadness on sufferers.

Most people, including health professionals, define death in a 'clinical' or 'biological' sense – that is, when clinical signs or symptoms signify that the event has occurred in the case of the former, or that there is an absence of cellular activity in the case of the latter (Sweeting and Gilhooly 1991). However, when biological or clinical death is preceded by a period or phase in the illness when a person has lost their connection with the living world, we have begun to understand it in terms of 'social death'. This is the time when a person is treated essentially as a corpse, though they are still clinically and biologically alive (Sudnow 1967). Mulkay suggests that

> the defining feature of social death is the cessation of the individual person as an active agent in others' lives ... Social death is the final event in a sequence of declining social involvement that is set in motion either by participants' preparation for, or by their reaction to, the advent of biological death.
>
> (Mulkay 1993: 33, 34)

In a review of the literature of the concept, Sweeting and Gilhooly (1991, 1997) demonstrate that the state of social death has regressed from being one where the body is revered and honoured to one of social exclusion and excommunication. Early anthropological accounts of burial traditions documented that people became socially dead only after the body had naturally disintegrated. Until that time, the dead were treated as though they were still alive, requiring food, company and conjugal rights (Sweeting and

Gilhooly 1997). However, with the increasing institutionalization of groups which society feared or had no use for, it has now come to be understood as a state of abandonment or revulsion. Sweeting and Gilhooly (1991, 1997) propose that there are three groups of patients for whom the concept may be most readily applicable. These are the very old, those in the final stages of a lengthy physical terminal illness and those suffering from loss of their essential personhood (e.g. through dementia or coma). Each has entered a phase in their illness or life which irredeemably affects their ability to interact normally with others.

Social loss

The concept was first described in relation to health care through the observations of social scientists and thanatologists in the 1960s as they presented their accounts of the ways in which health professionals interacted with patients according to their perceived social value (Glaser and Strauss 1964a; Sudnow 1967). These authors observed that the quality of care given to patients was dependent on such factors as their age, clinical value, importance in society, ethnicity, education, occupation, family status, social class, personality and accomplishment. Glaser and Strauss (1964a) observed that as nursing staff learned more about patients, they gradually developed a 'loss story' for each patient, which added and subtracted these factors to provide a social loss value. At certain times, for example, when the wards were busy and care had to be prioritized, low social loss patients received minimal or basic care, while high social loss patients often received special care. Social loss stories derived their meaning from the anticipated future. For example, a young person training to be a doctor would have a higher social value than an elderly person dying with a chronic illness. As a result, for low social loss patients (e.g. those suffering from a chronic illness), nurses had often lost interest in their stories after a relatively short time.

In his participant observation study of the social organization of death in two American hospitals, Sudnow (1967) observed that staff's efforts and interactions with the dying were associated with the extent to which patients were already perceived as socially dead. In addition, he observed that social death also predicted biological death because patients already labelled as such died sooner. His illustrations of the consequences which this situation entailed for persons also drew attention to the isolation of the dying. In a later study, Timmermans (1998) attempted to show that developments in health care policy and legislation now made Sudnow's earlier observations obsolete. He observed 112 resuscitations and interviewed 42 health care workers in two American trauma units. Though his method of analysis was not clearly described, he used a thematic account of his findings to argue that recent legislation had only affirmed Sudnow's earlier findings that patients of low social value were much less likely to be resuscitated aggressively than patients with a perceived high social value. While age was still the most obvious characteristic on which patients were valued, other measures of their social viability were the extent to which they were well-known and liked, whether staff identified with them or not (e.g. were the same age or had the same family circumstances) and whether or not they had established a relationship with them. These differences in value were manifested by the increased number of staff present, the involvement of the cardiologist, the breaking of protocols and greater evidence of teamwork apparent during the resuscitations of high value patients. In the case of low value patients, staff showed less vigour and sympathy, joked about the difficulty of inserting cannulae, stated time of death in advance and called the coroner before the patient was pronounced dead. While staff followed the protocol in these cases, they did it more slowly and often it became an end in itself. Similar strategies of social rationing have also been observed to apply at a much wider societal level and have implications for the outward display of mourning after the death and into bereavement (Prior 1989; Kastenbaum 2000).

Social exclusion

What is central to the notion of social death is others' (and mainly health professionals') behaviour and treatment, which enforces the physical and psychological segregation of those who have been labelled as deserving of such. Such behaviour, it is argued, stems partly from our own fears of death and our disinclination to be reminded of our own mortality, which closeness and intimacy with the dying person inevitably brings (Kastenbaum 2000). While Sudnow's definition of death was limited to death-related behaviour, subsequent definitions have been extended to non-person treatment. Sweeting and Gilhooly (1991) described the process by which patients in mental hospitals and other inmates of large institutions such as prisoners were stripped of their individuality and contact with the outside world as 'mortification', as they were forced to give up their possessions and undergo procedures of admission. In an attempt to distance themselves from the inmates, staff resorted to 'non-person' treatment when they pretended that they did not exist. The nursing literature talks about 'dehumanization' and 'warehousing' as patients are stripped of any social value (Sweeting and Gilhooly 1991).

Mulkay (1993) has argued that social death begins at retirement, at which point older people are gradually denied full participation in family life and society. He also suggests that the situation may be more evident in women, who not only live longer than men but who have also lost their central role in the mourning ritual as modern death has been removed to the confines of institutions and the hands of the professional. This exclusion is, therefore, imposed by a society which no longer values the inclusion of people without a valid role in that society. It can be extended and enforced by the physical separation which institutionalization entails (Sweeting and

Gilhooly 1991), for example in the hospital (Sudnow 1967), the residential home (Hockey 1990) and the hospice (Lawton 2000). 'This condition of social isolation, combined with the expectancy of death, is likely to lead others to think of the elderly as being as good as dead, or in other words, socially dead' (Sweeting and Gilhooly 1991: 263).

In a participant observation study comparing care in a residential care home and hospice, Hockey (1990) described how fitter residents in the residential home were distinguished from their frailer counterparts in an attempt to reaffirm their purpose and position in the home. Staff also enforced these differences by structuring the daily activities, physical space and their use of language around this distinction in a conspiratorial attempt to protect the one from the ultimate fate of the other. Kastenbaum (2000) talks of a similar 'hale and frail' distinction being evident in almost every medical setting which he has experienced, as staff attempt to segregate the dying from their own and others' consciousness. Elias (1985) argues that the confinement of death to institutions now means that when we are confronted with it, society no longer knows how to react or respond.

According to Mulkay (1993), what Hockey's (1990) study bore witness to was society's wider exclusion of the elderly: 'The ultimate outcome for the elderly is that they are systematically prevented from participating in this last culturally impoverished setting in much the same way that the elderly in general are excluded from the wider society' (p. 37). It also highlighted the residents' own perception of their path along this final journey. Residents perceived that they were no longer of any social value, and described themselves as 'rubbish to be swept up' or 'put out'.

Measuring social death

In one of the few empirical studies to attempt to quantify the concept of social death, Sweeting and Gilhooly (1997) measured the extent to which social death occurred before biological death among elderly people with dementia. According to these authors, the increasing degeneration of the patient with dementia fits all the criteria for the condition of social death. These criteria include incompetence, loss of control of bodily functions, loss of insight, changes in personality and an inability to communicate. Through interviews with 100 carers of these patients, they made ratings of the extent to which carers believed their relatives were 'socially' or 'as good as' dead. Though the term social death was never used, questions were devised to assess whether carers perceived the dementia sufferers in this way. References in the interview that alluded to social death were also recorded, including observing non-person treatment of the sufferer (e.g. ignoring their presence, perceiving their care as mechanical, discussing them as a dementia patient rather than as an individual and excluding them from household tasks or social visits).

Findings from this study showed that respondents could be categorized along two dimensions of believing and behaving into four categories. The first category included respondents who both believed and behaved as if the sufferer was socially dead. Here, sufferers were still cared for but only as non-person beings: 'We treat her mostly, unfortunately, as if she's not part of our world' (Sweeting and Gilhooly 1997: 104). The second category included respondents who believed the person to be socially dead without behaving as if they were – that is, still involving them in everyday activities but simultaneously acknowledging that they were 'as good as dead'. Such respondents expressed the relief they would feel if the sufferers died peacefully in their sleep. Third, and unusually, were respondents who behaved as if the dementia sufferer was dead without believing they were – that is, referring to them in a derogatory way while in their presence but acknowledging that they were not as good as dead. The respondents in the fourth category were categorized as neither behaving nor believing that the person was socially dead, because they were able to remember the person as they once were and their behaviour towards them remained unchanged: 'While he's there my feelings will never change ... and when he, if he ever was away, my feelings would never change' (Sweeting and Gilhooly 1997: 109).

Some respondents described the distress, confusion or numbness caused by having to deal with a healthy body from which the person has disappeared, the mechanical process of caring for an unresponsive stranger, the regression of the person they once knew to a child-like state, and the desire for the removal of the physical body. In contrast, relatives who maintained the social life of their relatives laid great store on the fact that their relatives continued to recognize them, that they were still enjoying a certain of quality of life and relationships were maintained through denial (Sweeting and Gilhooly 1997).

The impact of protracted dying

In a lengthy and often relentless disease trajectory such as cancer, the experiences of patients as they negotiate the physical and emotional effects of the disease process also highlight a whole range of conditions and circumstances that can serve to promote a state of social deadness. This process may be precipitated by the stigmatizing effects of their diagnosis and may be exacerbated by decreasing physical and social function and the separation which institutionalized care enforces. A state of social deadness may evolve as patients begin to withdraw from their social networks and environment in preparation for death. Conversely, they are gradually and insidiously excluded or ignored by staff and carers who can no longer relate to them socially, personally or sometimes physically. A situation of 'social death' can, therefore, be self-imposed or enforced by others.

Isolation

Glaser and Strauss (1964b) found that staff interacted with patients according to their awareness of the severity of the illness. They described four awareness contexts that guided and structured the social interaction between staff and patients according to what they were perceived to know about the prognosis (Glaser and Strauss 1964b). These awareness contexts have been described as: *closed awareness*, where the patient does not know he is dying though everyone else does; *suspected awareness*, where the patient has not been told but suspects and looks to others for confirmation of his dying status; *mutual pretense awareness*, where both parties know the prognosis but pretend to each other that they do not; and *open awareness*, where both parties openly acknowledge the prognosis. It appears that these contexts gradually evolved as patients took cues from their external environment as the disease progressed until most reached one of open awareness. However, during this process both staff and patients performed elaborate rituals of collusion and pretense in efforts to mask the reality of the situation from each other.

According to Field (1996), what these early studies of social interaction with the dying showed was the overriding attempt by staff to protect both themselves and patients from the truth of their prognosis, to avoid their own and patients' distress: 'Somehow it was believed that by not telling people they were dying could maintain the social fabric and allow things to continue as "normal"' (Field 1996: 257). However, in so doing, he argues, the dying became more isolated, alienated and abandoned. Later discussion will show that much recent evidence suggests that such behaviour may still govern our communication with the dying today and with the same consequences. This is borne out by studies of the way health professionals communicate with cancer patients, which have highlighted the distancing techniques they use to block open and effective communication with patients (Wilkinson 1991).

In a study of terminally ill cancer patients at home, in a hospital and in a hospice, Johnston and Abraham (2000) showed that the stigmatization of cancer and the fear it aroused in others meant that when patients were diagnosed, especially with a terminal prognosis, they found it difficult to express their fears to carers because of a need to protect them from further distress or a realization that this was not a subject they were comfortable in talking about. Patients, therefore, learned who among their social network would sanction its discussion and avoided it with others: 'I don't like to talk about [dying] too much. It depends who it is because some people don't like you talking about it too much' (Johnston and Abraham 2000: 491). However, carers in the same study also reported feeling similarly isolated by their inability to talk freely with patients because of a feeling that anything they would say would be inadequate in the circumstances or emotionally upsetting for the sufferer:

> I just can't get through to my wife to talk about what she wants to do, exactly what's to be done about things and what's to become of me when she dies. You see we've never discussed anything about after she dies, about how she wants to go or anything like that, you know. She doesn't want to discuss it.
>
> (Johnston and Abraham 2000: 492)

The result was that both parties felt increasingly estranged by their inability to communicate freely and effectively with each other. The very support that should have been mobilized at such a time was essentially paralysed. Such isolation has been long documented in the psycho-oncological literature when it seems that having knowledge of the existence of the disease serves to erect a psychological barrier between the sufferer and the non-sufferer, effectively blocking normal communication and relationships (Bertman 1991). Open awareness does not necessarily mean, therefore, that patients and their carers know how to cope with the prognosis and manage it effectively: 'No matter what happened to the father they were alive and would go on living. No matter how they might worry, exhibit concern or weep now, the tumour had divided him from them like a wall, and he remained alone on this side of it' (Solzhenitsyn 1968, cited in Bertman 1991: 40).

Lawton (2000) describes a similar process in her study of hospice patients as they became increasingly distanced from meaningful social relationships with their significant others. This, she argued, occurred not only because of their physical separation, but also as a result of the psychological and social ramifications of the disease – it was as if they were inhabiting two different worlds:

> Patients' experiences of social isolation could also be understood as resulting from the ways in which their social and temporal perceptions had ceased to be enmeshed with those of the people around them. Patients, in a sense, had become drawn into ways of seeing and experiencing the world with which family and friends could not empathize; the common ground between them had begun to dissipate and ebb away.
>
> (Lawton 2000: 148)

Such isolation may not be exclusive to the terminally ill. In a small phenomenological study, the experience of being diagnosed with colorectal cancer was explored in eight patients who had recently been given the bad news (Taylor 2001). Of six themes identified, one appeared to measure patients' experiences of 'feeling on their own'. Patients described a sense of being removed from everyday life and the 'here and now' as they contemplated their own mortality and life continuing without them. Four patients also reported feeling stigmatized and socially embarrassed by their diagnosis and increasingly excluded by their significant others as they talked 'about them' and 'it' but not to them. They compared the experience with having leprosy or AIDS and being 'branded' as a cancer patient. New ways of feeling and behaving because of changes to their body image also caused them to reconstruct their social identity. This social exclusion by others and patients' need to withdraw to assimilate the wider implications of the disease seemed to compound their feelings of social isolation. Taylor concluded that this generally related to an inhibition on the part of all parties to talk about cancer:

> And when we received this news I felt very alone . . . um because, however close people are to you, your wife, your children, whatever you call them. It's actually happening to you, not to them . . . what's going to happen is going to happen to my body, nobody else's body. And however . . . we use the word empathy . . . there are corners of you which think, 'You're on your own buddy'.
>
> (Taylor 2001: 656)

This emotional distancing can be compounded by the physical restraints that accompany admission to in-patient care. The physical separation involved in dividing one party from the other prevents relationships from continuing as normal. Johnston and Abraham (2000) reported that one woman described her husband's hospice ward as a goldfish bowl where normal relationships were not possible due to the lack of privacy and the constant stream of family visitors and health professionals. As a result, she felt that the precious time they had left together was being eaten away by others' intrusions:

> My husband and I are never together . . . And the other day I came in here and he started to cry, and everybody's looking on, and I just feel it's not right, we should be on our own when we're like this and he was trying to say he was really going to miss me. I just feel we're a peep show . . . it's like living in a goldfish bowl, everybody looking on . . . you do need time, I'm not going to have him for much longer.
>
> (Johnston and Abraham 2000: 492)

▌ Disengagement

Having knowledge of imminent death can also result in patients initiating and sustaining their own longer-term withdrawal from their social network and the societal constraints of everyday life by relinquishing their role to others. Disengagement theorists describe this process as the elderly purposefully starting to relinquish their social status, by handing over their role to others in preparation for the ultimate withdrawal of death. Such withdrawal, they argue, is a natural response to an increasing psychological inferiority. Although these theorists describe this process as positive, others consider that it is in fact socially inflicted by decreasing health and a declining social network (Pratt and Norris 1994). During a prolonged illness such as cancer, the same process also becomes apparent when it seems that patients are gradually disconnecting themselves from the living.

The following quote comes from the daughter of a woman dying of lung cancer who had been given a year's prognosis but now found it difficult to maintain her role and obligations within her family. To her daughter it seemed as though she was voluntarily opting out of life and had lost the will or motivation to carry on:

> She doesn't seem to be interested in all the kinds of things that mothers do. You know, they're so interested in you and what you do, it's just gone, and I think it's the illness. She doesn't want to know about any-one's families. I mean, she'll ask the token questions, but really you can see it in her eyes that she doesn't want to know and it's the illness it's coping with it all that's difficult ... Once you know [the prognosis] there's nothing you can do to help that. I mean I've said to her after the last time 'I hope you're going to think about Christmas, because if you turn around to me and say I've not bought you a Christmas present because you didn't think you'd be here, that's just not going to be good enough'. Because you have to keep pushing her towards the future, because she thinks it's all going to end next week.
>
> (Johnston and Abraham 2000: 492)

In such circumstances, carers have to work hard to keep patients going in the face of what they see as a future without purpose or point. Emotional conflict may occur when the two parties have different priorities or needs that cannot be resolved.

Anticipatory grief

Such emotional rifts can be intensified when patients appear to outlive their disease and its prognosis. In these circumstances, family members have said goodbye too soon, either because the prognosis has been miscalculated or because both parties have worn themselves out playing the deathbed scene in anticipation of a parting that has not occurred. Consequently, neither side now knows how to act, as everything has already been said and loose ends have been tied up. Patients can feel angry or cheated that connections have been severed prematurely and roles given up, and carers, who have become exhausted by their caring role, have eventually to abandon it to salvage relationships with other family members who are increasingly feeling neglected, forsaken and all out of sympathy. This process can lead to anticipatory grief as carers and patients in adjusting to the loss experience the phases of grief before the death has occurred (Fulton *et al.* 1996).

In her study of hospice patients, Lawton (2000) describes the case of Rose who had eluded death on a number of occasions and had had several admissions to the hospice. While her family had initially been attentive to her needs, they were now frustrated and somewhat embarrassed by her continued existence. Rose herself felt let down by staff who failed to provide her with a 'safe haven' and no longer felt part of the family in which she had previously had a central role.

It would appear, then, that during the final weeks of her life, Rose had entered into a state of social death wherein her family and others had started treating her as if she were as 'good as dead'. Rose herself expressed a clear lack of interest in continuing to live as it became apparent to her that she had ceased to have an active influence on the lives of the people she had known and cared about.

(Lawton 2000: 153)

Johnston (1997) describes a similar situation where a patient had sold her house and moved into a nursing home on hearing of her prognosis. Months later and apparently not deteriorating physically, she now felt bored and severely restricted in her new environment. Her continued well-being had also led her to question whether she was actually dying. Such protracted dying appears to leave patients and their carers in a sort of social and psychological limbo where their roles become both confused and inappropriate. A natural reaction is for both participants to withdraw as these roles become impossible to sustain: 'I think it's to do with self preservation, you do withdraw' (Johnston and Abraham 2000: 492).

In their review of the literature on the concept of anticipatory grief, Fulton *et al.* (1996) acknowledge that there are mixed views about the extent to which patients and carers are mourning present losses or a change to the future they had anticipated for themselves. While there is no doubt that patients are mourning current losses of change in health and status, it is also argued that they are lamenting future losses before they actually occur. Carers, therefore, fear the threat of abandonment and being left alone, while patients worry about death and the dying process (Fulton *et al.* 1996).

Loss of personhood

The link between this sense of loss and its relationship to individuals' sense of self appears inextricable. A further dimension of the impact of social death on patients with a chronic and debilitating disease such as cancer is their perceived loss of sexual and familial status, as the illness takes its toll on their ability to perform and maintain their previous roles within the family. In the presence of diminishing capacity, carers begin to relate to patients differently, as if they are no longer capable of being autonomous and independent and, as a result, patients begin to lose their own sense of purpose and self. They are no longer perceived by their significant others to be the people they once knew or to have the same status. Roles, therefore, start to shift as sufferers become dependents and previous dependents become carers. Carers, therefore, mourn the degenderization of patients or their regression to a sometimes child-like state (Lawton 2000). For example, the following quotes come from women who lamented the transition of their strong, masculine husbands from their role as bread winner and provider to that of needy dependent. These women spoke about the loss of their husbands long before their deaths:

> I feel cross with myself and I get cross with him because he's sometimes like a baby, needing this and needing that and calling for me for this and calling me for that. He's just so different, you know, but I suppose it's because he's frustrated and he just can't do anything, you know.
>
> (Johnston 1997: 158)

> He's no my man.
>
> (Johnston 1997: 152)

These stark examples of perceived role transition emphasize that people's ability to maintain normal functional status is linked to their ability to sustain their sense of self, which is largely defined through their relationships with others. When these relationships are jeopardized, sufferers find themselves confronted with social alienation and abandonment. Lawton describes how the breakdown of bodily functions in patients sometimes repel even the most dedicated of carers, so that patients become increasingly isolated and disconnected from meaningful relationships:

> patients encountered the harrowing situation of being left alone by family and friends after the boundaries of their bodies fell severely and irreversibly apart. Even those closest to a patient often found themselves repelled quite literally, by the smells and substances which oozed and seeped from his or her porous body. Patients, as a consequence, were often left in a situation of extreme social isolation.
>
> (Lawton 2000: 164)

In reviewing the relationship between the concept of social death and personhood, Sweeting and Gilhooly (1991) suggest that according to the belief in the sanctity of life, espoused by Christians, people should be valued simply because they are human. However, they go on to argue that the majority of definitions of personhood include socially based criteria that are not relevant for the groups most likely to be defined as socially dead. As a result, these persons may be relegated to non-person treatment and be treated as if their personalities have been taken away from them. Nevertheless, while loss of personhood may increase the risk of social death, they are distinguishable (Sweeting and Gilhooly 1991). The need to extricate the self from the body is crucial, then, in preserving the value of human life and preventing the labelling of persons as socially dead.

Interestingly, in a study of hospice nurses, Copp (1997) found an approach to coping with patients' imminent death which she describes as 'somotological nursing practice'. In this study, it appeared that as death approached, nurses referred to 'separating the body' from 'the self'. Only when the two were in harmony (i.e. body ready and self ready) were patients ready to die. Patients also made the same distinction. This appeared to enable staff and patients to ensure a sense of continuity of self and meaning after the death as opposed to the total annihilation caused by the body ceasing to exist.

Negating social death: reducing death anxiety

Kastenbaum (2000) suggests that part of our difficulty in dealing with death is that we separate out dying from any other normal function or previous life experience. Instead, he proposes a multi-perspective model that combines several theoretical perspectives describing the dying process where the underlying theme is to leave the 'dying out'. This novel approach to understanding the dying process encourages us to believe that dying is part of living and, conversely, that living is a significant part of dying. In suggesting, then, that no one model will be prescriptive or will completely fit an individual experience, and by counteracting the negative consequences of these models with strategies that will promote our understanding of the individual experience, we might be less inclined to exclude the dying from normal interactions in a way that the confines of a social death experience does.

The situation of social death is therefore largely imposed by strategies both staff and carers use to distance themselves from those for whom death is inevitable. Psychological and physical barriers are erected to separate them from the normal interaction of everyday life. These barriers, however, may also be constructed by those labelled as socially dead as they perceive others' withdrawal and initiate their own disengagement from the living. In a disease like cancer, this process may begin as early as diagnosis and may be prolonged and exacerbated with the physical and emotional impact of a lengthy and relentless disease trajectory. Behaviours that encourage others to be labelled as socially dead or their own self-labelling will only be addressed when we begin to view death as a normal part of living.

References

Bertman, S. (1991) *Facing Death: Images, Insights and Interventions. A Handbook for Educators, Healthcare Professionals and Counselors*. New York: Hemisphere.

Copp, G. (1997) Patients' and nurses' constructions of death and dying in a hospice setting. *Journal of Cancer Nursing*, 1(1): 2–13.

Elias, N. (1985) *The Loneliness of the Dying*. Oxford: Blackwell.

Field, D. (1996) Awareness of modern dying. *Mortality*, 1(3): 255–65.

Fulton, G., Madden, C. and Minichiello, V. (1996) The social construction of anticipatory grief. *Social Science and Medicine*, 4(9): 1349–58.

Glaser, B. and Strauss, A.L. (1964a) The social loss of dying patients. *American Journal of Nursing*, 64(6): 119–21.

Glaser, B.G. and Strauss, A.L. (1964b) Awareness contexts and social interaction. *American Sociological Review*, 29: 669–79.

Hockey, J. (1990) *Experiences of Death: An Anthropological Account*. Edinburgh: Edinburgh University Press.

Johnston, G. (1997) Assessing psychosocial and spiritual needs in terminally ill cancer patients. PhD thesis, Dundee University.

Johnston, G. and Abraham, C. (2000) Managing awareness: negotiating and coping with a terminal prognosis. *International Journal of Palliative Nursing*, 6(10): 485–94.

Kastenbaum, R. (2000) *The Psychology of Death*. New York: Springer.

Lawton, J. (2000) *The Dying Process: Patients' Experiences of Palliative Care*. London: Routledge.

Mulkay, M. (1993) Social death in Britain, in D. Clark (ed.) *The Sociology of Death*. Oxford: Blackwell.

Pratt, M.W. and Norris, J.E. (1994) *The Social Psychology of Aging*. Oxford: Blackwell.

Prior, L. (1989) *The Social Organization of Death: Medical Discourse and Social Practices in Belfast*. Basingstoke: Macmillan.

Sudnow, D. (1967) *Passing On: the Social Organization of Dying*. Englewood Cliffs: Prentice-Hall.

Sweeting, H. and Gilhooly, M. (1991) 'Doctor am I dead?' A review of social death in modern societies. *Omega*, 24(4): 251–69.

Sweeting, H. and Gilhooly, M. (1997) Dementia and the phenomenon of social death. *Sociology of Health and Illness*, 19(1): 93–117.

Taylor, C. (2001) Patients' experiences of 'feeling on their own' following a diagnosis of colorectal cancer: a phenomenological approach. *International Journal of Nursing Studies*, 38: 651–61.

Timmermans, S. (1998) Social death as a self fulfilling prophecy: David Sudnow's *Passing On* revisited. *The Sociological Quarterly*, 39(3): 453–72.

Wilkinson, S. (1991) Factors which influence how nurses communicate with cancer patients. *Journal of Cancer Nursing*, 16: 677–88.

18

No way in

Including the excluded at the end of life

Jonathan Koffman and Margaret Camps

The growth of palliative care and demands on services in the UK: is there a problem?

Palliative care now encompasses a wide range of specialist services, but commenced in the 1960s with the development of the modern hospice movement by Dame Cicely Saunders when she founded St Christopher's Hospice in Sydenham, London. The number of hospices and specialist palliative care services has increased rapidly since that time. In 1980, there were less than 80 in-patient hospices and 100 home support teams in the UK and the Republic of Ireland. By the end of the millennium, this had increased to 208 in-patient hospices comprising 3209 beds, 412 home care and extended home care support teams, and 243 day care centres (Hospice Information Service 2002). In addition, there are more than 260 hospitals with palliative care nurses or teams and many offer a shared model of care. While the actual supply of specialist palliative care plays a role in determining which patients with progressive disease and their families receive care, concerns have been raised about other factors that influence the accessibility of care at the end of life for those who might benefit from it. In this chapter, we examine the evidence, principally UK-based, to determine in what ways the 'socially excluded' – the poor, older people, people with learning disabilities and mental health problems, Black and minority ethnic communities, asylum seekers and refugees, those within the penal system and drug users – fare with respect to accessing specialist palliative care for advanced disease and at the end of life. While we have limited ourselves to these population groups, other socially excluded sectors of the population are not immune. They include those who are homeless or live in temporary or fragile accommodation, travellers and those who abuse alcohol – and this list is far from exhaustive. To date, however, little attention and therefore published research has focused on either their met or unmet palliative care needs, a testimony to their social distance from the mainstream.

What is social exclusion?

The concept of equity of access to health care is a central objective of many health care systems throughout the world and has been an important buttress of the UK National Health Service since its inception in 1948. In the early 1970s, Julian Tudor Hart coined the phrase 'inverse care law' to describe the observation that those who were in the greatest apparent need of care often had the worst access to health care provision (Hart 1971). Since that time, although a growing body of research evidence has accumulated to quantify the problem (Townsend and Davison 1982; Whitehead 1992; Department of Health 1998a; Goddard and Smith 2001), making care available to all has remained elusive. This has been no less an issue for those who require care at the end of life (Higginson 1993; Grande *et al.* 1998; Addington-Hall 2000; NCHSPCS 2000; O'Neill and Marconi 2001; Seymour *et al.* 2001, 2002). Renewed commitment to tackle health inequalities has been harnessed under the wing of 'social exclusion', a relatively new term in the UK policy debate to describe an old problem (Barratt 2001). It includes poverty and low income, but is broader and addresses some of the wider causes and consequences of social deprivation. The British Government has defined social exclusion as 'a shorthand term for what can happen when people or areas suffer from a combination of linked problems such as unemployment, poor skills, low incomes, poor housing, high crime, bad health and family breakdown' (Social Exclusion Unit 2001). This is a deliberately flexible definition, and the factors they suggest are only examples. Many other dimensions of exclusion could also be added. The most important characteristic of social exclusion is that these problems are linked and mutually reinforcing, and can combine to create a complex and fast-moving vicious cycle. The result is hugely expensive for society, not only in human but also in economic terms. Importantly, it can also lead to a society that is unpleasant for many. Although these problems are far from uniquely British, Britain has been instrumental in this research, because it has both severe problems and a long history of studying them (Editorial 2001).

Who are at risk of social exclusion?

Social exclusion is something that can happen to anyone. Some people, however, from certain backgrounds and experiences, are more likely to suffer. The key groups might typically include:

- the economically disadvantaged;
- those living in deprived neighbourhoods, in either urban or rural areas;
- those with mental health problems;

- older people;
- people with disabilities;
- Black and ethnic minority groups.

Older people are particularly at risk of social exclusion. Many are at disproportionate risk of falling into poverty. People from Black and minority ethnic communities are disproportionately exposed to risk of social exclusion. For example, they are more likely than others to live in deprived areas and in unpopular and overcrowded housing; they are also more likely to be poor and to be unemployed, regardless of age, sex, qualifications and place of residence. Pakistani, Bangladeshi and African-Caribbean people living in the UK are more likely to report suffering ill health than White people (Acheson 1998). None of these risk categories are mutually exclusive and may operate in combination with others at any point in time.

The causes of social exclusion

According to the Social Exclusion Unit in the UK, past British Government policies and structures have not coped well with helping socially excluded elements of society. Some of the reasons for this failure are specific to the nature of social exclusion. Others are more general difficulties in public services. Many social exclusion issues cut across the boundaries between services and government departments. This has a number of consequences, including:

- *'Orphan' issues.* Many of the problems currently tackled by the Social Exclusion Unit have been exacerbated in the past because no-one was in charge of solving them, either in government or on the ground. These include some very specific issues, such as refugees, as well as some much bigger ones for materially improving the infrastructure of socially deprived neighbourhoods.
- *Lack of 'joining up'.* Some services have been less effective because they are dealing with problems whose causes are partly outside of their remit.
- *Duplication.* With many organizations and government departments involved in an issue, efforts can end up being duplicated (Social Exclusion Unit 2001).

Broader problems

Attempts to tackle social exclusion in the past also suffered from some of the more general difficulties that can affect any government programme. These include:

- insufficient emphasis on working in partnership with businesses, local government, service providers, communities, and voluntary and faith groups, all of which have a huge amount to contribute;

- a focus on processes rather than on outcomes;
- a tendency to look at averages, which can mask the worsening position of those at the bottom;
- relying on short-term programmes, rather than sustained investment;
- focusing on the needs of service providers rather than the needs of their clients;
- imposing top-down solutions, rather than learning from individuals and communities, and harnessing their enthusiasm;
- weaknesses in the collection and use of evidence, whether statistics about the scale of the problem or evaluation of what works here and abroad

The cumulative effect of these factors led to weaknesses in prevention, reintegration and the delivery of basic minimum standards.

Social exclusion: the concept challenged

It has been suggested that the term 'social exclusion' is both misleading and misconceived, since it denotes being deliberately 'shut out'. Groups within society are only shut out as a result of the normal social processes society unconsciously subscribes to and abides by, but not as an act of deliberate social exclusion directed solely at them (Rose 1996). It might therefore be better to view these population groups as 'marginalized' or 'disenfranchised' groups (Morrell 2001). By understanding them as people in these terms, it becomes possible to better understand their needs in relation to society. Isolated and marginalized people do not enjoy the same opportunities as the rest of society. They lack fulfilment of personal potential, and dwell in a social space where there is a perceived distance between them and others. They also lack participation in social institutions, which springs from commonality in interests and a social sense of belonging.

Who are the 'excluded' at the end of life?

Palliative care has become more prominent within the UK's National Health Service during the last decade as more health care professionals become familiar with the lessons of caring for patients with advanced disease and their families (Koffman 2001). Nevertheless, it has still been very slow to reach certain patients who could benefit from it. Below we have focused on the available evidence on access to palliative care to poor and other disenfranchised population groups (see Figure 18.1). Our list of groups is admittedly restricted and we wish to reiterate that other vulnerable sectors of society may fare as badly.

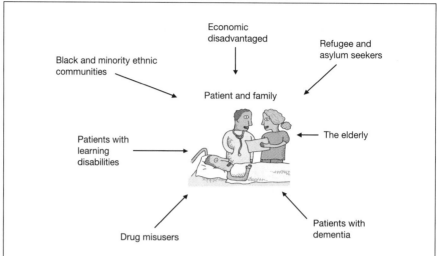

Figure 18.1   Factors that may influence access to palliative care by patients with advanced disease and their families.

The economically deprived

Britain leads Western Europe in its poverty, with twice as many poor households as Belgium, Denmark, Italy, Holland or Sweden. A quarter of men of working age were 'non-employed' in 1996, and a quarter of households existed on less than half of the national average income, after housing costs, in the early 1990s (Walker and Walker 1997). While overall personal income rose substantially in the 1980s and 1990s, the gap between the richest and the poorest has grown dramatically (Office for National Statistics 2000).

A recent systematic review of 15 studies in different developed countries, but primarily the UK, revealed that between 50 and 70 per cent of patients would prefer to be cared for at home for as long as possible, and to die at home (Sen-Gupta and Higginson 1998). In areas of high socio-economic deprivation, however, fewer people die at home (Higginson *et al.* 1994; Sims *et al.* 1997) (see Figure 18.2). They also die at younger ages (Soni Raleigh and Kiri 1997), often with a poorer quality of life (Cartwright 1992). Furthermore, services tend to require more resources to achieve the same level of care. A study in London compared the activity of home palliative care nurses in deprived and more affluent areas. It found that to achieve similar rates of home deaths, at least twice as many visits were needed in the deprived areas (Clark 1997). Clark also argued that it was difficult to raise voluntary funding for hospice and home care in deprived areas. An inverse law of hospice care is thus present, where provision is in indirect ratio to need (Clark 1993).

Several studies have shown that cancer patients who have had a better education or live in higher socio-economic areas of residence (McCusker 1983; Higginson *et al.* 1994) are more likely to die at home than other cancer patients. One US study showed this trend to be reversed only for people in

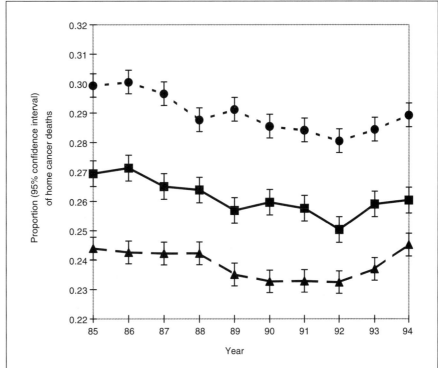

Figure 18.2 Trends in deaths at home from cancer by deprivation band (Source: Higginson *et al.* 1999). ●, low deprivation; ■, medium deprivation; ▲, high deprivation.

areas sufficiently deprived to warrant reimbursement of home care services (McCusker 1983). Data from one recent study (Sims *et al.* 1997) suggest that those in skilled occupations were more likely to die at home compared with both higher and lower occupational groups. However, lower occupational groups representing 61 per cent of the sample were considerably more likely to die in a hospital and less likely to die in a hospice. Figure 18.2 illustrates the wide variation in deaths at home by deprivation band (Higginson *et al.* 1999). It would appear that the lower occupational groups appear at a disadvantage both in terms of home death and in access to cancer-related services.

Older people

Fair access lies at the heart of good public services and this is no less true than for the provision of both health and social care to older people. However, in some health and social care services, older people and their carers have experienced age-based discrimination in access to and availability of services (Age Concern 1999). Furthermore, older people from Black and minority ethnic groups can be particularly disadvantaged (Department of Health 1998b).

In general terms, older people are less likely to be cared for at home and more likely to be in nursing and residential homes, where staff are often ill-equipped to manage the symptoms associated with advanced disease. In an evaluation of the adequacy of pain management in nursing homes in five states in the USA, Bernabei *et al.* (1998) found that pain was prevalent among nursing home residents and was often untreated, particularly among older patients and those from ethnic minorities. Similar concerns have been raised in the UK (Katz *et al.* 1999; Komaromy *et al.* 2000)

It has long been suggested that the palliative care movement has not afforded older patients adequate care, preferring to devote more of its resources to relatively younger people (Seymour *et al.* 2001). While some research has, in part, rebutted this accusation, the 1990 Regional Study of the Care of the Dying (RSCD) demonstrated that age is important when determining which patients receive hospice in-patient care (Addington-Hall *et al.* 1998) (see Box 18.1). Analysis of this large data set demonstrated that patients admitted to hospices with a cancer diagnosis were shown to be on average younger than those who were not. Although further examination of the data, controlled for the possibility that this may have been due to older patients being in residential or nursing homes, the difference still remained significant. A number of explanations may account for fewer older patients making use of this provision and they are presented in Box 18.2.

Many older patients do, however, experience significant distress from their illness and associated symptoms. Patients with cancer in particular and advanced disease in general should not be excluded from specialist palliative care input on the basis of their age alone.

Box 18.1   The Regional Study of the Care of the Dying (Addington-Hall and McCarthy 1995)

The Regional Study of the Care of the Dying (RSCD) made use of retrospective survey methods originally developed by Anne Cartwright in 1967. The RSCD was undertaken to provide a contemporary account of dying and bereavement in 20 health authorities (inner-city, semi-urban and rural) in England. Approximately 10 months after the patient's death, and following a letter of introduction, interviewers contacted the address of the deceased to identify the person best able to recount the deceased's last 12 months of life. They then conducted structured interviews that covered the deceased's health problems and restrictions, sources of formal and informal care, and the respondent's experience of caring for the deceased, the deceased's use of and satisfaction with health care services, information and communication with health care professionals, and the respondent's experience of bereavement and bereavement care.

Box 18.2   Why do older patients fail to make use of specialist palliative care?

1   Older cancer patients may be less troubled by their diagnosis than younger people
2   Many physical restrictions older patients experience may be due to the ageing process
3   Older cancer patients' physical symptoms may be due to other co-morbidities
4   Older cancer patients may be more accepting of death

People with learning disabilities

It has been argued that people with learning disabilities are among the most socially excluded and vulnerable groups in the UK today. Very few have jobs, live in their own homes or have real choice over who cares for them. Many have few friends outside their families and those paid to care for them (Secretary of State for Health 2001).

Learning disability includes the presence of a significantly reduced ability to understand new or complex information, to learn new skills (impaired intelligence), with a reduced ability to cope independently (impaired social functioning). The definition also covers adults with autism who also have learning disabilities, but not those with a higher level autistic spectrum disorder who may be of average or even above average intelligence, such as some people with Asperger's syndrome. Many people with learning disabilities also have physical and/or sensory impairments.

Producing precise information on the number of people with learning disabilities in the population is difficult. The White Paper, *Valuing People* (Secretary of State for Health 2001), suggests that there may be approximately 210,000 people described as having severe and profound learning disabilities, and approximately 1.2 million people with mild or moderate learning disabilities, in England.

Empirical knowledge of the general health needs of people with learning disabilities has increased in recent years. Research indicates that this client group have more demanding health needs than the general population and are also experiencing increased life expectancy, especially people with Down's syndrome (National Health Service Executive 1998). Increased life expectancy has in part been due to advances in medical treatments that are now available to this group of people. This, however, has resulted in the increased incidence of progressive disease, including myocardial and vascular disease, cancer and Alzheimer's disease (Jancar 1993). Surveys have increasingly demonstrated that many people with learning disabilities have undetected conditions that cause unnecessary suffering or reduce the quality or length of their lives. The accurate and timely diagnosis of a number of these problems can often be delayed for a variety of reasons, which include:

- People with learning disabilities and their carers usually have low expectations for their own health and of the services that they may receive. Many individuals and carers will tolerate poor health unnecessarily (Tuffrey-Wijne 1998).
- It has been shown that people with learning disabilities access primary care much less than they need to (Howells 1986).
- There appears to be a reluctance for people with learning disabilities to complain about symptoms; they may even be fearful of coming to the surgery.
- There are frequently serious communication difficulties with health care professionals, many of whom may be unfamiliar with their needs and the manner in which symptoms are presented (Keenan and McIntosh 2000).
- There appear to be many complexities of the present health care system and who assumes responsibility for care (Tuffrey-Wijne 1997, 1998).

Failure to diagnose advanced disease for this population group may mean that not only are treatment options limited, but also that the window for accessing palliative care becomes needlessly truncated. This prevents both patients and their care-givers from adequately planning and preparing for the final stages of their advanced illness (Brown 2000).

Once the opportunity for palliative care presents, problems continue. Very little is known about how people with learning disabilities experience pain and evidence suggests they may experience difficulties communicating its presence (Beirsdorff 1991). Other symptoms, for example nausea, fatigue or dysphagia, are similarly poorly communicated by individuals or poorly understood by health care professionals, and this may result in their sub-optimal assessment and management (Tuffrey-Wijne 1998).

Although the process of normalization of people with learning disabilities in recent years has meant that the philosophy of choice should be a right, many possess little control in their lives. Recent research has shown that only 6 per cent of people with learning disabilities have control over who they live with and 1 per cent over the choice of their carer (Secretary of State for Health 2001). This is an issue for those with advanced disease, as those who are cared for within group homes have limited opportunities to discuss, or realize, their preferred location of care and death – many continue to die in hospital or nursing homes (Tuffrey-Wijne 1998).

People with dementia

In recent years, dementia has become a major concern for all developed countries and greatly affects the use of health and social care services (Koffman *et al.* 1996; Koffman and Taylor 1997). People with severe mental illness require skilled professional care from health and social care professionals with expertise in their management. The focus on their mental health problems can lead to the under-diagnosis of life-threatening illnesses and to the under-recognition and under-treatment of symptoms. They may receive fragmented care, with responsibility for their physical health passed across agencies. Dementia can legitimately be seen as a terminal illness and patients die with this illness, if not directly of it (Addington-Hall 2000). The AIDS–dementia complex is an important cause of dementia in younger people. New variant CJD may also become a significant cause of dementia in younger people in the future. Patients with end-stage dementia often have significant unmet palliative care needs for symptom relief and for support for their informal carers (Addington-Hall 2000). Recent research has indicated that many patients with dementia have symptoms and health needs comparable with those who have cancer (McCarthy *et al.* 1997). Mental confusion, urinary incontinence, pain, low mood, constipation and loss of appetite were frequently reported symptoms, and many of these were experienced for longer periods than by patients with a cancer diagnosis (McCarthy *et al.* 1997). Respondents relaying the experiences of deceased patients with dementia reported levels of assistance required at home were far higher than for patients with cancer. Furthermore, they had been restricted for longer periods of time, 50 per cent having needed help for over a year with five or more activities of daily living compared with 9 per cent for cancer patients. These results indicate that many patients with dementia have unmet disease-related concerns, which, although they be met by generalist health and social services support are, nevertheless, amenable to specialist palliative care.

People from Black and minority ethnic groups

Ethnicity is difficult to define, but most definitions reflect self-identification with cultural traditions that provide both a meaningful social identity and boundaries between groups. People from minority ethnic backgrounds represent approximately 6.2 per cent of the population in the UK (see Figure 18.3). Although there is a significant lack of data about people from minority ethnic communities, the available data do confirm that some groups experience disproportionate disadvantage across the board, and others experience it in some areas.

Minority ethnic groups are more likely than the rest of the population to be poor. Twenty-eight per cent of people in England and Wales live in households with incomes that are less than half the national average, but this is the case for 34 per cent of Chinese people, over 40 per cent of African-Caribbean and Indian people, and over 80 per cent of Pakistani and Bangladeshi people (Berthoud and Modood 1997). Minority ethnic communities also experience a double disadvantage. They are disproportionately concentrated in deprived areas and suffer all the problems that affect other people in these areas. People from minority ethnic communities also suffer the consequences of overt and inadvertent racial discrimination, both individual and institutional; an inadequate recognition and understanding of the complexities of minority ethnic groups, and hence services that fail to reach them or meet their needs; and additional barriers like language, cultural and religious differences.

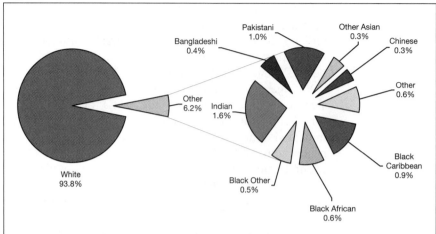

Figure 18.3 Ethnic composition of the United Kingdom (Source: Alexander 1999).

Minority ethnic social exclusion is complex and varies according to the economic, social, cultural and religious backgrounds of the particular people concerned. This complexity is not always understood or appreciated, partly because there is limited data available about different minority ethnic groups. Allegations of poor access and the use of health services by Black and minority ethnic groups are not new to health care in general (O'Neill and Marconi 2001) or the National Health Service in particular (Harding and Maxwell 1997; Secretary of State for Health 1997). A limited number of descriptive reports have levelled criticism of care at the end of life for these communities and poor access to appropriate care (Hill and Penso 1995). Low rates of cancer were seen as one explanation to account for low uptake of service provision, but the figures were likely to have been inaccurate because of inadequate ethnic monitoring (Aspinall 1995). The impact of ageing on Black and minority ethnic groups also now means larger numbers of older members within these communities will require health services for advanced disease.

Very few studies have addressed the needs and problems of patients with advanced disease in the last year of life, and their carers, in different communities. Most recently, a study in an inner-London health authority demonstrated that Black Caribbean patients with advanced disease experienced restricted access to some specialist palliative care services when compared with White deceased patients (Koffman and Higginson 2001), yet an analysis of local provision revealed no lack of palliative care services (Eve *et al.* 1997). This example of under-utilization of palliative care services by the Black Caribbean community at the end of life supports other recent research among minority ethnic communities (Farrell 2000; Skilbeck *et al.* 2002). The explanations to account for this are highlighted in Box 18.3.

Box 18.3 Minority ethnic social exclusion at the end of life: why does it occur?

Social deprivation
Low socio-economic status has been positively linked to an increased likelihood of hospital deaths, although this would apply equally to all population groups (Higginson *et al.* 1994, 1999).

Knowledge of specialist palliative care services and poor communication
There is a growing body of evidence that Black and ethnic minorities are not adequately aware of all local health (Watt *et al.* 1993) or specialist palliative care services available to them (Harron-Iqbal *et al.* 1995; Smaje and Field 1997; Camps 2001; Kurent *et al.* 2002). Problems of access to hospice and specialist palliative care provision can further be exacerbated by poor communication. Language problems between health care professionals and patients are a central component in perpetuating this barrier (Gerrish *et al.* 1996; Simmonds *et al.* 2001). Patients frequently rely on relatives, as this is often simpler than having to make use of an interpreter. However, this may disadvantage both patient and health care professional, as the family interpreter may filter, abbreviate or omit information and tell the doctor or the patient what he or she considers the health care professional may need to know or what the interpreter thinks should be said (Firth 2001).

Ethnocentrism
The demand for services may be influenced by the 'ethnocentric' outlook of palliative care services, discouraging Black and minority ethnic groups from making use of relevant provision (Smaje and Field 1997).

Attitudes to palliative care
Barriers to health care that the poor and the disenfranchised have traditionally encountered may affect their receptivity to palliative care. If patients perceive that they have been deprived of technologically advanced health care services during the course of their illness, they may be resistant to the idea of palliative care (Gibson 2001).

Dissatisfaction with health care
A number of studies not specifically related to palliative care support, for example the uptake of health and social services among Asian Gujarati and White elderly persons, have revealed significantly lower utilization of services in the former, not because of their better health, but because of their overall dissatisfaction of services (Lindsay *et al.* 1997).

Mistrust
There is some evidence from the USA to support the contention that Black and minority ethnic groups are less likely than White patients to trust the motivations of doctors who discuss end-of-life care with them (Caralis *et al.* 1993). This may be because health care institutions both historically and in the present have not always shown themselves to be worthy of trust. The Tuskegee syphilis study (Chadwick 1997) and segregated hospitals are still within the historic memory of many African Americans, and current treatment disparities between African Americans and White Europeans are extensively documented (Council on Ethical and Medical Affairs/American Medical Association 1990).

Gatekeepers
There is some evidence that general practitioners are more likely to act as 'gatekeepers' to services among minority ethnic groups, contributing to lower referral rates (Smaje and Le Grand 1995).

Refugees and asylum seekers

The UK, as a signatory to the 1951 Geneva Convention, is committed to offer asylum to people fleeing from persecution (Burnett and Fassil 2002). Estimating the total number of refugees and asylum seekers worldwide is difficult, as definitions differ widely. In the UK, refugees are defined as those who have been granted indefinite leave to remain or have permanent residence in the country. Asylum seekers are those who have submitted an application for protection under the Geneva Convention and are waiting for the claim to be decided by the Home Office. At the time of writing, there are in the region of 230,000 people in this category living in the UK and numbers continue to increase. Refugees and asylum seekers form significant minority populations in many UK towns and cities. The number of people seeking asylum has fluctuated over recent years and the UK ranks ninth in Europe in terms of asylum applications per head of population (Burnett and Peel 2001). It is extremely difficult to obtain demographic information on refugees and asylum seekers at the local level in the UK and this lack of information represents one of the difficulties in developing services that are accessible for these groups (Bardsley and Storkey 2000).

Although refugees and asylum seekers are often grouped together, they are not necessarily a homogenous group, and have varying experiences and needs (Burnett and Fassil 2002). Many refugees have health problems, including parasitic nutritional diseases (Jones and Gill 1998), and diseases such as hepatitis, tuberculosis, HIV and AIDS, which frequently overlap with problems of social deprivation. Their health problems are also amplified by family separation, hostility and racism from the host population, poverty and social isolation (Jones and Gill 1998; Bardsley and Storkey 2000; Kisely *et al.* 2002). Although asylum seekers and refugees are entitled to the full range of NHS services free of charge, many have difficulty in accessing health care services for a variety of reasons (see Box 18.4).

Individuals from sub-Saharan Africa, many of whom may be refugees and asylum seekers, make up the second largest group of people affected by HIV in the UK (Brogan and George 1999). They are more likely to be

---

Box 18.4 Asylum seekers and refugees: factors preventing access to care

1 Problems of understanding different languages and poor quality information on what services are available (Bardsley and Storkey 2000)
2 Special services available in areas with a high density of refugees are not always available to more dispersed groups
3 Many health care workers may be confused about the rights of refugees and asylum seekers to health care services, including the right to register with a general practitioner
4 Many general practitioners have difficulty in meeting the needs of refugees who may have complex social, psychological and physical needs (Hogan 1999)

socially disadvantaged and isolated, be much less aware of the health care to which they are entitled, and be more likely to present only when symptomatic. Experience has demonstrated that this patient group continues to require palliative care despite the advances made with highly active anti-retroviral therapy because they tend to present late with AIDS-related illnesses and have higher rates of tuberculosis, both of which are linked to a poorer prognosis. For many patients who do not have a general practitioner and are reluctant to register with one, the lack of a stable home environment and reluctance to access local services may mean that dying at home is not an option (Easterbrook and Meadway 2001). The advent of HIV/AIDS has in particular raised the need for cultural competence, since many of those affected by this disease are on the fringes of the usual health care system or even excluded from it (Alexander and Hoy 2001).

Prisoners

The prison population in the UK in 2000 was estimated to be in the region of 64,600, of whom 4540 were serving life sentences. England and Wales has the second highest rate (124) of prisoners per 100,000 of the population in Europe (Elkins and Olugundoye 2001). Prisoners are not typical of the general population with regards to their health needs. First, the prison environment is not conducive to healthy living. As a result, prison inmates have a disproportionately higher incidence of physical illness due to poor health behaviours, mental health problems and drug misuse, with suicide being significantly more frequent than in the general population (Finlay 1998).

Historically, prison health care has been organized outside the NHS. This has given rise to questions about equity, standards, professional isolation and whether the Prison Service has the capacity to carry out its health care function (Joint Prison Service/National Health Service Executive Working Group 1999). The government is now committed to developing a range of proposals aimed at improving health care for prisoners. These aims include ensuring that prisoners have access to the same quality and range of health care services as the general public receives from the NHS by promoting a closer partnership between the NHS and the Prison Service at local, regional and national levels.

The Working Group recommended that health authorities and prison governors work together to assess the health needs of prisoners in their area and develop Prison Health Improvement Programmes in line with those being developed in the NHS. They outline how the approach will address the current weaknesses in prison health care and ensure that real progress can be made in assessing the health needs of prisoners, in providing services to meet needs that are broadly equivalent to those received by the general population, and in getting better value from current resources.

To date, very little UK literature has focused on the palliative care needs of prisoners and that which is available is largely descriptive or relates to single case histories (Finlay 1998; Oliver and Cook 1998; Wilford 2001).

More research has taken place in the USA, where a number of palliative care programmes have been developed for prisoners, such as at the Louisiana State Penitentiary at Angola (Project for Dying in America 1998). This has been largely because in Louisiana, where the sentencing laws are tougher than in any other State in the USA, the courts hand out a disproportionate number of life sentences and few of these prisoners are granted parole. As a result, an estimated 85 per cent of Angola's 5200 inmates will grow old and will die there (Project for Dying in America 1998).

There are several problems in introducing palliative care into prisons, not least the mutual distrust between staff and prisoners. Effective symptom control, particularly adequate pain control, can be difficult under these circumstances. Drugs to manage pain control may be used for other illicit purposes. Also visiting from family and friends can be restricted, not least because the prison may be located at some distance from family members Evans *et al.* (2002). It has also been suggested that a reluctance to extend care to more prisoners is hampered by a belief that criminals do not deserve to die with dignity. There are also ethical concerns, which include the concept of patient autonomy, that might be difficult to uphold in a prison setting, as well as financial constraints.

Drug users

In England, during the year 2000–2001, the number of drug misusers reported as receiving treatment from both drug misuse agencies and general practitioners was approximately 118,500 (Department of Health 2001). Injecting drug misuse and its associated lifestyle carries a high risk of mortality. A variety of health issues are associated with injecting drug use, including HIV, hepatitis B and hepatitis C, which carry an increased risk of the development of cirrhosis, liver failure and primary liver carcinoma (Wodak 1998).

Although people who use recreational drugs have a right of access to health care in the UK, many are, however, isolated from health care and are not registered with general practitioners, relying inappropriately on accident and emergency departments as sites for primary treatment and access into health care (Brettle 2001).

There is very little literature on how drug misusers utilize specialist palliative care services. The limited literature that does exist focuses mainly on issues of pain control for this population. A single exploratory study in the USA explored the experiences of hospices providing care to intravenous HIV/AIDS drug users (Cox 1999). The survey revealed that the provision of community palliative care for these patients was frequently problematic because of patients' poor living conditions, many of which were considered unsafe to visit. Other challenges included health care professionals' concerns that patients might be resistant to hospice care if they perceived hospice as a barrier to their continued drug use.

It has been suggested that drug users require a modified health care system, which understands and considers the problems of drug users, but that the initiation and maintenance of contact may require a variety of initiatives (Brettle 2001). Morrison and Ruben (1995) similarly argue that services need to deliver care to these groups in imaginative and innovative ways, which are not judgemental and encourage contact without reinforcing traditional stereotypes. Without appropriate services, they argue, high levels of mortality among drug users will continue.

Conclusions

Since the introduction of the National Health Service, health care has been more widely extended to sections of the population, particularly women and children, many of whom were previously excluded from previous arrangements under the National Insurance Act. However, universal access to care and treatment remains elusive and care provided by the modern hospice movement, with laudable aspirations to extend care as widely as possible, has been shown to be inequitable on a number of fronts. We have shown that silent sections of the population are ignored or inadequately served at the end of life. This must remain a concern given that there is no second chance to improve the care of individuals who are dying, and it is practically and emotionally extremely difficult for these individuals with a progressive illness to raise concerns or to complain about the lack of services they receive. Solutions to the problems come in many forms, none of which will be successful in isolation.

First, there is an urgent need to raise public awareness of palliative care services and to provide public education about the care provided to reduce any misconceptions about services that may be influencing access. Information provided to NHS Direct and Primary Care Trusts may also be important. Second, health and social care professionals' knowledge and attitudes about engaging socially excluded populations must be improved (O'Neill and Marconi 2001). Multi-professional palliative care education offers exciting potential to explore these training needs (Koffman 2001). Third, regional implementation groups that look at and plan palliative care services in their own areas offer the potential to explore strategy at an epidemiological and corporate level. Examples include *Palliative Care in Wales: Towards Evidence Based Purchasing* (Welsh Office 1996) and *Palliative Care for Londoners: Needs, Experience, Outcomes and Future Strategy* (Higginson 2001), both of which have established a framework for the development of local policies and recommended closer links between agencies involved in the provision of care. Significantly, both documents advocate equity of access to high-quality care. Furthermore, they have recommended devoting more resources to research that explores the unmet palliative care needs of the socially excluded, given the paucity of evidence in certain areas. Without more comprehensive information, moving these complex agendas forward remains challenging.

Lastly, the charitable sector is uniquely suited to support new ideas that extend care and is able to elevate good ideas to the point where they can be integrated in society and become the social norm rather than the exception. Despite differences in the funding arrangements of care in the USA, the Robert Wood Johnson Foundation has been successful is pump-priming pilot projects to increase access to palliative care to socially deprived communities (Gibson 2001). The UK has followed suit (Box 18.5). Although specialist palliative care cannot completely remove the impact of progressive disease, approaches must be sought to extend its lessons to all those who stand to benefit from its increasing sophistication.

Box 18.5 Example of UK charitable sector-sponsored venture to manage social exclusion of patients with advanced cancer and their families

A 'Palliative Care Pathway', funded through the New Opportunities Fund, has recently been developed in north-west London focusing specifically on previously 'hard-to-access', socially excluded, patients with advanced cancer and their families. The aim of the project is to develop referral criteria, an interdisciplinary core assessment tool, and associated documentation for use by health and social care professionals to improve end-of-life decisions for pathway patients and their care-givers.

References

Acheson, D. (1998) *Independent Inquiry into Inequalities in Health Report*. London: The Stationery Office.

Addington-Hall, J. (2000) *Positive Partnerships: Palliative Care for Adults with Severe Mental Health Problems*. London: National Council for Hospices and Specialist Palliative Care Services.

Addington-Hall, J. and McCarthy, M. (1995) Regional study of the care of the dying: methods and sample characteristics. *Palliative Medicine*, 9: 27–35.

Addington-Hall, J., Altmann, D. and McCarthy, M. (1998) Which terminally ill cancer patients receive hospice inpatient care? *Social Science and Medicine*, 46(8): 1011–16.

Age Concern (1999) *Turning Your Back On Us: Older People and the NHS*. London: Age Concern.

Alexander, C.S. and Hoy, A. (2001) Palliative care in the age of HIV/AIDs: papers and recommendations from USA/UK meeting (workgroup 3: education). *Journal of the Royal Society of Medicine*, 94: 477–8.

Alexander, Z. (1999) *Study of Black, Asian and Minority Issues*. London: Department of Health.

Aspinall, P.J. (1995) Department of Health's requirements for mandatory collection of data on ethnic groups of inpatients. *British Medical Journal*, 311: 1006–9.

Bardsley, M. and Storkey, M. (2000) Estimating the numbers of refugees in London. *Journal of Public Health Medicine*, 22(3): 406–12.

Barratt, II. (2001) The health of the excluded. *British Medical Journal*, 323: 240.

Beirsdorff, K. (1991) Pain intensity and indifference: alternative explanations for some medical catastrophes. *Mental Retardation*, 29(6): 359–62.

Bernabei, R., Gambassi, G., Lapane, K. *et al.* (1998) Management of pain in elderly patients with cancer. *Journal of the American Medical Association*, 279: 1877–82.

Berthoud, R. and Modood, T. (1997) Ethnic minorities in Britain: diversity and disadvantage, in R. Berthoud (ed.) *The Fourth National Survey of Ethnic Minorities*. London: Policy Studies Institute.

Brettle, R.P. (2001) Injection drug use-related HIV infection, in M.W. Adler (ed.) *ABC of AIDS*, 5th edn. London: British Medical Journal Books.

Brogan, G. and George, R. (1999) HIV/AIDS: symptoms and the impact of new treatments. *Palliative Medicine*, 1(4): 104–10.

Brown, H. (2000) The service needs of people with learning disabilities who are dying. *Psychology Research*, 10(2): 39–47.

Burnett, A. and Fassil, Y. (2002) *Meeting the Health Needs of Refugees and Asylum Seekers in the UK: An Information and Resource Pack for Health Workers*. London: Department of Health.

Burnett, A. and Peel, M. (2001) What brings asylum seekers to the United Kingdom? *British Medical Journal*, 322: 485–8.

Camps, M. (2001) *A Palliative Care Needs Assessment of Bangadeshi People Living in Camden: A Pilot Study*. London: King's College.

Caralis, P.V., Davis, B., Wright, K. and Marcial, E. (1993) The influence of ethnicity and race on attitudes toward advanced directives, life-prolonging treatments and euthanasia. *Journal of Clinical Ethics*, 4: 155–65.

Cartwright, A. (1992) Social class differences in health and care in the year before death. *Journal of Epidemiology and Community Health*, 46: 54–7.

Chadwick, G.L. (1997) Historical perspective: Nuremburg, Tuskegee and the radiation experiments. *Journal of the International Association of Physicians: AIDS Care*, 3(1): 27–8.

Clark, C. (1997) Social deprivation increases workload in palliative care of terminally ill patients. *British Medical Journal*, 314: 1202.

Clark, D. (1993) Whither the hospice, in D. Clark (ed.) *The Future of Palliative Care: Issues for Policy and Practice*. Buckingham: Open University Press.

Council on Ethical and Medical Affairs/American Medical Association (1990) Black and white disparities in health care. *Journal of the American Medical Association*, 263: 2344–6.

Cox, C. (1999) Hospice care for injection drug using AIDS patients. *The Hospice Journal*, 14(1): 13–24.

Department of Health (1998a) *Inequalities in Health*. Report of an independent inquiry chaired by Sir Donald Acheson. London: The Stationery Office.

Department of Health (1998b) *They Look After Their Own, Don't They?* CI (98) 2. London: Department of Health.

Department of Health (2001) *Statistics from the Regional Drug Misuse Databases on Drug Misusers in Treatment in England, 2000/01. Statistical press release*. London: Department of Health.

Easterbrook, P. and Meadway, J. (2001) The changing epidemiology of HIV infection: new challenges for HIV palliative care. *Journal of the Royal Society of Medicine*, 94(442): 448.

Editorial (2001) Social exclusion: old problem, new name. *British Medical Journal*, 323.

Elkins, M. and Olugundoye, J. (2001) *The Prison Population in 2000: A Statistical Review*. London: The Home Office.

Evans, C., Herzog, R. and Tillman, T. (2002) The Louisiana State Penitentiary: Angola prison hospice. *Journal of Palliative Medicine* 5(4): 553–8.

Eve, A., Smith, A.M. and Tebbit, P. (1997) Hospice and palliative care in the UK 1994–5, including a summary of trends 1990–5. *Palliative Medicine*, 11(1): 31–43.

Farrell, J. (2000) *Do Disadvantaged and Minority Ethnic Groups Receive Adequate Access to Palliative Care Services?* Glasgow: Glasgow University.

Finlay, I.G. (1998) Managing terminally ill prisoners: reflection and action. *Palliative Medicine*, 12: 457–61.

Firth, S. (2001) *Wider Horizons*. London: National Council for Hospices and Specialist Palliative Care Services.

Gerrish, K., Husband, C. and Mackenzie, J. (1996) *Nursing for a Multi-Ethnic Society*. Buckingham: Open University Press.

Gibson, R. (2001) Palliative care for the poor and disenfranchised: a view from the Robert Wood Johnson Foundation. *Journal of the Royal Society of Medicine*, 94: 486–9.

Goddard, M. and Smith, P. (2001) Equity of access to health care services: theory and evidence from the UK. *Social Science and Medicine*, 53: 1149–62.

Grande, G.E., Addington-Hall, J.M. and Todd, C.J. (1998) Place of death and access to home care services: are certain patient groups at a disadvantage? *Social Science and Medicine*, 47(5): 565–79.

Harding, S. and Maxwell, R. (1997) Difference in mortality of migrants, in F. Drever and M. Whitehead (eds) *Health Inequalities*. Decennial Supplement Series DS No. 15. London: The Stationery Office.

Harron-Iqbal, H., Field, D., Parker, H. and Iqbal, Z. (1995) Palliative care services in Leicester. *International Journal of Palliative Nursing*, 1: 114–16.

Hart, J.T. (1971) The inverse care law. *The Lancet*, 1: 405–12.

Higginson, I.J. (1993) Palliative care: a review of past changes and future trends. *Journal of Public Health Medicine*, 15(1): 3–8.

Higginson, I.J. (2001) *Palliative Care for Londoners: Needs, Experience, Outcomes and Future Strategy*. London: London Regional Strategy Group for Palliative Care.

Higginson, I.J., Webb, D. and Lessof, L. (1994) Reducing hospital beds for patients with advanced cancer. *The Lancet*, 344: 409.

Higginson, I.J., Jarman, B., Astin, P. and Dolan, S. (1999) Do social factors affect where patients die: an analysis of 10 years of cancer deaths in England. *Journal of Public Health Medicine*, 21: 22–8.

Hill, D. and Penso, D. (1995) *Opening Doors: Improving Access to Hospice and Specialist Palliative Care Services by Members of the Black and Ethnic Minority Communities*. Occasional Paper No. 7. London: National Council for Hospice and Specialist Palliative Care Services.

Hogan, H. (1999) White paper will make access to health care more difficult. *British Medical Journal*, 318: 671.

Hospice Information Service (2002) *Directory of Hospice and Palliative Care Services*. London: St Christopher's Hospice.

Howells, G. (1986) Are the medical needs of mentally handicapped adults being met? *British Journal of General Practice*, 36(449): 453.

Jancar, J. (1993) Consequences of a longer life for the mentally handicapped. *American Journal of Mental Retardation*, 98(2): 285–92.

Joint Prison Service/National Health Service Executive Working Group (1999) *The Future Organisation of Prison Health Care*. London: Department of Health.

Jones, D. and Gill, P.S. (1998) Refugees and primary care: tackling the inequalities. *British Medical Journal*, 317: 1444–6.

Katz, J., Sidall, M. and Komaromy, C. (1999) Understanding palliative care in residential and nursing homes. *International Journal of Palliative Nursing*, 5(2): 58–64.

Keenan, P. and McIntosh, P. (2000) Learning disabilities and palliative care. *Palliative Care Today*, 9(3): 11–13.

Kisely, S., Stevens, M., Hart, B. and Douglas, C. (2002) Health issues of asylum seekers and refugees. *Australian and New Zealand Journal of Public Health*, 26(1): 8–10.

Koffman, J. (2001) Multi-professional palliative care education: past challenges and future issues. *Journal of Palliative Care*, 17: 86–92.

Koffman, J. and Higginson, I.J. (2001) Accounts of satisfaction with health care at the end of life: a comparison of first generation black Caribbeans and white patients with advanced disease. *Palliative Medicine*, 15(337): 345.

Koffman, J. and Taylor, S. (1997) The needs of caregivers. *Elderly Care*, 9(6): 16–19.

Koffman, J., Fulop, N.J., Pashley, D. and Coleman, K. (1996) No way out: the use of elderly mentally ill acute and assessment psychiatric beds in north and south Thames regions. *Age and Ageing*, 25: 268–72.

Komaromy, C., Sidell, M. and Katz, J. (2000) Dying in care: factors which influence the quality of terminal care given to older people in residential and nursing homes. *International Journal of Palliative Nursing*, 6(4): 192–205.

Kurent, J.E., DesHarnais, S., Jones, W. *et al.* (2002) End-of-life decision making for patients with end-stage CHF and terminal malignancies: impact of ethnic and cultural variables. *Journal of Palliative Medicine*, 5(1): 199.

Lindsay, J., Jagger, C., Hibbert, M., Peet, S. and Moledina, F. (1997) Knowledge, uptake and the availability of health and social services among Asian Gujarati and white persons. *Ethnicity and Health*, 2: 59–69.

McCarthy, M., Addington-Hall, J. and Altmann, D. (1997) The experience of dying from dementia: a retrospective study. *International Journal of Geriatric Psychiatry*, 12: 404–9.

McCusker, J. (1983) Where cancer patients die: an epidemiological study. *Public Health Reports*, 98: 170–6.

Morrell, P. (2001) Social exclusion (electronic letter). *British Medical Journal*, 323.

Morrison, C.L. and Ruben, S.M. (1995) The development of healthcare services for drug mis-users and prostitutes. *Postgraduate Medical Journal*, 71: 593–7.

National Council for Hospices and Specialist Palliative Care Services (2000) *The Palliative Care Survey 1999*. London: NCHSPCS.

National Health Service Executive (1998) *Signpost for Successful Commissioning and Providing Health Services for People with Learning Difficulties*. London: HMSO.

Office for National Statistics (2000) *Social Trends*. London: HMSO.

Oliver, D. and Cook, L. (1998) The specialist palliative care of prisoners. *European Journal of Palliative Care*, 5(3): 70–80.

O'Neill, J. and Marconi, K. (2001) Access to palliative care in the USA: why emphasize vulnerable populations? *Journal of the Royal Society of Medicine*, 94: 452–4.

Project for Dying in America (1998) Dying in prison: a growing problem emerges from behind bars. *PDIA Newsletter*, 3: 1–3.

Rose, G. (1996) *The Strategy of Preventative Medicine*. Oxford: Oxford Medical Publications.

Secretary of State for Health (1997) *The New NHS: Modern, Dependable*. Cm 3807. London: HMSO.

Secretary of State for Health (2001) *Valuing People: A New Strategy for Learning Disability for the 21st Century*. Cm 5086. London: HMSO.

Sen-Gupta, G.J.A. and Higginson, I.J. (1998) Home care in advanced cancer: a systematic literature review of preferences for and associated factors. *Psycho-Oncology*, 7: 57–67.

Seymour, J., Clark, D. and Philp, I. (2001) Palliative care and geriatric medicine: shared concerns, shared challenges. *Palliative Medicine*, 15(4): 269–70.

Seymour, J., Clark, D. and Marples, R. (2002) Palliative care and policy in England: a review of health improvement plans for 1999–2003. *Palliative Medicine*, 16(1): 5–11.

Simmonds, R., Sque, M., Goddard, J., Tillet, R. and Mount, J. (2001) *Improving access to palliative care services for ethnic minority groups*. London: St Catherine's Hospice.

Sims, A., Radford, J., Doran, K. and Page, H. (1997) Social class variation in place of death. *Palliative Medicine*, 11(5): 369–73.

Skilbeck, J., Corner, J., Beech, N. *et al.* (2002) Clinical nurse specialists in palliative care. Part 1. A description of the Macmillan nurse caseload. *Palliative Medicine*, 16(4): 285–96.

Smaje, C. and Field, D. (1997) Absent minorities? Ethnicity and the use of palliative care services, in J. Hockey and N. Small (eds) *Death, Gender and Ethnicity*. London: Routledge.

Smaje, C. and Le Grand, J. (1995) *Equity, Ethnicity, and Health Care*. Sheffield: University of Sheffield, Social Policy Association.

Social Exclusion Unit (2001) *Preventing Social Exclusion*. London: HMSO.

Soni Raleigh, V. and Kiri, A. (1997) Life expectancy in England: variations and trends by gender, health authority and level of deprivation. *Journal of Epidemiology and Community Health*, 51: 649–58.

Townsend, P. and Davison, N. (1982) *Inequalities in Health*. The Black Report. Harmondsworth: Penguin.

Tuffrey-Wijne, I. (1997) Palliative care and learning disabilities. *Nursing Times*, 93(31): 50–1.

Tuffrey-Wijne, I. (1998) Care of the terminally ill. *Learning Disability Practice*, 1(1): 8–11.

Walker, E. and Walker, C. (1997) *Britain Divided: The Growth of Social Exclusion in the 1980s and 1990s*. London: Child Poverty Action Group.

Watt, I., Howel, D. and Io, L. (1993) The health experience and health behaviour of the Chinese: a survey based in Hull. *Journal of Public Health Medicine*, 15: 129–36.

Welsh Office (1996) *Palliative Care in Wales: Towards Evidence Based Purchasing*. Cardiff: Welsh Office.

Whitehead, M., Black, Sir D. and Townsend, P. (eds) (1992) *Inequalities in Health: The Black Report and the Health Divide*. Harmondsworth: Penguin.

Wilford, T. (2001) Developing effective palliative care within a prison setting. *International Journal of Palliative Nursing*, 7(11): 528–30.

Wodak, A. (1998) Aspects of care for the hepatitis C positive patient. *Australian Family Physician*, 27(9): 787–90.

19

Ethical issues at the end of life

A very short introduction

Bert Broeckaert

Individual care-givers or institutions who care for terminally ill patients are inevitably confronted with serious ethical questions. Important decisions must be taken regarding the respective roles of the patient, the family and the care-givers in the decision-making process. What should the patient know? What should family members or friends of the patient know? To what extent can scientific research on terminal patients be justified? Can a patient be allowed to refuse life-prolonging treatment? How can the limited available resources be fairly distributed? The aim of this chapter on end-of-life ethical questions cannot be but modest. In view of space limitations, rather than merely summing up the wide range of ethical questions that arise at the end of life, I would like to try to delve more deeply into one specific issue – the important matter of life-shortening (or non-life-prolonging) treatment of terminal patients.

Dorothy is 82 and suffering from advanced dementia. She stopped recognizing her husband and children more than three years ago. In the past few months, she has spent a large part of each day in bed and lost virtually all her capacities to interact with the world around her. Three days ago, swallowing became totally impossible for her. The physician who has been treating her during the many years she has already spent in the nursing home decided not to start artificial nutrition. Although she thought artificial nutrition would probably lengthen the patient's life, in this case she considered it to be futile treatment and thus decided not to start it. A nurse who has known the patient for many years felt very uncomfortable with this decision and talked to the local newspaper. In a front-page article, the physician was accused of performing euthanasia.

At first sight, life-shortening medical treatment – whether it is a matter of withholding artificial feeding (as in the above example) or administering medication that could possibly shorten life – seems, to put it more mildly than the nurse in the case example, a bit strange. Of course, we can accept that there exist situations where medical treatment no longer brings about a cure, but we still tend to expect that if treatment does not prolong life, it will at least sustain it. Yet there are circumstances in which what health care workers consciously do has an accepted or even intentional life-shortening effect. I cannot deal extensively here with the various forms of life-shortening action and the ethical questions they give rise to. What I will attempt to do is offer nurses and other health care workers a conceptual framework that will permit them to develop further their own ideas about this complex and problematic field, and enter into dialogue about it. Without a shared set of words and concepts, any meaningful ethical discussion about this complicated matter is as good as impossible.

Euthanasia

When we speak of terminal patients, life-shortening medical treatment and ethics, then there is probably one word that immediately comes to mind: euthanasia. It is a term that is also a cause of controversy. For some, euthanasia is seen as a right, since it involves dying with dignity under undignified circumstances; for others, euthanasia is vilified as the very antithesis of palliative care, the opposite of a respectful and caring way to deal with dying patients. Nonetheless, in its original meaning 'euthanasia' gives little cause for such controversy. In ancient Greece, the word 'euthanasia' was used as a synonym for a gentle, fortunate and natural (certainly not medically induced) death without suffering, the sort of death that most people would hope for – *eu* (good) and *thanatos* (death): a good death. Though a shift of meaning can be observed already with Francis Bacon's use of the term in 1605 (the emphasis is more on what the physician does to reduce the dying person's suffering), it is only with people like Samuel C. Williams (1870) and Lionel A. Tollemache (1873) that the term 'euthanasia' acquires its contemporary meaning. It is only at the end of the nineteenth century that euthanasia is understood as 'suicide *by proxy*', or as 'suicide *in extremis*', where a physician intentionally administers lethal medication, at the patient's request, to relieve the patient of extreme and unendurable suffering.

Around the beginning of the twentieth century, various forms of euthanasia came to be distinguished, in reaction to the rise of the pro-euthanasia movement. For instance, an 1884 editorial in the *Boston Medical and Surgical Journal* already drew a distinction between active and passive euthanasia, rejecting the former (which was defended by people like Williams and Tollemache) and considering the latter – which amounted to withdrawing or withholding a possibly life-prolonging treatment – to be clearly acceptable. In 1899, *The Lancet* made another distinction, one which is still well known, between direct and indirect euthanasia, where indirect refers to the fact that a medical treatment (such as pain relief) can have side-effects that might shorten the patient's life, without this constituting the aim of the treatment: the actual (direct) aim is to bring the pain under control. Though the word 'euthanasia' in the Anglo-Saxon world is associated primarily with its voluntary character (the patient experiences life as unbearable and desires to escape from this suffering), the German discussion about the end of life was oriented differently from the outset. Long before the work of Binding and Hoche (1922), people such as Haeckel (1874) and Jost (1895) had already defended the killing of certain categories of incompetent patients.

The discussion about euthanasia that has been ongoing since the end of the nineteenth century has made the word into something very complex, a term that covers a multiplicity of meanings. Various adjectives were and still are added to the term to make it clear what sort of life-shortening or life-terminating action one is speaking about. Thus euthanasia is active or passive, direct or indirect, voluntary, involuntary or non-voluntary, and these adjectives can be used in all sorts of possible combinations. For instance, if one intentionally neglects to treat a lung infection with the aim of hastening the patient's death without the patient having requested this or given consent, then this could be seen as an example of direct passive non-voluntary euthanasia. In this way, the word 'euthanasia' becomes an umbrella term encompassing all possible forms of medical treatment (or non-treatment) that has a life-shortening effect.

The result of all this is that confusion reigns. One can present oneself as strongly for or against euthanasia and legalization or regulation of this practice, or state that euthanasia is illegal everywhere except the Netherlands and Belgium. One can give the word 'euthanasia' the specific meaning ascribed to it by people like Williams and Tollemache: the administration of

---

Box 19.1   Definitions of euthanasia

Euthanasia (broad definition):	a deliberate medical act or omission that shortens the life of a patient, with the restriction that this life-shortening effect is accepted or aimed at by the physician involved
Direct euthanasia:	the intention and direct effect of the treatment is the death of the patient
Indirect euthanasia:	the death of the patient is a foreseen but unintended side-effect of pain or symptom relief
Active euthanasia:	the death of the patient is the result of the administration of lethal medication
Passive euthanasia:	the death of the patient is the result of the withholding or withdrawing of life-sustaining treatment
Voluntary euthanasia:	the life of the patient is shortened to conform with his or her will
Involuntary euthanasia:	the life of the patient is shortened contrary to his or her will

lethal medication with the aim of ending the patient's life. Or one can use the word 'euthanasia' as an umbrella term, as I just described. But if one defends such a broad use of the term, then one must also accept the consequence that in most countries certain forms of euthanasia (the passive and the indirect variants) can be accepted medical practice. Then it would be simply wrong to state that euthanasia is illegal everywhere except in the Netherlands and Belgium.

The counterintuitive character of these conclusions shows that, in everyday speech, 'euthanasia' is usually used in a specific sense: people do not primarily think of *all* forms of life-shortening medical action, but of those specific cases where lethal medication is administered with the direct aim of ending the life of the patient. 'Euthanasia' in fact means active direct euthanasia. In delicate ethical discussions about the end of life, it would be ill-advised to employ a key term such as 'euthanasia' in both a broad and a narrow sense. A choice must be made. I would argue for using the narrow definition of euthanasia, not only because it is closer to everyday usage, to the idea immediately evoked by the term, but, more importantly, it is simply inopportune to use one and the same term for an entire series of actions that are judged quite differently, both ethically and legally. This would be tantamount to carrying out an unjustified conflation of the most controversial and often illegal practices with the most normal and perfectly legal (sometimes even legally required) acts. What is the benefit of talking about euthanasia in a case such as actively and intentionally ending the life of a quadriplegic patient (controversial) and using the same terminology in the case of not reanimating a terminal cancer patient (it is precisely reanimation that would be controversial here)? Is it really wise to use the term 'euthanasia' (with all the connotations it invokes) when the intention to end life is clearly absent, as in the second case? Is it not precisely this intentional, active ending of life that is far

---

Box 19.2　The Dutch and Belgian euthanasia laws

At this moment, two countries have legalized euthanasia: the Netherlands and Belgium. The fact that these are neighbouring countries doesn't imply that they have a similiar history as far as euthanasia is concerned. In the Netherlands, the recent euthanasia law (2002) is the result of a large-scale euthanasia discussion that has been going on for decades, which more than 10 years ago led to a very tolerant euthanasia policy. Belgium, on the other hand, was until 2002, at least as far as euthanasia was concerned, a perfectly 'normal' country. For an introduction to the two laws, with their similiarities and differences (i.e. the inclusion of assisted suicide, euthanasia for youngsters and the role of the nursing team in the euthanasia procedure), see the special issue of *Ethical Perspectives* (2002, Vol. 9(2)) on euthanasia in the Low Countries. A detailed and reliable overview of the Dutch debate is given in Griffiths *et al.* (1998). For an historical introduction to the little known Belgian euthanasia debate, see Broeckaert (2001).

removed from the healing and life-sustaining mission of the physician? Is it not this ending of life that creates all the controversy and thus deserves a term of its own?

Physician-assisted death

In opting for the strict sense of the term euthanasia, we will need to find a new umbrella term with which the diverse forms of life-shortening medical action might best be indicated. In 1990, when he took on the task of carrying out a large-scale empirical study of Dutch euthanasia practice, Paul van der Maas coined the term 'medical decisions concerning the end of life' or 'medical end-of-life decisions'. This new term comprises 'all decisions made by physicians about actions whose objective is to hasten the end of the patient's life, or where the physician can expect that the end of the patient's life will most probably be hastened as a result of such actions' (van der Maas *et al.* 1991). In other words, the term comprises all forms of life-shortening (or non-life-prolonging) medical action. Since then, the term has become standard usage in the Netherlands, and it regularly turns up in the international literature. I have, however, always tended to resist the use of this term, primarily for two reasons. In the first place, the term is misleading. According to his definition, van der Maas refers to the various forms of life-shortening action, so the meaning is actually the same as the term 'euthanasia' in the broad sense of the word (which I reject). The fact that what is at issue is the shortening of life or even the ending of life is not at all suggested by the phrase 'medical end-of-life decisions'. Why would the decision to permit someone to spend his or her final days at home, or the decision to prolong someone's life through a particular therapy, not be included in this category? Use of a term such as 'medical decisions concerning the end of life' only clouds the unique and troubling specificity – especially for physicians, who are assumed to seek a cure or at least to sustain life – of the kinds of acts one wishes to discuss (intentional shortening of life).

A second reason why I resist the use of the term 'medical end-of-life decisions' is the fact that it unjustly gives the impression that we are dealing here essentially with medical-technical decisions, decisions that can only, or should only, be made by physicians, since only they possess the required expertise. This suggestion, which is inherent in the use of the term, is especially misleading and dangerous. To give an example: a decision is made to withdraw artificial administration of food and fluids in a patient in a persistent vegetative state (PVS) who has been in a deep coma for 6 months. This is a clear example of a medical decision concerning the end of life. It is also clear that such a decision will have a life-shortening effect. But is it really a decision that is essentially *medical*? I think the answer is clearly no. Admittedly, this decision does have an unmistakable and inevitable medical component. Without a correct assessment of the patient's medical condition, and without a proper idea of the available medical evidence in this area, it is impossible to make an appropriate decision. Nevertheless, my point is that the ultimate decision involves much more than just these medical facts, however indispensable they may be. The more fundamental question being posed and answered here is whether the life of a PVS patient – a life that in principle can be prolonged, sometimes for several decades, until a natural death ensues – should be considered dignified and meaningful. Obviously, the decision to be made here is an *ethical* one and, in making essentially ethical decisions, I can think of no reason why the values and ideas of a single professional group (i.e. physicians) regarding what is dignified and meaningful should be the only ones that count. The ethical nature of many decisions and the fact that not everyone has the same ideas about what constitutes a meaningful human life are in themselves strong arguments in favour of involving other health care workers – and in the first place the patient and his or her family – in the decision-making process.

Out of dissatisfaction with terminology such as 'euthanasia' and 'medical end-of-life decisions', my search for a new umbrella term to encompass the various forms of life-shortening medical action yielded the term 'physician-assisted death'. One speaks of physician-assisted death when a medical action (or refraining from acting) has an acceptable or even sought-after life-shortening effect. The major benefit of this term is that it is honest and thereby perhaps somewhat confrontational; it is a term which clearly indicates what is at stake and which clearly exposes the physician's grave responsibility – one does not take the decision to shorten life lightly. It is a decision that can be the most appropriate one, but in any case it requires a clear justification.

It can easily be demonstrated with statistics that it would be unwise to limit the ethical discussion about life-shortening or life-ending medical action to euthanasia in the strict sense. While awaiting the forthcoming European figures from the Eureld E.C. study, I will cite the death certificate studies carried out in the Netherlands (1990 and 1995), Australia (1997) and Flanders (1998) (van der Maas *et al.* 1991, 1996; Kuhse *et al.* 1997; Deliens *et al.* 2000), since these give the most reliable and comparable figures regarding life-shortening medical acts (Table 19.1). Depending on the country, euthanasia (strict definition) accounts for between 1.1 per cent (Flanders) and 2.4 per cent (the Netherlands) of all deaths. The broader category, physician-assisted death (my definition), accounts for between 39.3 per cent (Flanders) and 64.8 per cent (Australia) of all deaths, which demonstrates

Table 19.1 Euthanasia and physician-assisted death as a percentage of all deaths (my definitions)

	Flanders (1998)	Australia (1995)	Netherlands (1995)	Netherlands (1990)
Euthanasia	1.1	1.7	2.4	1.7
Physician-assisted death	39.3	64.8	42.6	39.4

Sources: van der Maas *et al.* (1991, 1996), Kuhse *et al.* (1997) and Deliens *et al.* (2000).

that dying is frequently no longer 'natural'. More and more, the moment of death is determined, and the process of dying is controlled, by withholding or withdrawing life-prolonging measures or by performing actions that have a life-shortening effect. It would be regrettable if we were to overlook the important ethical dimension of these decisions and actions by focusing exclusively on a category that is relatively marginal from a statistical point of view.

Up to this point, I have been dealing with physician-assisted death in general and I have also said something about one specific form of physician-assisted death: euthanasia. In what follows, I would like to outline a typology of the various forms of physician-assisted death, not because I am so enamoured of divisions and categorization but because the various forms of physician-assisted death each raise specific ethical questions which risk being misconstrued if no distinctions are drawn. In the absence of the kind of conceptual and terminological clarification I propose here, we are trapped in a conceptual mist that impairs our vision and judgement, a conceptual mist in which the lack of any shared understanding of the basic terms renders ethical discussion impossible.

Withdrawing or withholding life-prolonging treatment

The simplest way of meaningfully dividing physician-assisted death into two categories is to draw a basic distinction between a life-shortening or life-ending measure that is essentially active in nature and one that is passive. In the former case, we are dealing with an active intervention that hastens death: death is accelerated or caused by the administration of medication with a life-shortening effect. In the latter case, the shortening or the ending of life is the result of the decision to suspend, or not to begin, a particular life-prolonging treatment. Let us first take a closer look at the second category.

Box 19.3   Physician-assisted death

Physician-assisted death is the result of a deliberate medical act or omission that shortens the life of a patient, with the restriction that this life-shortening effect is accepted or aimed at by the physician involved.

- *Active intervention*: administration of life-shortening medication
  - active termination of life
  - pain and symptom control with life-shortening effect

- *Passive intervention*: withdrawing or withholding life-sustaining treatment
  - at patient's request (integrity)
  - without patient's request (futility?)

Statistics from the Netherlands, Australia and Flanders show that in some cases – from 16.4 per cent (Flanders) to 28.6 per cent (Australia) of all deaths; the numbers from the Netherlands are slightly higher than in Flanders (17.9 per cent in 1990 and 20.2 per cent in 1995) – physicians believe that by withdrawing or withholding life-prolonging treatment they have hastened death (van der Maas *et al.* 1991, 1996; Kuhse *et al.* 1997; Deliens *et al.* 2000). It is immediately clear that, from a purely statistical point of view, we are dealing here with a very significant category, with a problem that confronts health care workers much more frequently than the question of euthanasia. Examples of withholding or withdrawing life-prolonging treatment are available in droves: not administering a necessary blood transfusion (because the patient is a Jehovah's Witness and refuses it); not administering antibiotics when a patient is in a coma and then develops pneumonia; withholding tube feeding when a severely demented patient develops swallowing difficulties that make normal feeding impossible; not starting with new chemotherapy even though this means that the patient's death will be hastened, and so on.

The motivation for withholding or withdrawing life-prolonging treatment can be two-fold: either it is done to respect the wishes of the patient or else it is done because further treatment would be futile, for medical and ethical reasons. Let us examine the first sub-category: life-prolonging treatment is withdrawn or withheld because the patient refuses treatment. Here, the textbook example is that of the Jehovah's Witness who refuses a needed blood transfusion, thus bringing certain death. There is growing international consensus that when a competent patient (such as a competent Jehovah's Witness) refuses a treatment, this refusal must be respected, even if such a refusal would lead to the patient's death. The relevant principle here is the principle of the right to physical integrity, a fundamental human right that can be found in the European Human Rights Treaty (article 8) and which is just as clearly present in the Convention on Human Rights and Biomedicine (Council of Europe 1997), where in article 5 one can read the following:

> An intervention in the health field may only be carried out after the person concerned has given free and informed consent to it. This person shall beforehand be given appropriate information as to the purpose and nature of the intervention as well on its consequences and risks. The person concerned may freely withdraw consent at any time.

When applied to the field of health care, the right to physical integrity implies that medical intervention – which undeniably has a clear impact on a person's body – can take place only when the patient has given explicit consent to such action. When a patient refuses or withdraws this consent, this refusal must in principle be respected, even if in the view of the health care workers such a refusal will have deleterious consequences for the patient's chances of healing or quality of life. As health care workers, we may find it particularly regrettable and irresponsible if a patient who is diagnosed with breast cancer refuses surgery when it is clear to everyone that surgery would increase her chances considerably. In such cases, health care workers certainly have the right and the duty to express their concerns to the patient and to point out the great risk she is taking. However, if after all this the patient sticks to her decision to refuse surgery, then this decision must be respected.

Life-prolonging treatment may also be suspended for yet another reason, one that is essentially unrelated to the patient's refusal of a specific action: when it is a matter of avoiding what is usually called *acharnement thérapeutique* in French or *therapeutische hardnekkigheid* in Dutch (avoiding 'therapeutic obstinacy' – there is no English equivalent). In Anglo-Saxon countries, one usually speaks of avoiding *futile treatment*. I would prefer to speak of withdrawing or withholding life-sustaining treatment *for medical-ethical reasons* and avoid using the term futile treatment in most cases, since the choices that need to be made here – for example, do we continue artificial feeding or not? – are only very rarely black-and-white choices where it would be perfectly clear what is 100 per cent meaningful and what is 100 per cent futile. Consider once again the example of the PVS patient. It would be too simple to claim that continuing to feed this patient artificially is futile. From a physical standpoint it is not futile at all: the patient's life is clearly prolonged, the patient remains alive due to the treatment. Second, what is considered to be a meaningful and dignified human life? How should one weigh prolongation of life against quality of life? These are clearly matters where no objective standard exists, but where much depends on one individual's values and assessments. This is why it is of prime importance to get the patient, family and nurses and other health care workers involved as much as possible in the choices that are made. Using the phrase futile treatment too easily tends to ignore and underestimate this important ethical and personal dimension.

Pain and symptom control with life-shortening effect

Let us now turn to those forms of physician-assisted death for which an active intervention on the part of the physician (i.e. the medication he or she administers) actually hastens death. At the active end of the wide spectrum of life-shortening medical action, there are two main choices: either we are dealing with intentional life-ending action (of which euthanasia is one sub-category) or it is a question of symptom or pain control to which life-shortening effects are ascribed. Let us first examine the latter sub-category. Unlike, for instance, euthanasia, nurses and physicians often regard pain relief as ethically unproblematic. The fact that the intention underlying pain control is said to be completely different from that of euthanasia ensures, it is often argued, an essential distinction between the two. Are we wasting our time, then, in looking more closely at the forms of pain and symptom control? I don't think so.

The following is a telling example. A survey carried out by the Pallium Group of the European and Israeli delegates to the Sixth Congress of the European Association of Palliative Care (Geneva 1999) revealed that only 5.3 per cent of the respondents thought that euthanasia should be permitted in palliative care under certain circumstances. On the other hand, 'the intentional shortening of life by raising opioid doses' commanded greater support: 15.4 per cent of the respondents stated that this action 'could be part of palliative care' (Janssens *et al.* 2002: 77). It is strange that suddenly three times as many people should say yes, simply because the controversial word euthanasia is avoided and talking about opioid doses suggests pain relief and the ethical qualities linked with it. 'The intentional shortening of life', however, can hardly be regarded as the ultimate purpose of pain control or, more generally, symptom control. What is typical of pain and symptom control, I would argue, is not only the physician's underlying subjective intention (treating symptoms, not shortening life), but the adequacy and proportionality of what is occurring at the objective level. For this reason, I define pain and symptom control as follows: 'the intentional administration of analgesic and/or other medication in such dosages and combinations as are required to adequately control pain and/or other symptoms' (Broeckaert 2000a: 100).

Striving for adequacy and proportionality – for a clear relation between the medication that is administered and the medication that is required – is absolutely essential for distinguishing pain control from forms of active termination of life (including euthanasia). This is not simply hair-splitting, as can clearly be shown by the Dutch and Flemish statistics on medical action with life-shortening effect. If we know that pain control is remarkably safe even when powerful medication is administered in extreme dosages [Bercovitch *et al.* (1999) are clear: 'high morphine dosage does not affect patient survival'], then we can conclude that when pain control is carried out according to the rules, it will hardly ever have a life-shortening effect and, as a result, will hardly ever count as a form of physician-assisted death. In light of this, it is quite astonishing to read that in Flanders, the Netherlands and Australia, according to the physicians involved, pain control led to a marked shortening of life in no fewer than 18.5, 19.1 and 30.9 per cent of deaths, respectively (van der Maas *et al.* 1996; Kuhse *et al.* 1997; Deliens *et al.* 2000). If we look more closely at these numbers, it turns out that in 3 per cent (the Netherlands in 1995) and even 5 per cent of deaths (Flanders in 1998), this pain control with life-shortening effect was administered 'in part with the aim of hastening the end of life'. One could reasonably conclude that in many of these cases the physicians were not very concerned about the aforementioned adequacy or proportionality of their dosages, and that they knowingly – precisely so as to shorten life – administered higher doses than were necessary to alleviate the pain. This very convincingly demonstrates the need for a good definition of pain and symptom control. A physician or nurse who deliberately and in full knowledge administers an overdose to shorten the patient's life, who is therefore unconcerned about adequacy and proportionality, is engaged in a form of actively ending life (euthanasia, if at the patient's request) and *not* pain and symptom control.

Palliative sedation: an exceptional form of pain and symptom control

In a landmark article dating from 1990, Ventafridda *et al.* asserted that more than 50 per cent of terminal cancer patients die with physical symptoms that can only be brought under control by means of (deep) sedation. Although the few more recent clinical studies of sedation in palliative care generally cite a much lower frequency (Morita *et al.* 1996, 1999; Stone *et al.* 1997; Fainsinger 1998; Porta Sales *et al.* 1999; Fainsinger *et al.* 2000a,b; Porta Sales 2001), in a considerable number of terminal patients (15–36 per cent in Fainsinger *et al.* 2000b) sedation still remains necessary to control a number of refractory symptoms (dyspnoea, delirium, etc.). For many working in palliative care, sedation has nothing to do with euthanasia. Indeed, as the ultimate therapy and most intense form of pain and symptom control, they believe sedation makes euthanasia superfluous. There are others, however, who think that sedation is nothing but 'slow euthanasia': a disguised, hypocritical and barely humane form of euthanasia or ending of life.

In dealing with a controversial practice like sedation, it is of upmost importance to determine what implicit and explicit messages and connotations are suggested by the terms used to indicate this practice.[1] One of the major problems with 'terminal sedation' – the most well known but also the most disputed term – is that it is too general, so that cases which are quite different from an ethical viewpoint get included in the same category, with all the concomitant risks of confusion and levelling out. Whether a patient is sedated with the intention of shortening his or her life (the same intention as with euthanasia) or out of a desire to treat a refractory symptom (i.e. pure symptom control), there is nothing about the term 'terminal sedation' to suggest that it could not be applied in both cases, though they are completely different from an ethical point of view. On the other hand, the term is too narrow, suggesting very clearly that this sedation leads to the end, that it is a sedation 'unto death' or, in any event, a sedation that is maintained until death. I think such a narrow conception of sedation is extremely dangerous, precisely because it tends to blur the boundaries between euthanasia and sedation. In light of these difficulties with the term 'terminal sedation', I opted to introduce the term 'palliative sedation' (Broeckaert 2000a). This term makes clear what sedation is essentially about: palliation, symptom control, an attempt to relieve patients' suffering. The term is also sufficiently broad that it can include the various different forms of sedation employed in palliative care (deep sedation, continuous sedation, temporary sedation, etc.).

Palliative sedation is not infrequently charged with being nothing more or less than a slow form of euthanasia. Although it is crucial to use a term that conveys the appropriate message, merely introducing a new term is of course not sufficient to refute this charge. Just like the term 'pain control', the term 'sedation' is used (or abused) in some cases to indicate (or camouflage) practices that should be regarded more as forms of euthanasia or ending of life without request. This is why a definition that clarifies what sedation in palliative care is and what it is not, one that explicates the meaning invoked by the term used, is a precondition for a meaningful debate on the relation between sedation and euthanasia. For some years now, I have defined palliative sedation as follows: 'the intentional administration of sedatives in such dosages and combinations as may be required to reduce the consciousness of the terminal patient in order to control one or more refractory symptoms in an adequate manner' (Broeckaert 2000b: S58).

The first thing to note about this definition is that palliative sedation is clearly an intentional medical act. It is clearly not a question of the many cases in which a terminal patient experiences reduced or diminished consciousness as a result of his or her illness or as a side-effect of a particular medication administered for some other purpose (pain control, for instance). Palliative sedation, according to this definition, is in the first place a (far-reaching) form of symptom control. In palliative sedation, everything revolves around bringing symptoms under control, in this case refractory symptoms that cannot be controlled in the traditional manner but only through consciousness reduction.[2] Now when a particular action is labelled 'symptom control', it not only means that the physician's underlying subjective intention is to control symptoms; it also means that what actually occurs on an objective level reflects this intention.

The upshot of all this can only be that, in a field where dosages and combinations are of crucial importance (if, for instance, too much is administered, then the risk of shortening life is very real), the dosages and combinations that are actually administered are proportional to the specific suffering that one is attempting to alleviate. It is for this reason that my definition places the emphasis on the adequacy and proportionality of what is done on the objective level. When a subjective intention to treat a refractory symptom does not get translated into an adequate and proportional action (i.e. administer as much as is needed), then either the intention in question was not the true intention or else it was genuine but got corrupted by other, competing intentions or by lack of experience or expertise. Any physician who deliberately and knowingly administers an overdose to shorten the patient's life must not try to delude himself or others. Whoever is not concerned with adequacy and proportionality is engaged in euthanasia or ending of life without request, not sedation. Whoever administers more than required because he is not sure what he is doing commits a medical error. It is clear that in neither case are we dealing with (adequate) palliative sedation. Though this conclusion does not, of course, resolve all the ethical questions regarding sedation, adequate palliative sedation is in any case not euthanasia, but rather an exceptional, far-reaching form of pain and symptom control.[3]

Box 19.4   Pain and symptom control

- (*Adequate*) *pain and symptom control*: the intentional administration of analgesics and/or other drugs in dosages and combinations required to adequately relieve pain and/or other symptoms
- (*Adequate*) *palliative sedation*: the intentional administration of sedative drugs in dosages and combinations required to reduce the consciousness of a terminal patient as much as necessary to adequately relieve one or more refractory symptoms

---

Active ending of life

The most controversial form of life-shortening medical action is labelled 'active ending of life'. Contrary to what was the case with forms of pain and symptom control (where shortening of life is a rare side-effect), all forms of active ending of life aim, by definition, to bring about the shortening or ending of life. The very purpose of the action, and of the one who performs the action, is to end the patient's life.

If, as we have done in the first part of this chapter, reject the term euthanasia in its broader sense, does it follow, then, that we see euthanasia as a synonym for this active ending of life? I am afraid not, for the Dutch (and Belgian) definition of euthanasia is even stricter than this. In the Netherlands, a country that for many years has followed its own path regarding euthanasia, the State Commission on Euthanasia in 1985 gave euthanasia the following strict but since then generally accepted meaning: *intentionally ending another person's life at that person's request*. This means that in the Netherlands since 1985, euthanasia is by definition active, direct and voluntary, though in this case 'voluntary' is actually not strict enough: euthanasia presupposes that the patient himself requests termination of life. So it is not a question of a patient's voluntary consent to a termination of life suggested by the physician. In its first recommendation in 1997, the Belgian Advisory Committee on Bioethics adopted the Dutch definition of euthanasia, and the recent Belgian Euthanasia Law (2002) includes exactly the same definition. The upshot is that this law, just like the Dutch euthanasia law, says nothing about forms of actively ending life without the patient's request (involuntary or non-voluntary 'euthanasia' remains illegal), or anything about passive or indirect 'euthanasia'. When I use the word 'euthanasia', it is always in this strict sense.

Active ending of life, then, can take three distinct forms (see Table 19.2), only one of these being labelled euthanasia. What is particular about the

Table 19.2 Active ending of life as a percentage of all deaths

	Flanders (1998)	Australia (1995)	Netherlands (1995)	Netherlands (1990)
Active ending of life	4.4	5.3	3.3	2.7
Euthanasia	1.1	1.7	2.4	1.7
Assisted suicide	0.1	0.1	0.2	0.2
Active ending of life without request	3.2	3.5	0.7	0.8

Sources: van der Maas *et al.* (1991, 1996), Kuhse *et al.* (1997) and Deliens *et al.* (2000).

first form, euthanasia in the strict Dutch and Belgian sense of the term, is the fact that the ultimately lethal action is taken by someone else. This means that when it is the patient who kills himself or herself (for example, by swallowing certain pills), then the word 'euthanasia' is not used. A further particularity of euthanasia is that it takes place at the patient's request. Of course, this presupposes that the patient is capable of making such a request – that is, that the patient is legally competent, or was legally competent: sometimes euthanasia can take place on the basis of an earlier request, written in a living will, rather than an actual request.

The distinction between euthanasia and assisted suicide does not lie in the fact that euthanasia applies in cases of terminal patients, while assisted suicide applies in cases of non-terminal patients (one could imagine the case of a quadriplegic patient with a normal life expectation who no longer finds life endurable). The only difference – and also the crucial difference – between the two is that in the case of euthanasia it is someone else who performs the ultimately lethal act, whereas with assisted suicide it is the patient who performs this act himself or herself. Whether or not one considers this distinction to be significant, it is a fact that in those few countries where euthanasia and/or assisted suicide is legally regulated, often the law does *not* lump them together. In Belgium, for instance, euthanasia is permitted under certain conditions. However, the Belgian Euthanasia Law says not a word about assisted suicide, so the legal status of assisted suicide is very unclear. In Switzerland and in the US state of Oregon, assisted suicide is permitted under certain conditions, but there is clearly not the same degree of permissiveness regarding euthanasia. Only the Netherlands allows both to an equal extent.

Apart from euthanasia and assisted suicide, there is still a third form of active ending of life. This comprises those cases in which death is a result of the intentional administration of lethal medication without the patient having requested it. Neither the Dutch nor the Belgian euthanasia laws make any provision for this ethically very problematic possibility (where there is no question of a request or even consent on the part of the patient). Nonetheless, it turns out that this does occur in practice, far more frequently than even the category of assisted suicide, which in absolute numbers is no more than marginal.

> **Box 19.5**　Active termination of life
>
> - *Euthanasia* (strict definition): intentionally terminating another person's life at that person's request
> - *Assisted suicide*: intentionally assisting a person to actively terminate his or her life at that person's request
> - *Active termination of life without request*: intentionally and actively terminating another person's life without that person's request

---

Conclusions

Physician-assisted death – or, viewed from the perspective of the nurse or other health care worker: life-shortening medical acts – is a daily reality that demands exceptional vigilance. Decisions are made that not only have radical effects, but that also are often essentially ethical in nature. Within the modest limits of this chapter, I have only been able to point out and explain a number of important distinctions. Further ethical reflection is needed about the different forms of life-shortening medical acts and, of course, about other important ethical problems at the end of life too.

Further reading

For an in-depth treatment of a number of ethical issues in palliative care, see Have, H. and Clark, D. (2002) (eds), *The Ethics of Palliative Care: European Perspectives*, Buckingham: Open University Press.

Notes

1　For an extensive discussion of terminology, see Broeckaert and Nuñez-Olarte (2002).
2　Refractory symptoms are symptoms that cannot be relieved normally without resorting to consciousness reduction (i.e. sedation). Which symptoms this refers to is left intentionally vague by my proposed definition. This means, of course, that not only physical but also mental symptoms can be refractory. Note that I speak here explicitly about refractory, not difficult, symptoms. See Broeckaert 2002.
3　The latter is also confirmed by the fact that on the basis of the scant available empirical evidence, it would appear that palliative sedation does not have the life-shortening effect that is so often ascribed to it. The literature shows that within the same environment, there is no observable difference in survival

periods between patients that have been sedated and those who have not (see Ventafridda *et al.* 1990; Stone *et al.* 1997; Thorns and Sykes 1999; Waller *et al.* 1999).

References

Bercovitch, M., Waller, A. and Adunsky, A. (1999) High dose morphine use in the hospice setting: a database survey of patient characteristics and effect on life expectancy. *Cancer*, 86(5): 871–7.

Broeckaert, B. (2000a) Medically mediated death: from pain control to euthanasia, in *Proceedings of the 13th World Congress on Medical Law*, Vol. 1, p. 100.

Broeckaert, B. (2000b) Palliative sedation defined or why and when terminal sedation is not euthanasia. *Journal of Pain and Symptom Management*, 20(6): S58.

Broeckaert, B. (2001) Belgium: towards a legal recognition of euthanasia. *European Journal of Health Law*, 8: 95–107.

Broeckaert, B. (2002) Palliative sedation: ethical aspects, in C. Gastmans (ed.) *Between Technology and Humanity: The Impact of Technology on Health Care Ethics*. Leuven: Leuven University Press.

Broeckaert, B. and Nuñez-Olarte, J.M. (2002) Sedation in palliative care: facts and concepts, in H. ten Have and D. Clark (eds) *The Ethics of Palliative Care: European Perspectives*. Buckingham: Open University Press.

Council of Europe (1997) Convention for the protection of Human Rights and dignity of the human being with regard to the application of biology and medicine: Convention on Human Rights and Biomedicine (ETS No. 164), Oviedo (http://conventions.coe.int/treaty/EN/cadreprincipal.htm)

Deliens, L., Mortier, F., Bilsen, J. *et al.* (2000) End-of-life decisions in medical practice in Flanders, Belgium: a nationwide survey. *The Lancet*, 356: 1806–11.

Fainsinger, R.L. (1998) Use of sedation by a hospital palliative care support team. *Journal of Palliative Care*, 14(1): 51–4.

Fainsinger, R.L., de Moissac, D., Mancini, I. and Oneschuk, D. (2000a) Sedation for delirium and other symptoms in terminally ill patients in Edmonton. *Journal of Palliative Care*, 16(2): 5–10.

Fainsinger, R.L., Waller, A., Bercovici, M. *et al.* (2000b) A multicentre international study of sedation for uncontrolled symptoms in terminally ill patients. *Palliative Medicine*, 14: 257–65.

Griffiths, J., Bood, A. and Weyers, H. (1998) *Euthanasia and Law in The Netherlands*. Amsterdam: Amsterdam University Press.

Janssens, R., ten Have, H., Broeckaert, B. *et al.* (2002) Moral values in palliative care: a European comparison, in H. ten Have and D. Clark (eds) *The Ethics of Palliative Care: European Perspectives*. Buckingham: Open University Press.

Kuhse, H., Singer, P., Baume, P., Clark, M. and Rickard, M. (1997) End-of-life decisions in Australian medical practice. *Medical Journal of Australia*, 166: 191–6.

Morita, T., Inoue, S. and Chihara, S. (1996) Sedation for symptom control in Japan: the importance of intermittent use and communication with family members. *Journal of Pain and Symptom Management*, 12: 32–8.

Morita, T., Tsunoda, J., Inoue, S. and Chihara, S. (1999) Do hospice clinicians sedate patients intending to hasten death? *Journal of Palliative Care*, 15(3): 20–3.

Porta Sales, J. (2001) Terminal sedation: a review of the clinical literature. *European Journal of Palliative Care*, 8(3): 97–100.

Porta Sales, J., Yllá-Catalá Boré, E., Estíbalez Gil, A. *et al.* (1999) Estudio multicéntrico catalano-balear sobre la sedación terminal en Cuidados Paliativos. *Medicina Paliativa*, 6(4): 153–8.

Stone, P., Phillips, C., Spruyt, O. and Waight, C. (1997) A comparison of the use of sedatives in a hospital support team and in a hospice. *Palliative Medicine*, 11: 140–4.

Thorns, A. and Sykes, N. (1999) Opioid use in the last week of life and the implications for end of life decision making, in *Proceedings of the 6th Congress of European Association of Palliative Care*. Geneva: EAPC.

van der Maas, P.J., van Delden, J.J.M., Pijnenborg, L. and Looman, C.W.N. (1991) Euthanasia and other medical practices concerning the end of life. *The Lancet*, 338: 699–74.

van der Maas, P.J., van der Wal, G. and Haverkate, I. (1996) Euthanasia, physician-assisted suicide, and other medical practices involving the end of life in the Netherlands. *New England Journal of Medicine*, 335: 1699–705.

Ventafridda, V., Ripamonti, C., deConno, F., Tamburini, M. and Cassileth, B.R. (1990) Symptom prevalence and control during cancer patients' last days of life. *Journal of Palliative Care*, 6(3): 7–11.

Waller, A., Bercovitch, M., Fainsinger, R.L. and Adunsky, A. (1999) Symptom control and the need for sedation during treatment in Tel Hashomer in-patient hospice, in *Proceedings of the 6th Congress of the European Association of Palliative Care*. Geneva: EAPC.

20

The impact of socialization on the dying process

Kay Mitchell

There are many aspects that are common across cultures (culture-common) rather than specific to one culture only (culture-specific) and there are certain values related to the dying experience that appear to be universally shared. This includes the hope that death will be achieved peacefully with minimal suffering and in the way preferred by the dying person (Kashiwagi 1991). However, the way this goal is achieved may differ between cultures and these differences may render some aspects of the death and dying experience 'culture-specific'. We are born, live and die within a social context and this chapter is an attempt to explore how socialization within such a context may impact on the dying experience. Here, I take culture to refer to the social context within which the person lives and works – the macro-culture of country of domicile, but also the institutions that form micro-cultures within each country, such as professional discipline, religion and ethnicity. The term 'society' is taken to refer to the wider social context, which may contain many micro-cultures.

Cultural relativism, a theory about the nature of morality, reminds us that many of our own beliefs probably owe more to cultural teaching than absolute truth (Rachels 1993). The social institutions that inform end-of-life care may be comparable on a macro level across many countries (e.g. the law, health, medicine and social values). However, the interpretation and application of philosophical values within these institutions may differ and it is here that the value of comparison becomes evident in exposing the culturally relevant perspective. Viewing seemingly different perspectives of two cultures through an ethnocentric lens, we may sometimes overestimate these differences.

Rachels (1993) uses the example of a very poor culture who believe that it is wrong to eat cows. Although people may starve, the cows remain untouched. The values in this culture appear very different from the values of a culture that puts the life of humans before the life of animals. However, the difference is in the significance of the cow. While one culture believes it is an animal less than human and to be used by humans, the other believes the cow may be the reincarnation of someone's dead grandmother. Both cultures agree – grandma should not be eaten. However, only one of the cultures believes that the cow could be grandma. The difference lies in our belief systems, not in our values (Rachels 1993). 'The realisation that different behaviors serve similar goals, and that *differences can be interpreted only in relation to the pursuit of those goals in different cultures* is one of the most important contributions that cross-cultural research has made (Brislin 1993: 86; emphasis added).

Differences in the way cultures 'do' dying are reported and thoughtfully challenge our own cultural beliefs. Discussing the differences between the psychological care of the dying in Japan and those in the West, Kashiwagi (1991) stated: 'Asiatic people [find] it difficult to express fear and anger in comparison to the West and . . . it [is] up to the physicians to develop Asiatic means of communicating to their people so that *their emotions are expressed*' (p. S99; emphasis added). By acknowledging that Asiatic people find it difficult to express emotion, Kashiwagi is exposing a culture-specific norm. However, by suggesting that the expression of emotion in dying is a goal worthy of pursuit, he is adopting the philosophy of a Western-developed institution (hospice) and applying it to a situation in his non-Western culture.

Along similar lines, until very recently the concept of brain death was not accepted in Japan and the harvesting of organs from persons with no cortical function obviously could not purposefully proceed. Elsewhere for many years such patients have been kept ventilated until the organs could usefully be taken. Cultural differences abound in end-of-life care from truth-telling with cancer diagnoses (Seale 1998) to the acceptance of morphine use for terminally ill patients (Zenz and Willweber-Strumpf 1993) or the provision of physician-assisted death (Leenaars and Conolly 2001).

Internationally, countries have taken their lead in end-of-life care from the seminal work of Dame Cicely Saunders and the early hospice movement (Saunders 2000). Palliative care for the terminally ill patient is seen as compassionate and appropriate care when symptoms are distressing. However, the cultural context within which the dying is occurring may see this 'culture-common' aspect of terminal care presenting with 'culture-specific' characteristics. When considering diversity in the field of death and dying, physician-assisted death provides a useful comparison between two seemingly opposing approaches to end-of-life care. Physician-assisted death is also a point where the socialization of the practitioner may impact on care offered. In this chapter, I do not argue for or against physician-assisted death as a practice. I merely use it as an example of how socialization may influence a practitioner's actions or a practitioner's discourse related to professional practice in end-of-life care. The terms 'physician-assisted death' and 'euthanasia' are used interchangeably, but both are taken to mean the intentional ending of the life of the patient as a result of actions taken by the physician.

Universally, the taking of innocent life has been frowned upon, but increasingly abortion (which can be argued as just such an action) and physician-assisted death (which is most certainly such an action) are accommodated if not encouraged in many countries. There is a difference *between* countries in their approaches to end-of-life decision making, but there is also a difference *within* countries that are peopled by representatives of many cultures, ethnic backgrounds and philosophical persuasions. Added to this, individualistic cultures such as the USA, New Zealand, Australia, the Netherlands and the UK encourage autonomy of thought and action, allowing for individual differences in approaches to decision making. In fact, the issue of patient autonomy in determining the manner and time of death became a focus of public concern in the Netherlands and in Oregon, and was instrumental in the subsequent formalization and ultimate legalization of physician-assisted death in those places (Griffiths *et al.* 1998; Oregon Public Health Services 2000). There were many societal 'forces' that came together to debate the legalization of physician-assisted death in Oregon and the Netherlands, including those of the government (state legislature in the case of Oregon), Church, judiciary, medical and lay opinion.

On an informal and *ad hoc* level, the same philosophical underpinnings related to personal autonomy, justice and patient preference preface the decision making of practitioners in other countries, leading some to consider that physician-assisted death should be available. But when society does not support this practice, a physician may find that, what is perceived to be the most compassionate option for some patients, is not legally available.

One doctor in New Zealand spoke of regret that one of his patients had been 'saved' from a suicide attempt when the need for death was clearly articulated by the patient and considered justified under the circumstances:

> But there is no doubt that there will be situations where people feel that this is their only option and I guess, I mean, thinking about it, you must accept that some people come to this decision and in some way you wonder if that should not be an option for such patients to have the right to have that. I mean, that would be a very very, small number but I think there is – I mean, a typical example is where a patient can't do anything for themselves any more, tetraplegics for example. And I mean, that's one of the situations where I can imagine that people would desperately try, and one of my patients recently desperately tried, a tetraplegic patient, to kill himself. A failed attempt, which was the only way he could manage which was running his wheelchair into a pond. Regrettably somebody jumped in after him and pulled him out. And I mean, for these people, if they make a conscious and open decision that this is their wish, I think if you think about self-determination, there might need to be the need to offer that option.
>
> (New Zealand pain specialist)

This highlights an anomaly that can occur for patients who suffer injuries that render them paralysed and incapacitated beyond what they can bear but who breathe independently, and those who suffer a similar fate and who require ventilation. Recently, such a patient in New Zealand requested his mechanical ventilation be removed after months of rehabilitation and counselling. He died at home shortly afterwards (NZPA 2000). However, the patient referred to by the physician above also clearly wanted to die but his physical disability restricted possibilities for suicide and under New Zealand law he could not receive active assistance to die, a situation at least one of his physicians clearly regretted.

Alternatively, if a physician does not support physician-assisted death (despite this being a legal option), what is perceived to be the most compassionate option for the patient is not *morally* available. In such contexts, the physician must (a) agree to physician-assisted death despite possible legal/moral consequences, (b) refuse physician-assisted death and continue with palliative care even when this may not meet patient need, or (c) agree to help the patient to die but formulate the actions taken in a way that preserves a societal or self-image that does not condone physician-assisted death.

Palliative care or euthanasia – a cultural semantic?

Traditionally, palliative care providers have spoken against physician-assisted death as contravening the core of ethical medical practice (Mount 1996). However, research among Dutch doctors (Mitchell 2002) suggests that those who have performed euthanasia believe that it is at the extreme end of the palliative care continuum. As one Dutch doctor put it:

> Euthanasia is only to be considered after all the other possibilities have been exhausted, after the best possible terminal care including palliative care. Euthanasia is certainly not something to choose as another choice opposed to palliative care. I see it on the same continuum. Not parallel, not one or the other, but one after the other.
>
> (Dutch general practitioner)

It is clear that this doctor is allying euthanasia with palliative care in his practice and this raises the question of how influential his cultural context has been in shaping his approach to end-of-life care. Elsewhere, discussions with a Dutch family about their experiences when a family member had received euthanasia indicated that the event had had a profound influence on the grandchildren of the family. Several years later, the grandson was at medical school and the granddaughter was doing her nursing training; each was positive about the euthanasia experience and saw a place for it in their future professional practice, if necessary. Whether such attitudes are a result of a true belief that euthanasia is a necessary option or as a result of a need to remember their grandfather's death in a positive way, is open for conjecture. Whatever the reason, euthanasia was legitimized as a way of doing death in that family just as it had been legitimized as a way of doing death in the wider social context – the availability of the action providing opportunity for socialization into another way of achieving death.

Traditionally, palliative care proponents have argued that efficient palliative care is sufficient to address patient suffering, making agreement to euthanasia unnecessary. When the patient's symptoms are difficult to control and suffering is intractable and unbearable, then terminal sedation is suggested as an option after careful assessment (Rousseau 1996). In most countries where physician-assisted death is illegal, terminal sedation is legal. Similarly, those who disagree with physician-assisted death and who practise in societies that condone this, can morally offer sedation to their patients given that the action is condoned under the principle of double effect and supported by hospice philosophy. However, the principle of double effect has received much scrutiny and criticism (Billings and Block 1996). One Dutch doctor suggested that knowing that death was the outcome of the action rendered it equivalent to euthanasia:

> Yes, but what's curing the problem for a lung cancer patient with very heavy dyspnoea. Huh? Morphine until he's unconscious? What are you doing? I think with morphine until unconscious, I believe that is the way to euthanasia.
>
> (Dutch nursing home doctor)

Living in a country where euthanasia is legal allows this physician to question openly the concept of terminal sedation, knowing that even if he, or society as a whole, decided that this is in fact 'euthanasia', it will still be possible to offer this option to those patients who may benefit from it. In a country where euthanasia is not legal, physicians may feel constrained by such open exploration of the ethics of the action, fearing that censure would prevent terminal sedation from being available when required. Furthermore, it is suggested that it may be in the best interests of the doctors not to endorse transparency of practice in making such decisions in order to pre-serve 'maximal wiggle room' (Brody 1996: 40). This will allow doctors who engage in such actions to present to themselves and others an account of these actions in a manner that preserves the ethical and moral assumptions of accepted medical practice within their society (Brody 1996). Similarly, the doctors will be able to present accounts of these actions in ways that preserve personal philosophy and belief systems related to end-of-life care.

Whatever position is adopted regarding terminal sedation, that it is palliative care or that it is 'slow euthanasia' (Billings and Block 1996), it may not always be a viable option as these two doctors have experienced. These accounts provide an interesting example of how the context within which the physicians practised (New Zealand and the Netherlands) may have impacted on the discursive representations of actions by the doctors concerned.

One experienced hospice doctor in New Zealand spoke of a patient who died within minutes of having drugs administered intrathecally to control unbearable pain after morphine and other drugs had been ineffective for over a week. This patient was dying with 'inordinate suffering'. Terminal sedation was attempted but could not be achieved. Midazolam and barbiturates, the drugs normally used for sedation, were ineffective, something this doctor had not experienced before:

> The most medically traumatic patient that I have cared for was a woman who was in her 30s with a breast cancer and had a particularly painful cancer and some cancers are particularly painful, and she had spinal metastases which gave most of the pain. And she had a lot of

intervention including an intrathecal catheter and a central line. And she, in retrospect, got ahh tolerance to morphine or that ahh morphine aggravated her pain, and ahh, and she was in the hospice and the pain control fluctuated wildly over the week . . . ahh there were times when we would have liked to have sedated her to relieve her of suffering but we couldn't. Ahh which was new to me and we used an awful lot of barbiturates and Midazolam without being able to sedate her which was obviously distressing for all that were concerned . . . she died within five or ten minutes of the administration of ahh local anaesthetic into the spine.

(New Zealand hospice doctor)

When he was questioned as to whether he felt comfortable that the action taken had not precipitated the patient's death, he stated that the local anaesthetic administered had stopped the pain, which had been acting as an 'antidote' to the morphine and other drugs administered. Once the pain had been stopped, the other drugs may have overwhelmed the patient and been implicated in death. When asked if he thought that the intervention had caused the death of the patient, the doctor struggled to answer, pausing frequently to consider his words.

Um . . . there's . . . um there's a feeling that the intervention um was the straw that broke the camel's back um and that the um . . . the pain relief that that brought may have brought all the other medications that had been lurking in the background that had been antidoted by the pain into um . . . play.

I said, 'Antidote to the morphine . . . would you like to just explain that?' The doctor continued:

Ahh . . . Although um, morphine is a sedative and a respiratory depressant, um, the effects of the morphine can be held off if somebody is really um, very anxious and there is a lot of emotional energy running around um, then the morphine will not be sedative or depressant and we run into trouble . . . And so pain would seem, ahh, the stimulating effects of pain would keep people awake. Does it keep people alive? Well, um . . . that's a discussion that we have. It would certainly keep people awake. And sometimes that consciousness means that people keep on struggling on.

(New Zealand hospice doctor)

This explanation for why the patient died within minutes of receiving an intrathecal infusion may be technically correct as far as pharmacodynamics are concerned. However, there does appear to be an element of rationalization present to prevent exploring the possibility that immediate death was caused by the last intervention. In a society where physician-assisted death is illegal, practitioners involved in such cases may not feel free to fully disclose and discuss cause and effect, fearing repercussions.

In addition to terminal sedation not always being technically possible to achieve, a Dutch palliative care physician suggested that terminal sedation is not always a compassionate or appropriate option for the patient.

I know of a young woman of not so long ago . . . she had had a very, very difficult life. We often think when you read in a book that it can't really be that bad, but sometimes life is really worse than you could ever think of . . . She was 22, and was dying of cancer. And for her, with her history, the idea of being asleep and of not being able to control her life which had been such an anxious and insecure life, she could not bear the idea. And so my colleagues could understand that this was impossible for her in this specific situation. The only possibility was euthanasia because that would be a way she could die quickly. So it all happened as it should happen, you know, telling the police. So that's why I say, 'never say never', because in this special circumstance, there was no choice. For me it was uncomfortable, but for her with her history, it was not. And then, well I had promised her to be there, and I saw it happen. It was frightening, but that was a consequence of the choice I made, it was a free choice. (I had promised I would be there! Always! Whatever happens!) [handwritten on transcript].

(Dutch nursing home palliative unit doctor)

Despite a personal belief against physician-assisted death, this doctor was legally able to explore this fully with her patient when she believed it was the most compassionate option. Working within a society where euthanasia is accepted as part of end-of-life care, discussions about individual cases between doctors and between doctors and their patients would be frank. In accordance with her promise, this doctor chose to stay with her patient while she received euthanasia, fulfilling one of the tenets of palliative care related to non-abandonment. This was an arguably courageous decision given the effect on the doctor, who found the experience 'frightening'. Elsewhere a Dutch hospice doctor reiterated that he would never perform euthanasia, in part because of fear of the personal effect on himself.

In very exceptional cases, I can imagine very well that euthanasia may be one of the possibilities . . . I would be very afraid to do this . . . Um, I think if I will get through this border, I will not be the same person. I will not be able to do this [hospice work]. Afraid of this. So I can accept that this border exists, and also have respect for people who are providing euthanasia, but I would be very reluctant to do this myself.

(Dutch hospice doctor)

This doctor expresses 'respect' for doctors who perform euthanasia. This expression came after his statement, 'Afraid of this', suggesting his respect may be for doctors who perform euthanasia despite the personal cost to themselves, rather than for doctors who perform euthanasia *per se*. The above comments from Dutch doctors are remarkable for their tolerance of disparate views related to the provision of physician-assisted death. Perhaps their shared enculturation within a society that has accepted euthanasia as a way of doing death has encouraged increased tolerance for the practice even among those who are opposed to it on moral, ethical or religious grounds. Whether this is evidence of a devolution or evolution in end-of-life care in the Netherlands is a matter for debate.

Just as individuals in the Netherlands would agree with the international view that physician-assisted death is ethically and morally wrong (Zylicz and Janssens 1998), there are individuals in societies that do not condone physician-assisted death who would agree that this is sometimes the most compassionate option for some patients (Quill 1993). However, the effect of providing assisted death clearly has a profound effect on the physician, which may be unexpected.

One Dutch doctor described the action as crossing a line proscribed by the Catholic Church and society. Crossing the line placed the doctor beyond the point that human beings can legitimately place themselves. He seems to suggest that he has 'played God' by performing euthanasia. It was not until he had performed the euthanasia that he was aware of these feelings, and they took him by surprise. He perceived that the 'line' he had crossed now became a barrier between him and any future relationship with the Church:

> I haven't been in church for nine years. I quit church. But at that moment I thought, you can't go back there either. You have crossed a line where the Catholic church says you can never cross that line, it is not for a human being, a human person to decide to cross that line. So, it, it took me by surprise. I wouldn't have thought that after all these years I would think in such a way about the line that you cross. Which is a line that is put upon you by church, but also by the normal Christian-Jewish morality which has been there for ages. The whole culture, the whole way of approaching ethics, morality, society as it runs, is based on some agreement that you do this and you don't do that.
>
> (Dutch nursing home doctor)

Agreeing to give someone euthanasia may be justified, but once it happens there is no going back. This doctor continued by portraying performing euthanasia as 'losing your innocence', emphasizing the exceptional nature of the event. Giving euthanasia made this doctor more aware that the practice should not be entered into lightly and should not be granted as a 'right' for patients. By likening performing euthanasia to losing virginity, he seems to imply that for the doctor there is a before-euthanasia state and an after-euthanasia state and that the latter is perhaps baser than the former. Although he *says* he does not regret the action, the doctor reiterates the exceptional nature of the act:

> And it is one of the agreements, maybe on good grounds, but it is one of the agreements you cross, it is like losing your innocence, or losing your virginity or something like that. It is very important, and one time it happens. You make it one time, and you never can go back. And it sharpened me in the way that I always thought it was a two way thing, but I am very – it sharpened my senses to say 'Don't talk about it too easily, don't think it is a right you can obtain access to'.

I said, 'Mmmm. Are you sorry you did it?' The doctor continued:

> No, I think I – I think it made me richer, but I have my doubts now and again. I think in that case, it was a good thing to do, but I think that it

should be the very extreme, and very careful decision. It shouldn't be part of the package. It shouldn't be the routine in the clinic every month, or every two weeks, or something like that . . . you should make a careful decision, and you can't do that every week or every month, you have to take your time. You can't turn back [emotional].

(Dutch nursing home doctor)

It is clear, therefore, that transparency of practice associated with such an action not only provides protection for the patient and their family, but also for the physician. Debriefing after the event and receiving support from colleagues for actions taken would perhaps assist in coming to terms with the death. This doctor struggled emotionally with what he had done, but was able to talk this through openly. Those who provide physician-assisted death in a society that does not condone such actions must act and 'recover', alone and in secret.

The above also raises another issue. Once the practice of physician-assisted death becomes part of the way a culture 'does' death, individuals may feel under some pressure to provide it when they believe it is the most compassionate option for the patient. Clearly, this doctor and the previous Dutch doctor who accompanied her patient while she received euthanasia had moral reservations about the action, but this did not prevent them going along with the patient – at considerable personal cost. Where physician-assisted death is not culturally accepted, physicians would not be exposed to such pressure. As one New Zealand doctor put it:

Maybe if I saw cases where . . . pain that we couldn't end and that was absolutely inadequately dealt with, then maybe it's time to get into that realm but . . . it extracts a huge huge moral price . . . It's easier to deal with that if it's not on the agenda and just say 'Sorry'.

(New Zealand general practitioner)

The cultural prohibition on physician-assisted death provides a protection for the practitioners who may proceed as conscience dictates without the added pressure of an expectation by patient and/or society that this should proceed. Each country must decide for itself whether it is comfortable leaving such decision making in the hands of individual practitioners, which is the *status quo* in all countries except the Netherlands and the state of Oregon in the USA. There is empirical evidence that physicians in other countries are providing physician-assisted death, despite the prohibition (Kuhse *et al.* 1997; Mitchell 2002).

Obeying the highest imperative

Across many countries, those who work in palliative and/or hospice care share a culture-common mandate to serve the dying and their families. However, any movement or discipline is made up of individuals and it is the individuals in combination who will ultimately determine the direction the discipline will take. The beliefs that individual care workers subscribe to are informed by the wider social context in which they live. They are also informed by the culture of the discipline within which they operate. As we have observed in the preceding case studies, sometimes the imperatives of one may conflict with the other. At times, what is perceived by the practitioner to be the most compassionate and just option for the patient is not available according to the tenets of society. For others, society may condone an action but the tenets of the discipline provide constraint. Some practitioners solve the dilemma by following their personal conscience. Others express relief that they do not need to do so, rather invoking the rules of the discipline, or the society, as reasons for their choice in practice. While the latter may feel comfortable maintaining the *status quo*, the former who act from personal conscience will be constantly challenged by the ethics, morality and/or legality of their actions. Such challenges may be uncomfortable and ultimately these practitioners may seek ways of resolving their dilemma by challenging society to re-think rules and laws. This is the way of social change and, in the field of death and dying, can be applied to physician-assisted death, truth-telling in cancer diagnosis and withdrawing life-sustaining measures.

Once a person is socialized into a culture, there is pressure to conform to the norms expressed in the culture (wider society or within discipline). Failure to conform may result in alienation from the group. Three ways that social influences control a person's behaviour are conformity, compliance and obedience. Social psychologists have demonstrated the effect of social influences on the individual. Group pressure to conform affects behaviour, so that individuals may question their own senses even when they perceive that they are correct (Asch 1952). Similarly, an individual may obey the instructions of authority figures even when these go against personally held beliefs (Milgram 1974).

A theory that investigates the nature and impact of social influence is the theory of social impact (Latane 1981). Latane suggests that social forces with predetermined characteristics operate to exert an effect on the individual (target). These characteristics relate to the strength or intensity of impact, the immediacy or absence of barriers to the target and the number of sources influencing the target. The theory proposes that the greater the strength, the more immediate the influence and the greater the number of sources exerting influence on a target, the stronger the impact and data typically bear this out (Latane 1981). We can apply such reasoning when considering, for instance, a request for physician-assisted death that is perceived to be justified by the doctor. If the request is considered justified because of intractable suffering (strength), and comes directly from the suffering patient for whom the doctor is caring (immediacy) and wider society condones and supports the action in such cases (number), the physician will be under some pressure to conform to the request. However, if the request comes from a similar patient with the same strength, same immediacy but not supported by wider society (less number), the pressure to conform will be weakened. As one New Zealand doctor commented previously,

'It's easier to deal with that if it's not on the agenda and just say "Sorry".' If the request for physician-assisted death occurs in a hospice situation (culture that does not support the practice), the strength and immediacy will be the same, but there will be no support within that context, even when that context is set within a wider society that supports physician-assisted death. Therefore, the impact of number will be weakened.

However, the individual is not passive in this process. The physician will also have an influence on the process via personal characteristics. Bhaskar (1979) discussed the transactional nature of any social situation by incorporating the influence of the individual in a transformational social impact model. When examining the individual and society considering physician-assisted death, we can overlay the social impact model with the transformational model and reflect the dynamic relationship between the individual and society, each becoming both source (of impact) and target (of impact). This can occur through:

- passive acceptance of the *status quo* (i.e. assisted death is tolerated or not tolerated);
- active resistance to the practice;
- support for the practice;
- participation in the practice.

The individual and society impact on each other, the relative force of the impact in either direction depending on the direction in which the intensity of strength, immediacy or number is moving. Thus we have some practitioners responding to requests as per the *status quo*, while some will be persuaded by other influencing forces according to their strongest personal imperative.

Conclusions

We are all culturally conditioned, creatures of our environmental context. Across many countries, those who work in palliative and/or hospice care share a culturally common mandate to serve the dying and their families. There may be different culturally specific values or belief systems that affect how that mandate is fulfilled. By embedding the different approaches to achieving the same end within a background of shared meaning of what the desired end is, we adopt the recommendation for effective cross-cultural understanding (Triandis 1994: 66). Or as Shweder (1991) suggests, to 'talk of differences one must first demonstrate likeness or equivalences' (p. 289).

Social impact theory provides a theoretical framework within which to examine how the individual and society impact on each other in the field of terminal care. Individuals are socialized into specific cultures and maintain societal structures even as those structures impact on and form the individual. However, the individual need not be passive and may apply pressure on society to promote change in the way we live and the way we die.

References

Asch, S.E. (1952) *Social Psychology*. Englewood Cliffs, NJ: Prentice-Hall.

Bhaskar, R. (1979) *The Possibility of Naturalism: A Philosophical Critique of the Contemporary Human Sciences*. Brighton: Harvester Press.

Billings, J.A. and Block, S.D. (1996). Slow euthanasia. *Journal of Palliative Care*, 12(4): 21–30.

Brislin, R. (1993) *Understanding Culture's Influence on Behaviour*. Fort Worth, TX: Harcourt Brace & Co.

Brody, H. (1996) Commentary on Billings and Block's 'Slow Euthanasia'. *Journal of Palliative Care*, 12(4): 38–41.

Griffiths, J., Bood, A. and Weyers, H. (1998) *Euthanasia and Law in the Netherlands*. Amsterdam: Amsterdam University Press.

Kashiwagi, T. (1991) Hospice care in Japan. *Postgraduate Medical Journal*, 67(suppl. 2): S95–S99.

Kuhse, H., Singer, P., Baume, P., Clark, M. and Rickard, M. (1997) End-of-life decisions in Australian medical practice. *Medical Journal of Australia*, 166: 191–6.

Latane, B. (1981) The psychology of social impact. *American Psychologist*, 36(4): 343–56.

Leenaars, A. and Conolly, J. (2001) Suicide, assisted suicide and euthanasia: international perspectives. *Irish Journal of Psychiatric Medicine*, 18(1): 33–7.

Milgram, S. (1974) *Obedience to Authority*. New York: Harper & Row.

Mitchell, K. (2002) Medical decisions at the end of life that hasten death. PhD thesis, University of Auckland.

Mount, B. (1996) Morphine drips, terminal sedation, and slow euthanasia: definitions and facts, not anecdotes. *Journal of Palliative Care*, 12(4): 31–7.

NZPA (2000) Death of a patient who begged to die. *The Dominion*, 16 November, p. 19.

Oregon Public Health Services (2000) Oregon's Death with Dignity Act: Three years of legalized physician-assisted suicide. Eugene, OR: Oregon Public Health Services (http://www.ohd.hr.state.or.us/chs/pas/ar-index.htm), accessed 23 November 2001.

Quill, T.E. (1993) Doctor, I want to die. Will you help me? *Journal of the American Medical Association*, 270(7): 870–4.

Rachels, J. (1993) *The Challenge of Cultural Relativism: The Elements of Moral Philosophy*, 2nd edn. New York: McGraw-Hill.

Rousseau, P. (1996) Terminal sedation in the care of dying patients. *Archives of Internal Medicine*, 156: 1785–6.

Saunders, C. (2000) The evolution of palliative care. *Patient Education and Counseling*, 41: 7–13.

Seale, C. (1998) Theories and studying the care of dying people. *British Medical Journal*, 317: 1518–20.

Shweder, R.A. (1991). *Thinking Through Cultures*. Cambridge, MA: Harvard University Press.

Triandis, H.C. (1994) *Cultural and Social Behavior*. New York: McGraw-Hill.

Zenz, M. and Willweber-Strumpf, A. (1993) Opiophobia and cancer pain in Europe. *The Lancet*, 341: 1075–6.

Zylicz, Z. and Janssens, M.J.P.A. (1998) Options in palliative care: dealing with those who want to die. *Baillière's Clinical Anaesthesiology*, 12(1): 121–31.

21

Palliative care in institutions

Jeanne Samson Katz

In the UK, palliative or hospice care is often synonymous with hospice buildings, where people with cancer are believed to go to die in their last weeks of life. However, end-of-life care takes place in many different situations and settings and, indeed, as Chapter 15 has identified, the longest period of the terminal phase is usually spent in one's own home. However, in the twenty-first century in Western industrialized societies, we have an ageing population and in the UK there are more people over the age of 60 than under 16 years of age (Office of National Statistics 2002). Unlike the nineteenth century, when most people died at home, changes in family and household composition have impacted on the site of care for dying people. In the UK, health and social care policies have resulted in a reduction in long- stay hospital beds for older people, yet hospitals are still the most likely site of death.

The development of palliative care in the UK is described in Chapter 2. Suffice it to note here that, unlike in the USA, palliative care services in the UK developed by focusing on 'buildings with in-patient provision'. With the opening of St Christopher's in 1967, the prototype of palliative care services was established in an 'institutional' base, although the intention was to ensure that the environment was un-institutional in a conventional sense. This meant that 'wards' were to be as home-like as possible, hospice staff would often refrain from wearing uniforms and an informal approach to relationships between hospice personnel and dying people (not patients) and their families would predominate.

Very shortly after the founding of St Christopher's, other palliative care services began in the UK and, partly for funding reasons, many of these services began as home care services, while funding was being sought to create a 'proper hospice' (e.g. North London hospice). So although this chapter focuses primarily on palliative care in institutions, the history, philosophy and practice of the kind of palliative care that takes place in institutions such as hospices and hospitals are intertwined with those in the community. This is less the case in prisons and care homes.

The way in which the services in in-patient hospices have developed has had a 'ripple effect' on all other palliative care services in the UK and elsewhere (Hockley 1997). For this reason, I first explore hospices and hospitals and then look in more depth at two other institutional settings, which, to date, are not wholly part of the palliative care network: prisons and residential and nursing homes.

Much has been researched and written about the efficacy of treatments available to people with palliative care needs. This includes the effectiveness of medication as well as other methods to relieve symptoms such as breathlessness (Corner 2001) and constipation (Bruera *et al.* 1994). Other studies have explored the extent to which, for example, volunteers have contributed to the running of hospice and palliative care services and their needs for training (Cummings 1999). Surprisingly, however, relatively little research has evaluated the provision of palliative care services according to type of service. In this chapter, I review the secondary evidence currently available about the quality of the services provided for dying people and their carers by statutory and voluntary health services and suggest areas for future enquiry.

Palliative care in hospices

The development of hospice and palliative care services in the UK was spearheaded initially by a push from voluntary groups to establish a 'hospice', a purpose-built or adapted building housing in-patient beds. The funding for the establishment and running of hospices varies even today; for example, finance may come exclusively from voluntary or independent organizations (registered charities), or in part from the National Health Service: NHS palliative care units or centres; Macmillan Cancer Care units, funded by the charity Macmillan Cancer Relief; and Marie Curie Centres and Sue Ryder homes, funded by the charities of the same names. The 2002 Hospice Directory lists 208 NHS and voluntary in-patient hospices; these include ten Marie Curie Centres and seven Sue Ryder Palliative Care Centre homes. Due to the initial unplanned development of in-patient units, they are spread rather unevenly throughout the UK, with the highest concentration in the south-east of England (Clark and Seymour 1999).

Twenty per cent of the free-standing specialist palliative care units are run by the NHS. Even where statutory provision is not available, most people in the UK requiring in-patient hospice care can be admitted to voluntary hospices (usually constituted as an independent charity) through contractual funding arrangements with health authorities.

Organizations delivering in-patient care for terminally ill people call themselves by a number of names, the most common of which are 'hospices', 'hospice wards' or 'dedicated specialist palliative care units'. They may be (a) wards within a general or specialist hospital, (b) free-standing buildings within the grounds of a hospital (general or specialist) or (c) not attached to any other particular hospital or medical/health setting (Doyle 1999). At the beginning of the twenty-first century, 80 per cent of in-patient provision in the UK is in the form of free-standing, geographically separate, independently funded hospices (Doyle 1999: 44).

Initially, hospice and palliative care services addressed, almost exclusively, the needs of people dying from cancer and, in many ways, these needs determined the nature of the services ultimately developed. As many hospices have foundations that explicitly state that services are exclusively for people with cancer, getting round these regulations has proven quite difficult to provide services for people with other diseases who also have palliative care needs. The focus on cancer has persisted – in 2000, of 40,000 new patients admitted to in-patient units, only 4 per cent did not have a cancer diagnosis; these non-cancer diagnoses include HIV/AIDS, motor neurone disease, heart disease and stroke.[1] (Children's hospices, however, focus on a much wider range of diseases, as children usually die of degenerative diseases. At the start of the children's hospice movement, hospices were established primarily to provide respite care for children and their families.) The average hospice unit in the UK accommodates 15 in-patients, although units range in size from two to 48 beds (Doyle 1999); three of every seven patients are discharged to another setting and the average stay in a hospice is 13.5 days.

In-patient hospices are designed with dying people in mind. Planning includes facilitating easy access to beds and facilities for carers as well as dying people themselves; in addition, where possible, the environment is emotionally warm and home-like. The physical location of a hospice building can influence the ways in which it operates; for example, a hospice on a hospital site might benefit from the advice of hospital personnel yet might have conflicts with hospital management (Doyle 1999). Hospices away from hospitals do not have the on-site availability of diagnostic facilities, or easy access to consultant advice. The composition of hospice staff is far from standard and this may influence the ethos of the hospice. Johnson *et al.* (1990) conducted a survey which indicated a difference in perspective between hospices with full-time medical personnel, who described their centres in a more technical way, and those without, who focused on different issues.

A unique feature of the modern hospice is the goal to achieve a complementary and non-hierarchical relationship between voluntary (unpaid) and professional (paid) staff. Some of the voluntary staff, particularly in the early days, were themselves qualified health professionals delivering care on a voluntary basis. There is considerable variation between units in staffing arrangements, although most units aspire to one nurse per 1.5 patients 24 hours a day and one consultant physician for every 10–15 patients (Doyle 1999). Medical and nursing staff with training in specialist palliative care are the backbone of the paid staffing of most hospices (see discussion about training in Chapter 35). Additionally, staff with palliative care qualifications or experience often include pharmacists, physiotherapists, occupational therapists, chaplains, social workers and complementary therapists. Other staff include domestic and administrative workers, gardeners, maintenance workers and often a large group of trained and regularly supervised volunteers providing many services, including befriending, home visiting, art and music therapy, and assisting in the general running of the hospice. Patients are usually admitted to an in-patient unit for one of three reasons: to achieve symptom control, to give dying people or their informal carers respite (a few days relief with assured quality of care) or for terminal care when dying people have reached the end stage. Over 65 per cent of hospice patients are over 65 and there is no significant difference between the sexes (Clark and Seymour 1999). As pointed out by Koffman and Camps in Chapter 18, ethnic minorities have been under-represented in hospice admissions, with several explanations being proposed to explain this anomaly: from GPs assuming that people from ethnic minorities would not want admission to a hospice to people from ethnic minorities not being offered this facility to the same extent as the host population.[2]

Hospices provide a range of services for dying people in addition to conventional in-patient services – for example, day care services, beauty therapy, complementary therapies and bereavement care. Day care services are an integral part of hospice provision in the UK, the first such service being established in 1975 at St Luke's Hospice in Sheffield (Myers and Hearn 2001). Current figures suggest that there are 243 day care units, which, on average, cater for 14 patients per day. Altogether, 32,500 patients are cared for annually by day care. Hospice palliative day care provides support in a variety of ways for dying people, ranging from sophisticated medical support (i.e. assessing appropriate drug dosage) and physical care to social, emotional and practical support. Activities provided for day care patients include stimulating them and encouraging them to participate in relaxation and other therapies. Supervised care of dying people also provides respite for home carers. As with other services, these are usually free.

Palliative care researchers have been trying to justify in-patient hospice care in the UK. Anecdotal evidence suggests that, for the past 20 years, the quality of life while dying in a hospice is considerably better than in other settings. After all, that is what hospices set out to do. Clark and Seymour (1999) note that, in the UK, information has been collected and evaluated in palliative care units to improve care. Attempts to demonstrate the value of in-patient hospice care usually make comparisons between hospice and other forms of care. Clark and Seymour (1999) observe that 'All the evidence so far reviewed suggests that those who receive hospice care value it particularly for the "human" approach it can offer, for the reductions in anxiety and improvements in communication it can achieve and for the standards and style of nursing care which it delivers' (p. 167). But Salisbury *et al.* (1999) note that measuring the impact of palliative care on patients' quality of life is not an easy task. Reviewing all the relevant studies, they found some, albeit dated, evidence that dying people in in-patient palliative care facilities receive better pain control than those receiving palliative care at home or in hospital.

In the UK, the 'hospice building' itself personifies 'palliative care' and is seen as an ideal type. James and Field (1992) courageously noted how 'routinization' and 'medicalization' had crept into hospice care and, indeed, reflected some of the concerns about conventional medical care in relation to caring for dying people. These critiques were sustained throughout the 1990s with further comments about the extent to which hospice care had been absorbed into mainstream health care and had lost its potential to lead and innovate (Corner and Dunlop 1997). In relation to in-patient hospice care, Lawton (2000) argues that 'contemporary inpatient hospices . . . are increasingly becoming enclaves in which a particular type of bodily deterioration and decay is set apart from mainstream society' (pp. 123–4). She demonstrates how in-patient hospice care has become super-specialized and, in many ways, has moved away from providing a setting for those with a variety of malignancies to die; instead, in-patient hospice care is now primarily for those with the most extreme physical symptoms or social conditions. Critiques, such as those already cited, emphasize the need for further research to demonstrate the value of in-patient hospice care and compare this with palliative care in other institutional settings as well as other approaches to caring for dying people.

Palliative care in hospitals

Although many dying people spend most of their last months in their own homes, they may be admitted to hospital on a regular basis or attend as out- or day-patients during that period. Those with cancer may be under the medical supervision of an oncology or radiotherapy team, who may have treated them during acute phases of their illness. Dying people may also be under the care of a number of other specialists, in particular general physicians or surgeons.

According to the Hospice Information Directory, the first hospital-based palliative care team was established in 1977 by St Thomas's Hospital in London; in 2002 in the UK, there were 221 hospital support teams. In contrast, in the USA, only 15 per cent of hospitals reported any end-of-life services and only 36 per cent reported pain management services (Pan *et al.* 2001). Hospital palliative care teams in the UK, sometimes known as support or symptom control teams, may include all or any of the following staff members: doctors (oncologists, specialist palliative care or general physicians), social workers, nurses and clergy. In addition, there are 100 support nurses who work on their own in hospitals.

Many hospital teams function in the same way as home care support teams working out of hospices or other settings. They spend much of their time in the community, in patients' homes, where they provide symptom control, pain relief and emotional and other support to dying people who are under the care of a hospital consultant, as well as supporting informal carers such as relatives and friends. They extend the same kind of support to in-patients and people attending out-patient appointments. These teams also play a particular role in the institution, providing expertise, information, support and advice to medical, nursing and paramedical colleagues. While home care teams and individual Macmillan nurses see part of their role as educating primary health care teams and other providers of health and social care in the community, providing palliative care services – in particular, undertaking an educational role in a hospital setting – is particularly challenging (Seymour *et al.* 2002).

Although there has been considerable movement towards embracing a concept of care in tertiary health care settings, the primary goal remains cure and this is the target towards which the health care team works, especially in specialist cancer wards. The death of a patient is still seen as a medical failure and, therefore, the presence of a group of people dedicated to a good death can be experienced as an irritant. This may be a partial explanation why these teams are often marginalized, as evidenced by their siting in inaccessible or inadequate accommodation.

In describing the demise of an early hospital-based support team, Herxheimer *et al.* (1985) illustrate some of the conflicts inherent in establishing the first teams, some of which may still be seen as irreconcilable with working in acute settings striving for 'cure'. They concluded that, for such a team to function adequately, in addition to substantial and realistic funding, leadership was essential, preferably from a hospital clinician (i.e. a physician), to give it the required status in the setting. Additionally, Herzheimer *et al.* noted that good communication between team members was essential. Many of these factors, identified nearly 20 years ago, are still relevant for the effective functioning of hospital palliative care teams. Yet we still do not have much evidence about the effectiveness of these teams in relation to the tasks they purport to perform. McQuillan *et al.* (1996) demonstrated that symptoms experienced by patients with cancer and HIV were indeed alleviated following the introduction of a palliative care service. A modified support team assessment schedule (STAS: Higginson 1993), used in a variety of forms in community palliative care teams to measure change in symptoms and functioning of 'patients', was used by Edmonds *et al.* (1998) to ascertain whether hospital palliative care teams improve symptom control. Their findings suggest that, other than depression, patients assessed three or more times using the STAS demonstrated improvement (in descending order) in psychological distress, anorexia, pain, mouth discomfort, constipation, breathlessness, nausea and vomiting. Another study in the hospital setting undertaken by the same research team (Edmonds *et al.* 2000) explored the palliative care needs of hospital in-patients. In addition to establishing that 12 per cent of the hospitals' medical and surgical patient population suffered from advanced disease, the study identified communication issues about discharge, relationships with community palliative care teams and primary care teams as problematic. They concluded that hospital palliative care teams can make a significant difference to patients' overall well-being, including pain and symptom control, and relationships with family and other professional carers.

A recently published survey by Higginson *et al.* (2002) searched databases to establish whether hospital-based palliative care teams really improve care for dying patients and their families. The outcome measures included quality of life, number of days spent in hospital and time allocated to a palliative care team. Many of the studies examined did not demonstrate strength in research methods, and none looked at different models of hospital teams. However, the skills and services that hospital palliative care teams provide do indicate some benefits (Higginson *et al.* 2002), but further research using similar and comparable tools is necessary to provide stronger evidence.

The impact of hospital palliative care teams or specialist nurses on the rest of the hospital community is one that is only now being researched. To date, it has been assumed that hospital medical staff (a) might resent the intrusion of these specialists or (b) might discount their 'skills'. Recent research by Jack *et al.* (2002), exploring the impact of a team in one large acute hospital, suggests that general nursing and medical staff might feel de-skilled by this service while empowering junior staff.

It is clear from the brief survey above that the jury is out about the effectiveness and functioning of hospital palliative care teams. Bearing in mind the enormous research endeavour in hospitals, it is somewhat surprising that this area is relatively under-researched. Action research, as well as experimental studies, is required to demonstrate the effectiveness of these teams as well as to understand their interrelationships with their host (acute settings) and palliative care teams operating in the community.

Palliative care in nursing and residential care

Large numbers of older people in Western societies reside and die in nursing and residential homes. For example, 20 per cent of all deaths in the USA occur in nursing homes (Buchanan *et al.* 2002) and 19 per cent in the UK die in residential care homes (not requiring nursing care), nursing homes and dual-registered homes (registered as both residential and nursing). Nursing homes in the USA tend to accommodate large numbers of residents (over 100), whereas the average size of old-age facilities in the UK is much smaller, usually ranging from 20 to 40 beds. Research within the field of gerontology has focused on many aspects of life in these facilities, but has rather neglected the condition of older people as they approach death. This reflects the lack of evidence, and many might claim lack of interest, in the plight of older people deteriorating and dying in all settings. In some ways, this is surprising given the fanfare that accompanied the palliative care movement's striving for a good death for everyone, as well as general concern about ageing, especially in Europe (including the UK) and North America (Peace *et al.* 1982, 1997; Willcocks *et al.* 1986). This is particularly marked in relation to residential settings, where other than some work in Australia (Maddocks and Parker 2001), there has been little interest in how and from what causes older people die, let alone discussion about the appropriateness of different settings as well as quality of living while dying for this age group. Most surprisingly, given the attention to dying children or people dying from AIDS, until very recently there has been little research into the applicability of palliative care strategies to caring for older people dying in nursing and residential homes. There has also been little debate about the appropriateness of palliative care for adults in all settings suffering and dying from diseases other than cancer (Addington-Hall and Higginson 2001).

Research studies have been undertaken in the USA and Australia, and to a lesser extent in the UK, on the quality of dying and management of death in residential and nursing home settings (Keay and Schonwetter 1998; Froggatt 2000, 2001a,b; Maddocks and Parker 2001). Many dying residents are transferred to hospital in their last days of life (Sidell *et al.* 1997). Decisions to transfer a resident are not necessarily taken in the spirit of palliative care where the dying person can express a preference, but usually are taken by the general practitioner who assesses the (in)ability of the home to address the needs of the dying resident. These decisions are often ratified by home staff who acknowledge their limitations in providing adequate care. Some residents who do remain in the homes have been observed to experience suffering and pain (Sidell *et al.* 1997). The primary care team is primarily responsible for the health care needs of residents. Unlike people residing in their own homes and also served by primary care teams, those dying in residential and nursing homes in the UK do not seem to access community palliative care services. Yet the impact of community palliative care provision – where it exists – has transformed the experiences of dying people and their carers; the most tangible outcome being a perceived opportunity to exercise choice to remain in their own domestic environments and avoid unwanted spells in hospital other than those requested by the dying person.

In the UK, there are nursing homes with dedicated terminal care beds paid for by the local health authority. Patients are transferred to these beds for the purpose of terminal care. However, 'specialist palliative care' services are not necessarily provided for these residents. In the Netherlands, there is a growing movement for homes for the elderly as well as nursing homes to have separate units for residents requiring palliative care. These units consist of between five and ten single rooms to which dying people with complex problems are transferred from other settings. Residents in these rooms are looked after by a multidisciplinary palliative care team of nurses, care-givers, nursing home physicians, social workers, psychologists, physiotherapists, ergo therapists, pastoral workers and volunteers (Francke and Kerkstra 2000).[3]

The question of whether community palliative care teams could or should become involved in caring for residents dying in these institutions has been debated primarily based on the argument that palliative care operates within a different paradigm from nursing home or residential home philosophy and that the latter may have its own 'successful' ways of accommodating dying residents' needs (Froggatt *et al.* 2001a). Avis *et al.* (1999) and Froggatt (2000) explored the potential input of community palliative care services in nursing homes in the mid-1990s, focusing in particular on how advice and training could be provided by these 'experts' to residential settings.

Sidell *et al.* (1997) examined the way in which death and dying were managed routinely in nursing, dual-registered and residential homes in England. This Open University study used a representative sample of all these homes and, therefore, investigated far more residential than nursing facilities (Sidell *et al.* 1997, 2000; Katz *et al.* 1999, 2000a,b; Komaromy *et al.* 2000). The same team undertook a second study in which they investigated staff training needs in caring for dying residents (Katz *et al.* 2001). Both studies found that caring for dying residents created stress for carers in these institutions and that delivery of high-quality care to dying residents was hard to achieve.

Factors internal and external to the home influence the quality of terminal care. The influence of the primary care team in making decisions about transferring residents to hospitals or other settings has already been mentioned. It is important to note that, until recently, there was little palliative care training in medical education and, consequently, general practitioners were unfamiliar with the principles and practices of palliative care, except in so far as they applied to younger people dying of cancer in their own homes (Katz *et al.* 1999). The general practitioners in Sidell and colleagues' study (1997) were loathe to introduce syringe drivers and other practices to residential and nursing homes. However, district nurses and specialist palliative care nurses are more willing to care for dying residents in these settings. In a recent study of clinical nurse specialists, Froggatt *et al.* (2001) demonstrated a concerted move towards educating, training and providing support for carers in the nursing and residential sector.

The most important internal factors for the care of dying residents are the quality of staff, their skill mix and their commitment to caring for dying residents (Sidell *et al.* 1997). Staff in care homes are traditionally very poorly paid, although there is some variation in pay scales across the UK (Dalley and Denniss 2001). Despite little training in delivering care in general and terminal care in particular to older people (Katz 2003), carers were keen to retain residents until death in what they believed were their own homes. However, they often felt ill-equipped to respond to residents' physical as well as their emotional needs. This related partly to their lack of training, but they perceived that the greatest difficulty related to staffing levels. Their demanding jobs meant that carers were unable to provide what they perceived to be appropriate 'nursing care', such as sitting with dying residents.

Staff in care homes, even including management, have limited understanding of the principles and practices of palliative care. Despite this, they shared a view of what constituted a good death, some of the components of which are embodied in the principles of palliative care. For example, little forward planning took place, mostly because it was rare for residents to be defined as dying in advance of the terminal phase. In reconstructing the care given to dying residents, home managers found it difficult to retrospectively reconstruct when or if they ever predicted that a resident was 'dying'. In contrast to younger people dying of cancer, defining older people as dying is particularly problematic because of the unpredictability of their health trajectories – residents were seen as in a chronic state of gradual decline, particularly those in nursing and dual-registered homes. Therefore, unless a particular medical event took place, managers found delineating the beginning of the dying trajectory meaningless. Yet following a tangible episode, be it refusal to eat or transient ischaemic attack, managers constructed a plan of action, which included notifying relatives and health staff external to the home.

Another factor internal to the home which affected the standard of care dying residents received was staffing levels: the availability of additional staff, whether bank (agency) or off-duty staff to ease the load when a resident became highly dependent. Many homes had minimal staffing at night with staff members caring for large numbers of residents, or assigned to particular areas of the home. As almost the same number of residents die at night as they do in the daytime, this created tremendous pressure for carers working at night who, in order to provide adequate care for the dying resident, *de facto* needed to 'neglect' other residents. This situation was exacerbated in the winter months when more residents died and staff were more likely to be off sick themselves.

The location and design of the home influenced the care received by dying residents. When homes were not close to public transport or primarily housed 'out-of-town' residents, relatives were less likely to be involved in 'caring' activities or in making decisions about treatment. The layout of the home, as well as the bedrooms, also impacted on the nature of terminal care. Many homes were converted from domestic dwellings and did not have spacious bedrooms allowing easy access to both sides of the bed for carers.

Official and semi-official documents in the UK have noted a poor quality of dying in residential settings. The Centre for the Policy on Ageing had, in the 1980s, produced a document entitled *Home Life* (1984) in which little was said about caring for dying and bereaved residents. However, its updated version *A Better Home Life* (1996), which examined issues about the quality of death as well as life, included specific recommendations about ways to improve the care of dying residents. It noted: 'The fact that most residents die in the homes they are living in rather than returning to their own homes or being moved into hospital does not mean that dying and death should be routine and commonplace' (p. 113). And they suggested that:

Consideration should be given to:

- Physical, medical and nursing care (especially with regard to comfort and pain relief)
- Spiritual and emotional aspects
- Cultural and religious beliefs and practices

- Legal issues and other formalities to do with death
- Relatives' and friends' involvement
- The communal life of the home and the involvement of other residents
- Support for staff

(Centre for the Policy on Ageing 1996: 114)

The recommendations of the Centre for Policy on Ageing were supported by research findings published shortly thereafter (Sidell *et al.* 1997; Avis *et al.* 1999) as well as government directives. The two Open University studies (Sidell *et al.* 1997; Katz *et al.* 2000a), while focusing on some of the practicalities involved in providing better terminal care for dying residents, noted the importance of introducing concepts of palliative care into these settings. Care staff receive very little preparatory or on-the-job training and, despite some provision across the UK, to date there is little information about the quality of this training and, therefore, one can only assume that standards vary (Dalley and Denniss 2001). Training for carers in managing dying and bereaved residents is extremely rare; many carers receive minimal training in 'caring and assessment skills'. The situation should change in the UK by 2005, by which time 50 per cent of carers in residential and nursing homes will be required by the National Minimum Standards for Care Homes to hold National Vocational Qualifications in Social Care at Level Two. Introducing training to care staff is a target of the Care Standards Act 2002. Care Standard 11, acknowledging this, specifies that 'Care and comfort are given to service users who are dying, their death is handled with dignity and propriety, and their spiritual needs, rites and functions observed.' The concept of dignity and privacy is also enshrined in the National Service Framework for Older People (2001), which acknowledges the importance of 'fitting services around people's needs'.

In conclusion, it is relevant to note the differences between the UK and the USA where, through medical insurance schemes, 'hospice services' are bought in to an increasing, but still proportionately small, number of nursing homes and, where this occurs, they take over a substantial proportion of the residents' total care. In the Netherlands, as noted earlier, there is a trend towards moving dying people into nursing homes or homes for the elderly and then apply the US model by bringing in specialist palliative care teams.

Caring for dying prisoners: the US experience

Research into the care of prisoners dying from disease, as opposed to violent deaths, has been neglected by palliative care researchers in most countries. However, voluntary organizations in the USA have fostered growing interest in this field and philosophers have considered the conflicts between the Hippocratic oath and custodial personnel's commitment to the penal harm movement which seeks to inflict pain on prisoners.

In the UK, a few reports have been published about the need for humane palliative care services to be available for dying prisoners. An example of bad practice where a prisoner was shackled to his bed described by Finlay (1998) was counteracted by good practice presented by, for example, The Wisdom Hospice (Oliver and Cook 1998). The prison population in the UK includes older people likely to die of chronic diseases. However, the number of prisoners dying of natural causes (about 45 per annum; personal communication) is about half the number of those dying violent deaths. The prison population is growing older, particularly male sex offenders who are unlikely to be released as they approach death. Personal communication with the prison health service suggests that prisoners are entitled to receive community palliative care services, including hospice admission in the same way as the general population. Where feasible, prisoners are given compassionate release on the grounds of deteriorating health. Inevitably, however, considerations such as the safety of the public and staffing issues influence the extent to which prisoners receive the services to which they are entitled.

Certain principles of palliative care, such as bereavement support, could help to reduce the use of drugs to cope with difficult emotions (Finlay and Jones 2000). Prison authorities say (personal communication) that officers have training in communication skills and are supported by chaplaincy teams and voluntary groups. Individual prisoners have a personal officer who acts as their key worker, and distressed prisoners have constant access to 'listeners', fellow prisoners trained by the Samaritans. Dying prisoners are cared for by local specialist palliative care teams referred by the hospital consultant.

In the USA, the need of prisoners for palliative care has been raised and researched over a number of years. The National Prison Hospice Association recognizes some of the particular problems faced in caring for prisoners. For example, in the USA – as in the UK – the volunteer is pivotal in delivering hospice care; however, when dealing with potentially dangerous prisoners, finding external volunteers is somewhat problematic. Price explores some of these issues:

> The basic concepts of a prison hospice are the same as those for a community hospice. The differences are only procedural. How will you train volunteers? How will you allow inmates movement? To what degree do you allow special circumstances to supersede segregation time? To what extent do you change rules for visits by the family? How do you give inmates control of their own care? And how do you define your team?

She cautions:

> if you forget the concepts of pain control, patient autonomy, multi-disciplinary team, patient and family as unit of care, volunteer – you can call your programme comfort care, but don't call it hospice.
>
> (Price 2002)

In recent years in the USA, the Grace (Guiding Responsive Action for Corrections in End-of Life) Project has been ongoing, 'promoting compassionate End-of-life Care in Prisons and Jails'. This is supported by the Robert Wood Johnson Foundation, which has links with many prison, health and palliative care organizations in the USA and is administered by the Volunteers of America. It incorporates an on-line resource centre to distribute information about existing programmes and others being developed by other jails and prisons and to support embryonic projects. (This includes an annotated updated bibliography about palliative care in correction facilities available through its website.) The Grace Project is connected to many correctional organizations in the USA, as well as hospice organizations.

Ratcliff (2001), in reviewing the Grace Project, notes that in the USA more than 2500 inmates died of natural causes (including AIDS) but few actually died in prison for the following reason:

> Traditionally, there has been great discomfort and reluctance in allowing death to occur on-site for fear that the death would be equated with neglect. Often, to avoid potential legal, ethical, and medical complications, facilities have found it easier to send all dying patients out of the facility. As one correctional professional explained, 'inmates are expected to go to the hospital "in shackles" to die, and not die behind bars'.
>
> (Ratcliff: 2001: 13)

However, for many prisoners, particularly after long periods of incarceration, the prison has become their home and their community and other inmates their family (Ratcliff 2001; Tillman 2001).

Ratcliff describes some of the challenges to providing good end-of-life care in prisons. These include: a focus on conforming to administrative rule rather than enabling individual choice; crowded conditions that mitigate against treating dying people as individuals and involving their families in their care; concern about pain control and symptom relief medications being abused; problems in relation to liability and litigation with regard to heroic treatments; the need to involve prison staff whose primary responsibility is to ensure security and efficiency; and, lastly, problems posed by inmate classification. Through visiting prisons, the Grace Project identified the most important issues to be addressed in prisons to enable prisoners to die there. These include:

- *Pain and symptom management*. The challenges include the attitude of health care and security personnel about the use and abuse of narcotics, prison formularies that severely limit available medications, possibility of theft and trafficking, and assurance of effective dosages.
- *Family visitation and involvement*. The challenges include the identification and reunification of families, the definition of other inmates as 'family' and arrangement for their visitation, visitor access to inmates who are unable to be transported to visitation areas (especially for children) and extended and off-hours visitation.
- *Training*. The challenges include orienting and training a diverse group that includes medical and nursing staff, security, and other administra-

tive staff and volunteers: changing negative staff attitudes; adjusting staff assignments; and conflicting demands for staff time.

- *Inmate isolation*. The challenges include care for high-security inmates, transfer of inmates from one facility to another to access the programme, and lack of family or inmate family.

- *Volunteer involvement*. The challenges include securing administrative approval and security staff support for involvement of inmates as volunteers, as well as community volunteer engagement.

- *Attitude*. The challenges include creating what Tanya Tillman refers to as a neural zone, where anger, fear and prejudice of inmates and staff can be set aside (Ratcliff 2001: 14).

Based on these challenges, the Grace Project produced End-of Life Care Standards of Practice in Correctional Settings, which resemble some of the palliative care core standards developed in the UK but are developed in much greater detail. The categories, which are divided into standards and then subdivided into practices, are care, safety, security, justice, programme and activity, administration and management.[4] In summary, the most important standards include:

- involvement of inmates as volunteers;

- increased visitation for families, including inmate family;

- interdisciplinary team, including physician, nurse, chaplain and social worker, at a minimum;

- comprehensive plans of care;

- advance care planning;

- training in pain and symptom management;

- bereavement services;

- adaptation of the environment and diet for comfort (Ratcliff 2001: 15).

Hospice programmes are now operational in 20 federal or state jurisdictions in the USA and they work in a variety of ways. For example, the Louisiana State Penitentiary Hospice Programme provides palliative care to the state's men-only maximum security prison at Angola, Louisiana (Tillman 2001). This prison houses over 5000 inmates, most of whom will die behind bars. The hospice programme established in 1998 is part of the prison health system. A 40-bed ward in the prison infirmary is the setting where dying prisoners receive care from a multidisciplinary team, known as an interdisciplinary team in the USA. One innovative aspect of this team is the extensive use of inmate volunteers who undergo intensive training delivered by external as well as internal experts. Security personnel have also been taken on board in an attempt to reduce the mutual distrust and suspicion between them and prisoners. Prisoners are admitted to the programme through personal choice but only if they meet stringent criteria, including knowledge of diagnosis and prognosis (not more than 6 months). The programme is very comprehensive and even includes a formal bereavement assessment early on to anticipate future needs of family members and surviving inmates. Annual memorial services held to commemorate hospice patients are planned by inmate volunteers and future plans include attendance from patients' families in the newly completed chapel (Tillman 2001). The goals of the hospice team at the Louisiana State Penitentiary – comprising the medical staff, security personnel and inmate volunteers – are as follows:

- to provide quality, compassionate end-of-life care to patients and their families;
- to redirect efforts at end of life to palliate distressing symptoms rather than extend life (at all costs) as indicated by vital signs;
- to improve the institution's previous practice of withholding a patient's right to make health care choices for himself;
- to recognize and acknowledge those relationships formed by the patient that he finds meaningful and life-affirming (Tillman 2001: 18).

The USA has led on hospice care in prisons and other correctional facilities, partly because of its large prison population. The voluntary sector has promoted palliative care in prison and, although many of these programme are still to be evaluated, their results will prove to be interesting and of potential use to other countries with ageing prisoners with health problems.

Conclusions

In exploring palliative care in institutions, I have demonstrated that, although there is some agreement about the goals of palliative care, the nature of the setting can determine the quality of palliative care delivered. Relationships between team members and the composition of 'teams' working in palliative care also vary from setting to setting – volunteers play a major role in hospices and prisons and less so in residential and nursing homes and hospitals. There is need for further information to be gathered about the types of palliative care different organizations strive to deliver as well as in-depth research to ascertain whether their goals are met. The fact that hospices have been operational for 35 years in the UK is no grounds for complacency; it is clear that existing programmes in other settings have much to learn from newer hospice programmes such as those in US prisons.

Notes

1   See the Hospice Information website (www.hospice.information.com).
2   See the audio-cassette produced by the Open University (Addington-Hall 2000).

3   See the European Association of Palliative Care website (www.eapcnet.org).
4   See the Grace Project website (www.graceproject.org).

References

Addington-Hall, J. (2000) Cassette tape for the Open University, *K260: Death and Dying Course*. Milton Keynes: The Open University.

Addington-Hall, J.M. and Higginson, I.J. (eds) (2001) *Palliative Care for Non-Cancer Patients*. Oxford: Oxford University Press.

Avis, M., Jackson, J.G., Cox, K. and Miskella, C. (1999) Evaluation of a project providing community palliative care support to nursing homes. *Health and Social Care in the Community*, 7(1): 32–8.

Bruera, E., Suarez-Almazor, M., Velasco, A. *et al.* (1994) The assessment of constipation in terminal cancer patients admitted to a palliative care unit: a retrospective review. *Journal of Pain and Symptom Management*, 9(8): 515–19.

Buchanan, R.J., Choi, M., Wang, S. and Huang, C. (2002) Analyses of nursing home residents in hospice care using the Minimum Data Set. *Palliative Medicine*, 16: 465–80.

Centre for Policy on Ageing (1984) *Home Life*. London: Centre for Policy on Ageing.

Centre for Policy on Ageing (1996) *A Better Home Life*. London: Centre for Policy on Ageing.

Clark, D. and Seymour, J. (1999) *Reflections on Palliative Care*. Buckingham: Open University Press.

Corner, J. (2001) Management of breathlessness in advanced lung cancer: new scientific evidence for developing multidisciplinary care, in M.F. Muers, F. Macbeth, F.C. Wells and A. Miles (eds) *The Effective Management of Lung Cancer*. London: Aesculapius Medical Press.

Corner, J. and Dunlop, R. (1997) New approaches to care, in D. Clark, S. Ahmedzai and J. Hockley (eds) *New Themes in Palliative Care*. Buckingham: Open University Press.

Cummings, I. (1999) Training of volunteers, in D. Doyle, G.W.C. Hanks and N. MacDonald (eds) *Oxford Textbook of Palliative Medicine*. Oxford: Oxford University Press.

Dalley, G. and Denniss, M. (2001) *Trained to Care? Investigating the Skills and Competencies of Care Assistants in Homes for Older People*. Centre for Policy on Ageing Report No. 28. London: Centre for Policy on Ageing.

Department of Health (2001) *National Service Framework for Older People*. London: Department of Health.

Doyle, D. (1999) The provision of palliative care, in D. Doyle, G.W.C. Hanks and N. MacDonald (eds) *Oxford Textbook of Palliative Medicine*. Oxford: Oxford University Press.

Edmonds, P., Stuttaford, J.M., Penny, J. *et al.* (1998) Do hospital palliative care teams improve symptom control? Use of a modified STAS as an evaluation tool. *Palliative Medicine*, 12: 345–51.

Edmonds, P., Karlsen, S. and Addington-Hall, J. (2000) Palliative care needs of hospital inpatients. *Palliative Medicine*, 14(3): 227–8.

Finlay, I.G. (1998) Managing terminally ill prisoners: reflection and action. *Palliative Medicine*, 12(6): 457–61.

Finlay, I.G. and Jones, N.K. (2000) Unresolved grief in young offenders in prison. *British Journal of General Practice*, 50(456): 569–70.

Francke, A.L. and Kerkstra, A. (2000) Palliative care services in The Netherlands: a descriptive study. *Patient Education and Counselling*, 41: 23–33.

Froggatt, K.A. (2000) *Palliative Care Education in Nursing Homes*. London: Macmillan Cancer Relief.

Froggatt, K.A. (2001a) Palliative care in nursing homes: where next? *Palliative Medicine*, 15: 42–8.

Froggatt, K.A. (2001b) Life and death in English nursing homes: sequestration or transition? *Ageing and Society*, 21: 319–32.

Froggatt, K.A., Poole, K. and Hoult, E. (2001) *Community Work with Nursing Homes and Residential Care Homes: A Survey of Clinical Nurse Specialists in Palliative Care*. London: Macmillan Cancer Relief.

Herxheimer, A., Begent, R., MacLean, D. *et al.* (1985) The short life of a terminal care support team: experience at Charing Cross Hospital. *British Medical Journal*, 290: 1877–9.

Higginson, I. (1993) Clinical audit: getting started and keeping going, in I. Higginson (ed.) *Clinical Audit in Palliative Care*. Oxford: Radcliffe Medical Press.

Higginson, I.J., Finlay, I, Goodwin, D.M. *et al.* (2002) Do hospital-based palliative teams improve care for patients or families at the end of life. *Journal of Pain and Symptom Management*, 23(2): 96–106.

Hockley, J. (1997) The evolution of the hospice approach, in D. Clark, J. Hockley and S. Ahmedzai (eds) *New Themes in Palliative Care*. Buckingham: Open University Press.

Jack, D., Oldham, J. and Williams, A. (2002) Do hospital-based palliative care clinical nurse specialists de-skill general staff? *International Journal of Palliative Nursing*, 8(7): 336–40.

James, N. and Field, D. (1992) The routinization of hospice: bureaucracy and charisma. *Social Science and Medicine*, 34(12): 1363–75.

Johnson, I.S., Rogers, C., Biswas, B. and Ahmedzai, S. (1990) What do hospices do? A survey of hospices in the United Kingdom and the Republic of Ireland. *British Medical Journal*, 300: 791–3.

Katz, J., Sidell, M. and Komaromy, C. (2001) Dying in long-term care facilities: support needs of other residents, relatives and staff. *American Journal of Hospice and Palliative Care*, 18(5): 321–6.

Katz, J.S. (2003) Managing dying residents, in J.S. Katz and S.M. Peace (eds) *End of Life in Care Homes: A Palliative Care Approach*. Oxford: Oxford University Press.

Katz, J.T., Komaromy, C. and Sidell, M. (1999) Understanding palliative care in residential and nursing homes. *International Journal of Palliative Nursing*, 5(2): 58–64.

Katz, J.T., Sidell, M. and Komaromy, C. (2000a) *Investigating the Training Needs in Palliative Care*. Unpublished Report for the Department of Health.

Katz, J.T., Komaromy, C. and Sidell, M. (2000b) Death in homes: bereavement needs of residents, relatives and staff. *International Journal of Palliative Nursing*, 6(6): 274–9.

Keay, T.J. and Schonwetter, R.S. (1998) Hospice care in the nursing home. *American Family Physician*, 57: 491–4.

Komaromy, C., Sidell, M. and Katz, J.T. (2000) The quality of terminal care in residential and nursing homes. *International Journal of Palliative Nursing*, 6(4): 192–204.

Lawton, J. (2000) *The Dying Process*. London: Routledge.

Maddocks, I. and Parker, D. (2001) Palliative care in nursing homes, in J.M. Addington-Hall and I.J. Higginson (eds) *Palliataive Care for Non-Cancer Patients*. Oxford: Oxford University Press.

McQuillan, R., Finlay, I., Roberts, D. *et al.* (1996) The provision of a palliative care service in a teaching hospital and subsequent evaluation of that service. *Palliative Medicine*, 10: 231–9.

Myers, K. and Hearn, J. (2001) An introduction to palliative day care: past and present, in J. Hearn and K. Myers (eds) *Palliative Day Care in Practice*. Oxford: Oxford University Press.

Office of National Statistics (2002) *Social Trends*. London: The Stationery Office.

Oliver, D. and Cook, L. (1998) The specialist palliative care of prisoners. *European Journal of Palliative Care*, 5(3): 79–80.

Pan, C.X., Morrison, R.S., Meier, D.E. *et al.* (2001) How prevalent are hospital-based palliative care programmes? Status report and future directions. *Journal of Palliative Medicine*, 4(3): 315–24.

Peace, S.M., Kellaher, L.A. and Willcocks, D. (1982) *A Balanced Life: A Consumer Study of Life in 100 Local Authority Old People's Homes*. CESSA Research Report No. 13. London: Polytechnic of North London.

Peace, S.M., Kellaher, L. and Willcocks, D. (1997) *Re-Evaluating Residential Care*. Buckingham: Open University Press.

Price, C. (2002) To adopt or adapt? Principles of hospice care in the correctional setting. *National Prison Hospice Association News*, Issue 6, Boulder, CO.

Ratcliff, M. (2001) Dying inside the walls, in M.Z. Solomon, A.L. Romer, K.S. Heller and D.E. Weissman (eds) *Innovations in End-of-life Care*. New York: Mary Ann Liebert.

Salisbury, C., Bosanquet, N., Wilkinson, E.K. *et al.* (1999) The impact of different models of specialist palliative care on patients' quality of life: a systematic literature review. *Palliative Medicine*, 13(1): 3–17.

Seymour, J., Clark, D., Hughes, P. *et al.* (2002) Clinical nurse specialists in palliative care. Part 3. Issues for the Macmillan nurse role. *Palliative Medicine*, 16: 386–94.

Sidell, M., Katz, J.T. and Komaromy, C. (1997) *Dying in Nursing and Residential Nursing Homes for Older People: Examining the Case for Palliative Care*. Report for the Department of Health. Milton Keynes: Open University.

Sidell, M., Katz, J.S. and Komaromy, C. (2000) The case for palliative care in residential and nursing homes, in S. Dickenson, M. Johnson and J.S. Katz (eds) *Death, Dying and Bereavement*. London: Sage.

Tillman, T. (2001) Hospice in prison: the Louisiana State Penitentiary Hospice Programme, in M.Z. Solomon, A.L. Romer, K.S. Heller and D.E. Weissman (eds) *Innovations in End-of-life Care*. New York: Mary Ann Liebert.

Willcocks, D.M., Peace, S.M. and Kellaher, L. (1986) *Private Lives in Public Places*. London: Routledge.

PART THREE

Loss and bereavement

22

Overview

Sheila Payne

Most books present death as a clear junction between being alive and being dead. Similarly, being bereaved is regarded as a state that occurs following death. Therefore, the discussion of death and bereavement is usually relegated to the final chapter of a textbook. In this book, we have chosen to devote much more space than other nursing texts to loss and bereavement. We regard death not as a single event, but as a process in which nurses often have an important role to play (Quested and Rudge 2003). They manage and orchestrate the dying period, by controlling physical symptoms such as pain or a dry mouth. Nurses work by containing and shaping the behaviours of the onlookers, for example by calling patients' relatives, medical staff or chaplains to the bedside at key times. Nurses also help to transform the newly dead body, making it presentable to family members, by washing and dressing the body, removing clinical equipment and any evidence of last resuscitation attempts. I start, then, at the time of death, focusing on nursing work with the person who has died.

I then move on to discuss the impact of death on those who survive. Instead of explaining bereavement theories as entities to be proved or disproved, I regard them as discourses – ways of talking about loss and conceptualizing the experience of bereavement. I then review three major groups of discourses: those which arise from psychological or psychiatric understanding of loss; those which arise from theories of stress and coping; and, lastly, those which are derived from sociological understandings of transitions in relationships and social networks. There are, of course, many other ways to understand bereavement which are located within major 'world-views', such as the main religions or philosophical accounts of human beings. These are likely to be modified by the culture, social class and life experience of those experiencing the loss. I will emphasize that it is the experience of loss that is important in life-threatening illness. Importantly, families and friends will have encountered many losses throughout the person's illness. Bereavement may be thought of not as a single loss, but as a culmination of losses and changes to their previously taken-for-granted way of living.

I then go on to explore the types of services and resources that are available to support bereaved people. I make no assumption that all people need additional support. There is evidence that most people are very resilient and manage major life changes with their own resources and support from their families and communities. However, for some people bereavement presents such a challenge that they seek additional support from community-based organizations such as Cruse (a charity concerned with providing counselling and bereavement support), faith groups, hospice and specialist palliative care bereavement services, and other health and social care services. I review the evidence about the efficacy of interventions designed to support bereaved people. I conclude the chapter by reviewing the content of the seven chapters that make up Part Three, helping the reader to make links with the theories of loss and providing a framework for understanding the structure of this part of the book.

Caring for the dead

In many cultures throughout history, women have cared for the dead. It is a common mark of respect that the newly dead are treated with dignity. As the place of death in developed countries has moved more commonly into institutional environments, usually hospitals, it has generally been the role of nurses rather than family members to care for the newly dead. The nursing procedures and practices for performing the 'last offices' are thought to have changed little over the last 100 years (Wolf 1988). In an analysis of the procedure manuals of an Australian hospital, Quested and Rudge (2003) argue 'that to move from alive to dead involves a transition during which the individual is reconfigured conceptually, physically, socially and culturally through the care practices inflicted on the dead body' (p. 559). They highlight how nurses manage the newly dead person's body in ways that contain the physicality of the body as it changes colour, leaks urine or faeces, smells, stiffens and cools. It has been argued that nurses, especially those working in hospices and specialist palliative care services, collude in creating the image of the 'good death' (McNamara *et al.* 1994). Prior to death, the myth of peaceful dying is engineered by the use of sedation and, subsequently, nurses' actions help to create the impression that the person is asleep. This supports wider societal discourses that seek to pretend that the dead are merely asleep. This myth is exemplified in the use of metaphors like 'at peace' and 'the long sleep'. In the UK, a study of medical and nursing records indicated that, however traumatic and distressing the actual death was and whatever symptoms were present near the end, the patient was described as having 'a peaceful death' and the words 'rest in peace' were usually written by the physician who certified the death (Birley 2002).

While the dead person might be presented as though asleep, their body tends to be treated in very different ways from the bodies of living people. Quested and Rudge (2003) described how personal ornaments like jewellery are normally removed, the body is stripped of clothing, washed, dressed in a shroud, labelled and placed in a body bag or sheet. All these practices serve to remove the identity of the former living person from the now dead body. Even the way the person's body is spoken about positions them as different from the bodies of the living (see Box 22.1).

In Chapter 24, Sque and Wells highlight how the language used to describe the removal of organs from donors, described as 'harvesting', can be experienced as deeply distressing by relatives who are somewhat uncertain about the status of the 'deadness' of their loved ones. In this special case, death is defined by brainstem death testing and the normal transitions in the physical body, such as discoloration and coolness, are not present because these people are generally maintained on life-support machines until their organs are removed. As Sque and Payne (1996) have argued, it requires considerable faith in medical staff to believe that their loved ones are really dead. They found that although intellectually people realized that a dead person cannot experience pain, some family members believed that the newly dead body retained some sentience.

Deaths enacted in intensive care units provide another good example of uncertainty as patients hover between living and death. In a detailed ethnographic study in the UK, Seymour (2001) provides accounts of how death is managed and contested between medical staff, nurses and family members in the intensive care unit. In patients with multiple organ failure, the treatment of each organ may become the work of different teams of medical experts – for example, renal failure may be treated by nephrologists, respiratory failure by chest physicians and heart failure by cardiologists. As previously discussed by Seymour and Ingleton in Chapter 10, the work of the medical team is directed at assembling a case to justify the withdrawal or continuation of life-prolonging medical treatment, while the nursing team attempts to provide integrated care that serves to maintain the integrity of the person as a whole individual (see Box 22.2).

Box 22.1   Words used to describe the newly dead person's body

Mortal remains
The body
A 'stiff'
Corpse
The deceased
Cadaver

Box 22.2   'Nursing care only' (adapted from Seymour 2001)

The data from Seymour's study suggest that 'nursing' in intensive care is constituted dually. First, by the technical-medical work of medicine: this is the context within which 'nursing' operates and within which nurses must fashion their relationships with patients and their companions. And, second, by strategies which incorporate 'whole person work' into what is an essentially depersonalized context. Achieving and sustaining a balance between these constituents is a central, and inherently difficult, feature of nursing work in intensive care. The period during which nurses care for individuals who are approaching death is a time in which the contradictions associated with sustaining 'whole person' work become highly visible and highly problematic for nurses. A common feature of the case studies was the subtle change in emphasis, away from medicine and towards nursing, for both those individuals 'known' to be dying in a 'technical' sense *and* those 'felt' to be dying in a 'bodily' sense. 'Technical' dying is used here to represent a judgement informed by the collection of physiological data, while 'bodily' dying refers to 'intuitively' based clinical judgement. The common sense concept of 'nursing care only' was used to describe this time period.

An example from the case study concerns a young man, Richard, who had been fatally injured in a road traffic accident one week previously. In Richard's case, bodily dying started to outpace technical death. However, in spite of Richard's moribund appearance, there was a lengthy delay before active medical treatment was withdrawn. During this time, his nurse was largely left alone by the medical staff, who were conducting 'behind the scenes' negotiations about a withdrawal of drug therapies. The nurse described in her follow-up interview how:

> . . . we had to continue making up all his drips, washing him and cleaning, just doing the usual care that you give to other patients but I knew by looking at him . . . it was like 'Why am I doing this?' I knew I was doing it because they hadn't decided to withdraw but I just wanted to get someone in to look at him and say to them: 'How would you like your relative to look like this?' and: 'You're doing all this treatment but you're not doing anything'.

The dissonance between the requirement to care for the 'already dead' body and the ideology of the 'whole person' seemed to be solved by an attribution to the young man, 'Richard', of particular personal qualities by the nurse. Thus it became possible for her to describe him as 'fighting', as 'still living' and later:

> . . . he was strong and trying to say: 'I'm not giving up' although his body was saying: 'You can't survive with this', I felt his heart and his brain was fighting everything.

In this way, this particular nurse achieved a sense of meaning in her nursing work, albeit at considerable personal cost. She recalled how his image remained in her mind long after his death:

> Yes, Richard, really, I was – erm – I couldn't stop thinking about him. I can still see him.

Definitions of terms in bereavement

It has been argued elsewhere that definitions of terms are closely related to the way loss is understood and the theories used to explain bereavement (Small 2001; Payne and Lloyd-Williams 2003). However, for the purposes of this text, it might be useful to offer some broadly accepted definitions. Stroebe *et al.* (2002: 6) have provided brief definitions of the key concepts:

- *Bereavement* is understood to refer to the objective situation of having lost someone significant.
- *Grief* is the reaction to bereavement, defined as a primarily emotional (affective) reaction to the loss of a loved one through death.
- *Mourning* is the social expressions or acts expressive of grief that are shaped by the practices of a given society or cultural group.

Scholars have debated whether grief is universal. There is plenty of evidence that humans and other animals react to the loss of significant others in their environment but the nature of the expression and duration of grief are more likely to be contingent upon the meaning placed upon the loss (Lofland 1985). So grief tends to refer to what is *felt*, while mourning refers to what is *done*. It is important for nurses and others working with bereaved people to realize that they should not infer the depth or intensity of grief from the overt behaviours displayed. Wailing at the bedside may be culturally sanctioned by some groups, while other social groups value stoicism and public emotional reserve, and both responses may be gender related (Walter 1999).

It is generally agreed that there are no single 'correct' or 'true' theories that explain the experience of loss or account for the emotions, experiences and cultural practices that characterize grief and mourning (Payne *et al.* 1999; Hockey *et al.* 2001). A post-modern position suggests that individual diversity is paramount and that within broad cultural constraints each of us develops our own ways of *doing* bereavement (Walter 1999). The following is an example of the diversity of expression of grief and memorialization practices within a family after the loss of a child: the grandparents may find comfort in religious rituals and prayer; the parents may react differently, the mother by retaining photographs, special items of clothing or toys, the father by 'burying' himself in work; and siblings may create a memory box, be disruptive at school or be 'super' good (see Riches and Dawson 2000). These examples of different responses to loss accord well with many nurses' experiences of relatives following a bereavement and their awareness of the variability of grieving. Some ways of talking and thinking about bereavement have become so popular that many people are unaware of their origins and they have become part of our taken-for-granted knowledge about bereavement – for example, the stage/phase models of loss. Although there may not appear to be strict social rules on how to behave when bereaved in mainstream White British society, Hockey (2001) has highlighted that there are more subtle injunctions: 'that the individual shall express their emotions, shall acknowledge the reality of their loss and shall share their thoughts and feelings with appropriate others' (p. 208). Many bereavement support services operate with these basic requirements of their clients.

Understanding loss and bereavement

Much of the patients' and families' experience of advancing illness can be understood as coming to terms with a series of losses. These losses may be related to all aspects of a person's life, including their functional abilities to walk unaided, to talk and to be continent. In some conditions, such as Parkinson's disease, emotional expression may be blunted or emotional control may be lost such as in some dementias and following stroke. Advancing illness also impacts on social relationships and roles; for example, paid employment may be lost, leading to loss of self-esteem, financial hardship and loss of identity. Therefore, advancing illness provides a cascade of losses for both the ill person and their family members. Moreover, with open communication about the probable outcome of disease and greater awareness of prognosis, people in these circumstances may start to anticipate a series of losses that they have yet to experience. This has been described as anticipatory grief (Evans 1994). It has been argued that when life-threatening illness is very protracted as in dementia, family members may start to withdraw from the ill person before their death. Sudnow (1967) described social death as a loss of personhood and the dying person being treated as if they were already dead.

Theories of loss and bereavement

In the following section, I introduce three groups of theories used to understand loss and bereavement. My aim is to provide the reader with sufficient information to evaluate critically the following chapters. Guidance on how to obtain more detailed information about each of these theories is available from 'Recommended reading' at the end of the chapter. I have categorized the theories into three conceptual groups based on their major emphasis: (1) intra-psychic processing, (2) transactional and (3) social aspects of loss.

The ordering of the theories does not imply anything other than their historical emergence. Of course, the major religions and philosophies of the world also provide important accounts of loss and bereavement, which shape the way loss is understood and experienced for many people (Parkes *et al.* 1997). These positions will not be discussed here because in an increasingly secular society, especially in the UK and some parts of Europe, religious teachings are arguably no longer the dominant way that loss is conceptualized.

Theories that emphasize intra-psychic processing

Over the last century, the most influential perspective on loss has been to focus on the experience of distressing emotions and the accompanying cognitions (thoughts) and behaviours. These ways to construe bereavement and grief have been derived from medical discourses, especially those that arise from psychiatric and psychological understandings. Attention has been directed predominantly to what happens inside people's heads (hence 'intra-psychic') and bereavement has been likened to an illness from which the person eventually recovers (Engel 1961). Thus there has been an emphasis on describing the physical and psychological manifestations of grief as 'symptoms' and there has been an assumption that the typical trajectory of bereavement is from high distress to little or none. The time span of this trajectory has been variously estimated from weeks to years. However, the outcome of bereavement has been construed in terms of 'recovery' or 'resolution', rather like getting over a bad illness. The trajectory of bereavement has often been conceptualized as a series of stages or phases through which the person must progress (hence 'process'). Thus the theories have similarities to developmental models used by psychologists to explain how children adapt to the world. The content and number of stages/phases vary but they tend to define the emotions and thoughts that are necessary to achieve 'resolution'. The tendency to map bereavement in terms of stages/phases has also given rise to notions of 'normal' and 'abnormal' grief (also may be described as complicated, complex and conflicted grief). This language of grief, therefore, suggests that there are 'right' and 'wrong' ways to grieve. For the last 20–30 years, most bereavement support workers have attempted to guide bereaved people along the 'right' path according to these models (Worden 1982, 1991, 2001; Parkes *et al.* 1996).

Freud (1917) is usually credited with the initial ideas that helped to shape the development of the phase/stage models of loss. Freud contributed much to twentieth-century thought and his psychoanalytic theory has been very influential in shaping our ways of understanding people. Writing during the turmoil and huge loss of life during the First World War in Europe, Freud was the first to point out the similarities and differences between grief and depression in his classic text *Mourning and Melancholia* (Freud 1917). His paper offered one of the first descriptions of normal and pathological grief. The thoughts discussed in it underpin psychoanalytic theory of depression and provide the basis for many current theories of grief and its resolution. In the light of the impact of Freud's theory of grief on subsequent theoretical developments, it is surprising to acknowledge that grief, as a psychological process, was never Freud's main focus of interest. Moreover, Freud's personal experiences of bereavement were not even compatible with his theoretical position. In *Mourning and Melancholia*, Freud argued that people became attached to others who are important for the satisfaction of their needs and to whom emotional expression is directed (cathexis). Love is conceptualized as the attachment of emotional energy to the psychological representation of the loved object (person). It is assumed that the more important the relationship, the greater the attachment. According to Freudian theory, grieving represents a dilemma because there is a simultaneous need to relinquish the relationship so that the person may regain the energy invested and a wish to maintain the bond with the love object. However, this is acknowledged to be painful work and so the bereaved person tends to hold on to an image of the dead person for as long as possible, until inevitably they have to face the reality of the loss and their new situation. According to Feud, the bereaved individual needs to accept the reality of the loss so that the emotional energy can be released and redirected. The process of withdrawing energy from the lost object is called 'grief work' (decathexis). He regarded this intra-psychic processing as essential to the breaking of relationship bonds with the deceased, to allow the reinvestment of emotional energy and the formation of new relationships with others. Arguably, Freud's most important contributions to loss have been:

- introducing a developmental perspective (his personality theory emphasized early childhood development);
- introducing the 'grief work' hypothesis; and
- defining the difference between grief and depression.

His ideas were taken up and developed by many other people working within the psychodynamic tradition, such as Lindemann (1944), Fenichel (1945) and Sullivan (1956).

In the second half of the twentieth century, Bowbly (1969, 1973, 1980) proposed a complex attachment theory to account for the formation of close human relationships, especially between mothers and their babies, and to account for what happened when these relationships were interrupted, either temporarily or permanently. He suggested that through the process of human evolution, there had developed a need for mothers and infants to be in close proximity for survival and that this was achieved through an interactional process involving reciprocal behaviours and feelings between mothers and babies called attachment. Temporary separation was marked by characteristic behaviours and feelings such as distress, calling and searching, which usually resulted in the coming together of both people. He suggested that the nature of distress for infants and young children varied sequentially in the following ways (described as stages):

- *Protest* – marked by anger and loud crying, with constant searching for the lost mother and a hypervigiliance anticipating her return.
- *Despair* – marked by withdrawal and less vigorous crying.
- *Detachment* – marked by an outward display of cheerful behaviour but the child remains emotionally distant.

Separation anxiety was thought to be an unpleasant state for infants. Therefore, infants quickly developed behaviours such as crying, which brought their mothers nearer to them, and other social behaviours that also served to maintain contact, such as smiling and later talking or physically clinging to their mother. Based on his knowledge about young children, Bowlby thought that permanent loss, such as bereavement, also triggered these feelings of intense distress and the same immediate behavioural responses of crying, searching, clinging, giving way to despondency, depression and later detachment. Bowlby proposed that the intensity of the grief was related to the closeness of the attachment relationship. For example, he predicted that we would be more distressed by the loss of a parent or sibling than a distant cousin because we had invested more emotional energy in that relationship. In writing about the experience of loss, Bowlby was careful to emphasize that the phases were not discrete entities and that people may oscillate between phases, although over the course of time it was anticipated that people would move through the phases. The four phases following loss were described by Bowlby (1980: 85) as:

1   Phase of numbing that usually lasts from a few hours to a week and may be interrupted by outbursts of extremely intense distress and/or anger.

2   Phase of yearning and searching for the lost figure lasting some months and sometimes for years.

3   Phase of disorganization and despair.

4   Phase of greater or lesser degree of reorganization.

Because the experience of loss was related to the type of attachment, Bowbly suggested that 'abnormal' attachment patterns were likely to be associated with 'abnormal' grieving. For example, he noted that relationships that were very unequal, such as highly dependent or domineering relationships, were more likely to result in difficulties during bereavement. Like Freud, Bowlby emphasized the emotional aspects of loss and the need to 'work through' the loss (think about the experience which is called 'grief work') to achieve an outcome where there was no longer any emotional investment in the dead person ('letting go'). Bowlby's ideas about attachment have been taken up by health and social care services, for example in encouraging early contact between mothers and babies after birth. Bowlby's, ideas were also influential in the development of Parkes's (1996) theories of loss. Both Bowlby and his colleague Parkes were psychiatrists and were in contact with patients struggling to understand the impact of their bereavements.

Parkes (1971, 1993, 1996) suggested that bereavement should be considered as a major psychosocial transition, which challenged the taken-for-granted world of the bereaved person. He argued that most people think of their world as relatively stable, in which they make assumptions of perceived control. Death, especially sudden death, challenges this, as people have to adapt to changes in relationships and social status (for example, from being a wife to a widow) and economic circumstances (having less money). He, like Bowlby, proposed that people progress through phases in coming to terms with their loss: numbness, pining, depression and recovery. Overall, there was a linear progression over time, although he acknowledges that there is great individual variability and that not everyone progresses at the same rate or that all phases are experienced. Parkes's ideas of 'normal' phases of grief have changed somewhat through the three editions of his influential book, *Bereavement* (Parkes 1972, 1986, 1996). The latest version of his theory emphasizes the emotional reactions experienced following the loss (Parkes 1996) rather than discrete phases. Parkes based his ideas on several research studies undertaken in the UK and the USA, as well as his clinical psychiatric work. Parkes was also influential in establishing one of the first hospice-based bereavement support services at St Christopher's Hospice, London, in which volunteers were trained to offer support to bereaved people.

Finally, there are two well-known models that are widely applied in specialist palliative care. Kubler Ross (1969), a psychiatrist working in the USA who was heavily influenced by psychoanalytic ideas, proposed a stage model of loss in relation to dying that has been applied to bereavement. This model emphasizes changing emotional expression throughout the final period of life. Her model has become hugely popular with health professionals and aspects of it are now part of common lay taken-for-granted assumptions about how bereavement is experienced. It has been heavily critiqued over the years because it assumes that bereavement can be conceptualized as a series of sequential stages, and it focuses on emotional aspects of loss and largely ignores the social aspects (for a more detailed critique, see Payne *et al.* 1999). Despite the criticisms of her model, it continues to be dominant in the education of nurses, bereavement support workers and others.

Worden (1982, 1991, 2001) based his therapeutic model on phases of grief and what he called 'tasks of mourning'. According to Worden (1991), the goals of grief counselling, are to:

- increase the reality of the loss;
- help the counsellee deal with both expressed and latent affect;
- help the counsellee overcome various impediments to readjustment after the loss; and
- encourage the counsellee to say an appropriate goodbye and to feel comfortable reinvesting back into life.

By the latest edition, he has modified the final task to suggest a less final break with the dead person (Worden 2001). He suggested that grief was a process not a state and that people needed to work through their reactions to loss to achieve a complete adjustment. Worden's books have been widely used as texts to guide counsellors and others working with bereaved people. It is therefore noteworthy that much of the language used presents bereavement as a medical condition and bereaved people as in need of therapy. He also describes pathological aspects of bereavement, highlighting how bereavement workers might identify different types of 'abnormal' grief.

Parkes, Kulber Ross and Worden have modified and developed their ideas over time and the accounts presented here do not do justice to the complexity of their thinking. All these theories have been critiqued and challenged, especially in relation to notions of a linear progression through phases or stages and the need for 'grief work' (see Wortman and Silver 1989). However, many of these stage/phase theories are widely taught to student nurses and others working in health and social care. Moreover, they are frequently presented in a simplified form with little acknowledgement of the criticisms. In fact, the pervasiveness of psychological stage/phase models of grief means that they have largely been incorporated into everyday taken-for-granted assumptions about how people should feel and behave following a loss. In the following sections, two other ways of understanding loss will be introduced.

Transactional models

While the theories of loss highlighted in the previous section emphasize what is happening inside the person's head, a more recent model of loss has concentrated on explaining grief as a transaction between the cognitive appraisal of the individual (how they understand their world) and what is happening in their environment. These ideas build upon psychological theories of stress and coping rather than the psychodynamic ideas of Freud. Psychological and medical research has explored how people react to stress and develop coping responses (Selye 1956). Early ideas tended to be based on an assumption that if certain things, called stressors, were present in sufficient amounts or intensities, they would trigger a stress response (Selye 1956). This response could be both physical and psychological. Early research tended to see the stressor as independent of the person exposed to the stress. It was recognized that people varied in their resilience to stressors. However, it was thought that humans were able to adapt to most things in the environment; it was those things that challenge the adaptation process that were considered to be stressful (Bartlett 1998). A number of models have been proposed for how stress can be conceptualized. The most important model for the purposes of understanding loss is the transactional model of stress and coping developed by Lazarus and Folkman (1984). They proposed that any event may be perceived as threatening by an individual, and it is the meaning of the event for that individual which determines its stressfulness. They suggested that each event was thought about (called cognitive appraisal) to estimate its degree of threat (primary appraisal) and to determine and mobilize resources to cope with it (secondary appraisal). Coping may focus on dealing with the threat directly or may emphasize the emotional response. These different ways to respond are called 'problem-focused' and 'emotion-focused' coping.

Stroebe (1992) challenged some aspects of the grief work hypothesis. While she recognized the cognitive processing element of the grief work hypothesis, she considered that it was limited because it focused attention on just the loss of the dead person and not all the subsequent changes that are likely to arise for a bereaved person. She also challenged the notion that the lack of cognitive processing was potentially pathological by highlighting psychological research which showed that excessive rumination may also be harmful (Nolen-Hoeksema 2002). So just dwelling upon the loss may not be adaptive. She also argued that part of the experience of bereavement is coming to terms with psycho-social changes. In particular, she criticized the emphasis of the grief work hypothesis on intra-psychic processing and its neglect of interpersonal relationships. Stroebe and Schut (1999) developed these ideas to form a new model, which they called 'the dual processing model'. They proposed that, following a death, people oscillate between 'restoration-focused' coping (e.g. dealing with everyday life), and 'loss-focused' coping (e.g. by expressing their distress). Examples of 'loss-focused' coping activities include thinking about the dead person, crying and talking about the loss. Examples of 'restoration-focused' activities include making new relationships, attending to everyday demands like parenting, 'forgetting' or being distracted from thinking about the loss, and returning to employment. They suggest that people move between these two forms of coping with grief depending upon their personality, age, gender and social roles, although many of the coping responses become progressively more 'restoration-focused'. From these ideas, they developed therapeutic interventions to help people address both types of coping to achieve a balance, especially for those people who have a tendency to retain loss- or restoration-focused modes of coping. For example, if a person is so overwhelmed by grief that they spend all their time crying, they may not be able to engage in everyday self-care activities such as cooking a meal or attending to the needs of their children. Similarly, some people may 'bury' themselves in activities such as paid employment, which functions well to distract their attention from their loss; however, in such cases, there is a danger that the emotional impact of the loss may not be fully acknowledged.

Social aspects of loss

In this section, I turn my attention to the writers who have emphasized the social aspects of bereavement and loss (e.g. Klass *et al.* 1996; Walter 1999). Most of these writers bring sociological or anthropological perspectives to the topic of bereavement. They emphasize the changes to social roles and relationships that bereavement precipitates. Social roles are very important in defining identity (as explained in Chapter 1). Moreover, in modern society, identity is usually not fixed but is constantly renegotiated throughout the life span. Therefore, social factors such as age, gender, social class and ethnicity all impact on the meaning of loss and the way bereavement is enacted (Field *et al.* 1997). From this perspective, grief is not merely a set of psychological responses that are largely biologically determined (as Bowlby has argued), as patterns of grief and possibilities for its expression are largely influenced by social and cultural factors (Reimers 2001; Field and Payne 2003). Historians and anthropologists have also noted the diversity of expressions of loss, in terms of the rituals associated with death, and the differing impact that different types of loss may have depending upon social status, age and gender. It is these social discourses about loss and bereavement that I explore next.

Lofland (1985) has drawn attention to the effects of the meaning of loss in different societies. She argues that the 'painful, debilitating and relatively long-lasting' (Lofland 1985: 172) grief typical of contemporary experience in North America and the UK arise from social conditions in which the majority of losses are experienced. Typically in the USA and the UK, deaths occur in older age and, therefore, spousal bereavement is common. In addition, the partner usually dies after a long joint relationship and, because of differences in male and female mortality, it is usually women who are left as widows with often little opportunity to form new partnerships. Some features of contemporary Western family structure and personal relationships – such as high investment in small numbers of children, high rates of divorce and marital separation, geographical mobility for education and employment, and increased numbers of people living in single-person households – may mean that, relative to other societies, older people are not very socially enmeshed in their local communities. Therefore, when bereavement occurs in older age, it may be experienced in relative isolation. The solitary widow living alone in the former family home may have plenty of opportunity to be constantly reminded of her lost partner.

Deaths that occur in younger people are almost always regarded as untimely and a tragedy. There are few agreed social responses to the loss of children in developed countries, so they tend to be regarded as highly abnormal and threatening (Riches and Dawson 2000). In addition, cultural expectations that bereavement should be an intensely personal and distressing experience are perpetuated through influential personal accounts (e.g. Lewis 1966) and by the self-help and popular literature, which tends to present a psychological and emotional account of grief (the types of information leaflets provided by hospices and specialist palliative care services are good examples). Lofland (1985: 181) argues that contemporary Western grief is expressed as it is because of four aspects of modern life:

- a relational pattern that links individuals to a small number of highly significant others;
- a definition of death as personal annihilation and as unusual and tragic except among the aged;
- selves which take very seriously their emotional states; and
- interactional settings that provide rich opportunities to contemplate loss.

Several writers have commented upon how the personal meaning of loss influences reactions to bereavement. Reimers (2001) highlights how Swedish society debated the 'proper' reaction to a major disaster, the sinking of a passenger ferry with the loss of 852 lives in 1994. Public debate centred on whether the bodies of the dead should be retrieved to permit burial or remain entombed in the sunken ship. Reimers argued that the public debates, which concluded that the bodies ought to be left in the ship, served to construct social discourses about 'normal' grieving. She concluded that this example demonstrated 'a societal ambition to discipline and control eruptions of strong sentiments, such as grief. One way to do this is to delineate the boundaries for what is to be considered as normal and permissive and to pathologise those who do not remain within those boundaries' (Reimers 2001: 244).

Other societies choose to memorialize certain deaths and not others. For example, memories of the many deaths that occurred during the First World War continue to haunt Britain and other countries (Hockey 2001). In the UK, the rituals associated with remembering the deaths of young soldiers in the First World War have increased rather than diminished in importance over the last few years, although few people remain alive who witnessed these events almost a century ago. In comparison, no attempt is made to memorialize those killed in industrial accidents over the last century.

Perhaps one of the most difficult types of bereavement for Western people at the present time is the death of a child (Riches and Dawson 2000). Low rates of infant mortality and the prevention and treatment of many acute medical conditions mean that the probability of babies, children and young people dying are generally very low in most developed countries. There are thus few socially accepted accounts to provide a meaning for these deaths. According to Riches and Dawson (2000), bereaved family members struggle to find a meaning for the death and differences between family members may give rise to different responses and ways of coping with grief. The devastating impact of child loss is not inevitable. Evidence from countries such as Brazil, where infant mortality rates are much higher, attest to different reactions, with some mothers describing their dead infants as angels returned to heaven and who are therefore safe and should not be mourned (Shepherd-Hughes 1972). Historically, the death of at least some children within large families was anticipated, but it is important not to attribute a lack of grief to parents in such circumstances. In modern society, childhood deaths are considered to be devastating to the parents, because with smaller families relatively more emotional and material resources are invested in each child.

Riches and Dawson (2000) show that the death of a child challenges many of the taken-for-granted aspects of everyday life. Certain roles, such as being a parent, can only be enacted in the presence of a child; therefore, the death of an only child removes the possibility of this social role. Parenting is a highly valued social role from which the individual receives not only personal satisfaction but social esteem from others. Parents generally invest a great deal of themselves in the lives of their children and on the death of a child their role of protector and provider is taken away. The death of a child disrupts the sense of identity, not only because the person may feel guilt but because other people react to them in different ways. The loss of a sibling when family sizes are small leaves gaps that are hard or impossible to fill. Families are complex social structures in which there are reciprocal roles and shared identities, which are maintained over time by mutual support, collective memories and goals (Kissane and Bloch 2002). Families are also dynamic and may not be mutually supportive (as discussed in Chapter 1). Families are situated in cultural contexts that may frame the meaning of the loss, such as the major religions. They are also situated in social contexts that may constrain the possibilities and behaviours open to them. For example, stillbirth and neonatal deaths may not be openly recognized by some societies and the mourning rituals associated with them may not be similar to the rituals following the death of an adult. Thirty years ago in Britain it was unusual for hospitals to return miscarried foetuses and stillborn infants to their parents for burial. Hospitals tended to dispose of the infant in the way they would deal with unwanted biological material, without exploring the wishes of the parents. It is now more common practice for parents to arrange burial or cremation themselves.

Walter (1996) in the UK and Klass *et al.* (1996) in the USA have challenged the notion that successful resolution of grief involves 'moving on' and 'letting go' of the deceased person. Their views are based on the assumption that people wish to maintain feelings of continuity and that, even though physical relationships will end at the time of death, these relationships become transformed but remain important within the memory of the individual and community. Walter (1996, 1999) has proposed a biographical model of loss in which he suggests bereaved people seek to create a narrative that describes both the person who has died and the part they played in their lives. He argues that these narratives are socially constructed. Drawing upon his own personal experiences of grief, Walter argues that because post-modern societies are so fragmented and compartmentalized, people relate to others in different ways depending upon the social roles they occupy at any one time. For example, a person may be known to work colleagues as a hard driven boss, to his children as a kind but distant and largely absent father, to his wife as a generous but moody provider of finances, and to his Saturday morning golfing friends as a relaxed and easy going man. The palliative care team may know this person as a difficult and demanding person. Each role and aspect of this person's identity may not be known to others because societies are no longer enmeshed. We may know little about the different aspects of the life of our loved ones because much of our lives are spent apart in paid employment, separate leisure pursuits and in travelling. Klass *et al.* (1996) also proposed a similar idea and illustrated this in relation to different types of loss. They argued that, for many people, adapting to loss involves incorporating some aspect of their previous relationship with the deceased person into their current lives but in a way that is tolerable and not distressing.

Walter (1996) proposed that the purpose of grief was to construct a durable biography in which the 'whole' person was revealed and this became integrated into the memory of survivors. Thus a grandchild would be told stories of what their dead grandfather did and what he was like as a person. In this model of grief, memories and relationships with the dead person are fostered and developed in ways that are helpful and supportive in the life of those still living. Walter (1999) has protested against counselling practices that urge people to 'let go' or 'break the bonds' of relationships with the deceased. From his perspective, it is thought that continuing to have a relationship with deceased friends and family members is helpful. These relationships are largely construed as taking place in shared memories or discussion about the dead person, but they may also be expressed in retained precious objects, photographs or mementoes from the dead person. He rejects the notion that 'holding on' to these aspects of the dead person represents a failure to resolve grief or is in anyway pathological. While Walter's analysis is helpful in challenging the dominance of psychological perspectives on loss, it is based on his autobiographical accounts rather than a body of empirical research. Walter is an articulate academic for whom words (in narrative accounts) come easily; it should not be assumed that others have a similar facility with language.

How have these models influenced our thinking and resources to help bereaved people?

Most bereaved people manage the experience of loss by drawing upon their personal resources, in terms of their personality and coping styles, and by mobilizing their social resources. These resources include family and friendship relationships in which grief can be acknowledged and shared, and faith groups and wider social structures that provide opportunities to express grief and perform mourning rituals. In the past, social concern for bereaved people largely focused on supplying financial help to widows and making arrangements for the care of orphans. Such endeavours continue to be vitally important in some areas of the world, as in parts of Africa for example, to help the bereaved following deaths from AIDS. In the latter half of the twentieth century in the UK, a number of self-help groups such as Cruse began to offer emotional support to bereaved people. By the end of the century, there had been a large increase in these types of groups, funded by charitable giving and catering for many different types of loss (e.g. by suicide) and different age groups (e.g. childhood bereavement services; see Chapter 29). Bereavement services associated with health care provision are unusual in the UK, the exceptions being specialist palliative care (predominantly funded by the charitable sector), a few accident and emergency departments and a few obstetric units. Statutory provision for bereavement support in the UK was largely confined to the activities of hospital chaplains and a few concerned individuals; however, following public inquiries into the common practice of organ retention by pathology departments at British hospitals, the Department of Health has made recommendations that acute general hospitals should provide bereavement services, although there is little guidance on what services should be provided. Most bereavement support services in the UK remain outside the remit of statutory health and social care services.

From its early beginnings, hospice philosophy encompassed the care of patients and their families, which continued after death into bereavement.

Most UK hospices and palliative care units regard the provision of bereavement support as integral to their services, although there is little consensus about the nature of the services that should be provided or how they should be delivered or allocated (Wilkes 1993; Payne and Relf 1994). For a number of reasons, bereavement support has been marginalized and, arguably, remains the least well-developed aspect of hospices and specialist palliative care services (Payne and Relf 1994; Payne 2001a). Most services are based on an assumption that bereavement is a major stressful life event and that a minority of people experience substantial disruption to their physical, psychological and social functioning (Parkes 1996). Parkes (1993) has argued that offering support to people who have adequate internal and external resources can be disempowering and be detrimental to coping. This suggests that blanket provision of services to all bereaved family members may be at best wasteful of resources and, at worst, threatening to the coping responses of most people.

There is much that we do not know about what happens in hospice and specialist palliative care bereavement services and what constitutes good practice. There have been few methodologically rigorous evaluations of general bereavement support services and even fewer in relation to hospices (Payne *et al.* 1999). In 2003, a postal survey was conducted of all bereavement support services located in hospices and specialist palliative care units in the UK that were listed in the Hospice Directory (Payne *et al.* 2003). There were 253 replies from bereavement coordinators (a response rate of 83 per cent). Almost half of the services (47 per cent) had been in existence for 10 years; 65 per cent provided services just for those already associated with the hospice or specialist palliative care unit. Bereavement services employed paid workers from the following professional backgrounds: nurses (53 per cent), social workers (45 per cent), counsellors (45 per cent), doctors (16 per cent), psychologists (9 per cent), psychiatrists (2 per cent) and others such as chaplains. The survey shows there is less input from medical staff than in other aspects of specialist palliative care services. Typically, bereavement services have a median of two paid staff and a median of seven volunteers. In 66 per cent of services, volunteers played an important role in supporting bereaved people. Volunteers may enhance the range of services offered and address the need to make services culturally appropriate by involving local people and those from different minority ethnic groups. However, there is controversy about the extent to which volunteer labour is valued and how the needs of volunteer workers are met (Payne 2001b). Volunteers require careful recruitment, selection, training and supervision. Relf (1998) has pointed out that providing for the needs of volunteer workers in bereavement support is a demanding and skilled activity.

Bereavement support may include a broad range of activities such as social evenings, befriending, one-to-one counselling and support groups. Figure 22.1 presents information about the types of activities offered by UK hospice bereavement services. The data show that individual support in the form of befriending, one-to-one counselling or other personal contact was provided by virtually all services, while drop-in centres were the least likely

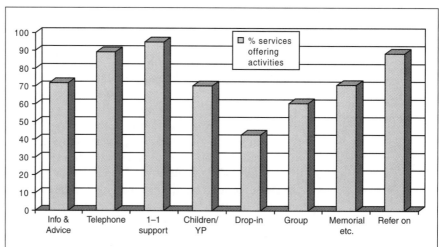

Figure 22.1   Types of activities provided by UK hospice bereavement support services (adapted from Payne *et al.* 2003).

to be provided. The average service provided 160 people with one-to-one support per year. Bereavement support may start before the death, when families are put in touch with volunteer workers who may befriend them and maintain contact with them following the death. Such services offer the opportunity for relationships to be built up over time, and for newly bereaved people to be spared the difficulty of making new relationships when they are at their most vulnerable. However, most bereavement services only offer post-death contact and support. I have summarized some of the activities that nurses caring for newly bereaved people in institutional settings may wish to consider (see Box 22.3).

All bereavement services need to set up systems to identity which clients need help and most have to make decisions about their use of resources. In the UK survey described previously, approximately a third of services adopted formal assessments using questionnaires and checklists, combined with clinical judgements to assess how likely it is that a bereaved person will have an adverse outcome and is likely to benefit from the offer of services. This figure represents a small increase from the 25 per cent reported using formal assessments in a survey conducted in 1993 (Payne and Relf 1994). The use of formal risk assessment relies on well-recognized attributes of the person, their environment and the nature of the death, which allow predictions to be made about which people need help (Saunders 1993). For example, a person with previous mental health problems experiencing concurrent losses, such as their job or home, and witnessing a traumatic sudden death of their young child in a car accident, is likely to be more vulnerable than a person bereaved of their elderly grandmother after a chronic illness. Although risk assessment measures are available, none are perfect and most services continue to allocate bereavement support based on clinical judge-

---

Box 22.3 Suggestions for supporting people immediately after a death

- Tell the family member that the patient has died.
- Obtain medical confirmation and certification of death as soon as possible.
- Ask if the family member wishes to see the deceased person. Offer to accompany them to the room if the dead person is still on the ward or to view the body elsewhere.
- Warn them what their dead family member may look like, especially it they have visible injuries, bandages, etc. Many people have never seen a dead person and may be fearful.
- Offer to remain with them until they feel comfortable in the presence of the deceased person, and then offer to withdraw.
- Make it clear that they can touch the deceased person, kiss and caress them, and talk to them if they wish.
- Allow them as much time as they wish to remain with the body. Do not appear to be rushing them to leave.
- Enable family members to take mementoes of the deceased such as a lock of hair. For babies and young children, some parents wish to take photographs, hand or foot prints.
- Ask if family members wish to have a priest or faith advisor to pray with them or perform religious rituals.
- Enable family members to perform any cultural or religious practices that are meaningful for them.
- Help families to leave the hospital or hospice when they are ready. Ensure that they are able to get home, assist with arranging transport and, if they wish, offer to contact friends or other family members who are able to offer support.
- Provide written information about procedures such as collection of the deceased's property, how to register the death and arrange a funeral.
- If there is to be a post-mortem examination and if body parts need to be removed for examination, request permission and obtain written consent. Make clear the reasons for any legal procedures such as an inquest.
- Provide family members with a contact telephone number in case they have questions they later wish to ask about the care of their loved one prior to or at the time of death.
- There are no 'right' words to say immediately after a death, but having the time and ability to listen to whatever the newly bereaved person may wish to talk about is generally valued.

---

ment. Hospice bereavement support services also need to be able to identify when clients have such difficult and complex problems that they exceed their capacity to deal with them. Close and well-established links with other mental health services, such as liaison psychiatry or clinical psychology, are needed but may be difficult to access.

Providing bereavement services is difficult and demanding work. The emotional demand placed on those who witness grief and support bereaved people requires skill, knowledge and sensitivity (Payne 2001b). The paradoxical nature of bereavement support, which demands both professional standards of knowledge and skill and the warmth of human understanding and sensitivity, represents a challenge for all. There is a dilemma in training volunteers and professionals that the compassion and empathy, which lead them into this work, becomes constrained by a framework imposed by models of bereavement. Exposure to repeated distress needs to be acknowledged as potentially difficult to deal with. In our recent UK survey, 67 per cent of services provided specialist training in addition to general induction programmes. Approximately two-thirds of services (61 per cent) provided regular supervision to paid bereavement workers and 60 per cent of services employing volunteers provided them with regular supervision. It is generally considered to be good practice to ensure that supervision is available to bereavement care workers, in which emotional off-loading and discussion of difficult circumstances can be dealt with on a regular basis (Payne *et al.* 1999). By drawing on the data from the survey, we have provided a 'snapshot' of the nature of hospice bereavement support in the UK in the early part of the twenty-first century, but much remains that is not known about the efficacy of services.

▌Overview of chapters in Part Three

In the remainder of this chapter, I will introduce the following seven chapters. The aim is to guide the reader by providing a conceptual framework to understand the content. The themes of loss and the consequences of care at the time of death and during bereavement incorporate a number of perspectives. Authors of the following chapters draw on research, clinical practice and experience of bereavement support services from several domains.

In the first chapter, Komaromy focuses on nursing care during the process of dying. In doing this, she draws on a large ethnographic study of older people dying in residential and nursing care homes in the UK. Froggatt (2001a,b) has described the plight of older people in care homes as 'disadvantaged dying'. Komaromy and her colleagues have done much to expose this plight by revealing how difficult it is to achieve high-quality nursing care for dying people in these institutions. There are a cluster of factors that appear to conspire against optimal care. There is, of course, great diversity in the quality of residential and nursing homes for older people in the UK and in other countries. In 2001 in the UK, there were approximately 29,850 care homes for older people with 594,431 beds. Recent trends have been for a reduction in statutory provision for long-term care of frail and disabled older people, and a large increase in privately run (for-profit) homes. While some of these homes offer excellent care and facilities, many do not. In particular, there have been concerns about the quantity and quality of care staff. Typically, care homes have relatively few qualified nursing staff and the majority of the personal care is provided by care assistants who may have had very little skills training or specialist knowledge about older people or how to care for dying people. Many homes experience difficulties in recruiting and retaining staff. Care staff are likely to be on low wages and many work part-time. These employment characteristics present particular problems in providing continuity of care and in offering additional education and skills training. The hierarchical nature of the organizational structure of many care homes may inhibit staff from developing their practice, using evidenced-based care guidelines or challenging organizational cultures (Wicke *et al.* in press).

The protracted nature of dying for older people may also make it difficult for nurses to realize when they are dying and to predict when the death is likely to occur (Seymour *et al.* 2001). As Komaromy argues in her chapter, it is important for nurses to be able to predict when the person is dying to elicit additional resources and, if necessary, make a referral to a specialist palliative care team. Recognition of impending death also allows care to be modified; for example, regular pressure area care may involve disturbing the patient and contribute to pain and discomfort, and is not necessary if the person is in the final stages of dying. Changes to medication, food and fluid intake may all be appropriate as the person approaches death. The signs of dying may be harder to detect in very old people whose health declines slowly over many years. It may also be difficult for nurses in care homes to initiate discussions about dying with these people and their family members, if open discussion is not part of the culture of care. To achieve this they may need additional communication skills training and support from other staff members. Komaromy's chapter offers an illumination of these and other issues for nurses caring for those at the time of death.

Chapter 24 by Sque and Wells concerns a health technology that spans the boundaries between life and death. Organ donation and organ transplantation have become available for those with severe end-stage organ failure. The technical surgical procedures and the medical management of associated immune reactions have been pioneered over the last 30 years. Organ transplantations offer the potential for life enhancement, improved quality of life and greatly extended survival for many people who would otherwise have died or had seriously compromised quality of life, such as those using haemodialysis. However, cadaveric organ donation is only possible because another person has died and their family has agreed to donation.

Organ donation, therefore, raises important moral and ethical issues. It also challenges our taken-for-granted notions of what being dead means, because parts of the dead person continue to live on in other people. There has been much debate about how the end-of-life care of those who become organ donors is managed. For example, the extent to which normal physiological functions are artificially maintained (such as by mechanical ventilation) to ensure lungs and other organs are 'healthy' and well perfused prior to removal, even though the person has been certified as brainstem dead. Sque and Wells note the ambivalence experienced by families as they come to realize that their loved one, while appearing to be warm, pink and breathing (all normal signs of life), is in fact dead because their brain has been irreparably damaged. They show that paradoxical beliefs about awareness of death (and, therefore, agreement for organ donation) can run alongside lingering doubts about the sentience of the newly dead body.

In the future, it is likely that health technologies will increasingly impact on how death and dying is managed (Seymour *et al.* 2002) both for the benefit of the dying person and for the benefit of what they may donate to others. Sque and Wells argue that discussion of organ and tissue donation in palliative care promotes patients' autonomy and choices. Others may argue that it is insensitive and potentially exploitative of vulnerable people. By including this topic in our book, we wish to open up debate about the role of organ and tissue donation in palliative care. What evidence there is suggests that families may welcome the opportunity to consider corneal and other types of donation in palliative care contexts (Carey and Forbes 2003).

The remaining chapters in Part Three focus on families and friends of the deceased person, who rapidly change their status in the minds of health and social care workers from 'carers' to become 'the bereaved'. In Chapter 25, Cobb writes about the role of nurses immediately after a death has occurred. He highlights the individuality of the experience of loss and the inadequacy of any one theoretical model to provide a template.

Much general palliative care is delivered by general practitioners (GPs) and community nurses. It is therefore appropriate that we consider how bereavement support is provided in primary health care. In Chapter 26, Birtwistle focuses on the role of the primary care team and in particular community nurses in providing bereavement support. He argues that because in largely secular societies such as the UK people lack religious frameworks and spiritual advisors to support them in times of crisis, people increasingly construe their bereavement problems as within the remit of health care services. In the UK, access to primary health care services is readily available and free at the point of contact. Primary care services have responded to increased demands from bereaved people in a number of ways, including the use of proactive bereavement follow-up protocols, informal bereavement visits by community nurses and referral to practice-based counsellors. There is little consensus about what should be the proper role of primary care team members or evidence about the efficacy or cost-effectiveness of proactive bereavement support. It is not clear to what extent GPs regard this as an appropriate role, and even whether they have sufficient time and the appropriate expertise to engage in prolonged supportive interventions (Harris and Kendrick 1998; Main 2000).

Over the last decade, there has been a rapid growth in the provision of counselling services based in or associated with British primary health care. By 1999, 51 per cent of practices had counselling provision (Foster 2000). This growth has arisen from various British government policy initiatives and recognition that the many patients who consult GPs with psychological problems may be better served by referral to those with counselling skills. However, there is evidence of great variation in the skills, training and therapeutic approaches of counsellors employed in general practice (Wiles 1993). Dealing with loss, and more specifically bereavement, seems to form a substantial proportion of counsellors' caseloads (Sibbald *et al.* 1993). Evidence from a study conducted in primary care settings in southern and south-western England indicated that GPs primarily saw their role as identifying 'risk factors' for abnormal bereavement and making referrals to counsellors (Payne *et al.* 2002). Counsellors perceived bereavement as just one type of loss for which they had skills in working with clients. Most drew upon psychological phase/stage models in guiding their interventions with bereaved clients (Wiles *et al.* 2002).

Health care is increasingly being construed as the management of risk and public health messages are often conveyed in terms of reducing health risks associated with lifestyle choices such as smoking or eating high-fat foods. Relf applies the perceived logic of risk management in Chapter 27 to her discussion of risk assessment in bereavement. She details the history of the use of standardized measures that predict the likelihood of poor bereavement outcome. This method has been used to allocate bereavement care to those most likely to benefit from it. It is argued that risk assessment not only targets costly and limited resources appropriately, but ensures that low-risk individuals are not disempowered by implying that they may not be able to cope with their loss and thus create dependency. Relf is critical of the notion of risk assessment and argues that it is embedded in a positivitist paradigm and is derived from the psychological/psychiatric models of bereavement. She explains how later models, introduced earlier in this overview, have challenged concepts such as 'recovery' and 'resolution' of grief. She concludes pragmatically by indicating the weaknesses and the strengths of using formalized risk assessment procedures. The debates about risk assessment in this chapter raise important issues for consideration in designing bereavement support services.

In Chapter 28, Kissane provides an overview of bereavement support activities provided by hospices and specialist palliative care services. He proposes that support should be conceptualized at three levels:

- a general culture of support and understanding provided by all the members of the health and social care team in collaboration with the wider community;
- identification of those at risk and offers of support to prevent adverse outcomes; and
- recognition of those with existing problems and referral for psychotherapeutic interventions.

Kissane describes the common activities and interventions that fit the different requirements of these categories of support. He considers the evidence base for the various activities and offers a summary of how nurses might engage in providing different types of support. Kissane and his colleagues are best known for developing family-focused grief support interventions (Kissane and Bloch 2002) in Australia. He draws upon his wide experience in making recommendations in this chapter. Working with families facing death and during bereavement is complex, as family members may respond in very different ways. Gender roles may determine expectations about how individuals may react and the resources both within and outside the family that they can access. For example, it might be easier for men to use the distraction of paid employment to 'take time off' from grieving. Family members may also be protective of each other and seek to minimize the distress of others by concealing their own feelings. This may be misconstrued as a lack of feeling. In multicultural societies, it cannot be assumed that partners share the same cultural or religious backgrounds. The differences in accepted cultural mourning practices may mean that the wider family misunderstands the grieving responses of the unrelated partner. Working with families, therefore, requires a high degree of skill and sensitivity (Riches and Dawson 2000; Kissane and Bloch 2002).

A focus on families and childhood bereavement is the topic of the final chapter in Part Three by Rolls. We have decided to include this chapter on childhood bereavement services in a book predominantly concerned with adult palliative care because adults are parents of children and therefore may use these family-orientated services. Also, the terminal illness and death of an adult may impact upon children in their family system, including grandchildren. In Chapter 29, Rolls considers not only the characteristics of childhood bereavement services in the UK and how they work with children and families, but their wider role in society. She argues that, in the past, loss and bereavement affecting children was contained within the family and was treated as a private matter for parents to deal with. One response to this was that death was hidden from young children who were not encouraged to participate in mourning rituals like funerals and open discussion of the death was not allowed. Contemporary responses to death affecting children have become 'professionalized' with the introduction of grief counsellors into schools and the rapid increase in the number of childhood bereavement services. Why is it that these services have emerged in developed countries when the probability of children being exposed to sibling or parental death is so low and decreasing? It is perhaps for these very reasons that there are few social frameworks for providing meanings for these deaths and each family may have little opportunity to meet with others who share their experiences (Riches and Dawson 2000).

▌ Recommended reading

Hockey, J., Katz, J. and Small, N. (eds) (2001) *Grief, Mourning and Death Ritual.* Buckingham: Open University Press.

Payne, S., Horn, S. and Relf, M. (1999) *Loss and Bereavement.* Buckingham: Open University Press.

Stroebe, M.S., Hansson, R.O., Stroebe, W. and Schut, H. (eds) (2002) *Handbook of Bereavement Research: Consequences, Coping and Care.* Washington, DC: American Psychological Association.

Walter, T. (1999) *On Bereavement.* Buckingham: Open University Press.

References

Bartlett, D. (1998) *Stress*. Buckingham: Open University Press.

Birley, J. (2002) How ward doctors and nurses record that a patient is 'dying'. Unpublished MMedSci dissertation, University of Sheffield.

Bowlby, J. (1969) *Attachment and Loss, Vol. 1: Attachment*. London: The Hogarth Press.

Bowlby, J. (1973) *Attachment and Loss, Vol. 2: Separation*. London: The Hogarth Press.

Bowlby, J. (1980) *Attachment and Loss, Vol. 3: Loss: Sadness and Depression*. London: The Hogarth Press.

Carey, I. and Forbes, K. (2003) The experiences of donor families in the hospice. *Palliative Medicine*, 17: 241–7.

Engel, G. (1961) Is grief a disease? *Psychological Medicine*, 23: 18–22.

Evans, A. (1994) Anticipatory grief: a theoretical challenge. *Palliative Medicine*, 8(2): 159–65.

Fenichel, O. (1945) *The Psychoanalytic Theory of Neurosis*. New York: Norton.

Field, D. and Payne, S. (2003) Social aspects of bereavement. *Journal of Cancer Nursing*, 2(8): 21–5.

Field, D., Hockey, J. and Small, N. (1997) *Death, Gender and Ethnicity*. London: Routledge.

Foster, J. (2000) Counselling in primary care and the new NHS. *British Journal of Guidance and Counselling*, 28(2): 175–90.

Freud, S. (1917) *Mourning and Melancholia*. London: The Hogarth Press.

Froggatt, K.A. (2001a) Life and death in English nursing homes: sequestration or transition? *Ageing and Society*, 21: 319–32.

Froggatt, K.A. (2001b) Palliative care and nursing homes: where next? *Palliative Medicine*, 15: 42–8.

Harris, T. and Kendrick, A.R. (1998) Bereavement care in general practice: a survey in South Thames Health Region. *British Journal of General Practice*, 46: 1560–4.

Hockey, J. (2001) Changing death rituals, in J. Hockey, J. Katz and N. Small (eds) *Grief, Mourning and Death Ritual*. Buckingham: Open University Press.

Hockey, J., Katz, J. and Small, N. (eds) (2001) *Grief, Mourning and Death Ritual*. Buckingham: Open University Press.

Kissane, D.W. and Bloch, S. (2002) *Family Focused Grief Therapy*. Buckingham: Open University Press.

Klass, D., Silverman, P.R. and Nickman, S.L. (1996) *Continuing Bonds*. Philadephia, PA: Taylor & Francis.

Kubler-Ross, E. (1969) *On Death and Dying*. New York, Macmillan.

Lazarus, R.S. and Folkman, S. (1984) *Stress, Appraisal and Coping*. New York: Springer.

Lewis, C.S. (1966) *A Grief Observed*. London: Faber & Faber.

Lindemann, E. (1944) Symptomatology and management of acute grief. *American Journal of Psychiatry*, 101: 141–8.

Lofland, L.H. (1985) The social shaping of emotion: a case of grief. *Symbolic Interaction*, 8(2): 171–90.

Main, J. (2000) Improving management of bereavement in general practice based on a survey of recently bereaved subjects in a single general practice. *British Journal of General Practice*, 50: 863–6.

McNamara, B., Waddell, C. and Colvin, M. (1994) The institutionalization of the good death. *Social Science and Medicine*, 39: 1501–8.

Nolen-Hoeksema, S. (2002) Ruminative coping and adjustment, in M.S. Stroebe, R.O. Hansson, W. Stroebe and H. Schut (eds) *Handbook of Bereavement Research: Consequences, Coping and Care*. Washington, DC: American Psychological Association.

Parkes, C.M. (1971) Psychosocial transitions: a field for study. *Social Science and Medicine*, 5(2): 101–14.

Parkes, C.M. (1972) *Bereavement*. London: Routledge.

Parkes, C.M. (1986) *Bereavement*, 2nd edn. London: Routledge.

Parkes, C.M. (1993) Bereavement as a psychosocial transition: processes of adaptation to change, in M.S. Stroebe, W. Stroebe and R.O. Hansson (eds) *Handbook of Bereavement*. Cambridge: Cambridge University Press.

Parkes, C.M. (1996) *Bereavement*, 3rd edn. London: Routledge.

Parkes, C.M., Relf, M. and Couldrick A. (1996) *Counselling in Terminal Care and Bereavement*. Leicester: BPS Books.

Parkes, C.M., Laungani, P. and Young, B. (1997) *Death and Bereavement Across Cultures*. London: Routledge.

Payne, S. (2001a) Bereavement support: something for everyone? *International Journal of Palliative Nursing*, 7(3): 108.

Payne, S. (2001b) The role of volunteers in hospice bereavement support in New Zealand. *Palliative Medicine*, 15: 107–15.

Payne, S. and Lloyd Williams, M. (2003) Bereavement care, in M. Lloyd-Williams (ed.) *Psychosocial Issues in Palliative Care*. Oxford: Oxford University Press.

Payne, S. and Relf, M. (1994) The assessment of need for bereavement follow-up in palliative and hospice care. *Palliative Medicine*, 8: 291–7.

Payne, S., Horn, S. and Relf, M. (1999) *Loss and Bereavement*. Buckingham: Open University Press.

Payne, S., Jarrett, N., Wiles, R. and Field, D. (2002) Counselling strategies for bereaved people offered in primary care. *Counselling Psychology Quarterly*, 15(2): 161–77.

Payne, S., Field, D., Relf, M. and Reid, D. (2003) *Evaluating the Bereavement Support Services Provided to Older People by Hospices, Phase 1*. Unpublished report, Trent Palliative Care Centre, University of Sheffield.

Quested, B. and Rudge, T. (2003) Nursing care of dead bodies: a discursive analysis of last offices. *Journal of Advanced Nursing*, 41(6): 553–60.

Reimers, E. (2001) Bereavement – a social phenomenon? *European Journal of Palliative Care*, 8(6): 242–5.

Relf, M. (1998) Involving volunteers in bereavement counselling. *European Journal of Palliative Care*, 5(2): 61–5.

Riches, G. and Dawson, P. (2000) *An Intimate Loneliness: Supporting Bereaved Parents and Siblings*. Buckingham: Open University Press.

Saunders, C.M. (1993) Risk factors in bereavement outcome, in M.S. Stroebe, W. Stroebe and R.O. Hansson (eds) *Handbook of Bereavement*. Cambridge: Cambridge University Press.

Selye, H. (1956) *The Stress of Life*. New York: McGraw-Hill.

Seymour, J. (2001) *Critical Moments – Death and Dying in Intensive Care*. Buckingham: Open University Press.

Seymour, J.E., Clark, D. and Philp, I. (2001) Palliative care and geriatric medicine: shared concerns, shared challenges (editorial). *Palliative Medicine*, 15(4): 269–70.

Seymour, J.E., Clark, D., Gott. M., Bellamy, G. and Ahmedzai, S. (2002) Good deaths, bad deaths: older people's assessments of risks and benefits in the use of morphine and terminal sedation in end of life care. *Health, Risk and Society*, 4(3): 287–304.

Shepherd-Hughes, N. (1972) *Death Without Weeping. The Violence of Everyday Life in Brazil*. Berkeley, CA: University of California Press.

Sibbald, B., Addington-Hall, L., Brenneman, D. and Freeling, P. (1993) Counsellors in English and Welsh general practices: their nature and distribution. *British Medical Journal*, 306: 29–33.

Small, N. (2001) Theories of grief: a critical review, in J. Hockey, J. Katz and N. Small (eds) *Grief, Mourning and Death Ritual*. Buckingham: Open University Press.

Sque, M. and Payne, S.A. (1996) Dissonant loss: the experience of donor relatives. *Social Science and Medicine*, 43(9): 1359–70.

Stroebe, M. (1992) Coping with bereavement: A review of the grief work hypothesis. *Omega: Journal of Death and Dying*, 26: 19–42.

Stroebe, M. and Schut, H. (1999) The dual process model of coping with bereavement: rationale and description. *Death Studies*, 23: 197–224.

Stroebe, M.S., Hansson, R.O., Stroebe, W. and Schut, H. (2002) *Handbook of Bereavement Research: Consequences, Coping and Care*. Washington, DC: American Psychological Association.

Sudnow, D. (1967) *Passing On*. Englewood Cliffs, NJ: Prentice-Hall.

Sullivan, H.L. (1956) The dynamics of emotion, in H.L. Sullivan (ed.) *Clinical Studies in Psychiatry*. New York: Norton.

Walter, T. (1996) A new model of grief: bereavement and biography. *Mortality*, 1(1): 1–29.

Walter, T. (1999) *On Bereavement*. Buckingham: Open University Press.

Wicke, D., Coppin, R. and Payne, S. (in press) Team working in nursing homes: a focus group study of qualified nurses. *Journal of Advanced Nursing*.

Wiles, R. (1993) *Counselling in General Practice*. Southampton: Institute for Health Policy Studies, University of Southampton.

Wiles, R., Jarrett, N., Payne, S. and Field, D. (2002) Referrals for bereavement counselling in primary care: a qualitative study. *Patient Education and Counselling*, 48: 79–85.

Wilkes, E. (1993) Characteristics of hospice bereavement services. *Journal of Cancer Care*, 2: 183–9.

Wolf, Z. (1988) *Nurses' Work: The Sacred and the Profane*. Philadelphia, PA: University of Pennsylvania Press.

Worden, J.W. (1982) *Grief Counselling and Grief Therapy: A Handbook for the Mental Health Practitioner*. New York: Springer.

Worden, J.W. (1991) *Grief Counselling and Grief Therapy*, 2nd edn. New York: Springer.

Worden, J.W. (2001) *Grief Counselling and Grief Therapy*, 3rd edn. New York: Springer.

Wortman, C.B. and Silver, R.C. (1989) The myths of coping with loss. *Journal of Consulting and Clinical Psychology*, 57(3): 349–57.

23

Nursing care at the time of death

Carol Komaromy

'We're expected to be able to cope with anything really. Sometimes you just have to pretend to be OK. 'Cos –you know –it's expected of you. You are it –the one who copes –while everyone else falls about' (Mary, sta ff nurse). This quote from Mary (whose name has been changed), a nurse in a care home for older people, is representative of the type of response that I commonly heard during the fieldwork on a project into the management of death and dying in these settings in the UK (Sidell *et al.* 1997). Indeed, nurses, as frontline workers, have to cope with death in a variety of settings –hospitals, hospices, domestic homes as well as residential care homes. In this chapter, I explore what happens at and around the time of death from a sociological point of view and how this impacts upon nursing care.

I begin with a discussion of the importance of being able to predict when death will occur and go on to ask what it is about death that makes it such a special event. I follow this discussion with an exploration of the different ways in which death is constructed and how this impacts upon the moment of death. I challenge the assumptions that underpin the notion of a 'good' death, both from the point of view of the possibility of being able to define what this means as well as its achievement. I conclude with a discussion of the body after death and its immediate impact upon any family and friends of the deceased.

Where and when death occurs

The time, setting and place of death all have the potential to impact upon the way that professionals are able to provide care at the time of death. One of the key factors in being able to provide care is knowing that someone is dying and when his or her death is likely to occur. The importance of being able to predict death and dying was something that Glaser and Strauss

(1965) explored in a seminal ethnographic study based on the observations that they made in hospital wards in San Francisco. They found that, to be able to plan terminal care, hospital staff needed to be able to predict when deaths might occur. However, these predictions were complex, needed to be updated and even 'renegotiated'. For example, they categorized predictions into three main types:

1   First, they found that it was possible to be virtually certain about when the death would occur.

2   Second, for those patients for whom there was less certainty about the time of death, it might be possible in the future to establish a time when there could be certainty.

3   The third and final category, and the one that staff found most difficult to cope with, was that in which the time of death was 'uncertain' and there was no clear time when any certainty could be established. In other words, there were patients for whom it was unlikely that staff would be able to predict the time of death.

Perhaps in the 1960s the need for predictions about death could be viewed as part of the more instrumental treatment of dying people. But the need for accurate predictions of the time of death is even greater as a result of changes in practice from general non-disclosure of diagnosis and prognosis to the current situation in which fuller disclosure is the norm. 'Hospice pioneers advanced a model of care in which patients were informed frankly and openly of their condition, and were actively encouraged to participate in all the decisions surrounding their treatment and care' (Abel 1986, cited in Lawton 2000: 42).

Underpinning this philosophy is the assumption that predicted deaths can be managed in the 'best' setting, that being the one that the dying person has chosen. Realistically, however, many people have little choice, even the small percentage of people for whom hospice care is available. The elite nature of palliative care has been well documented (Clark *et al.* 1997; Addington-Hall *et al.* 1998), but there are people for whom this shared disclosure of death is not available or part of the normal approach to their care. Seymour (2001), for example, in her ethnographic account of end-of-life care, discussed the 'uncertain' deaths that occur in intensive care units. Similarly, death occurs in settings in which it can be classified as being 'out of place', such as accident and emergency departments (Tinnermans 1998).

The reality seems to be that for everyone who is involved in death and dying, there is a premium upon being able to predict when the death is likely to occur. Being able to make an accurate prediction of death affects the ability of those involved to be able to choose the place of death and the manner of that death. But there are other reasons that explain why it is important to be able to predict death and it is to some of these that I turn next.

The meaning of death

Bauman (1992) argues that in a post-modern society death does not carry the same significance that it did in the past – for example, in the fifteenth century, when people were more likely to believe that reward or punishment in the 'next' life was a result of their behaviour in this one. Bauman also suggests that the general decline in the belief in life after death in Western culture has reduced the power of creeds to dictate how we behave in this life. The result of this, he claims, is that in a post-modern society people are more likely to focus upon the intrinsic value of this life rather than postponing any investment in an 'afterlife'.

There are dangers in this type of generalized statement, not least because it fails to acknowledge the varied terrain of beliefs. It might be reasonable to claim that, in Western culture, there is no longer a unified belief in an 'afterlife' or in the belief that admission to an afterlife is granted by some sort of moral or spiritual gatekeeper. But Davies (2002) argues that many people believe in a continuation of life after death and that, 'Death rites are as much concerned with the issues of identity and social continuity as with the very practical fact that human bodies decay and become offensive to the sight and smell of the living' (p. 6).

With the focus for individuals on their social identity, it is difficult to imagine a world in which we do not continue to exist in some way and even more difficult to remove ourselves from the influences in society that shape the way that death is treated. This makes what happens at the time of death significant, albeit to varying degrees. Furthermore, the practical fact of the decay of the material body that Davies refers to above does not mean that the body at the time of death is unimportant. For some who believe in a transition from one existence to another, the body plays a significant part. Davies (2002) argues that just as the living body is subjected to social rules or norms of behaviour, we also invest the corpse with meaning and feelings that reflect the values of society.

But the body has different meanings associated with it and I would add that the body is also a container of death and as such is a 'taboo' object. When the bodies of residents in care homes are removed, their exit is mostly concealed from other residents. Staff and funeral directors collude in conferring a dangerous status onto the body by covering the corpse with sheets or placing them into thick, black plastic bags. These covered up, enclosed bodies represent death in the form of a tightly wrapped corpse . . . Having produced something unsightly it must be concealed' (Komaromy 2000: 311).

This diversity in beliefs about the meaning of death places a high premium on effective communication about what needs to happen at the time of death, as well as the need to be able to predict the moment of death. Such diversity also suggests the potential for a lack of any clear understanding about what those needs might be. With so much invested in the significance of the moment of death, nurses, as key players at the time of death, face a potential minefield of inconsistent spiritual, emotional and physical needs, all of which are in a relationship with each other and the dying person and any family and friends.

The moment of death

The significance of the moment of death arises at several different levels: the medical, legal, spiritual, cultural and social. The impact of what happens at the moment of death is part of the understanding of the way that people are able to grieve. Institutional and social practice require action to be taken at the moment of death in part arising from the professionalization of death. Perhaps it is unsurprising that there is a lot of anxiety about being present at the moment of death and doing the 'right' things at that moment. This places a burden upon those professionals who are involved at the time of death to get it 'right', because there is no second chance. Nurses present at the moment of death need to understand the significance of this moment on all of these levels.

Medical and legal context

The need for information to be able to certify death is a legal requirement and one which places a great demand on being present at the moment of death. Rosenblatt *et al.* (1976) argue that the medicalization of death is itself a form of ritual that involves medical people as the specialists who witness death. The medical construction of death defines it as a precise moment in time. The medicalization and legalization requires there to be a precise time given to the moment of death, even though there are ambiguities to this diagnosis (Turner 1987). Certainly, having the power to define a moment of death carries its own ritualistic power. Particularly so when within the medical paradigm where there are categories of death. For example, the status of the 'ventilated corpse' has been created to define the status of the body in the stage between the definition of brain death and the removal of organs for transplantation.

But what happens in the emergency resuscitations and the ambiguity of a cardiac arrest and the patient or person for whom the moment of death is one from which there is the possibility of recovery and who might be resuscitated? For people whose hearts are defined as having 'arrested', death is deemed to be 'out of place' and there are likely to be attempts made to resuscitate them. In their ethnographic study of a resuscitation team in a large teaching hospital, Page and Komaromy (2000) note the ritualistic aspects of cardiopulmonary resuscitation (CPR): 'However, it is perhaps not difficult to see how a CPR event might be viewed in terms of a symbolic ritual, which, as van der Woning (1997) suggests, involves living out the myth of the superhuman, the heroic and "in control" and as such is illuminative of the culture in which it occurs'. They also claim that this ritual is an enactment of the power of medicine to be able to intervene and even possibly reverse death.

Spiritual and cultural context

Any spiritual or religious belief system will invest meaning in the moment of death. If death is believed to be the time at which there is a transition from one existence to another, there might be rituals that have to be carried out so that the passage is successful. For example, for some Jewish people the Rabbi should be present at the moment of death to say a confessional prayer and recite the fundamental affirmation of faith (Samson Katz 2001). Some Muslims need to sit up and face Mecca and the family needs to be able to perform certain bedside rituals, such as moistening the dying person's mouth and repeating their words. Some Buddhists might need a reading from the Book of the Dead to be performed by a Tibetan Monk so that their spirit might be guided, while Hindus might need to be placed on a mat on the floor to die and to have a few drops of water of the River Ganges placed on their lips from a basil leaf to the accompaniment of hymns and holy songs (Parkes *et al.* 1997).

Social context

Parkes *et al.* (1997) argue that alongside death, as an event that is increasingly postponed in the Western world, is an associated inability for people to face death. They also argue that the need for rituals associated with death (such as those outlined above) have correspondingly declined. Rituals that surround death can be of different orders. But it could be argued that there are different forms of social ritual, such as the professionalization and medicalization of death that serve the purpose of guiding people through the moment of death. Medical rituals include the need for staff involved in deaths to be able to 'perform' (Goffman 1959). This means that everyone involved needs to be seen to be concerned to get things right and must give a convincing performance of this, whatever their personal feelings. Goffman claims that 'impression management' is central to an understanding of what is taking place. In applying this idea to the moment of death, it seems that the 'impression' is 'managed' according to routines and rituals that structure how staff members behave. To take the analogy of performance further, these 'scripts' are often written into organizational procedures and protocols as codes of behaviour. It is as inappropriate for professionals to be too upset as it is for them to appear to be unaffected (Walter 1999).

Family and friends often want to be present at the moment of death and might participate in a bedside vigil, or request to be notified when a death is imminent. The need to say 'goodbye' could be regarded as greater if there is no belief in the likelihood of meeting in another life. Whatever the need at a personal level, this is part of his or her social role when someone is dying.

The role of nurses at the moment of death

It is not easy for nurses involved in end-of-life care and death moments to provide care that is appropriate at the time of death for individual dying people. There are dangers inherent in all of the interpretations of the purpose of death and the needs of dying people and their families. For example, it is dangerous to assume that people who belong to particular ethnic or religious groups will all share the same needs and conform to the expectations of that group at the moment of death. Similarly, there is a corresponding danger in not understanding the needs associated with someone's religious and cultural needs. These needs might conflict with the routines and rituals that are associated with the setting in which the death takes place. One care home manager told me of the resistance by her staff to leave a dead resident sitting in a chair for several hours while the family said their 'goodbyes' (Sidell *et al.* 1997). She recounted how the staff tried to pressurize her into putting the resident to bed, straightening the body and getting the undertakers to remove the body. As head of home she had the power to resist, but it is difficult to imagine this happening in many institutional settings.

In an ideal situation, the dying person should be invited to articulate their needs in advance of death so that the care staff would understand their needs and try to meet them. This would allow for people who need to be present at the death to be invited to do so and for those things that need to be done to be performed. The difficulty arises when dying people are unable to make their wishes known and nursing staff have to make a judgement on their behalf. All of this discussion about the significance of the moment of death carries assumptions about the type of death that people could achieve and this is the subject of the next section.

The 'good' death

Achieving a 'good' death clearly depends upon being aware of the imminence of death and the opportunity for the dying person to express their wishes as well as the capacity for care staff to be able to carry these out. The concept of a 'good' death is not new. Neither is it a straightforward concept. Its meaning has varied over time and between social and cultural groups. Bradbury (2001) has categorized the concept of a 'good' death into three types: the medicalized, the sacred and the natural. For example, a 'good' medicalized death might be one that is anticipated and pain-free, but this may conflict with the criteria associated with the natural dimension of a 'good death'. What the definition of the concept in this way ignores is the answer to the question 'good for whom?' As early as 1972, Weisman had introduced the concept of 'appropriate deaths', which took much more account of the relational aspects of death and the fact that people do not die as isolated individuals but as members of a social group. But, however the concept is defined there is a danger in its suggestion that death can be well managed and controlled.

In a study into physicians' emotional responses to the way that people in their care die, Good *et al.* (2002) took account of the technological changes that have impacted upon end-of-life care. Their findings suggest that 'dying is difficult, particularly in the modern hospital where there are so many treatment options and where relationships are short, discontinuous, without a perspective on the patient as a person, and with little time to acquire it. "Good deaths", if they exist, take place in the context of relationships in which the patient's personhood is known and valued' (p. 23).

In homes for older people, death is much more likely to be construed as a 'natural and timely' event, coming as it does at the end of a long life. But there are still problems and concerns associated with death in old age. The care staff in homes for older people have to manage the difficult boundary between life and death. The staff in these settings to whom I talked described a 'good death' as one that was 'peaceful', 'pain-free' and 'accompanied'. 'Good death is neither protracted nor sudden, its shape constituting a straightforward trajectory from deterioration to death' (Komaromy and Hockey 2001: 75). Even when the 'ideal' death was achieved, deathbed scenes were still construed by staff as dramatic events, seemingly conferring significance on a life when the quality of that life had been lost (Komaromy 2000).

Concerns about the quality of the care of dying people in acute and community settings and the focus upon medical care and saving life regardless of its quality gave rise to the demand for a more holistic approach to death and dying. The hospice movement pioneered the approach that aimed to incorporate death and dying back into life through the high-quality care of dying people. To do this, the forms of distress of dying people had to be recognized and relieved. The hospice approach and palliative care have become synonymous with best quality care for dying people. Even so, a hospice death is proscribed by moral ethics, which means certain wishes such as euthanasia (a 'good death') would not be granted. Palliative care offers itself as a viable alternative to the need for euthanasia. 'Palliative care professionals have, for a long time, been able to argue that the provision of palliative care relieves suffering to such an extent that euthanasia is no longer wanted by many people, even those who have previously been its advocates' (Oxenham and Boyd 1997: 284).

Dignity as part of a 'good death' is not easily defined. In a qualitative study of the way that dying people define dignity, Chochinov *et al.* (2002) discuss the way that the term 'dignity' is used in clinical and philosophical discourse in an ambiguous manner. Responses from patients in the study that specifically relate to the time of death seemed to highlight what the authors call 'death anxiety' and which included concerns about what the terminal phase of the illness would be like. Several of the patients who are quoted in this study wanted a 'quick' ending.

Sudden deaths as bad deaths

Most of the discussion of the achievement of a 'good death' has so far implied that there is a possibility of preparation for death. As discussed above, not everyone wants to be able to prepare for death through a period of protracted dying. Some people would prefer to die quickly. But there are deaths that cannot be anticipated and these create their own problems. The way that sudden death can complicate bereavement is well documented (Walter 1999; Eyre 2001; Howarth 2001). However, the main focus of these studies has been the effect of sudden death on bereaved people, with comparatively little attention being paid to the effect of sudden death upon the professionals involved, apart from the context of violent death and disaster (Eyre 2001). Most significantly, for those settings in which death is anticipated for all residents and considered to be 'natural' and 'timely', such as care homes for older people, sudden death has an enormous impact on the care staff and sometimes other residents depending upon their awareness of what has taken place. Key concerns for care staff in homes for older people include coping with the shock of the unexpected death, informing the family and reporting such deaths to the coroner. Deaths that are not expected – often classified as 'sudden' deaths – cause equal distress to the professionals and any family and friends involved.

The impact of the manner of death on bereavement

Anderson (2000), writing about the therapeutic response to grief, describes the event of death as something that is at the 'hub' of the stories of grief that are told during bereavement counselling and grief work. What he means by this is that all accounts lead to and from the event of the death. In grief counselling, people who are grieving are encouraged to talk about events that are categorized as being 'before' and 'after' the event. The death, then, is foregrounded as the most significant event in the grief process. This serves to focus more strongly on the moment of death and how this is managed.

Emerging and future issues

How the moment of death is managed impacts upon the experience of everyone involved in death and dying. The increasing ambiguity about when death occurs and the diversity of meanings that are attached to the significance of death makes caring for people at the moment of death a highly complex task. Nurses who are frequently involved in these moments need to be able to understand the wishes of the dying person and any family and friends. This involves more than being able to obtain answers to questions about what needs to be done at the time of death. Nurses also need to challenge some of the assumptions that underpin how the moment of death is routinely managed. Part of this challenge involves their awareness of the significance of the moment of death to them.

Conclusions

In this chapter, I have argued from a sociological point of view that the moment of death carries heavy responsibilities for nurses as the most likely professionals to be present. This is because the moment of death is affected by a number of key factors, including:

- the meaning of death, which includes the medical and legal, the spiritual, religious and cultural significance;
- the manner of death;
- the quality of death and how that is translated;
- the setting of death; and
- the social significance of death and how the performance of death is carried out.

All of these factors are related to each other and provide the context in which death occurs. The premium on 'getting it right' is high given that the immediate aftermath of death affects the grief-work of those who are bereaved.

References

Abel, E. (1986) The hospice movement: institutionalising innovation. *International Journal of Health Services*, 16(1): 71–85.

Addington-Hall, J., Fakhoury, W. and McCarthy, M. (1998) Specialist palliative care in non-malignant disease. *Palliative Medicine*, 12(6): 417–27.

Anderson, M. (2000) 'You have to get inside the person' or making grief private: image and metaphor in the therapeutic reconstruction of bereavement, in J. Hockey, J. Katz and N. Small (eds) *Grief, Mourning and Death Ritual*. Buckingham: Open University Press.

Bauman, Z. (1992) *Mortality, Immortality and Other Life Strategies*. Oxford: Polity.

Bradbury, M. (2001) The good death?, in D. Dickenson, M. Johnson and J. Samson Katz (eds) *Death, Dying and Bereavement*. London: Sage.

Chochinov, H.M., Hack, H.T., McClement, S., Kristjanson, L. and Harlos, M. (2002) Dignity in the terminally ill: a developing empirical model. *Social Science and Medicine*, 54: 433–43.

Clark, D. (1996) *The Future for Palliative Care*. Buckingham: Open University Press.

Clark, D., Hockley, J. and Ahmedzai, S. (1997) *New Themes in Palliative Care*. Buckingham: Open University Press.

Davies, D.J. (2002) *Death, Ritual and Belief*. London: Continuum.

Eyre, A. (2001) Post-disaster rituals, in J. Hockey, J. Katz and N. Small (eds) *Grief, Mourning and Death Ritual*. Buckingham: Open University Press.

Glaser, B.G. and Strauss, A. (1965) *Awareness of Dying*. Chicago, IL: Aldine.

Goffman, E. (1959) *The Presentation of Self in Everyday Life*. London: Penguin.

Good, M., Gadmer, N.M., Ruopp, P. *et al.* (2002) Narrative nuances on good and bad deaths: internists' tales from high-technology work places. *Social Science and Medicine*, Working Paper No. 198, November.

Howarth, G. (2001) Grieving in public, in J. Hockey, J. Katz and N. Small (eds) *Grief, Mourning and Death Ritual*. Buckingham: Open University Press.

Komaromy, C. (2000) The sight and sound of death: the management of dead bodies in residential and nursing homes for older people. *Mortality*, 5(3): 299–315.

Komaromy, C. and Hockey, J. (2001) 'Naturalising' death among older adults in residential care, in J. Hockey, J. Katz and N. Small (eds) *Grief, Mourning and Death Ritual*. Buckingham: Open University Press.

Lawton, J. (2000) *The Dying Process: Patients' Experiences of Palliative Care*. London: Routledge.

Oxenham, D. and Boyd, K. (1997) Voluntary euthanasia in terminal illness, in D. Clark (ed.) *The Future for Palliative Care*. Buckingham: Open University Press.

Page, S. and Komaromy, C. (2000) Lonely death: the case of expected and unexpected death. Paper presented to the *Fifth International Conference on Death, Dying and Disposal*, Goldsmiths College, London, September.

Parkes, C.M., Laungani, P. and Young, B. (1997) *Death and Bereavement Across Cultures*. London: Routledge.

Rosenblatt, P., Walsh, R.P. and Jackson, D.A. (1976) Grief and mourning in cross-cultural perspectives, cited in Davies, D. (2002) *Ritual and Belief*. London: Continuum.

Samson Katz, J.T. (2001) Jewish perspectives on death, dying and bereavement, in D. Dickenson, M. Johnson and J. Samson Katz (eds) *Death, Dying and Bereavement*. London: Sage.

Seymour, J. (2001) *Critical Moments in Death and Dying in Intensive Care*. Buckingham: Open University Press.

Sidell, M., Katz, J.T. and Komaromy, C. (1997) *Death and Dying in Residential and Nursing Homes for Older People: Examining the Case for Palliative Care*. London: Department of Health.

Tinnermans, S. (1998) Resuscitation technology in the emergency department towards a dignified death. *Sociology of Health and Illness*, 20: 144–67.

Turner, B.S. (1987) *Medical Power and Social Knowledge*. London: Sage.

van der Woning, M. (1997) Should relatives be invited to witness a resuscitation attempt? A review of the literature. *Accident and Emergency Nursing*, 5: 215–18.

Walter, T. (1999) *On Bereavement: The Culture of Grief*. Buckingham: Open University Press.

Weisman, A. (1972) *On Dying and Denying*. New York: Behavioural Publications.

24

Organ and tissue donation

Helping patients and families to make choices

Magi Sque and Joanne Wells

Introduction

Human organ and tissue transplantation has proven to be an economically viable and successful therapy that extends life expectancy and improves the quality of life of individuals with certain severe medical conditions or irreversible organ failure. The demand for cadaveric organs is growing worldwide, to give health benefits to certain individuals. The supply of organs and tissues for transplantation has not kept pace with demand and the medico-surgical success of transplantation is limited by the low availability of organs, giving rise to an escalating number of preventable human deaths. Concomitantly, innovations in mechanical and bioengineered organ replacements remain problematic and protracted. In part, the shortfall in donations reflects an increase in the number of individuals who could benefit from a transplant. In this chapter, we draw mainly from UK data and practices.

On 30 March 2003, there were 5653 people in the UK waiting for suitable organs, while there had only been 772 cadaveric donors during the previous 12 months.[1] Corneal donations throughout the UK have fallen by 30 per cent since 1995, forcing the cancellation of sight-saving operations.[2] Over the next few years, it has been estimated that there will be a 30 per cent increase in the number of patients with end-stage renal failure (Royal College of Surgeons 1999). Roderick *et al.* (1998) predict that renal replacement costs will increase by up to one-third by 2011 and that there will be an increase in the liver transplant waiting list from 11 per million to 14–18 per million. There are two reasons to increase organ and tissue donation rates. First, to halt unnecessary deaths and to improve the quality of life of certain individuals. Second, to stem the increased demand on British National Health Service (NHS) resources as the population ages and more people are added to transplant waiting lists.

The cost to the NHS of alternative therapies (e.g. renal dialysis), which is greater than the cost of maintaining a transplanted patient, are set to rise further. Other researchers (Salih *et al.* 1991; Gore *et al.* 1992; New *et al.* 1994; Randhawa 1995; Smith-Brew and Yanai 1996) state that the basis of the current organ shortage is not merely a problem of inadequate numbers of potential donors, but is exacerbated by suboptimal use of the available donor pool and the failure of health professionals to identify potential donors and initiate the donation process. Patients and relatives of potential organ and tissue donors are the most critical link in maintaining supply, as they must express they have no objection before organ retrieval may take place. The close and continuous proximity of nurses to potential donors and their families makes them important contributors to this process, especially in palliative care settings where tissue donation is most appropriate.

In this chapter, we discuss issues that surround the decision to donate organs and tissues and explain how patients and families can be helped to make decisions that are right for them. The chapter is divided into three sections:

- organ and tissue donation as a sociocultural process;
- organ and tissue donation in palliative care; and
- understanding families' decision making and bereavement.

The first section seeks to contexualize decisions about donation by showing how the history of human dissection may still impinge upon our understanding of the transplant process. The second section explores the importance of the patient's involvement in the donation decision within the palliative care setting. Finally, evidence drawn from a recently completed study (Sque *et al.* 2003) is used to explain families' decision making and bereavement.

Organ and tissue donation as a sociocultural process

Historical context

The transplantation of organs and tissues is not a new phenomenon. Myths and tales date back to the second century B.C. when the Chinese were believed to have transplanted organs and tissues into humans (Smith 1990). The first acknowledged transplantation in the West was in 1905 when a pioneering corneal graft was successfully completed to restore a person's sight (Doering 1996). Although claimed as a biomedical prerogative, organ transplantation is a wider cultural issue. It is a procedure that engages in both the physical and symbolic manipulation of human bodies, thereby transforming ideas about what constitutes a dead body (Lock 1995) and personal identity, because of the ability to interchange body parts (Kroenig and Hogle 1995; Sharp 1995; Postgraduate Update 1998; Sanner 2001), and hence raises issues that influence Western ideas of death (Douglas 1966). Donotransplantation[3] also offers the opportunity to challenge ideas about what is natural, the use of health technology and how it is integrated into Western ways of thinking. The ability to interchange human organs and tissues has promoted many philosophical debates, but theoretical insight is lagging behind. Certainly, the perceived existential implications of dissection for transplant purposes cannot be overlooked in the ability to dispose of a body, but to know that the deceased is still contributing to life elsewhere.

To date, research has focused predominantly on physiological issues, with the above sociocultural and psychological aspects of the process receiving less attention (Sanner 1995). The ability to transplant human organs raises questions about: the moral obligation of society and individuals towards donation and the replacement of organs and tissues; the impact of health technology on sustaining a legally dead but functioning body on ventilatory support; the importance of perceptions of deadness following death certified by brainstem death testing and the consequent mutilation of the ventilated corpse; and the sentiments attached to the interchangeable body parts. Some of these issues can be contextualized within the long historical past of the dissection of the human dead.

Since the Renaissance, the bodies of the dead have been dissected to treat the living by exploring and learning how the body worked and how it was affected by illness. Prior to the Tudor period (1485–1603) in the UK, there was no legal stipulation on how bodies for dissection were obtained or treated (Richardson 1996). In 1540, Henry VIII bestowed upon the companies of Barbers and Surgeons the annual gift of four hanged felons (Anno32 Henrici Octavi c.42 1540, cited by Richardson 1989). This limited source of bodies led to illegal and immoral methods of obtaining corpses, as supply was not meeting demand. The law and the public viewed dissection as a mutilation, a post-mortem punishment and a terrible aggravation of the death penalty. Society perceived dissection as a fate worse than death, leading Richardson (1996) to suggest that the loathing of dissection may have derived from fears that the process either damaged the soul or prevented resurrection, reasons still given for refusing the donation of organs in today's society.

While no major religion opposes donation and transplantation of organs and tissues (Randhawa 1995), British cultural protection of the dead body has been drawn from judicial adoptions of punishments to the corpse (Richardson 1989). Richardson (1996) believes that the historical premise of dissection has spawned many of the current problems in obtaining organs and tissues for transplantation. Dissection represents not only the exposure of nakedness, the possibility of assault upon and disrespect towards the dead, but also the deliberate mutilation or destruction of identity. The consensus attaching deep importance to post-mortem care and the respectful, integral disposal of the corpse still holds deep cultural meaning within British society (Richardson 1989). Donotransplantion challenges society's beliefs about deadness, requiring a conceptual reconstruction of what constitutes a dead body or organ and what can be regarded as a surgical procedure (i.e. organ retrieval as opposed to mutilation of the corpse).

Organ and tissue donation processes in the UK today

In the UK, individuals express their desire to donate their organs and tissue after death by an 'opt in' system, either by carrying a donor card or by registering their wish with the NHS National Organ Donor Register. However, New *et al.* (1994) showed that 70 per cent of the UK population were in favour of donation but only 19 per cent carried donor cards.

Nurses and doctors act as 'gatekeepers' and control access to potential donors, as well as providing broad-based consultation (Sque and Payne 1994; MORI 1995; Evanisko *et al.* 1998; Kent 2002; Wells and Sque 2002; Sque *et al.* 2003). Yet little is known about the importance of the nature of their contact with families in maintaining the availability of organs and tissues. Consequently, little information exists that could contribute to an understanding of the donotranplant process.

More information is needed about the relationship between donor families and 'the gatekeepers' to the donotransplant process. Gatekeepers' first duty of care to the deceased person is to ensure that, even in death, no act or omission results to their detriment (Sque *et al.* 2000). This could mean a commitment to explore with the next of kin the wishes of the deceased in relation to organ donation. They also need to optimize the recipient's chance for survival and offer a good quality of life post-transplant. Their objective is to achieve the process without social or psychological harm to donor families, the recipient and their significant others. Gatekeepers must identify potential donors, initiate the discussion about organ donation with families, screen for biologically acceptable organs, and make the decision as to which organs are retrieved and to whom they are given. Gatekeepers are also the managers of information that may be required by donor and recipient families.

While several studies have indicated the important role health professionals play as 'gatekeepers' of the donation process (Siminoff *et al.* 1994; Sque and Payne 1994; Politoski *et al.* 1996), there is little evidence of the potential conflicts and difficulties faced by them in initiating optimal circumstances for discussion about donation and sustaining the transplant process. A major criticism of previous studies is that they have been very general, accessed health professional groups in isolation (Kent and Owens 1995; Evanisko *et al.* 1998) or focused entirely on the perceptions of the nurse (Sque *et al.* 2000; Kent 2002). And none of these studies took into account the broader sociocultural contexts in which any of these groups function.

No studies to date have identified the potential impact and interplay between a particular hospital's polices with regard to donotransplantation and health professionals' perceptions, experiences, practices and interactions with their clients and other health professionals. Nor has any study investigated how health professionals work together within their own belief systems to create a culture in which to provide effective delivery of donotransplant care within their own hospital trusts. MORI (1995) and Caplan (1988) provide some indication of the importance of such cultural influences; for instance, families not being approached about organ donation simply because of a medical consultant's preference. As a precursor to any attempt to increase donation discussions with families, it is imperative to identify the culture that exists within a hospital, and to evaluate its impact on the urgency and importance given to organ and tissue donation. Sque (1996) allowed for further exploration of these concerns by providing a theoretical explanation of how donor families perceived and dealt with such issues as death certified by brainstem testing and organ retrieval. She identified particular bereavement needs in coming to terms with the concept of a relative's organ continuing 'to live' in a different body. However, such depth of explanation does not exist for the health professionals who need to provide support and care for families involved in donotransplantation. Richardson (1989) argues that the clinical detachment required by health professionals to suspend or suppress, to facilitate and perform the normally repugnant tasks of dissection of the body during organ retrieval represents a cultural detachment or reorientation of no small dimension.

In addition, most of the research undertaken has focused on the concerns of organ donation and not tissue donation. The little research conducted in this area suggests that awareness of and experience in tissue donation is less than that of organ donation. Furthermore, research undertaken by Kent and Owens (1995) and Wells and Sque (2002) demonstrates that while many of the difficulties for staff in raising the issue of donation with families are the same for organ and tissue donation, tissue donation does raise specific concerns. For example, with corneal donation, concerns have been raised over disfigurement and the beliefs of a need for the deceased 'to see into the next life' (Sque 1996).

Dissonant loss: families' experiences of organ and tissue donation

Consideration of organ donation predominantly arises following critical injuries that lead to premature and sudden death. Sudden death robs relatives of the opportunity for anticipatory grief, and is known to potentially lead to poor bereavement outcomes (Saunders 1993; Wright 1996). This is of concern, as it has implications for the scale of human suffering and, ultimately, health care provision.

Sque and Payne's (1996) seminal UK study used a cross-sectional approach to investigate the critical care experiences of donating relatives. They showed that the impact of sudden death and donation could create a need for bereavement support, but the mechanisms for assessment of need were *ad hoc* and there was disparity in the provision of such support between NHS Hospital Trusts. Sque and Payne also found that nurses and general bereavement counsellors appeared ill-prepared to help these families. There appeared to be a need for training development. However, the study was limited by being merely cross-sectional and including only those who agreed to donation. Relatives who did not agree, and whose experiences could well have had an impact on their bereavement outcomes and donation rates, were not investigated.

Sque and Payne (1996) further suggested that the experience of organ donation could be explained as a series of complex decisions that create conflicts and distress for the relatives involved. Some of these conflicts were: coming to terms with the loss of a relatively young person who was robbed of a future; deciding about giving consent for organs to be removed from a relative who, because they remained on ventilatory support, still appeared to be alive; saying goodbye to a relative who did not appear to be dead; and coming to terms with disposing of a body when their relative's organs were responsible for improving the quality of a recipient's life. Within the study, bereaved adults also described the factors that created resolutions to their conflicts and helped them to move through the phases of the donation process. A theory of 'dissonant loss', defined as a bereavement or loss that is characterized by a sense of uncertainty and psychological inconsistency, was developed to explain donor relatives' experiences. However, the work was limited to donor families' experiences and was unable to 'complete the picture' of the donotransplant process by explaining the perspectives of the health professionals involved at the interface with families.

Organ and tissue donation in palliative care

The hospital intensive care unit is generally considered the place where the discussion about retrieval of organs and tissues takes place. This assumption is supported by a lack of literature published on organ and tissue donation in areas other than intensive care units. Although patients who die in the palliative care setting can donate heart valves, tracheas, kidneys and skin (Feuer 1998), the most common tissues to be donated are corneas. This is due to few donor contraindications and the convenience of entire retrieval taking place within palliative care units or at undertakers (Wells and Sque 2002).

Statistics from UK Transplant show that the need for corneas is rising. In December 2001, the waiting list figure was 479. Within 2 months the figure had risen to 534. The UK Transplant report (2002) showed that in 2001 there were 1715 cornea donors, 354 (21 per cent) of whom died from cancer. Bearing in mind the statistics from the Hospice Information Service (2000), which indicate that approximately 30,000 deaths from cancer occur in palliative care units each year, this would suggest there is only limited donation from this source.

One of the main aims of palliative care is respecting the views and autonomy of the patient (Woodward 1998). Health professionals within palliative care pride themselves on their ability to communicate with families and to help them in their bereavement (Feuer 1998). Although this is the case, there appears to be little evidence of corneal donation being offered as an option for patients and families to consider. Spivey (1998) supports this lack of evidence in a study on tissue donation in palliative care. Of the 83 (55 per cent) palliative care units in England that responded to a questionnaire, 33 units believed that donation was appropriate, 17 believed it was inappropriate and 32 did not know or gave reasons for not participating. Of the 33 units that believed that donation was appropriate, only two reported that they routinely discussed donation with patients and families. The remainder only participated when the patient or family initiated the enquiry.

An exhaustive literature search only identified two published studies that have explored organ and tissue donations in palliative care (Peters and Sutcliffe 1992; Wells and Sque 2002). Peters and Sutcliffe (1992) presented an account of 12 asystole kidney donors who died at St Christopher's Hospice, London between January 1990 and October 1991. The positive effects for patients and families were discussed and issues raised for staff explored. All the discussion related to patients', families' and staff's feelings, and opinions were drawn from the authors' own experiences and personal views.

A more recent study by Wells and Sque (2002) explored why the commitment to tissue donation in palliative care was so low. Eight nurses and doctors employed within two palliative care units were invited to participate in semi-structured interviews to explore their views, feelings and experiences of tissue donation within the palliative care setting. The findings showed that health professionals in palliative care are in a unique position in that their patients are often aware that they are dying, as are the patients' families. This awareness enables the patient to be involved in the decision-making process about end-of-life issues. In this context, tissue donation becomes highly relevant and the patient can be involved in any decisions about what should happen to their own body. Anecdotal information suggests that patients may regard donation as a positive outcome to what may have seemed meaningless suffering.

Sque (2000) analysed post-bereavement correspondence between donor families, recipients, their transplant coordinating centres and the National Donor Family Council in the USA. She suggested that the donation and use of corneas could be helpful to relatives in their grief. As a husband wrote:

> The knowledge that her eye tissue is helpful is all I need. Just two short weeks after M's death and tissue donation I received a booklet for donor families along with a letter from (name) . . . of the . . . Eye and Tissue Bank. This letter was of great importance to me. In the letter she states that two people have had their sight restored through corneal transplantation. This was very helpful to me during a very dark period in my life.

Wells and Sque (2002) suggest that the patient's ability to be involved in decision making has many implications and concerns for health professionals that are explained by a theory of 'living choice' (Figure 24.1). Living choice is defined as 'the ability of terminally ill patients within the palliative care environment to make choices about donation that have an impact on the knowledge and role of health professionals'. The dominant, pervasive core-variable is 'patient choice', which influences the other categories: 'professional role', 'donation process', 'concerns' and 'knowledge'. These categories will be examined further below.

Discussing donation forces health care professionals to broach the finality of the patient's death, an area of communication that even palliative

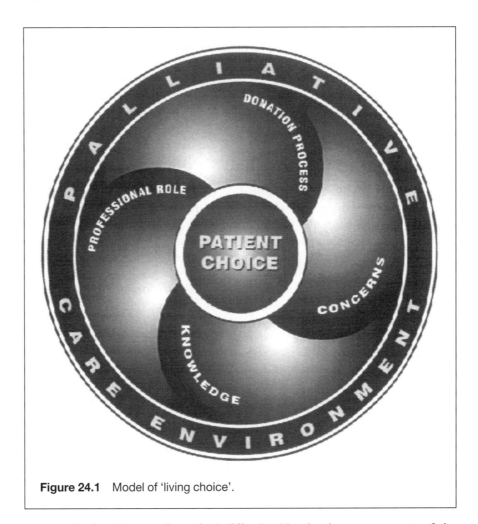

Figure 24.1 Model of 'living choice'.

care professionals sometimes find difficult. Clearly, the management of the 'donation process' raised certain 'concerns' for health professionals, in particular that such a discussion should cause no harm to patients or their families. All participants in the above study believed that it should be the health professional who developed a trusting relationship with the patient and family, who should discuss donation with them. This ability also depended on their 'knowledge'. Participants who routinely discussed donation believed that had they not had training and information initially, they would not have felt comfortable or confident to discuss donation.

Although a small qualitative study, it highlighted many areas for discussion as well as pinpointing the differences between intensive care and palliative care with regard to donation, in particular, the ability of the patient, in the palliative care setting, to be involved in the decision-making process. Patients can expect to be given a choice and to be informed of all their options when facing a terminal illness, obliging health professionals to find out more about donation and develop it within their practice framework.

The study also highlighted the importance of health carers needing to recognize and appreciate the difficult and emotional position families are in when a relative is terminally ill and the need for them to know the wishes of their sick relative, to facilitate their donation wishes after their death.

There is no prior research to ascertain if the effects of donating tissues is the same for families who donated in intensive care units, compared with the very different palliative care setting. This is particularly true in relation to a long illness compared with a sudden death, which is more commonplace in an intensive care environment. Further exploration needs to involve palliative care patients and relatives as well as the many health professionals, working within palliative care, who have both a stake and a role to play in organ and tissue donation (e.g. individuals working in tissue retrieval and transplant coordination). Wells (2001) has questioned the potential philosophical clash that might exist between palliative care promoting 'the tame' natural death, while the donotransplant process is steeped in medico-surgical interventionist practices. Could this philosophical conundrum contribute to the low commitment to donation within the palliative care setting?

Understanding families' decision making and bereavement

Families need to be aware of the option of donation or their post-mortem choices will be limited and they may be deprived of fulfilling the donor's wish (Finlay and Dallimore 1991; DeJong *et al.* 1998; Sque 2001), or from finding some meaning in their often tragic loss (DeJong *et al.* 1998; Sque 2000; 2001). One factor contributing to the difficulty in discussing donation with families is health professionals' lack of knowledge or confidence in broaching the subject (Salih *et al.* 1991; Kent 2002).

Evidence suggests that potential donor families are not as unreceptive to organ and tissue donation as many health professionals believe; indeed, many find the donation process very positive (Randhawa 1995; Sque *et al.* 2003). The experiences and benefits for families of a request for donation is well documented and is of major importance when considering whether organ and tissue donation is appropriate to be discussed. Pelletier (1992) found that it was evident that facilitating organ donation reflected a strong respect for the dead relative's wishes and to positively change the meaning of the death. Clearly, there appears to be a mismatch between the views of health professionals and potential donor families that warrants detailed investigation.

Factors relevant to the family refusing organ donation include low socio-economic status, poor education, cultural beliefs and the number of family members present when donation is discussed (Burroughs *et al.* 1998; DeJong *et al.* 1998). A finding associated with ethnic groups and younger adults is the fear of mutilation and the importance of the body remaining whole after death (Martinez *et al.* 2001).

The way that relatives are treated at the time donation is discussed has been shown to affect their donation decisions (DeJong *et al.* 1998; Sque *et al.* 2003). Norton and Sukraw (1990) suggest that when the facts about organ and tissue donation are presented at the right time and in the right way, relatives are helped to make the best choice that is closest to their own values and beliefs. Limited research (Burroughs *et al.* 1998) has shown that rather more donating and non-donating families regret their decisions than was previously thought. Sque *et al.* (2003) have shown that relatives who are comfortable with their decisions about donation may be less likely to have a complicated bereavement with unresolved grief reactions. Prior to this study, no longitudinal studies had shown how these regrets affected relatives' bereavement outcomes, and no information was available about the possible benefits of decisions with which families remain satisfied.

Positive beliefs and attitudes of nurses have been significantly correlated with requests and consents for organs. Therefore, success in organ donation may depend on nurses' awareness and integration of knowledge about the donotransplant process. Through their experience, bereaved families become informal educators about organ donation (Sque 1996). This means that adequate bereavement support for relatives could positively affect donation rates. Presently in the UK, the care of donor families is patchy and incomplete, as there is limited evidence to explain the process of donation and its outcomes (Sque *et al.* 2003).

In a three-year longitudinal study of the bereavement experiences of 49 families who had donation discussed with them, Sque *et al.* (2003) have expanded the theory of dissonant loss and confirmed that Sque's (1996) earlier model of conflict and resolution as the predominant emotional land-scape for donating families remains relevant. Four main categories were identified that provide a framework to illustrate the issues that influenced families' ability to agree or decline donation, their overall support for organ donation and their perception of the decision-making process (Sque *et al.* 2003) (see Figure 24.2). These categories will now be discussed in further detail.

The first category explicated concerns about the concrete or discursive knowledge of the deceased's donation wish. Participants made decisions in line with the wishes of the deceased where these were known, whether this was a positive decision or a negative decision. The evidence suggests that participants who knew the wishes of the deceased did not appear to have to make a decision, as it was more important to fulfil the wishes of the deceased as shown by the following quote: 'It just seems a really odd thing to do if you know what the person who's died wants. Why would you want to do anything different?' Some participants knew that their relative carried a donor card or had signed their passport and this was seen as concrete evidence of their wish to donate (Figure 24.2). When the views of the deceased were not known, participants recalled the attributes of the donor (Figure 24.2), the donor's perceived neutral stance with regard to donation and the possible benefits to others, all of which influenced their decision. For example, recycling was a way of life for one family and this extended to donation.

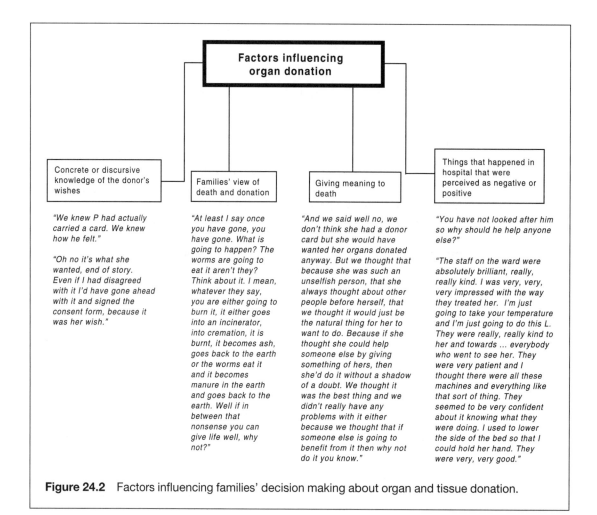

Figure 24.2   Factors influencing families' decision making about organ and tissue donation.

The second category concerned the neutral or positive views held by the family about death and organ and tissue donation. The third category highlighted the opportunity for families to give meaning to the death (Figure 24.2). The fourth category concerned events that occurred in the hospital that were perceived as either positive or negative, an example being the care given to the donor and the family.

In the case of two non-donating participants, family conflict, communication with hospital staff and a perceived lack of care of the deceased were linked with not knowing the deceased's wishes and led to the decision not to donate:

We had had the most appalling seven days in hospital while he had surgery. No one was ever available to talk to us and on one occasion I saw the sister tell the consultant that we wanted to see him and we saw him leave the ward. I had to ambush him in the corridor later and he was just incapable of communicating. I just could not believe that a man in his position could get away with not being able to speak to people. We never really knew what was going on, in fact I read about the diagnosis in a textbook and learned more in five minutes than I had learned on the ward in four days.

One young man, who had surgery, had to return to theatre for a drain to be inserted after which he suffered brain swelling and brainstem death. When asked about donation, the family responded to this perceived negative experience as follows: 'You have not looked after him so why should he help anyone else?' (Figure 24.2).

All the donating participants had concerns about the retrieval operation. Most had very little knowledge about what would happen (even participants with medical backgrounds) and how the deceased would look afterwards. Their reports of their concerns were peppered with words such as 'rip', 'chop' and 'tear out'. One family was very concerned about whether their relative had felt anything. Very little was known about brainstem testing, how recipients were selected and the time-scales involved. Some participants did not know that their relative would go to theatre still connected to the ventilator.

Once the decision was made about donation, participants were encouraged to say goodbye to their relative. The majority of participants left the hospital after saying goodbye before the deceased had gone to the operating theatre. Spending uninterrupted time with the deceased was important to all the participants.

> But there was plenty of time to say goodbye. They never rushed us or anything, even though I'm sure they would have, you know, wanted to get on quicker, they never rushed us or anything like that. You know they gave us time with P.

The image of the deceased still warm and on ventilatory support made parting particularly difficult: 'Even though S was breathing, she was warm and she was soft to the touch, she clinically was dead at that point. It was still hard to leave her there on her own.'

Four participants waited to see the deceased after the retrieval operation. Some found this a positive experience:

> Then after the operation I went into the Recovery Room and I just put his one set of teeth in. And he just looked so peaceful, he had a sort of smile on his face as if to say you bugger, I'm on me holiday.

But for some it was a negative experience.

> It was horrible, it was absolutely horrible. He was white. He had no colour. It just it didn't look like M. I mean there he was, had a cover on, I mean we didn't see anything that was, but he just looked terrible. By this time his lips were purple. His colour was terrible. He was frozen, it was absolutely nothing, which basically he was just a shell, that was really, really bad.

The majority of participants choose to see their relative in the Chapel of Rest or at the undertakers. A minority wanted to remember them as they were. For those who did see their relative, most were apprehensive about how they would look, but felt that it would confirm death for them. Some had a positive experience:

> Well I walked in there he was sort of lying on the table or whatever and he had a very beautiful satin embroidered sheet over him. And then he had an awful frilly nightdress underneath. I lifted this sheet up so nobody could see it, I just thought if he could see this he would just turn. So that made me chuckle but it was horrible because I'd never seen anybody dead before.

Others did not:

> Was just awful it was horrible, it just didn't look like L, he was laying on like a table, a high table, and had like a purple robe sort of thing right up to his neck and he looked yellow and it was horrible.

Sque (1996) proposed that decisions about donation might have consequences that affect the rest of donor relatives' lives. For instance, even as time goes by, the effects of the donation were perpetuated in the desire for continuing information about the recipients (Sque and Payne 1996; Sque 2000; Sque *et al.* 2003).

The anonymity that surrounds the relationship between donor and recipient is there, in part, to protect the recipient from the possible searching behaviour described by Bowlby (1980) and *mislocations*, where the deceased is seen as manifest in another person (Bowlby 1980). Donor families did attribute importance to their relatives 'living on', and the continuation of the donor's life was mentioned as a reason for donation (Sque 1996, 2000). Other donor families regarded recipients as their relative's keeper (Sque 2000). Mislocations could lead to damaging effects both for the bereaved and the recipient. For example, notions of incarnations of the dead person could become attached to the recipient. La Spina *et al.* (1993) showed how deleterious the collapse of this incarnation could be to donor relatives. However, our present state of knowledge only allows us to speculate about the damage or comfort manifest in such thoughts and projections about the deceased and donor relatives' relationship with recipients, although Sque (2000) reported the benefits of donor and recipient families meeting.

Klass *et al.* (1996) theorized that, generally, bereaved people experience a strong need for continuation of a relationship with the dead person. It is possible that the way the relationship with the deceased continues to play a central role in donor relatives' lives, manifested in the often sustained yearning for information about recipients, is because of the attachment they feel for the part of the donor that 'lived on'.

Similarly, Walter (1996) views the purpose of grief as a time during which the survivor constructs a durable biography of the deceased, allowing the living to integrate the memory of the dead into their ongoing lives. The process hinges on talking about the dead person and moving on with them in a new relationship. Walsh and McGoldrick (1991) share this perspective. They explain grieving as a transactional process involving the deceased and the survivors in a shared life cycle, which acknowledges the finality of death as well as the continuity of life. Walter's (1996) concept highlights the inter-personal nature of grief and the importance of social support that Little-wood (1992), Payne *et al.* (1999) and Riches and Dawson (2000) view as a critical buffer to the stress of bereavement. Social support has an ameliora-tive impact on the intensity of grief symptoms and the ultimate outcome of bereavement.

Parkes (1993) and Payne *et al.* (1999) suggest that the best people to help are those that share the common experience of a certain type of loss, as only they can provide the support of friends who have some insight into the experience. Parkes (1993) further suggests that special bereave-ment services are more effective if they are integrated with the services provided by members of the caring professions. Collaboration with pro-fessionals tends to ensure that volunteers receive the expert assistance in training to be counsellors, while avenues are provided for dealing with individuals whose problems need professional skills. Could this be the way donor families found help and social support by writing about their organ donation and grief experiences to the US National Donor Family Council, an organization they felt would understand their situation (Sque 2000)?

Sque (1996) and Sque and Payne (1996) showed that donor families have two main concerns about donation: the mutilation of the body and the possible suffering the relative might sustain as a result of the retrieval oper-ation. It was very important to donor families that retrieval was carried out with dignity, propriety and with utmost care and gentleness. Donor families found the knowledge that retrieval was carried out as a proper surgical procedure reassuring. There was another type of suffering which partici-pants worried about. They felt that the relative had already suffered so much – a horrible death and invasive medical procedures. Was it fair to subject them to further indignities by allowing their organs to be removed? Sque (2000) and Sque *et al.* (2003) have shown that follow-up information about recipients provides donor families with a sense of reassurance about the continued achievement of the donor to make a positive difference to the life of the recipient, fostering a sense of wholeness that made the mutilation of retrieval worthwhile.

Could this also explain the deep regret felt when the desired communica-tion was not forthcoming from recipients? When these families did not receive information about the achievements of the donor, they were unable to know that their gift was appreciated and valued, and did not receive thanks on behalf of the donor. They could not achieve closure by complet-ing the biography of the donor and thus were denied the opportunity, as Klass *et al.* (1996) and Walter (1996) suggest, of constructing a new relation-ship, integrating them into their ongoing life. Finally, they were denied the knowledge that the organ had achieved a human wholeness and safety in another body.

Conclusions

In this chapter, we have discussed evidence that underpins the sociocultural process of organ and tissue donation by drawing on historical perspectives and explaining the current position in the UK. Focusing on a number of relevant studies, we have highlighted the particular issues pertinent to donation in the palliative care setting, discussed families' experiences and offered insights into their difficult decisions and their bereavement. Important aspects of care for palliative nurses to consider include:

- The need for the donation of organs and tissues and the valuable contributions that they can make to the quality of recipients' lives.

- The need to be aware of their own feelings about cadaveric organ and tissue donation, as nurses need to be comfortable, knowledgeable and confident to facilitate this sensitive discussion. Therefore, they may require additional training and education.

- The need to make the donation discussion part of their care of the dying and the bereaved, to increase their choices, facilitate their requests and potentially give them some comfort in their dying or bereavement through this achievement.

- Initiating a discussion about donation as part of palliative care could enhance patients' choice by giving them the opportunity to be involved in decisions about their own body and thus substantially decrease the difficulties faced by family members in making a decision following their death.

- The success of donation discussions, whatever the outcome, has been shown to depend on good relationships and rapport with patients and their families.

- The timing of the discussion will need careful assessment of the individual's needs and emotional responses to the ongoing situation.

- The appropriate use of visual aids or written information that explains the positive contribution of donation and the relevant procedure has been shown to be helpful in facilitating discussions.

As yet, little evidence exists within the palliative care setting of the potential conflicts and difficulties faced by patients and families who choose to donate or not to donate and how best to help them to make choices that are right for them and will not be regretted. Decisions that may have some benefit to them in their dying or bereavement. The questions that need to be answered here are: What are the conflicts and resolutions in the palliative care setting that result in patients and families choosing to donate or not to donate organs and tissues? How can these individuals be helped to make decisions that are right for them and will not be regretted?

Notes

1   Statistics prepared by UK Transplant Statistical Services, Bristol, from the National Transplant Database maintained on behalf of the UK transplant community, April 2003.
2   Personal communication, Dr Armitage, Scientific Director, Bristol Eye Bank, 13 May 2002, at the Third Regional Transplant Symposium, Eastleigh, Hants.
3   Donotransplantation includes organ and tissue donation, retrieval and transplantation.

References

Bowlby, J. (1980) *Attachment and Loss, Vol. 3: Loss, Sadness and Depression.* London: The Hogarth Press.

Burroughs, T.E., Hong, B.A., Kappel, D.F. and Freedman, B.K. (1998) The stability of family decisions to consent or refuse organ donation: would you do it again? *Psychosomatic Medicine*, 60: 156–62.

Caplan, A.L. (1988) Professional arrogance and public misunderstanding. *Hastings Center Report*, April/May, pp. 34–7.

DeJong, W., Franz, H.G., Wolfe, S.M. *et al.* (1998) Requesting organ donation: an interview study of donor and nondonor families. *American Journal of Critical Care*, 7: 13–23.

Doering, J. (1996) Families' experiences in consenting to eye donation of the recently deceased relative. *Heart and Lung*, 25: 72–8.

Douglas, M. (1966) *Purity and Danger: An Analysis of the Concepts of Pollution and Taboo.* London: Routledge.

Evanisko, M.J., Beasley, C.L., Brigham, L.E. *et al.* (1998) Readiness of critical care physicians and nurses to handle requests for organ donations. *American Journal of Critical Care*, 7: 4–12.

Feuer, D. (1998) Organ donation in palliative care. *European Journal of Palliative Care*, 5: 21–5.

Finlay, I. and Dallimore, D. (1991) Your child is dead. *British Medical Journal*, 302: 1524–5.

Gore, S.M., Cable, D.J. and Holland, A.J. (1992) Organ donation from intensive care units in England and Wales: two year confidential audit of deaths in intensive care. *British Medical Journal*, 304: 349–55.

Hospice Information Service (2000) *Hospice Facts and Figures.* London: St Christopher's Hospice.

Kent, B. (2002) Psychological factors influencing nurses' involvement with organ and tissue donation. *International Journal of Nursing Studies*, 39: 429–40.

Kent, B. and Owens, R.G. (1995) Conflicting attitudes to corneal and organ donation: a study of nurses' attitudes to organ donation. *International Journal of Nursing Studies*, 32: 484–92.

Klass, D., Silverman, P.R. and Nickman, S.L. (eds) (1996) *Continuing Bonds: New Understanding of Grief.* London: Taylor & Francis.

Kroenig, B.A. and Hogle, L.F. (1995) Organ transplantation (re)examined. *Medical Anthropology Quarterly*, 9: 393–7.

La Spina, F., Sedda, L., Pizzi, C. *et al.* (1993) Donor families' attitude toward organ donation. *Transplantation Proceedings*, 25: 1699–701.

Littlewood, J. (1992) *Aspects of Grief: Bereavement in Adult Life*. London: Routledge.

Lock, M. (1995) Transcending mortality: organ transplants and the practice of contradictions. *Medical Anthropology Quarterly*, 9: 390–3.

Martinez, J.M., Lopez, J.S., Martin, A. *et al.* (2001) Organ donation and family decision-making within the Spanish system. *Social Science & Medicine*, 53: 405–21.

MORI Health Research Unit (1995) *Report of a Two Year Study into Reasons for Relatives' Refusal of Organ Donation*. London: Department of Health.

New, B., Dingwall, M.S. and McHale, J. (1994) *A Question of Give and Take: Improving the Supply of Donor Organs for Transplantation*. London: King's Fund Institute.

Norton, D.J. and Sukraw, J. (1990) Helping patients give a gift of life. *RN*, 53: 30–4.

Parkes, C.M. (1993) Bereavement as a psychosocial transition: processes of adaptation to change, in M.S. Stroebe, W. Stroebe and R.O. Hansson (eds) *Handbook of Bereavement: Theory, Research and Intervention*. Cambridge: Cambridge University Press.

Payne, S., Horn, S. and Relf, M. (1999) *Loss and Bereavement*. Buckingham: Open University Press.

Pelletier, M. (1992) The organ donor family members' perception of stressful situations during the organ donation experience. *Journal of Advanced Nursing*, 17: 90–2.

Peters, D. and Sutcliffe, J. (1992) Organ donation: the hospice perspective. *Palliative Medicine*, 6: 212–16.

Politoski, G., Coolican, M. and Casey, K. (1996) Perspectives on communication issues among transplant and procurement professionals, transplant recipients, and donor families. *Journal of Transplant Co-ordination*, 6: 78–83.

Postgraduate Update (1998) Tolerance in ambiguity: supporting the donor family. *Nursing Inquiry*, 5: 194–6.

Randhawa, G. (1995) Organ donation: social and cultural attitudes. *Nursing Standard*, 9: 25–7.

Richardson, R. (1989) *Death, Dissection and the Destitute*. London: Penguin.

Richardson, R. (1996) Fearful symmetry: corpses for anatomy, organs for transplantation?, in S. Youngner, R. Fox and L. O'Connell (eds) *Organ Transplantation: Meanings and Realities*. Madison, CT: University of Wisconsin Press.

Riches, G. and Dawson, P. (2000) *An Intimate Loneliness: Supporting Bereaved Parents and Siblings*. Buckingham: Open University Press.

Roderick, P., Clements, S., Diamond, I., Storkey, M. and Raleigh, V.S. (1998) Estimating demand for renal replacement therapy in Greater London: the impact of demographic trends in ethnic minority populations. *Health Trends*, 30: 46–50.

Royal College of Surgeons (1999) *The Report of the Working Party to Review Organ Transplantation*. London: The Royal College of Surgeons.

Salih, M.A., Harvey, I., Frankel, S. *et al.* (1991) Potential availability of cadaver organs for transplantation. *British Medical Journal*, 302: 1053–5.

Sanner, M. (1995) Attitudes toward organ donation and transplantation. *Social Science and Medicine*, 38: 1141–52.

Sanner, M. (2001) Exchanging spare parts or becoming a new person? People's attitudes toward receiving and donating organs. *Social Science and Medicine*, 52: 1491–9.

Saunders, C.M. (1993) Risk factors in bereavement, in M.S. Stroebe, W. Stroebe and R.O. Hansson (eds) *Handbook of Bereavement: Theory, Research and Intervention*. Cambridge: Cambridge University Press.

Sharp, L. (1995) Organ transplantation as a transformative experience: anthropological insights into the restructuring of the self. *Medical Anthropology Quarterly*, 9: 357–89.

Siminoff, L.A., Arnold, R. and Miller, D.S. (1994) Differences in the procurement of organs and tissues by health care professionals. *Clinical Transplantation*, 8: 460–5.

Smith, S.L. (1990) *Tissue and Organ Transplantation*. St. Louis, MO: Mosby.

Smith-Brew, S. and Yanai, L. (1996) The organ donation process through a review of the literature. Part 2. *Accident and Emergency Medicine*, 4: 97–102.

Spivey, M. (1998) Organ tissue donation within the palliative care setting. BA (Hons) dissertation, University of Luton, Luton.

Sque, M. (1996) *The experiences of donor relatives and nurses' attitudes, knowledge and behaviour regarding cadaveric donotransplantation*. PhD thesis, University of Southampton, Southampton.

Sque, M. (2000) *'A Story to Tell': Post Bereavement Correspondence Between Organ Donor Families, Recipients, Their OPOs and the National Donor Family Council – An American Investigation*. Report of a study funded by the General Nursing Council for England and Wales Trust. Guildford: University of Surrey.

Sque, M. (2001) Being a carer in acute crisis: the situation for relatives of organ donors, in S. Payne and C. Ellis-Hill (eds) *Chronic and Terminal Illness: New Perspectives on Caring and Carers*. Oxford: Oxford University Press.

Sque, M. and Payne, S. (1994) Gift exchange theory – a critique in relation to organ donation. *Journal of Advanced Nursing*, 19: 45–51.

Sque, M. and Payne, S.A. (1996) Dissonant loss: the experiences of donor relatives. *Social Science and Medicine*, 43: 1359–70.

Sque, M., Payne, S. and Vlachonikonis, I. (2000) Cadaveric donotransplantation: nurses' attitudes, knowledge and behaviour. *Social Science and Medicine*, 50: 541–52.

Sque, M., Long, T. and Payne, S. (2003) *Organ and Tissue Donation: Exploring the Needs of Families*. Final report of a study for the British Organ Donor Society and the National Lottery Community Fund. Southampton: University of Southampton.

UK Transplant (2002) *Transplant Activity 2001*. Bristol: UK Transplant.

Walsh, F. and McGoldrick, M. (eds) (1991) *Living Beyond Loss: Death in the Family*. New York: W.W. Norton.

Walter, T. (1996) A new model of grief: bereavement and biography. *Mortality*, 1: 7–26.

Wells, J. (2001) 'Living choice': the commitment to tissue donation in palliative care. MSc thesis, University of Surrey, Guildford.

Wells, J. and Sque, M. (2002) 'Living choice': the commitment to tissue donation in palliative care. *International Journal of Palliative Nursing*, 8: 22–7.

Woodward, V. (1998) Caring, patient autonomy and stigma of paternalism. *Journal of Advanced Nursing*, 28: 1046–52.

Wright, B. (1996) *Sudden Death: A Research Base for Practice*, 2nd edn. New York: Churchill Livingstone.

25

The care and support of bereaved people

Mark Cobb

Introduction: in the company of the bereaved

Being present at the moment of someone's death is a familiar experience for many nurses and other health care professionals. Bearing witness to the consequence of fatal pathological events is an inevitable part of clinical practice and there are protocols and procedures to guide the necessary practicalities of dealing with a dead body (Mallett and Dougherty 2000). This unexceptional biological reality, however, is an incomplete description because death is more than a clinical punctuation. In the presence of death, we face the significance of human absence and loss, the deprivation of future possibilities, and the emptiness of an embodied space once filled with life. Most immediately, nurses find themselves in the company of the bereaved wanting to care and console, fearful of making matters worse, and aware that death imposes a loss that must be lived with.

Most people begin their bereavement in the company of health professionals and in the unfamiliar environment of health care institutions (Office for National Statistics 2001). Many of these deaths will occur in acute care settings of hospitals and be the result of diseases of the circulatory system and respiratory system as well as neoplasms. Consequently, while informal and *ad hoc* bereavement care may exist, largely as a result of the interest of individual staff, consistent and well-resourced bereavement care is unlikely to be available because it is not a common feature of most hospitals beyond the practicalities necessary for the disposal of deceased patients (Department of Health 1992, 1997; Kissane 2000). In addition, professional boundaries, the discontinuities between care settings, and the relatively brief encounters bereaved people often have with health professionals may contribute to both a neglect and paucity of bereavement care.

It can be argued that bereavement has no part to play in health services and that nurses have no obligation to offer care to the bereaved beyond everyday compassion and the human desire to alleviate the suffering. There is also the criticism that as medicine provides a dominant framework to order death (Seale 1998), so bereavement may become subject to an equivalent regulation and expert clinical lore (Walter 1999). But bereavement has far-reaching consequences for people that can be detrimental to their well-being and health (Parkes 1998). While people may not choose to die in health care settings, the current reality means that many bereaved people have contact with and access to nurses both initially and following the death, a situation that also exists in the community through primary care teams and domiciliary services (see Chapter 26). What this suggests is that nurses should be prepared for their encounters with people who are bereaved and should understand what role they may have in offering care and support. This is a position familiar to those working in palliative and hospice care, but it is an area that has received minimal attention in National Health Service (NHS) hospitals in the UK. However, a number of public inquiries have highlighted the need for high-quality services for all bereaved people and the provision of a professional bereavement service is a recent recommendation for NHS Trusts (Department of Health 2002). In addition, aspects of bereavement care are also featuring in specific service frameworks (Department of Health 2001; NHS Executive 2001).

Views of bereavement

> Being bereaved is not a career, like teaching or acting. I can see that. But I wish it were. How much more comfortable if it were a recognised profession . . . I would like to be *engaged* in bereavement. An exacting job but a rewarding one, after the arduous period of preliminary training. Or even if it isn't a career there must be some ideal way of doing it.
> (Bayley 2002: 213)

This chapter is premised on a palliative care philosophy that encompasses the bereaved within an overall remit of care that continues beyond a disease trajectory to encompass those who have to live with the consequences of death and the experience of bereavement (NCHSPCS 1995). The exploration is based on an understanding of bereavement as a life event that requires people to revise and renegotiate the world (Parkes 2000). Many of the expectations, assumptions and meanings by which we navigate our lives and orientate ourselves can be invalidated as a result of bereavement. It therefore becomes necessary to relearn the world, not simply to take account of the absence of the person who has died, but because the death of an individual can have a pervasive impact upon whom we are and how we live. This requires attending to more than our internal world and may involve relearning the physical, temporal, spiritual and social aspects of our world (Attig 1996).

Relearning implies changing and this can be a creative, positive and fruitful journey. However, bereavement can also be a challenging or stressful transition in that it makes demands upon people beyond their resources as they attempt to deal with loss and renegotiate a meaningful life without the deceased. A recent empirically based model suggests that people may alternate between confronting the reality of loss and attending to the consequences of loss. This 'dual process' model proposes that bereaved people have to deal with two broad types of stressors – loss-orientated and restoration-orientated – and it recognizes that this dynamic process may include beneficial times in which people choose not to face or avoid aspects of loss (Stroebe and Schut 1999). This theoretical model integrates a range of existing ideas about bereavement and supports the differences and individuality that are evident in people's grieving. It is a model that informs the broad approach adopted in this chapter and it avoids some of the problematic assumptions, prescriptions and frameworks used by earlier models and theories (Wortman and Silver 2001)

In offering bereavement care and support we should be aware that we are guided and influenced not only by theories, but also by our own experiences, training, beliefs, attitudes and assumptions (Saunderson and Ridsdale 1999). In this sense, we have to acknowledge that while we stand in the company of the bereaved as professionals, we are also living with the losses characteristic of life, some of which may be the result of death. Nurses need to develop and maintain a level of self-awareness and self-knowledge about areas of their own lives that are potential sources of difficulty or conflict in the context of bereavement. People who are bereaved may become subject to the needs of nurses who are living out, through either conscious or unconscious processes, their own bereavement. Equally, nurses may develop strategies and practices that avoid or minimize the possibility or impact of caring for the bereaved when painful personal loss is evoked. There is a need, therefore, for nurses to be aware of the implicit boundaries in which care and support is offered. At one extreme boundaries become effective barriers and at another they become shaped by personal interests with a potential for a betrayal of trust, respect or intimacy that may be considered an abuse of the practitioner–client relationship (Nursing and Midwifery Council 2002). For these reasons, nurses should ensure that their practice of bereavement care and support is the subject of clinical supervision, preceptorship or mentorship in which it can be safely and honestly explored.

Respecting the diversity of individuals

All people have a finite future and death is an event that will apply to everyone. Bereavement, as the objective condition resulting from loss, can also be understood as a ubiquitous category. Standardized in this way people who are bereaved can be expected to make conventional responses to loss and react to death in ways that can be reduced to explanatory theories and models. The logical consequence of this schema is that people who do not fit the accepted standard models present complications and abnormalities requiring interventions to resolve their deviant behaviour. However, the objectivity of death and bereavement required for their investigation and conceptualization is a limited and depersonalized perspective. The objective may appear to provide a vantage point in the care and support of the bereaved, but it cannot provide an adequate position from which to appreciate the subjective value, meaning and impact of a particular death for the bereaved person.

In offering care and support to people who are bereaved, we need to take the fullest possible account of the subjective view. However, if a theoretical view is necessarily insensitive to any individual, so a focus on the subjective view may not recognize any external references. People can also share much in common and their lives are inscribed through their social and cultural interactions and the contexts in which they live. Therefore, we may consider that a bereaved person is neither a predetermined abstract category nor a self-defining identity but an individual facing loss. A person in these circumstances will, therefore, draw upon his or her own unique understanding and experience that is embedded within a wider shared world in which people die. For these reasons, becoming involved with bereaved people requires of us a broad understanding of the impact of loss upon personhood that is sensitive not only to psychological insights but also to other significant aspects of the person, including history, gender, ethnicity (Field *et al.* 1997) and culture (Rees 2001).

Sharing the story

Loss and change are unavoidable aspects of life and, consequently, people have to negotiate many types of disruptions and dislocations to their worlds over the years. In this sense, bereavement is a normal situation that people find themselves in and which most will cope with and go on to reconstruct and revise their worlds. They do this without any particular professional intervention but they may often receive support and care from people they associate with and in whose circles they move. Family and friends, because of their proximity, can often be well placed to care for someone in their bereavement, providing accessible practical help as well as understanding companionship and a sympathetic ear. Such people can also be well placed to share in the storytelling about the loss and the person who has died. This narrative process may help people in transition to make some sort of sense and find meaning in their irreversibly changed world and lives. This human tendency to tell stories (in spoken and written form) can be both loss-orientated and restoration-orientated and Neimeyer and Anderson (2001) outline three types of narratives that seem to operate in accounts of loss:

- *External narratives*: these are accounts, descriptions and reports of what has happened. The objective form of these narratives provides ordered versions of external events from a personal perspective and therefore also relate to the storyteller. Descriptions of how the person died, reporting the actions of individuals and recounting what happened at the funeral are examples of external narratives.

- *Internal narratives*: these focus upon the affective responses to the death as experienced by the narrator or biographer. These self-expressions of what it feels like to experience the loss are emotion-based narratives and articulate the internal world of the bereaved person.

- *Reflexive narratives*: these build upon the primary narratives, recalling what happened or expressing feelings and provide a secondary narrative of interpretation and reflection. Exploring the significance of the death, why it happened and what the death means to the storyteller are examples of reflexive narratives.

Narratives of loss are ongoing projects and people who are bereaved may revise and revisit them individually and in association with others. Health professionals may also share in the stories of the bereaved because they may be part of the story. A person may need to establish a coherent account of how someone became ill and died with those who hold records of such events. A bereaved person may also feel confident in describing their feelings to someone who they expect might understand how people respond to loss. In this way, a bereaved person may be checking out their own position and seeking validation for their feelings and thoughts. Finally, health professionals may also be turned to by a bereaved person in reflecting upon the meaning of the experience in terms of the past, present and future. A nurse involved in the care of the person who has died (directly or vicariously) may be considered by the bereaved person as someone who understands the context of loss and who therefore may be able to assist in conserving what has gone while negotiating what it means to live in the changed world.

The idea of storytelling can be considered a helpful approach to supporting bereaved people. Most people can tell stories and those who listen to stories do not require any particular expertise or specialist training, just the ability and time to listen. Stories can be told in the absence of other people through the written word and the internet provides a virtual worldwide space within which to share stories. But we must enter a caveat to this attractively simple proposition of support because some people will choose to remain solitary in their grief, a narrative may not be formed in spoken or written words, and silence may be just as important to someone as dialogue. If death imposes an absence, then for some people bereavement may not require anything to be said about it other than what is evident. Storytelling must not be an imperative to fill the silence. Equally, we must resist the social convention of making people talk and we should question a professional convention that automatically refers the inarticulate to counsellors and therapists. Phillips suggests that the mourning process tends to make people more self-absorbed as well as in need of other people. However, he cautions that:

If grief doesn't have a shareable story, if there is no convincing account of what happens to people when someone they know dies, grief will always be singular and secluding: as close as we can get to a private experience without it sounding nonsensical. When someone dies something is communicated to us that we cannot communicate. Hence the urgency that goes into making death a communal experience . . . The only taboo, where grief is concerned, is not experiencing it: not feeling it and performing it appropriately. There are no grief scandals in the way that there are sex scandals; there are only scandalous absences of grieving.

(Phillips 2000: 257–8)

Follow-up contact and aftercare

Most people do not die suddenly and from diagnosis to death both patients and carers may receive the support of professionals. Even death resulting from acute events and undiagnosed conditions can often be accompanied by a host of people paid to care. However, as noted at the start of this chapter, many health services come to a halt following a death. The exceptions to this are usually to be found in specialist services, of which palliative care is a particular example, and community services which are more likely to have to deal with long-term consequences of bereavement. What is evident is that some people who are bereaved experience the ending of what can be intensive support and some may be offered support from new sources and for the first time.

Health services generally do not have the resources to offer more than a minimal amount of care and support to the bereaved. What care is offered is often targeted at those who are considered to be vulnerable to adverse bereavement outcomes and a risk assessment measure is used to identify susceptible people (Aranda and Milne 2000; see Chapter 27). However, in the immediate period following a death, there are many tasks that require the involvement of the bereaved, principally the funeral, which brings them to the attention of others and which can establish a transient cluster of support and people to turn to for help and advice. But within weeks, this support has usually been withdrawn and bereaved people may experience a further ending of care.

What may help bereaved people through these significant transitions of care and supportive company are relatively simple follow-up contacts. These can take the form of domiciliary visits, telephone calls, letters and cards. The purpose of these contacts include: the expression of concern into the well-being of the bereaved; an opportunity for the bereaved to say something of their current feelings and experiences; the opportunity to raise questions or concerns either about the death or the bereavement; the provision of information about sources of bereavement support in the community; the offer of further follow-up; and a means of ending the involvement of a service. Follow-up contacts should form part of a systematic approach to bereavement by services so that they are coordinated and adequately supported by staff. A bereavement aftercare programme introduced into one emergency department aimed to be easily absorbed into existing workloads, beneficial and unobtrusive as possible to the bereaved, and offering some continuity with staff present at the time of the person's death. The follow-up aspect of this programme involved sending a handwritten sympathy card to the closest relative and a follow-up phone call at one week (to assess needs) and at six weeks (which relatives could decline). The hospital received much positive feedback from those enrolled on the programme who had appreciated that staff cared about them. It was also considered to be a beneficial process for the staff involved, as it allowed them to demonstrate a more human side of health care (Williams *et al.* 2000). In a study of the impact of a supportive telephone call, the bereaved people contacted mainly perceived the contact as positive in that it provided them with emotional support as well as the opportunity to ask questions about the illness and death (Kaunonen *et al.* 2000).

Bereavement counselling and therapy

Bereavement results in diverse reactions in people with considerable variability in the manifestations of grief. Within this spectrum it is recognized that, for some people, bereavement may affect their health and well-being to such an extent that there may be a justification for psychological or pharmacological interventions. Prolonged or extreme reactions to bereavement may be considered abnormal or complicated and diagnostic criteria have been proposed for bereavement-related pathologies and disorders (Horowitz *et al.* 1997). Historically, links have been made between bereavement phenomena and the psychological and somatic symptoms associated with syndromes such as depression and anxiety. However, more recent studies have cautioned against oversimplification and Middleton *et al.* (1997) have concluded that '[t]he bereaved can experience considerable pain and yet be coping adaptively, and they can fulfil many depressive criteria yet at the same time be experiencing phenomena that are not depressive in nature' (p. 451).

People may be identified before a death has occurred as being in a high-risk category in terms of developing morbidities and disorders post-bereavement (see Chapter 27). Screening for adverse outcomes may result in referrals to professionals who offer medical or psychological interventions. However, it may be much later after the death that a bereaved person feels that they are in difficulty or that they present to a health professional with symptoms of complicated grief. A common source of help for these people is counselling, which may be available through general practitioners (GPs), voluntary agencies and private practices in the UK. A review of counselling in primary care in England concluded that current evidence suggests it is useful in the short-term treatment of mild to moderate mental health problems, but that in the long term (8–12 months) outcomes between counselling and usual GP care cannot be differentiated (NHS Centre for Reviews and Dissemination 2001). In another systematic review of studies of interventions for complicated grief, results were mostly positive and lasting, but the effects were modest (Schut *et al.* 2001). Finally, it should be acknowledged that individuals, as a result of a bereavement experience, may wish to take time to review and explore aspects of their lives to understand themselves better. A self-referral, for example to a psychotherapist, can be a creative response towards difficulties encountered in bereavement and it can be considered as a way of sharing stories about an individual's life that is both interesting and helpful.

Support and care beyond health professionals

I have considered some of the general ways in which those who care for the dying may also care for the bereaved. There are some unique benefits that may be associated with professionals who become involved with people prior to death being able to offer some support to them in their bereavement. However, most people leave behind care settings, or services withdraw, and they face their bereavement not in the company of professionals but in the context of family, friends and the social networks provided in places of work, residence and the communities with which they associate. Health professionals need to be aware of the resources of support and care that may be available to bereaved people once they have returned to the places in which their lives continue.

Formal (paid) care of the bereaved may be provided through social care workers, including professionally qualified social workers. Bereavement can be a significant aspect of social care services either because service users have experienced loss in this way or there is need for social care input as a result of a death (Currer 2001). However, much of the support available to bereaved people comes from voluntary and non-statutory organizations. One of the most well-known voluntary community services in the UK is provided by the national charity Cruse Bereavement Care,[1] which offers support through a network of over 170 branches and 6000 trained volunteers. Cruse offers free information and advice to anyone who has been affected by a death; provides support and counselling one to one and in groups; offers education, support, information and publications to anyone supporting bereaved people; and increases public awareness of the needs of bereaved people through campaigning and information services.

Many national and local bereavement care resources have been established to meet the needs of specific groups. Winston's Wish[2] is a charity offering support throughout the UK to bereaved children and young people through a national telephone helpline, practical resources and publications, and training and consultancy services for those working with bereaved families and those wishing to set up a grief support service in their own area. More information about childhood bereavement services can be found in

Chapter 29. Another example is The Way Foundation,[3] which provides a self-help social and support network to people bereaved under the age of 50 and their children.

Bereaved people frequently come into contact with religious and cultural communities for the practical reason of arranging a funeral. These communities provide rituals, ceremonies and customs around death but many also offer some form of bereavement support. In Judaism, for example, the first seven days of intense mourning (*Shiva*) is a period in which the bereaved are exempt from the requirements of daily life and the Jewish community demonstrates practical care and condolence in the provision of meals (Rees 2001). In addition, there are Jewish support networks and counselling services. Christian churches, whose ministers conduct the majority of funerals, provide pastoral care to bereaved people and there are church-based bereavement visiting schemes offering community support through trained volunteers (Billings 2002).

Finally, the virtual community of the internet provides access for many people to a wealth of information and advice to help them in their bereavement as well as a route to obtain personal support. The style, quality and up-to-date nature of the contents varies widely (see Chapter 34). There are sites provided by statutory agencies such as the UK government's own online website,[4] which contains a section on death and bereavement. In contrast, there are sites developed from personal experiences that many people will find helpful. ifishoulddie.co.uk[5] was created following the death of the author's father. The site provides much practical information, including details about the legal requirements following a death, organizing a funeral and a section on understanding and coping with grief. Merrywidow.me[6] is a web-published guide for bereaved women needing clear practical advice based upon the author's experience following the death of her husband at the age of 37.

Conclusions

This chapter has brought together two major themes. The first derives from the fact that people die in health care services and that therefore these services have a responsibility for providing care and support to people who are bereaved. The second is derived from the changing views of scholars and clinicians who recognize that, in response to the death of someone significant to them, a bereaved person becomes involved in a dynamic process of relearning a changed world and reconstructing meaning in order to live with the experience of loss. Together these themes suggest a creative and challenging agenda for nursing and its important contribution to the care and support of bereaved people in terms of training, practice, service development and research. If most people begin their bereavement in the company of nurses, then nurses are uniquely placed in relationship to the care of bereaved people and the contexts in which death occurs.

Storytelling can play an important role in the lives of bereaved people in their search to 'make sense' of what has happened and to assimilate their experience of loss into their life story. The challenge is that, '[l]ike a novel that loses a central character in the middle chapters, the life story disrupted by loss must be reorganized, rewritten, to find a new strand of continuity that bridges the past with the future in an intelligible fashion' (Neimeyer 2000: 263). The biographical nature of this narrative indicates each person's unique and varied response to bereavement. Storytelling reminds us that bereavement has a social context and involves other people. By implication, an important question for nurses concerns what narratives inform their understanding of bereavement and the care they offer bereaved people. Equally, we need to pay attention to whose language prevails: the person facing loss or the nurse who frames bereavement with professional and personal meanings?

Whatever the particular interests and skills of individual nurses, professional and service boundaries can impose their own disruption and discontinuity upon bereaved people. People who are bereaved can therefore find themselves estranged from both the context in which death has taken place and those professionals who they may expect to understand what it is that they are experiencing. Follow-up programmes, even of a basic form, that have been well thought through and properly organized may offer an important element of continuity to bereaved people. However, it is also important that nurses should be actively aware of the resources available in the community to support bereaved people and be able to access relevant advice and information. None of this is to suggest that the care and support of bereaved people is a responsibility that nurses alone should be expected to bear, but neither is it one that they should neglect.

Notes

1   See Cruse website (http://www.crusebereavementcare.org.uk).
2   See Winston's Wish website (http://www.winstonswish.org.uk).
3   See Way Foundation website (http://wayfoundation.org.uk).
4   See the UK government's own website (http://www.ukoline.gov.uk).
5   See If I Should Die website (http://www.ifishouldie.co.uk).
6   See Merrywidow website (http://www.merrywidow.me.uk/).

References

Aranda, S. and Milne, D. (2000) *Guidelines for the Assessment of Complicated Bereavement Risk in Family Members of People Receiving Palliative Care.* Melbourne, VIC: Centre for Palliative Care.
Attig, T. (1996) *How We Grieve: Relearning the World.* New York: Oxford University Press.

Bayley, J. (2002) *Widower's House*. London: Abacus.

Billings, A. (2002) *Dying and Grieving: A Guide to Pastoral Ministry*. London: SPCK.

Currer, C. (2001) *Responding to Grief: Dying, Bereavement and Social Care*. Basingstoke: Palgrave.

Department of Health (1992) *Patients Who Die in Hospital*, HSG (92)8. London: Department of Health.

Department of Health (1997) *Patients Who Die in Hospital*, HSG (97)42. London: Department of Health.

Department of Health (2001) *National Service Framework for Older People*. London: Department of Health.

Department of Health (2002) *Learning from Bristol: The Department of Heath's Response to the Report for the Public Inquiry into Children's Heart Surgery at the Bristol Royal Infirmary 1984–1995*. London: The Stationery Office.

Field, D., Hockey, J. and Small, N. (1997) *Death, Gender and Ethnicity*. London: Routledge.

Horowitz, M.J., Siegel, B., Holen, A. *et al.* (1997) Diagnostic criteria for complicated grief disorder. *American Psychiatric Association*, 154(7): 904–10.

Kaunonen, M., Tarkka, M.-T., Laippala, P. and Paunonen-Ilmonen, M. (2000) The impact of supportive telephone call intervention on grief after the death of a family member. *Cancer Nursing*, 23(6): 483–91.

Kissane, D.W. (2000) Neglect of bereavement care in general hospitals. *Medical Journal of Australia*, 173(9): 456.

Mallett, J. and Dougherty, L. (eds) (2000) *The Royal Marsden Hospital Manual of Clinical Nursing Procedures*. Oxford: Blackwell Science.

Middleton, W.F., Raphael, B.F., Burnett, P. and Martinek, N. (1997) Psychological distress and bereavement. *Journal of Nervous and Mental Diseases*, 185(7): 447–53.

National Council for Hospice and Specialist Palliative Care Services (1995) *Specialist Palliative Care: A Statement of Definitions*. London: NCHSPCS.

Neimeyer, R.A. (ed.) (2000) *Meaning Reconstruction and the Experience of Loss*. Washington, DC: American Psychological Association.

Neimeyer, R.A. and Anderson, A. (2001) Meaning reconstruction theory, in N. Thompson (ed.) *Loss and Grief: A Guide for Human Services Practitioners*. Basingstoke: Palgrave.

NHS Centre for Reviews and Dissemination (2001) *Counselling in Primary Care*. York: University of York.

NHS Executive (2001) *Manual of Cancer Service Standards*. London: NHS Executive.

Nursing and Midwifery Council (2002) *Patient–Client Relationships and the Prevention of Abuse*. London: NMC.

Office for National Statistics (2001) *Mortality Statistics: General 1999*, Series DH1 No. 32. London: HMSO.

Parkes, C.M. (1998) Coping with loss: bereavement in adult life. *British Medical Journal*, 216: 856–9.

Parkes, C.M. (2000) Bereavement as a psychosocial transition: processes of adaptation to change, in D. Dickenson, M. Johnson and J.S. Katz (eds) *Death, Dying and Bereavement*. London: Sage.

Phillips, A. (2000) *Promises, Promises*. London: Faber & Faber.

Rees, D. (2001) *Death and Bereavement: The Psychological, Religious and Cultural Interfaces*. London: Whurr.

Saunderson, E.M. and Ridsdale, L. (1999) General practitioners' beliefs and attitudes about how to respond to death and bereavement: qualitative study. *British Medical Journal*, 319: 292–6.

Schut, H., Stoebe, M.S., van den Bout, J. and Terheggen, M. (2001) The efficacy of bereavment interventions: determining who benefits, in M.S. Stroebe, R.O. Hansson, W. Stroebe and H. Schut (eds) *Handbook of Bereavement Research: Consequences, Coping, and Care*. Washington, DC: American Psychological Association.

Seale, C. (1998) *Constructing Death: The Sociology of Dying and Bereavement*. Cambridge: Cambridge University Press.

Stroebe, M. and Schut, H. (1999) The dual process model of coping with bereavement: rationale and description. *Death Studies*, 23: 197–224.

Walter, T. (1999) *On Bereavement: The Culture of Grief*. Buckingham: Open University Press.

Williams, A.G., O'Brien, D., Laughton, K.J. and Jelinek, G.A. (2000) Improving services to bereaved relatives in the emergency department: making healthcare more human. *Medical Journal of Australia*, 173: 480–3.

Wortman, C.B. and Silver, R.C. (2001) The myths of coping with loss revisited, in M.S. Stroebe, R.O. Hansson, W. Stroebe and H. Schut (eds) *Handbook of Bereavement Research: Consequences Coping, and Care*, Washington, DC: American Psychological Association.

26

Bereavement support

The perspective of community nurses

Jon Birtwistle

In the UK, a typical general practice with a patient list of 8000 will have around 80 patient deaths per year. Although an estimated 75 per cent of people die in an institution (i.e. hospital, hospice or nursing home), general practitioners (family doctors) and community nurses frequently care for patients with terminal illness in their homes and carry out bereavement visits to families of patients they have cared for. In a survey of community nurses in the UK, Hatcliffe *et al.* (1996) reported that 69 per cent had cared for between one and ten patients dying from cancer or AIDS in the past year. However, there is a paucity of published literature about the practice of community nurses in bereavement support. Most published literature is aimed at informing nurses about the theoretical aspects of bereavement, or provide descriptions about dealing with bereaved people. Other research has addressed bereavement issues from the hospital perspective (e.g. bereavement on the ward or within the accident and emergency department) or from specialist areas such as obstetrics or paediatric medicine.

In recent years, the professional role and responsibility of nursing has been expanded and the skill base extended. In the UK, the community nurse is one of the key providers of palliative care (Audit Commission 1999) and in a recent editorial Payne (2001) suggested that bereavement support had become a fundamental aspect of palliative care. At present in the UK, many community nurses carry out bereavement follow-up visits and some provide bereavement counselling or other bereavement services. Some have suggested that when community nurses have provided palliative care in the community they are ideally placed to offer bereavement care as they are multiskilled, in the right place (patient's home) and there at the right time (time of death) (Koodiaroff 1999). Furthermore, some suggest that they also have a key role in assessing the needs of the bereaved person, detecting any abnormal pathological grief, helping the individual with the pain of grief, and offering advice, support and information (Costello 1995; Monroe and Smith 1997). However, little is known about the extent of community nurses' involvement in bereavement support, or their level of training, skills or knowledge of bereavement.

In this chapter, I examine some of these issues. I start by defining the roles of community nurses and district nurses from the UK perspective. I provide evidence for the impact of bereavement on health and discuss the practical implications for community nurses. I also explore practical and professional issues that may affect the support that community nurses provide to bereaved people. I draw upon evidence from a recently published self-completed postal questionnaire of community nurses in the central southern coastal area of Britain, which focused on community nurses' current practice and perceived roles in supporting bereaved people (Birtwistle *et al.* 2002).

The community nurse in the UK

In its broadest sense, a community nurse within the UK can be described as any nurse who works with patients in the community and outside medical institutions. These include the community mental health nurses, community learning disability nurses, community midwives, school nurses, health visitors, practice nurses, district nurses, occupational health nurses and specialist nurses, such as Macmillan nurses, paediatric district nurses, diabetic nurses, asthma and stoma care nurses.

Recently in the UK, the title of district nurse and community nurse has become synonymous, although at present to use the title of district nurse requires the nurse to hold a mandatory post-registration qualification specifically in district nursing. However, this is not a nursing registration as defined by the UK's Nursing and Midwifery Council. Typically, a district nurse is a senior nurse who leads a team of nurses including other district nurses, community staff nurses and unqualified 'auxiliary' or support staff. The district nurse forms part of the core primary health care team, which is comprised of general practitioners (GPs), practice nurses, district nurses, health visitors, practice managers and administrative staff. For the purpose of this chapter, the district nurse and qualified members of the team (e.g. community staff nurse) will be treated as one entity and for simplification the term community nurse will be used.

Although any community nurse may deal with a death or bereavement as part of their professional role, they differ in the types of death encountered and the frequency of dealing with death and bereavement. For example, community mental health nurses may deal with a disproportionately higher number of client suicides and the subsequent family bereavements compared with other community nurses. Within the UK, health visitors tend to deal with deaths in children and young people and bereaved parents, while community nurses deal with older clients. However, this is not always the case, as there are specialized areas within district nursing such as paediatric district nurses who may deal with terminally ill children and in some general practices health visitors specialize in the care of older people.

Fortunately, the reduction in infant mortality over the last century has meant that although the death of a baby or child is a very traumatic event, it is now relatively rare. With the reduction of infant mortality, the main bereavement (following that of parents and grandparents) is the loss of a spouse or partner, which affects women to a greater extent than men.

The importance of communication skills

Dealing with patients on a daily basis in a variety of situations requires that all nurses develop effective communication skills. However, when patients are in their own home, it is different to dealing with them on a hospital ward. There is a subtle shift in control and power as the nurse is a guest within the home of the patient, rather than the patient being 'admitted' onto the ward. Dealing with bereaved people requires effective communication and empathic listening skills.

Evidence suggests that health professionals are sometimes poor communicators (Audit Commission 1993). Many cancer patients and carers suggest that health care professionals should receive better communication skills training (National Cancer Alliance 1996). There is inadequate training in how to communicate with terminally ill patients or bereaved people, which may reflect a lack of priority in health care, or alternatively, the difficulty of teaching such a sensitive subject (Field and Kitson 1986; Faulkner 1992; Jeffrey 1994, Lloyd-Williams and Lloyd-Williams 1996). Breaking bad news and dealing with bereaved people can be a particularly stressful event and it is important that nurses develop the appropriate skills in dealing with this. Occasionally, a community nurse may be present at the death or the patient may already be dead when the nurse arrives. Although death is usually expected in palliative care, those present may still feel shocked by the news. Being informed about the death of someone close may be so overwhelming that it can result in a state of shock, which can in some people cause cardiac changes that can increase the risk of sudden cardiac death. Brandspiegel *et al.* (1998) described a 70-year-old woman who was being monitored in hospital with an electrocardiograph machine. Upon hearing of her husband's death, she showed acute cardiac arrhythmias and a subsequent blood analysis found elevated cardiac enzymes. The shock could have killed her. In addition, the recipient can occasionally react to the news in unexpected ways, with outbursts of anger that can be distressing for all concerned.

The pragmatics of death in the community

The death of a person is a major event, which can cause great emotional distress and social upheaval for those who are bereaved. However, many people have never dealt with the death of someone they are close to and are unsure about what to do. There are the immediate practical problems, which can raise some difficult questions. For example, who to call for help – the doctor, the community nurse, the police, the undertaker? There are also several questions which may be asked depending on culture and religious beliefs, such as when and why a postmortem would be required, who has 'legal ownership' of the body, when the family will be allowed to have the deceased prepared for a wake and who has responsibility for removal of the body? For some people even expected deaths can be a shock, while for others it may sometimes be a happy release. In either case, following a death there are a number of practical legal issues to sort out, such as arranging a funeral, deciding on a burial or cremation, registering the death, obtaining a death certificate and sorting out legal and financial matters. Following an expected death at home, the GP or community nurse is usually the first health professional to arrive on the scene. If that happens, they may be involved in the practical aspect of dealing with the death and offering immediate support to the family.

The role of the community nurse in bereavement support

If bereavement is to be expected and grief is a normal reaction to bereavement, what is the role, if any, of the community nurse in supporting bereaved people who, in essence, are not ill? Although bereaved people may have an increased risk of health problems, unless they actually have a medical condition they are not technically ill and one must question whether 'uncomplicated' bereavement should be viewed as a 'medical' problem, requiring community nurse input. Prior to death, the family/partner/carer of the patient may build up a strong relationship with the community nurse, but following the patient's death bereaved people are not part of the community nurse patient caseload. The professional relationship between bereaved people and the community nurse will therefore change from the time of death.

The bereavement visit

The death of a patient does not necessarily mean the end of community nurse involvement (Baly *et al.* 1987). It is usual for the community nurse to visit at least once following the death to offer condolences and to arrange for the collection of any medical equipment (e.g. infusion pumps), which may be required by other patients. Occasionally, the GP or other members of the primary health care team may also visit, to assess how the person is coping following their loss.

The increased health risks following bereavement have led some GPs to advocate a proactive bereavement protocol for the primary care team

(Charlton and Dolman 1995). However, others have questioned the advisability of adopting such protocols unreservedly, without evidence that active follow-up in primary care improves outcomes (Woof and Carter 1995). General practitioners are sometimes unsure about how to approach their bereaved patients. A survey of GPs to ascertain their bereavement support and practice activity following patient deaths found responders were equally divided over whether bereavement support should be proactive or reactive. One of the reasons for not following up bereaved relatives proactively was a concern not to 'over-medicalize' grief (Harris and Kendrick 1998).

There are no published guidelines for bereavement support within primary care. General practitioners who keep a death register and/or who have a special interest in palliative care are more likely to offer routine bereavement support (Harris and Kendrick 1998). Some bereaved people see bereavement support as an important role of the GP (Main 2000). Some community nurses offer long-term bereavement support, although this varies by nursing team and is influenced by several factors, including the personal views of the nurse, the presence of community nurse involvement prior to the death, the amount of available time, the nurse's interest and knowledge of bereavement, and their training and experience of bereavement support.

Birtwistle *et al.* (2002) carried out a survey of a representative sample of district nurses to ascertain their current practice and perceived role in supporting bereaved people and to identify factors that influence their practice. A self-completed postal questionnaire was distributed anonymously to 522 district nurses in the central southern coastal area of Britain. The response rate was 62 per cent.

A number of factors appear to be associated with whether a community nurse is likely to follow up a bereaved person with a series of visits. Birtwistle *et al.* (2002) used logistic regression to assess which factors best predicted post-bereavement follow-up visits. Essentially, logistic regression is a statistical method used to select factors that predict one of two possible outcomes (e.g. death or survival, pass or fail). In this example, the two possible outcomes for the nurses were that they always or frequently did post-bereavement visits or occasionally or never did bereavement visits. Three factors were independently associated with an increased likelihood of visiting: the location of the community nurse's place of employment (based on the geographical boundaries or 'districts' of employment), the age of the nurse and academic qualification of the nurse. The older the nurse, the more likely they were to do follow-up visits, as were those with better academic qualifications such as a degree or diploma. Certain general practices were associated with an increased likelihood of visiting, which probably reflects the culture of the nursing team and the general practice ethos regarding bereavement support. There may also be influences from local hospices that sometimes have close links with the community nurses and GPs in their locality and provide training to community nurses.

Lack of guidelines or protocols means that there is much variation in the structure of bereavement support, both in terms of the content of the bereavement visit and the timing of bereavement visits. In the survey by Birtwistle *et al.* (2002), the length of time community nurses remained in contact with bereaved people ranged from 2 weeks to over 12 months. Some reported a specific structure with visits at particular times, such as immediately after the death, after the funeral and then at 3, 6 and 12 months (the anniversary of the death). The timing of these visits revolved around the funeral and the availability of family support afterwards. However, the majority of respondents suggested that post-bereavement contacts should not be prescriptive but tailored to individuals' needs and circumstances. There is little evidence that bereavement visits are counselling sessions *per se*; most appeared to be an opportunity for the person to 'chat about the deceased' with the nurse over a cup of tea.

Not all aspects of bereavement support have been welcomed and the professionalization and medicalization of bereavement is a contentious issue. Walter (1999) has suggested that as society becomes increasingly secularized, bereaved people who once turned to their families, community and religious advisors for support are turning to health professionals, which has important implications for the primary care services.

Community nurse involvement prior to death

Community nurses are frequently involved in the care of patients immediately prior to death and could therefore provide support to bereaved relatives. Previous contact and knowledge of patients and their families appears to be a key factor in deciding whether nurses carry out bereavement visits. In the survey by Birtwistle *et al.* (2002), 95 per cent of responders believed their role should involve visiting bereaved relatives and carers of patients they had nursed, but only 19 per cent believed they should visit bereaved people when the deceased was not their patient (43 per cent of community nurses were uncertain whether a visit should be made and 38 per cent felt that no visit should be made). This probably reflects difficulties due to the lack of an established prior relationship and the unpleasant prospect of visiting a complete stranger to discuss aspects of their recent loss.

There are many deaths where there has been no prior contact with community nursing services. These include sudden deaths, deaths in hospital and hospices. Occasionally following a bereavement visit from the GP, the community nurse may be asked to visit to 'keep an eye on' their patient, particularly if they are old and vulnerable. In addition, the author is aware of at least one general practice where there is a coordinated bereavement service run by the senior nurse who contacts any bereaved patient belonging to the practice, irrespective of prior community nurse involvement, to offer condolences and support. However, this is not widespread and at present there is no evidence to indicate if this is the best practice.

Is bereavement visiting a good use of community nursing resources?

There is some evidence from the UK that GP consultations may increase following bereavement (Parkes 1964, Tudiver *et al.* 1995; Charlton *et al.* 2001). Any increase in GP consultation following bereavement has cost and resource implications for primary care services. Evidence presented by Parkes (1964) suggests that older widows are more likely to consult GPs with physical health problems, while younger widows are more likely to consult with mental health problems. At present, there has been scant research within primary care into possible interventions to identify and reduce post-bereavement consultation (see Chapter 28 regarding bereavement support provided by palliative care services). A Canadian study by Tudiver *et al.* (1995) compared newly bereaved widowers attending a 9-week intervention (focusing on mutual peer group support and health promotion) with those who remained on a waiting list for support. Following the intervention, there was a significant reduction in the number of consultations with the family doctor compared with the non-intervention (waiting list) control group, suggesting that a mutual support programme with newly bereaved men may help to reduce the overall use of primary health care resources.

Any discussion of increased primary care interventions is likely to be resisted by the medical profession, which is understaffed and hard pressed to cope with current health care demands. In February 2002, the British Medical Association (BMA) published a discussion document in which they proposed a model of health care designed to overcome the shortages of GPs. In this document, they suggest that community nurses should have an expanded clinical role, involving them undertaking a wider range of interventions. The practical implications of the BMA proposal would involve a radical change to the boundaries of the nursing role. Bereavement support may be one area of nurses' skills base that needs to be expanded, to reduce the increased use of health care services after bereavement and to identify people with bereavement-related physical and mental health problems. At present, it is unclear what effect, if any, there is from community nurse led bereavement support.

Community services are under a great deal of pressure and any expansion or extension of the community nurse role potentially adds to that pressure. A report from the Audit Commission (1999) outlined a number of problems faced by the district nursing services in the UK. Two-thirds of primary care trusts reported a fall in the number of qualified district nurses, one in ten district nurses were above the age of retirement and the numbers entering training have shrunk by one-third since 1990. Overall, this has reduced the capacity of the service. Added to this has been the increased demand on the service from an increasing older population, of whom 50 per cent over 85 years see a district nurse, and an increase in early hospital discharge with specialist care (e.g. palliative care), which is increasingly being carried out within the home (Audit Commission 1999).

How interested and informed are community nurses about bereavement?

In the survey by Birtwistle *et al.* (2002), 69 per cent of respondents expressed an interest in bereavement and 80 per cent an interest in palliative care, with 67 per cent expressing interest in both. One interesting finding was that 12 per cent of respondents expressed an interest in palliative care but not bereavement support. This reflects the way that some community nurses compartmentalize these aspects of care. Most current training in palliative care recommends that bereavement support is part of the continued care and support of the family and these findings have important implications for the education and training of nurses as undergraduates and postgraduates.

Eighty-nine per cent of nurses in the survey reported their main education about bereavement came from experiential learning 'on the job', 82 per cent reported they gained it from reading the nursing literature, and 75 per cent reported they had gained it from post-registration training. However, only 25 per cent reported their undergraduate training as a source of bereavement education. Less than half felt they had received sufficient training in dealing with newly bereaved people, which raises questions whether nurses have sufficient knowledge, appropriate training or the necessary skills to offer bereavement support.

What can community nurses do to support bereaved people?

In practice, there is wide variation in the bereavement support provided by nurses and few community nurse teams provide an actual bereavement service. Much current practice could be described as unstructured, for example the 'cup of tea and a chat' approach. However, the lack of research to indicate a positive impact on bereavement outcomes does not in itself condemn bereavement support. There is much that a nurse can offer a bereaved person, including the comfort of just being there to listen. They can also offer practical support, such as the provision of information about grief and bereavement. In addition, being skilled in the assessment of patients' health and social needs they may be best placed to assess and identify risk factors and refer to specialist services.

Just 'being there'

Anecdotal evidence suggests that an important role of the GP and community nurses is often simply to 'be there' and listen to the bereaved person and to recognize grief as a painful but normal process. Making contact with the bereaved person can be appreciated and remembered. Sometimes the nurse has cared for the deceased patient over a long period of time, sometimes years, and may have developed a close relationship with both the patient and their family. Community nurses provide much practical and emotional support to the family and can become like one of the family. However, there is a downside to this close relationship both for the nurses and their relatives. Occasionally, nurses may develop a close relationship that is beyond the boundaries of their professional status, developing into 'friendship'. Lyttle (2001) reported that bereaved people referred to their community nurse as a 'friend' or person with whom they had a special relationship. This raises a number of professional and personal boundary issues that need to be explored.

The nurse must deal with the emotional context of the situation, since the 'demand for friendship' and role ambiguities are major stressors for community nurses involved in palliative care (Wilkes *et al.* 1998). In such circumstances, long-term follow-up visits to bereaved people may reflect the needs of the nurse in addition to that of the bereaved person. Structured visits, peer support, debriefing, quality clinical supervision and access to counselling may be ways of reducing stress in community nurses by maintaining role boundaries and a sense of professionalism (see Chapter 32).

When the patient dies, the family are at a vulnerable stage and there is a potential risk of bereaved people becoming dependent on the nurse. Some feel a sense of loneliness and loss when this support network is removed. The ending of that relationship with the community nurse can also be perceived as another loss, a 'double bereavement', to those already vulnerable or lonely. That is particularly so when the bereaved person is older with a poor social and family network.

For bereaved adults, having friends or neighbours to turn to seems to be a protective factor against emotional problems such as depression, loneliness and worry. When social isolation is the main problem, the community nurse may be able to refer to social services and provide information about local groups (e.g. lunch clubs, community centres, charities) that may provide social support to the bereaved person.

Provision of information

One of the roles of the community nurse is to promote health (Baly *et al.* 1987), which includes the provision of information about health problems and services available. However, the results of the survey by Birtwistle *et al.* (2002) do not support this in practice, as 44 per cent of nurses indicated that no information was provided to bereaved people about the emotional impact of grief and 11 per cent did not know. However, community nurses were slightly better at providing information on the practical aspects of bereavement (53 per cent) and services available (64 per cent), but about 25 per cent were unaware of the availability of written information. There are currently several useful publications aimed at informing bereaved people and community nurses alike, including *What to Do After a Death in England and Wales* (Department of Social Security 2000) and various publications from organizations such as the Royal College of Psychiatrists and charities such as Cruse and Help the Aged.

Assessment of health risks

There is some evidence that bereaved carers of cancer patients who die at home may experience higher psychological distress than carers of patients who die elsewhere (Addington-Hall and Karlsem 2000). Community nurses could potentially play a key role in assessing the needs of the bereaved person, helping them with the pain of grief, offering advice, support and information (Costello 1995; Monroe and Smith 1997) and helping to prevent any breakdown in health. Community nurses may be well placed to assess for potential health problems during bereavement visits and to refer at-risk people to more specialized services (Baly *et al.* 1987; Costello 1995). In addition, an assessment of risk in vulnerable bereaved people should be seen as an essential aspect of professional practice (see Chapters 27 and 29).

The UK Nursing and Midwifery Council (2002) code of professional conduct for nurses states that a registered nurse or midwife must:

- protect and support the health of individual patients and clients; and
- protect and support the health of the wider community.

As with any major stressor, bereaved people may experience a general deterioration in health or an exacerbation of symptoms following bereavement. Typical non-specific physical symptoms including fatigue, insomnia, aches and pains (e.g. headaches, musculoskeletal), tightness in the chest and throat, loss of appetite, weight loss, gastrointestinal symptoms (e.g. nausea, vomiting, indigestion, constipation, diarrhoea) and an increased incidence of infections (e.g. colds and sore throats). A consistent finding from bereavement research has been the significant association between bereavement and an increased risk of mortality from cardiovascular disease, suicide and alcohol-related diseases.

Cardiovascular disease

In general, most studies of bereavement have found an excess mortality from cardiovascular disease (Mellstrom *et al.* 1982; Mergenhagen *et al.* 1985; Jones 1987). The concept of the death from a 'broken heart' has influenced both romantic fiction and entered into the realms of research. The latter mainly as a result of Parkes *et al.* (1969), whose paper entitled 'Broken heart' followed up the work of Young *et al.* (1963) on widowhood, and reported an increase risk of death from arteriosclerotic and degenerative heart disease. A recent prospective study by the West of Scotland Coronary Prevention Study Group (Shepherd *et al.* 1997) found widowhood to be a predictor of their primary endpoint of 'definite coronary heart disease death or nonfatal myocardial infarction'. The risk of this was over one and a half times greater in those who were widowed.

It is not uncommon for bereaved people to develop symptoms or even mannerisms of the deceased, such as a widow complaining of chest pain after her husband has died from a heart attack. From the community nurse perspective, it is important to differentiate the physical aspects of grief from serious or even life-threatening conditions, which may be overlooked. It is important to treat any complaint of poor health as a potential medical problem unless investigations have found otherwise. Bereavement *per se* does not exempt people from dying from the same conditions as the deceased patient and should not always be put down to the symptoms of grief or anxiety. It is useful to remember that spouses shared the same living environment and often had similar lifestyles, which may have exposed them to the same environmental risk factors that could be linked to a disease. In most cases, the community nurse will have been involved with the care of the deceased and through the relationship have built up a general knowledge of the health and social needs of the family. While the nurse is visiting it may be appropriate to offer a quick assessment of the bereaved person's physical health including vital signs (e.g. blood pressure, pulse, respiration) and some tactful enquiries about current medication and medical history may help in deciding whether it may be worthwhile asking the doctor to call round.

Pearce (1996), who carried out a series of interviews with GPs and bereaved people in the UK, provides a useful reminder to be vigilant for medical symptoms that may be overlooked as a 'psychosomatic' grief reaction. In one case, a widow whose husband had recently died from a gastro-intestinal cancer went to see her GP complaining of bowel disturbance. In addition, she had also developed a 'nervous sniff' which her husband always had. Both could have been assessed as psychosomatic. However, the GP correctly referred her to a specialist for the bowel problems, which was diagnosed as cancer requiring major bowel surgery.

Assessment of mental health problems

The expression of grief is complex and varies greatly between cultures and between individuals within the same culture, so it is difficult to define 'normal' grief. The work of Bowlby (1980) and Parkes (1971) among others has been particularly influential in determining how grief is conceptualized within Western culture, and their ideas have been central to the development of models that include stages or phases of grief, through which the bereaved person is thought to move as they adapt to their loss. Although there are a number of different phase models of grief, they all share similar perspectives. Bowlby (1980) describes typical grief as having four main stages: numbness, yearning, despair and recovery. Such psychological responses are not usually perceived as clinical problems unless they are 'abnormal' or 'complicated' in some way, for example being excessive (unable to function normally) or prolonged (more than 6 months). In fact, in Western culture the absence of grief is seen as abnormal.

The main mental health problems that community nurses are likely to find in bereaved people are depression, anxiety and substance abuse, particularly alcohol and occasionally sedatives (e.g. benzodiazepines). Very rarely there are also individuals who are at an increased risk of suicide. The GP and/or the mental health specialists and not the community nurse usually carry out assessments of mental health problems. Many community nurses do not feel competent to assess, although they may be able to identify the general signs and risk factors associated with mental health problems. Most bereaved people experience low mood for several months following their loss, although most are able to cope and the symptoms do not develop into full-blown depression or anxiety disorders.

The results of the survey by Birtwistle *et al.* (2002) suggest that community nurses do assess bereaved people during their post-bereavement visits, although the depth and objectivity of the assessment remains unclear. Few, if any, use an assessment tool, and the assessment tends to be based on 'gut feelings' and intuition. Prior knowledge of the family can help the community nurse assess changes in behaviour following the death and to refer to the GP or the community psychiatric nurse for a more in-depth assessment. Risk factors for a poor outcome are discussed in Chapter 27. However, one of the key risk factors for mental health problems following bereavement is a current or previous mental health problem.

Depression

Depression is a psychiatric condition and bereavement does not automatically result in depression. However, those who are widowed or divorced have a greater risk of depression than those who are married or single (Bebbington 1987), and the risk of developing an affective (mood) disorder is greater in widowed men (van Grootheest *et al.* 1999). Symptoms of anxiety and depression generally peak during the first 6 months of bereavement and improve afterwards, with most people being comparable to their pre-bereavement state after the first year. Zisook and Shuchter (1991) compared the frequency of depressive syndromes among those who had lost their spouse and those who had not. In those who were bereaved, the percentage that met the criteria for a depressive episode was 24 per cent at 2 months, 23 per cent at 7 months and 16 per cent at 13 months. In comparison, the prevalence in a group of married people was 4 per cent. Factors that predicted depression were younger age, a past history of major depression and still grieving 2 months after the loss (see Chapter 14).

Anxiety

> No one ever told me that grief felt so much like fear. I am not afraid, but the sensation is like being afraid. The same fluttering in the stomach, the same restlessness, the yawning. I keep on swallowing.
>
> (Lewis 1961: 5)

Parkes (1998) suggests that anxiety is the most common response to bereavement. Jacobs *et al.* (1990) found the risk of panic disorder and generalized anxiety disorder in the second 6 months of bereavment to be about double that rate in the first 6 months of bereavement. The main predictor of panic disorder was a past history of panic disorder, while the predictors of generalized anxiety disorder were younger age, past history of anxiety disorders and past history of depression. There were also associations with depression and 56 per cent who had anxiety disorder also reported a depressive syndrome.

Community nurses may care for bereaved people who have developed a fear of going out of the house, a possible indication of agoraphobia. This may not be identified unless the nurse asks the bereaved person about their social contact. However, there are effective pharmacological and psychological therapies for these anxiety disorders, which could be explored with the bereaved person and the GP. Community nurses may occasionally care for bereaved patients with post-traumatic stress disorder, who require post-hospital treatment following a major accident in which there was a death. However, this will be relatively rare. A diagnosis of post-traumatic stress disorder requires that a person experiences or witnesses a traumatic event (e.g. a major accident or physical assault). The three main symptom clusters are: intrusive recollections (thoughts, nightmares, flashbacks); avoidant behaviour, numbing of emotions and hyperarousal (increased anxiety and irritability, insomnia, poor concentration); and hypervigilence (being constantly on edge). People with post-traumatic stress disorder require support from a mental health specialist and it would be fruitful for any community nurse dealing with bereaved people suffering from this condition to liaise with those services.

Alcohol, nicotine and substance misuse

In a study of 68 widows in Harvard, Massachusetts, Glick *et al.* (1974), found they consumed more tranquillizers, alcohol and tobacco following their loss. Bereaved people who previously drank alcohol and or smoked sometimes increased their consumption as a means of 'self-medication', to help them cope with the grief. The negative impact on health from smoking is well documented and the community nurse may be in a position to identify the increased consumption and to offer health advice. However, it should be noted that nicotine has antidepressant properties and there is an association between cigarette smoking and depression (Glassman 1993; Covey *et al.* 1998), so smoking cessation at stressful times can sometimes result in a depressive relapse (Covey *et al.* 1997). That said, the role of the community nurse is still one of promoting health and preventing illness and so bereaved people should still be counselled about the health risks of smoking and advised on smoking cessation programmes.

Parkes (1998) suggests that dependence on alcohol is a real danger after bereavement and excess mortality from alcohol-related disorders has been found for widows and widowers (Helsing *et al.* 1982; Martikainen and Valkonen 1996; Johnson *et al.* 2000), suggesting that for some bereaved people excessive alcohol consumption is a problem. There are clear associations between alcohol misuse and mental health problems, including anxiety and depression. The risk may be greater in men, as there is evidence that some widowers increase their consumption of alcohol (Byrne *et al.* 1999), but for most newly bereaved people the quantity may not be significant and may in most cases be seen as alcohol use (to aid sleep and to take the 'edge' off grief) rather than constitute abuse. However, some bereaved people may show signs of alcohol abuse and the community nurse may tactfully explore the issue if they can smell alcohol, or notice signs such as tremor, sweating or slurring of speech, particularly in the morning. Evidence presented by Byrne *et al.* (1999) suggests that men with previously established drinking patterns are at increased risk. With this in mind, one community nurse who helped with the author's research said when she suspected a widower of drinking alcohol in excess, she found it more appropriate for a male health professional (community nurse colleague, GP, bereavement support worker) to have a 'man-to-man' talk about the drinking as her advice was generally ignored.

In the past, GPs would frequently prescribe diazepam as a means of relieving the pangs of grief, helping with sleep and depression, but the fear of addiction has resulted in a more cautious attitude to prescribing these types of benzodiazepines. In one study, a fifth of all those referred to a drug abuse programme for withdrawal from dependence on benzodiazepines had started them following a bereavement (Hamlin and Hammersley 1993). The risk associated with long-term use of benzodiazepines and the availability of safer antidepressant drugs has resulted in a change in the type of prescriptions offered by doctors to their depressed patients, which has resulted in a shift to safer antidepressants, particularly those with anxiolytic (anti-anxiety) properties such as the serotonin selective re-uptake inhibitors.

Suicide

Compared with the general population, there is an increased risk of suicidal gestures, completed suicide and death from accidents following the death of a spouse or a parent (Charlton 1995; Martikainen and Valkonen 1996) with young men at particular risk (Mergenhagen *et al.* 1985) and the risk being is greatest immediately following the loss.

Although the risk of suicide is raised in bereaved people, it is a rare event and is usually associated with other risk factors such as personality, early loss of parents and a history of mental health problems. Those with a history of deliberate self-harm are at the greatest risk. Harris and Barraclough (1997) estimated that when a person has previously attempted suicide, they are 42 times more likely to commit suicide compared with members of the general population. Any nurse dealing with a bereaved person who has a history of deliberate self-harm (suicide and self injury), a history of mental health problems, alcohol abuse or poor health should be aware of the potential risk and refer to a GP or mental health specialist. Some people may have access to a ready means of suicide, especially if their loved one has been treated with potentially dangerous drugs (e.g. opioids). It is important, therefore, that community nurses assess the risk of self-harm and remove the potential source as soon as possible. Most nurses feel reluctant to discuss self-harm with bereaved people, as there is the misconception that discussing suicide with vulnerable people may actually be suggestive. The evidence is to the contrary, however, as asking about suicidal thoughts and plans is one of the key assessments of suicide risk used by mental health specialists and is beneficial in reducing the risk (Hirschfeld and Russell 1997).

Coping with loss

Through their prior experience and relationship with bereaved people, community nurses may be a good judge of people's ability to cope. Of all the post-bereavement assessments carried out by community nurses, 94 per cent reported assessing the bereaved person's ability to cope alone (Birtwistle *et al.* 2002). Ability to cope is a rather vague notion but includes being able to cook, having the means to obtain sufficient food and general self-care. Knowledge of the person prior to the bereavement is invaluable in deciding if they are looking run down and not caring for themselves or looking after their home. Self-neglect is usually a sign of depression or simply giving up the will to live.

Self-referral bereavement support agencies (e.g. Cruse) may be beneficial for some bereaved people and may reduce their reliance on GP services (Relf 1997). Studies of palliative care bereavement services suggest that professional services and professionally supported volunteer and self-help services are best targeted at those who are at high risk and unsupported and may help reduce the consumption of drugs, alcohol and tobacco by reducing anxiety and tension.

For some older people with limited mobility, access to shops may be a problem. In addition, some bereaved people simply cannot be bothered to cook for one person, and there is evidence that older bereaved people may be at an increased risk of under-nutrition (Todorovic 2001), which can increase the risk of poor health. During a post-bereavement visit, community nurses are ideally placed to assess for potential problems, such as poor mobility and the risk of poor nutrition, and to offer advice and refer to other support agencies. The author is aware of one community nurse service that provides details of a local restaurant that delivers nutritious meals to bereaved people at home at a discounted rate.

Loneliness and isolation is a problem for many bereaved people, particularly older people who may have no family and a poor support network. Many community nurses report concern for older people who are lonely and vulnerable. Some report doing 'bereavement visits' and occasional drop-in visits as a means of checking that they are coping alright. Unfortunately for most community nurses, their workload prohibits frequent visits for social support. However, there are a number of useful community resources that could be considered as a means of providing social support to bereaved people. These include the local church or place of worship, which could provide pastoral care and support, lunch clubs and also various charities. For some, enrolling on an adult education course at the local college may provide a network of social support, teach useful life skills and encourage reintegration into the community. One example would be encouraging widowers who are not used to preparing meals to attend a basic cooking course.

Conclusions

Overall, there has been limited research about bereavement support from the community nurse perspective, which may in turn reflect the low priority afforded to bereavement issues in medicine and nursing. However, based on the limited findings, it would appear that most community nurses believe that the provision of bereavement support to relatives is one of their roles following the death of a patient they have cared for. Prior contact with the relatives of those they cared for and the established relationship and knowledge of the family, built up during the care of the patient, have been reported as key factors in the type of bereavement support provided.

It is widely recognized that bereavement can have a negative impact on mental and physical health, particularly in the old and vulnerable. It is the role of the primary care system to recognize and treat such health problems at the earliest opportunity. However, most community nurse services have limited time and resources to deal with bereaved people. In addition, there is a wide variation in the way community nurses organize bereavement support and most bereavement visits lack structure and appear to be more of an occasional social visit for a 'cup of tea and a chat' to ensure the bereaved person is coping. About half of all community nurses don't provide information about bereavement issues and few bereaved people receive any formal health assessments. In general, most community nurses appear unsure about the scope of their involvement with bereaved people who are not perceived to be their patient. This lack of clarity is not surprising, as there are practically no research or professional guidelines on which to base their practice.

At present, it is too early to assess whether the development of an expanded bereavement role would be a welcome or useful development to the community nurse services. Limited evidence indicates that community nurses could play an important part in the provision of information about bereavement and suggests that community nurses are valued by bereaved people for the 'friendship' and emotional support they provide mainly through simply 'being there'. Few community nurses are trained or experienced in dealing with bereavement-related problems such as complicated grief, or mental health problems. However, with adequate training they may undertake assessment of bereaved people for potential health risks, with the aim of referring them on to other specialist health care services (e.g. GP, community psychiatric nurse, clinical psychologist, psychiatrist, counsellor) and appropriate community resources such as the local church and local clubs.

References

Addington-Hall, J. and Karlsem, S. (2000) Do home deaths increase distress in bereavement? *Palliative Medicine*, 14: 161–2.

Audit Commission (1993) *What seems to be the matter? Communication between hospitals and patients*. National Health Service Report No. 12. London: Audit Commission.

Audit Commission (1999) *First Assessment: A Review of District Nursing Services in England and Wales*. Oxford: Audit Commission Publications/Bookpoint Ltd.

Baly, M.E., Robottom, B. and Clark, J.M. (1987) *District Nursing*. London: Butterworth-Heinemann.

Bebbington, P. (1987) Marital status and depression: a study of English national admission statistics. *Acta Psychiatrica Scandanivica*, 75: 640–50.

Birtwistle, J., Payne, S.A., Smith, P. and Kendrick, T. (2002) The role of the district nurse in bereavement care. *Journal of Advanced Nursing*, 38(5): 467–78.

Bowlby, J. (1980) *Attachment and Loss, Vol. 3: Sadness and Depression*. London: Hogarth Press.

Brandspiegel, H.Z., Marinchak, R.A., Rials, S.J. and Kowey, P.R. (1998) A broken heart. *Circulation*, 13: 1349.

Byrne, G.J., Raphael, B. and Arnold, E. (1999) Alcohol consumption and psychological distress in recently widowed older men. *Australian and New Zealand Journal of Psychiatry*, 33(5): 740–7.

Charlton, J. (1995) Trends and patterns in suicide in England and Wales. *International Journal of Epidemiology*, 24(1): S45–S52.

Charlton, R. and Dolman, E. (1995) Bereavement: a protocol for primary care. *British Journal of General Practice*, 45: 427–30.

Charlton, R., Sheahan, K., Smith, G. and Campbell, I. (2001) Spousal bereavement – implications for health. *Family Practice*, 18(6): 614–18.

Costello, J. (1995) Helping relatives cope with the grieving process. *Professional Nurse*, 11(2): 89–92.

Covey, L.S., Glassman, A.H. and Stetner, F. (1997) Major depression following smoking cessation. *American Journal of Psychiatry*, 154(2): 263–5.

Covey, L.S., Glassman, A.H. and Stetner, F. (1998) Cigarette smoking and major depression. *Journal of Addictive Diseases*, 17(1): 35–46.

Department of Social Security (2000) *What to Do After a Death in England and Wales: A Guide to What You Must Do and Help You Can Get*. Booklet D49. London: HMSO.

Faulkner, A. (1992) The evaluation of training programmes for communicating skills in primary care. *Journal of Cancer Care*, 7: 175–8.

Field, D. and Kitson, A. (1986). Formal teaching about death and dying in UK nursing schools. *Nurse Education Today*, 6(6): 270–6.

Glassman, A.H. (1993) Cigarette smoking: implications for psychiatric illness. *American Journal of Psychiatry*, 150(4): 546–53.

Glick, I., Parkes, C.M. and Weiss, R.S. (1974) *The First Year of Bereavement*. New York: Wiley.

Hamlin, M. and Hammersley, D. (1993) Benzodiazepines following bereavement, in S. Jacobs (ed.) *Pathologic Grief: Maladaptation to Loss*. Washington, DC: American Psychiatric Press.

Harris, E.C. and Barraclough, B. (1997) Suicide as an outcome for mental disorders. *British Journal of Psychiatry*, 170: 205–28.

Harris, T. and Kendrick, T. (1998) Bereavement care in general practice: a survey in South Thames Health Region. *British Journal of General Practice*, 46: 1560–4.

Hatcliffe, S., Smith, P. and Daw, R. (1996) District nurses' perceptions of palliative care at home. *Nursing Times*, 92(41): 36–7.

Helsing, K.J., Comstock, G.W. and Szklo, M. (1982) Causes of death in a widowed population. *American Journal of Epidemiology*, 116: 524–32.

Hirschfeld, R.M. and Russell, J.M. (1997) Assessment and treatment of suicidal patients. *New England Journal of Medicine*, 337(13): 910–15.

Jacobs, S., Hansen, F., Kasl, S. *et al.* (1990) Anxiety disorders during acute bereavement: risk and risk factors. *Journal of Clinical Psychiatry*, 51: 269–74.

Jeffrey, D. (1994) Education in palliative care: a qualitative evaluation of the present state and the needs of general practitioners and community nurses. *European Journal of Cancer Care*, 3(2): 67–74.

Johnson, N.J., Backlund, E., Sorlie, P.D. and Loveless, C.A. (2000) Marital status and mortality: the National Longitudinal Mortality Study. *Annals of Epidemiology*, 10: 224–38.

Jones, D.R. (1987) Heart disease mortality following widowhood: some results from the OPCS longitudinal study. *Journal of Psychosomatic Research*, 31(3): 325–33.

Koodiaroff, S. (1999) Bereavement care: a role for the community nurse. *Collegian*, 6(2): 9–11.

Lewis, C.S. (1961) *A Grief Observed*. London: Faber & Faber.

Lloyd-Williams, M. and Lloyd-Williams, F. (1996) Communication skills: the house officer's perception. *Journal of Cancer Care*, 5(4): 151–3.

Lyttle, C.P. (2001) Bereavement visiting: older people's and nurses' experiences. *British Journal of Community Nursing*, 6(12): 629–35.

Main, J. (2000) Improving management of bereavement in general practice based on a survey of recently bereaved subjects in a single general practice. *British Journal of General Practice*, 50: 863–6.

Martikainen, P. and Valkonen, T. (1996) Mortality after death of a spouse in relation to duration of bereavement in Finland. *Journal of Epidemiology and Community Health*, 50: 264–8.

Mellstrom, D., Nilsson, A., Oden, A., Rundgren, A. and Svanborg, A. (1982) Mortality among the widowed in Sweden. *Scandinavian Journal of Social Medicine*, 10: 33–41.

Mergenhagen, P.M., Lee, B.A. and Gove, W.R. (1985) Till death do us part: recent changes in the relationship between marital status and mortality. *Sociology and Social Research*, 70: 53–6.

Monroe, B. and Smith, P. (1997) The value of a single structured bereavement visit. *British Journal of Community Nursing*, 2(5): 225–8.

National Cancer Alliance (1996) *Patient Center Cancer Services – What Patients Say*. Oxford: National Cancer Alliance.

Nursing and Midwifery Council (2002) *Code of Professional Conduct*. London: NMC.

Parkes, C.M. (1964) Effects of bereavement on physical and mental health – a study of the medical records of widows. *British Medical Journal*, 2: 274–9.

Parkes, C.M. (1971) The first year of bereavement: a longitudinal study of the reaction of London widows to the death of their husbands. *Psychiatry*, 33: 444–66.

Parkes, C.M. (1981) Evaluation of a bereavement service. *Journal of Preventative Psychiatry*, 1(2): 179–88.

Parkes, C.M. (1998) *Bereavement: Studies of Grief in Adult Life*. London: Penguin.

Parkes, C.M., Benjamin, B. and Fitzgerald, R.G. (1969) Broken heart: a statistical study of increased mortality among widowers. *British Medical Journal*, 1: 740–3.

Payne, S. (2001) Bereavement support: something for everyone? *International Journal of Palliative Nursing*, 7(3): 108.

Pearce, V.M. (1996) The giving and receiving of bereavement care: an assessment of this process in general practice. Unpublished master's thesis, University of Birmingham.

Relf, M. (1997) How effective are volunteers in providing bereavement care?, in F. de Conno (ed.) *Proceedings of the IVth Congress of the European Association for Palliative Care*, pp. 244–9.

Shepherd, J., Cobbe, S.M., Lorimer, A.R. *et al.* (1997) Baseline risk factors and their association with outcome in the West of Scotland Coronary Prevention Study. *American Journal of Cardiology*, 79(6): 756–62.

Todorovic, V. (2001) Detecting and managing undernutrition of older people in the community. *British Journal of Community Nursing*, 6(2): 54–60.

Tudiver, F., Permaul-Woods, J.A., Hilditch, J., Harmina, J. and Saini, S. (1995) Do widowers use the health care system differently? Does intervention make a difference? *Canadian Family Physician*, 41: 392–400.

van Grootheest, D.S., Beekman, A.T.F., Broese van Groenou, M.I. and Deeg, D.J.H. (1999) Sex differences in depression after widowhood: do men suffer more? *Social Psychiatry and Psychiatric Epidemiology*, 34: 391–8.

Walter, T. (1999) *On Bereavement*. Buckingham: Open University Press.

Wilkes, L., Beale, B., Hall, E. *et al.* (1998) Community nurses' descriptions of stress when caring in the home. *International Journal of Palliative Nursing*, 4(1): 14–20.

Woof, R. and Carter, Y. (1995) Bereavement care. *British Journal of General Practice*, 45: 689–90.

Young, M., Benjamin, B. and Wallis, C. (1963) Mortality of widowers. *The Lancet*, 2: 454–6.

Zisook, S. and Shuchter, S.R. (1991) Depression through the first year after the death of a spouse. *American Journal of Psychiatry*, 148: 1346–52.

27

Risk assessment and bereavement services

Marilyn Relf

It has long been thought that grief is associated with illness, to the extent that some people may even die of a 'broken heart'. Research provides some support to these beliefs. Stroebe and Stroebe (1987), in a comprehensive review of the empirical research, conclude that there is substantial evidence that bereavement is associated with serious health risks. However, experiences of bereavement vary and while health is frequently affected in the short term, only a minority of people suffer lasting poor health. One line of enquiry has focused on identifying the factors that influence the course of grief. If it is possible to predict those whose health may be 'at risk', then it may be possible to intervene to prevent 'pathological' grief, a concept that is framed in terms of health deterioration. In this chapter, I explore the concept of risk in relation to bereavement, risk factors and their use in palliative care. Is it possible to predict those who may need help? If so, what are the implications for bereavement services and how transferable are methods of risk assessment pioneered in palliative care?

Bereavement and risks to health

The relationship between health and illness is increasingly explained in terms of risk (Petersen and Lupton 1996). A major focus has been on identifying personal characteristics, behaviour and environments that predispose individuals to ill health. The health consequences of bereavement are well documented. Bereaved people frequently experience short-term health problems arising from changes in everyday behaviour, such as loss of sleep, altered nutrition and increased use of alcohol and tobacco. Bereavement may also affect the endocrine (Kim and Jacobs 1993) and immune systems (Bartrop *et al.* 1977; Schleifer *et al.* 1983), particularly among those who are depressed (Irwin and Pike 1993). A substantial minority of bereaved people suffer serious health consequences (Stroebe and Stroebe 1987), including an increase in mortality rates (particularly among younger widowers), depression, anxiety disorders and continuing poor general health. It is not surprising that bereaved people visit doctors more frequently and increase their consumption of psychotropic drugs.

Lasting poor health is viewed as an indicator that grief has become 'pathological' (Parkes 1990) or 'complicated' and a major theme of bereavement research has been to discover the factors that influence the course of grief. The influential Harvard Bereavement Study (Parkes and Weiss 1983) identified a number of such factors and Parkes hypothesized that these could be used to predict outcome. He developed a risk index, using a numerical scoring system to divide widowed key carers into 'high'- and 'low'-risk groups. This index was first used at St Christopher's Hospice to identify people who should be offered ongoing bereavement counselling by trained volunteers. Parkes (1981) conducted a randomized controlled trial to test both the index and the effectiveness of volunteer support. He concluded that nurses can assess risk and that support significantly reduces bereavement-related health risks. In Australia, Raphael (1977) used similar factors to identify a high-risk group of widows and conducted a randomized controlled trial to test the efficacy of intervention, this time offered by herself, a psychiatrist. Like Parkes, she found significant differences between the health outcomes of the intervention and control groups. She argued that it was not necessary to be a psychiatrist to provide effective intervention and that non-specialists, such as nurses or volunteers, would be able to do so as long as they had training and supervision from appropriately qualified people.

These early studies indicated that it is possible to assess vulnerability and that intervention can reduce the risks to health from high to low. There is little evidence supporting the efficacy of untargeted bereavement services (Parkes 1980; Niemayer 2000). Indeed, offering counselling to people who have adequate resources may be counterproductive, as it may cause them to question their capacity to cope (Parkes 1996). Parkes (1981, 1993a) has argued that risk assessment should be an integral part of bereavement services and his index, or variations of it, are widely used in palliative care, in the UK (Payne and Relf 1994), in Australia (Gibson and Graham 1991) and in the USA (Beckwith *et al.* 1990; Levy *et al.* 1992), where hospices are required to make formal assessments (Lattanzi-Licht 1989). Generally, nurses have responsibility for making assessments and volunteers are the main providers of support (Lattanzi-Licht 1989; Payne and Relf 1994). In addition, risk factors may be used to assess the needs of people seeking help after bereavement.

The practice of risk assessment was developed within a philosophical framework, or paradigm, that conceptualized vulnerability to bereavement as predictable and intervention as a preventive health care measure that would limit the incidence of complicated grief. This is a positivist approach and suggests a 'medical model' of grief. It may be argued that traditional models of grief are also framed within this paradigm (Silverman and Klass 1996). Such models view 'healthy' adjustment as dependent on the capacity of the individual to 'work through' a 'normal' grief process encompassing working through emotional pain and detaching from the deceased (Bowlby 1961; Averill 1968; Bowlby and Parkes 1970). Both failure to engage (absent or delayed grief), and failure to disengage (chronic grief), with this process are conceptualized as dysfunctional and predictive of poor health (Parkes and Weiss 1983). According to this view, intervention should encourage people to confront and work through their grief (Worden 1983). This approach has been criticized in recent years (Wortman and Silver 1989; Stroebe 1992; Klass *et al.* 1996). However, before exploring the implications of new theoretical developments for risk assessment, I shall first provide an overview of the risk indicators identified by empirical studies.

Risk factors

There have been several reviews of the extensive literature on risk factors (Stroebe and Stroebe 1987; Sanders 1993). It is not my intention to repeat these reviews but to summarize the key findings. There are three groups of factors: situational, individual and environmental.

Situational factors

These factors reflect the circumstances surrounding the death. They are concerned with what happened, how prepared key carers felt, how distressing they found the death and the impact of concurrent life events.

Circumstances of the death

There is conflicting evidence about the importance of the mode of the death. Some studies suggest that sudden, untimely or violent bereavements may be more difficult than those that are expected. Sudden death is associated with persisting feelings of shock, disbelief and anxiety (Parkes and Weiss 1983; Stroebe *et al.* 1988). Violent or accidental deaths may cause post-traumatic stress disorder with very high levels of anxiety, flashbacks and nightmares. Suicide is associated with high levels of anger and guilt and the associated stigma may decrease the availability of social support.

It is often argued that anticipated losses are less problematic because a period of forewarning provides a context for understanding that loss is inevitable and the opportunity to make amends, to take a gradual leave-taking and to begin to grieve and adjust. When death occurs, it is 'the result of an understood, if hated, process' (Parkes and Weiss 1983: 94) rather than a sudden event. Giving support and nursing care also may leave positive feelings and the death may bring feelings of relief that the patient's suffering has ended. However, some studies have found that forewarning is not related to outcome (Maddison and Walker 1967; Cleiren *et al.* 1988) and that a protracted terminal illness, such as cancer, is also associated with increased health risks (Maddison 1968; Vachon *et al.* 1977; Sanders 1983). Nursing a relative over many months may limit social contact and may be physically and emotionally demanding, especially if the disease causes disfigurement or personality changes.

Foreknowledge is not always associated with 'anticipatory grief'. Caregivers may cope by refusing to accept that their partner is terminally ill (Vachon *et al.* 1977) and impending separation may cause relationships to intensify rather than to begin a process of detachment (Parkes and Weiss 1983). Duke (1996) found that grieving for the inevitable losses and life changes associated with advanced cancer is perceived by family members to be qualitatively different from their experience of grief after bereavement. Parkes and Weiss (1983) argue that grief begins with the actual loss. Foreknowledge, therefore, appears to be too general to be useful as an indicator of risk alone. It ignores important factors such as coping strategies and the availability of social support. It is not surprising that Cleiren (1991), in comparing the impact of road traffic accidents, suicide and long-term illness, concluded that the mode of death was not as important as other factors.

Concurrent life events

People facing multiple crises, such as other losses or financial difficulties, may experience more stress-related health problems (Parkes 1975; Sanders 1993). It is difficult, however, to disentangle the relationship between bereavement, socio-economic factors and health because of the main effect of low socio-economic status on poor health in the general population.

Individual factors

These factors are concerned with what the individual brings to the experience – their life experience, history and personality.

Age

In the general population, as people get older they experience more ill-health. However, bereavement studies indicate that younger widows and widowers have higher mortality rates and increased morbidity. These differences may be explained by the concept of 'timeliness' (Parkes 1996); bereavement later in life may be less distressing because it fits societal expectations about longevity. Older people may also meet with more understanding because members of their social networks are more likely to have experienced bereavement. However, there is evidence that older people may also experience psychological problems (Gallagher-Thompson *et al.* 1993). For example, Sanders (1981) found that while younger people react to bereavement with greater shock and emotional intensity, older people experience problems later, arising from feelings of isolation and loneliness.

Gender

In the general population, women report more illness and make more use of health care and men have higher mortality rates. Many studies of bereavement have focused exclusively on widows with the result that it is often erroneously assumed that women are at higher risk than men. Studies that compare widows and widowers with non-bereaved married people conclude that widowers are at greater risk. These studies consistently reveal significant differences between the health of widowers and married men but not between widows and married women. These finding are usually explained by gender differences in access to, and use of, social support. Widowers may have smaller friendship circles (Berardo 1970), may have relied on their partners to maintain social contacts (Stroebe and Stroebe 1983) and may be more likely to have strained relationships with adult children and to find it difficult to seek support (Wortman *et al.* 1993). Moreover, men may have been socialized to hide distress to conform to ideals of masculinity (Riches and Dawson 1997).

Relationship to the deceased

The loss of a close relationship, such as that with a spouse, parent or child, is related to greater risks to health. However, the subjective meaning of the lost relationship may be more important than the degree of kinship (Niemayer 2000).

Pre-existing health

Poor physical and psychological health may be exacerbated by the stress of bereavement. People who commit suicide after bereavement are likely to have had a previous psychiatric illness (Bunch 1972) and alcoholics may be at increased risk of suicide following the loss of a significant relationship (Murphy and Robins 1967).

Personality

Relatively few studies have focused directly on the relationship between personality and grief. This is surprising, as personality factors are likely to influence the course of grief. There is evidence to show that people who are insecure, over-anxious, have low self-esteem (Parkes and Weiss 1983), low self-trust (Parkes 1990) or who cope by denial (Sanders 1981) or extreme self-reliance (Parkes 1990) are likely to find bereavement more problematic. Personality factors indicative of resilience include the ability to communicate feelings and thoughts to others, high self-esteem and personal competency (Lund *et al.* 1993).

Personality traits influence the quality of individual relationships. Two types of relationship are related to vulnerability to bereavement: overly dependent and highly ambivalent relationships (Lopata 1979; Parkes and Weiss 1983; Gallagher-Thompson *et al.* 1993). Parkes describes intense clinging as being associated with a 'grief prone personality' and protracted high levels of distress or 'chronic' grief (Parkes and Weiss 1983). People in dependent relationships may have little support outside the primary relationship and high initial distress is associated with poor social functioning (Cleiren 1991). Grief may be 'conflicted' following the loss of an ambivalent relationship. Feelings of relief may be accompanied by guilt at not having been able to resolve difficulties. According to attachment theory (Bowlby 1980), the security of childhood attachment bonds has a powerful influence on personality, the nature of adult relationships and vulnerability to loss. Parkes (1995), in a retrospective study of people referred to psychiatric care for bereavement therapy, provides some evidence to support these claims.

Environmental factors

Environmental factors reflect the social and cultural context within which the individual experiences loss. This includes the family and wider social network and the influence of culture on attitudes and beliefs about grief that may influence the availability of support.

Social support

There is general agreement that the perception that social support is inadequate is a robust indicator of bereavement outcome (Stroebe and Stroebe 1987; Sanders 1993). There is convincing documentation of the distress experienced by bereaved people who feel compelled to keep their mourning private by the insensitivity, lack of empathy and ignorance they encounter (Maddison and Raphael 1975). Several factors may influence the availability of social support following bereavement:

- Bereavement may deprive individuals of their main, perhaps only, source of emotional support (Stroebe and Stroebe 1987).
- Geographical mobility may mean that family and close friends live at some distance and are not easily accessible (Stroebe *et al.* 1988).
- Members of social networks do not necessarily grieve in similar ways or at the same rate. Contact with kin may be much less than anticipated (Machin 1996) and they may lack the emotional energy to help each other (Stylianos and Vachon 1993), particularly following a long terminal illness. Family members may avoid talking about problems because they do not want to burden each other (Cleiren 1991) and family discord is a common source of additional stress (Lopata 1979; Littlewood 1987). Bereavement may precipitate a social network crisis:

  > The vacuum created through the loss of a significant relationship . . . will draw the entire group into distress. The joint experience of suffering may render network members unable to support the individual for whom the loss is most immediate and profound.
  >
  > (Stylianos and Vachon 1993: 397)

- Although grief is universal, the way it is experienced and expressed varies across cultures (Parkes *et al.* 1997). In post-modern societies, such as the USA and the UK, a decline in ritual is believed to contribute to a lack of shared understanding about how long, and how much, to grieve and is associated with anxiety and adjustment problems. The prevailing norm is to keep grief private and great value is placed on self-reliance, independence and autonomy (Walter 1999). Revealing feelings is equated to weakness and bereaved people, particularly men, may feel expected to suppress emotions and hide distress. These norms influence the behaviour of both men and women (Riches and Dawson 1997; Martin and Doka 2000).

- The lack of shared understanding means that bereaved people may be pressured to behave in particular ways and this may cause further distress (Lopata 1979; Silverman 1986). For example, Maddison and Walker (1967) found that widows with poor outcome were more likely to experience others blocking their desire to talk about their grief. Instead, they were encouraged to focus on the present or future. Lehman *et al.* (1986) report that bereaved people are more likely to be given advice than empathy. This may be related to anxiety-inhibiting helping behaviour in interactions with bereaved people:

  > The potential supporter may be so conscious of what is happening, and so worried about responding inappropriately, that natural expression of concerns may be unlikely to occur. Several specific strategies, such as minimising the problem or blocking expressions of feelings, may stem primarily from the support provider's desire to control his or her own anxiety in a situation which is very stressful.
  >
  > (Lehman *et al.* 1986: 443)

- The need to grieve may be unrecognized if the relationship is not widely acknowledged or socially sanctioned, such as following the loss of a lover or same-sex partner. When a loss is not generally acknowledged, grief may be more difficult and described as 'disenfranchised' (Doka 1989). For example, same-sex partners may be excluded from family rituals such as the funeral (Sanders 1993).

- The ability to mobilize or use social support may be influenced by pre-existing personality traits (Cleiren 1991; McCrae and Costa 1993). Bereaved people who are angry, or seemingly inconsolable and depressed, may be less likely to seek support and may alienate or exhaust supporters (Stroebe and Stroebe 1987). Some people attract warmth and compassion, while others perceive hostility when none is intended and feel that their needs are not being met despite the good intentions of others. Helpers are likely to withdraw if they feel their support attempts are not helpful (Schilling 1987).

Summary

Risk factors may be divided into three groups: situational, individual and environmental (Figure 27.1). The relative strength of individual risk factors is unclear. Age and kinship may be less important than the availability of

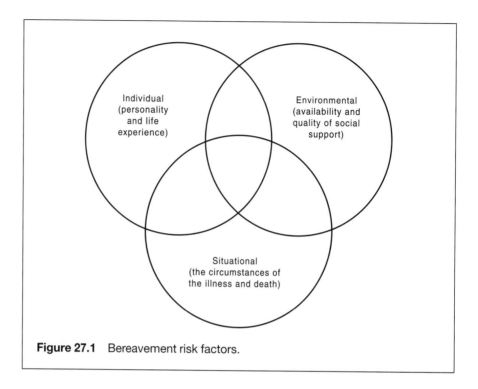

Figure 27.1   Bereavement risk factors.

social support and the quality and meaning of the relationship with the deceased (Cleiren 1991). Cultural factors such as norms that influence the expression of grief and gender appropriate behaviour are also important.

Methods of risk assessment

Risk assessment involves considering the cumulative impact of the situational, environmental and individual factors that influence the course of grief. The key questions for each group are shown in Box 27.1. Parkes emphasizes the interrelationship of risk factors in his much-quoted summary of the research:

> In short, statistical studies confirm what common sense leads one to suspect – that secure people whose experience of life has led to a reasonable trust in themselves, and others, will cope well with anticipated bereavements, provided they are well supported by a family who respects their need to grieve. However, multiple or unexpected and untimely losses of people on whom one depends or who depended on the survivor can overwhelm the most secure person and lack of security and support can undermine a person's capacity to cope with all types of bereavement.

(Parkes 1990: 309)

Box 27.1   Key questions when assessing risk

Situational
- How did the individual experience and react to the illness and death?
- Are there any concurrent life events that may cause additional stress?

Individual
- Who has been lost? What is the meaning of the lost relationship?
- How is the individual's life experience and personality affecting their reactions and way of coping?
- Are there any pre-existing psychological or physical health problems?

Environmental
- How much support is available and to what extent is it perceived as helpful?

Figure 27.1 provides a simple diagram to indicate this interrelationship and to illustrate how the cumulative presence of risk factors may be used to indicate the level of support needed. Thus, those in the centre are more likely to need therapeutic counselling, those in other overlapping areas may be offered supportive counselling and those where there are relatively few factors may not need regular help but may welcome other strategies of support such as social groups or memorial services.

Little is known about how risk assessment is undertaken in practice. Although the literature emphasizes using formal methods, in the UK informal methods are more widespread. In a national survey, Payne and Relf (1994) found that 31 per cent of palliative care units use assessment forms to make decisions about ongoing support, whereas 37 per cent rely on clinical experience and 'gut feelings' and a quarter offer support to all. Seven per cent provide support only if requested. This is in marked contrast to the USA, where the majority use formal methods (Lattanzi-Licht 1989). One factor may be the availability of resources to provide support. The use of formal measures is more common among units that have coordinated bereavement services (Lattanzi-Licht 1989; Payne and Relf 1994).

The literature on risk assessment has focused on adult grief. The factors that influence children's grief have only relatively recently become a focus of research and there is no consensus on how to identify children who would benefit from intervention. In a review of the literature, Lowton and Higginson (2002) describe the cumulative impact of pre-existing, current and subsequent events on children, describing developmental, family and social factors.

Problems with current methods of risk assessment

First, it has been increasingly recognized that experiences of bereavement vary. To be responsive to diverse needs, bereavement services in the UK are urged to offer a multiplicity of supportive strategies (London Bereavement

Network 2001). There may be a tension between providing choice and accessible services and the need to make decisions about the use of limited resources. Formal methods of risk assessment may be viewed as limiting access. For example, Payne and Relf (1994) found that concerns about withholding services influenced the decision to offer support to all. There is a need to study the use of risk assessment within comprehensive multi-faceted bereavement services.

Second, risk assessment relies on nurses' knowledge and understanding of families and care-givers as well as patients. However, there is evidence that pre-bereavement work with family members may be limited by constraints on time, skills and resources. Attending to psychosocial needs may be given low priority (Field *et al.* 1992) and staff may not always assess relatives' needs accurately. Pottinger (1991), for example, found that those who wanted support, but did not receive it, showed marked feelings of anxiety and intense grief. The time available to work with relatives as well as patients may be limited. By the 1990s, the mean length of in-patient specialist palliative care in the UK was 12 days (Eve and Jackson 1994) and admissions are becoming shorter (Eve *et al.* 1997). Lack of time may mean that the focus of care is inevitably the patient rather than the family, making it difficult to make assessments.

Third, risk assessment relies on care-givers being prepared to talk about themselves at a time when their energies are often focused on the patient. In addition, nurses may find asking questions pertaining to risk assessment to be intrusive (Payne and Relf 1994).

Fourth, two studies, conducted in the USA, have found only limited support for the reliability of Parkes's original risk index as a predictive tool. Beckwith *et al.* (1990) found that the index was predictive of outcome 3 months after bereavement but not at 1, 6 or 12 months. Levy *et al.* (1992) found that the index had low internal consistency and concluded that it is flawed. In the UK, Relf (2000) assessed nurses' ability to predict risk using a revised version of Parkes's index. Overall, the evidence supported nurses' ability to assess need (see Box 27.2). However, while nurses could identify accurately those who were in particular need, under- and over-scoring led to the conclusion that, although the index is helpful, it is not a reliable predictor of outcome.

The lack of reliability may reflect a number of factors. Following Parkes, assessment tools often include difficult-to-rate concepts such as 'unusual' levels of anger. The tools reflect subjective opinions; what one nurse considers 'unusual' may be 'normal' to another. As described earlier, the original index was derived from the Harvard Bereavement Study (Parkes and Weiss 1983). This study was conducted in the USA and focused on an atypical group of young widows and widowers (mean age 45). It may lack sensitivity for use across cultures, with older people or with non-spouses. Similarly, many influential studies of the relationship between bereavement and health have focused on the experiences of younger widows, often obtaining low response rates and relying on self-report. These problems with the reliability of research findings have been described elsewhere (Payne *et al.* 1999). Lastly,

Box 27.2 Focus on research

Relf (2000) evaluated the effectiveness of a palliative care bereavement service offering volunteer support to people identified as high risk. The study included:

- a comparison of the health of a volunteer intervention group and a control group at 14 and 22 months after bereavement;
- users' views;
- an exploration of how volunteers provide support;
- nurses' ability to assess risk accurately.

The study demonstrated that support is associated with lower anxiety and significantly reduced use of health care, particularly GPs. Bereaved people appreciated talking to a neutral person who listened, understood and who was knowledgeable about grief.

Relf adapted Parkes's original risk index (Parkes and Weiss 1983). Following Parkes (1981), nurses could specify those for whom it would be unethical to withhold support. At risk assessment, care-givers were assigned to one of five groups: very high risk referred to professionals for bereavement support (A); urgent need referred to volunteers (B); high-risk intervention group referred to volunteers (C1); high-risk control group (C2); or a low-risk group (D). The control and low-risk groups were given written information only. During the study, 385 care-givers were assessed. Almost half (184, 48 per cent) were considered to be 'high risk', of whom 26 were referred to professionals (A). The research sample (269) was drawn from all groups and 160 people agreed to be interviewed.

Parkes's Post-Bereavement Health Questionnaire (Parkes and Weiss 1983) was used to measure outcome. Following Parkes (1981), the accuracy of the nurses' predictions were assessed by comparing the mean overall outcome scores of the high-risk control (C2) and low-risk (D) groups. If the prediction was accurate, the control group should have had significantly higher overall scores than the low-risk group. The scores of those who had most concerned the nurses (groups A and B) would provide a further indication of the nurses' ability to assess risk.

The trend was in the expected direction; either group A (professional support) or the control group had the higher scores for each measure of outcome. However, the difference between the control and low-risk groups was not significant (chi-square 2.40, degree of freedom = 1, $P = 0.11$).

If intervention reduces the risks to health from high to low, the scores of the intervention and low-risk groups should be similar. However, those in the intervention group (C1) were significantly less likely to increase their use of health care ($P = 0.01$). This difference was accounted for by six people with scores just below the high-risk cut-off point and there was evidence of under-scoring.

Relf concluded that nurses could identify those in greatest need of support but that risk assessment was unreliable. This may reflect (a) the use of a numerical scoring system and the rather arbitrary cut-off delineating high and low risk, and (b) that nurses did not always have sufficient information to make accurate assessments.

assessment tools may be limited in scope. Risk indices focus on indicators of pathology and neglect indicators of resilience (Payne and Relf 1994).

Despite these problems, experience at one hospice shows that assessment can be remarkably consistent. At Sobell House, a palliative care unit in Oxford, UK, a scored assessment form has been used for over 15 years. The form (Relf 2000) includes a genogram, contact details and space for the nurses' comments as well as a vulnerability questionnaire. The proportion of key carers assessed as 'high risk' has been approximately 40 per cent per annum with approximately 70 per cent accepting offers of support (Sobell House Annual Reports). This consistency may reflect the commitment to risk assessment and the use of the form as part of a process that includes providing training for new staff members, weekly multi-professional discussions of bereavement assessments and regular contact between the bereavement service and the wider team. As Lattanzi-Licht (1989) argues, the assessment and referral process is a significant part of the work of the bereavement service coordinator.

To summarize, making decisions about who may be vulnerable after bereavement is a complex process that relies on nurses' knowledge of risk factors and having the time and skills to work with family members as well as patients. While the need to target ongoing support is widely accepted, current methods are problematic and formal tools may lack reliability. Suggestions for improving assessment tools include incorporating measures of resilience and methods of self-assessment (Payne and Relf 1994).

Implications for practice

Given these problems, how should risk factors be used? One solution would be to abandon attempts to assess risk and either offer support to all or to wait for people to seek support. Offering support to everyone, however, ignores the evidence that not all people need ongoing support and that counselling has only been found to be effective when targeted (Parkes 1980; Niemayer 2000). Moreover, systematically contacting all bereaved people involves assessment decisions (such as deciding who to contact in a family) and, given the high number of deaths each year in specialist palliative care, would be resource consuming. Rather than abandoning the practice, there are powerful reasons for seeking to improve assessment procedures.

First, it is important to clarify the place of risk assessment within practice. As described earlier, both assessment and intervention have been framed within a positivist paradigm that views behaviour as measurable and predictable. However, this view is simplistic. Many factors influence the way individuals express grief and pathological grief can no longer be thought of as a unitary concept. Models that conceptualize grief as primarily an emotional, linear process of stages or phases are too narrow. It is now accepted that 'normal' grief is multi-dimensional (Shuchter and Zisook 1993; Parkes *et al.* 1996; Martin and Doka 2000). Bereavement affects cognitive processes as well as emotions, is experienced within a social context and may influence behaviour, social interaction, role performance, self-esteem and spiritual beliefs. These theoretical developments have changed our understanding of normal and complicated grief and 'risk'.

Studies of childhood and parental grief have demonstrated that adjustment does not depend on severing attachment bonds (Klass *et al.* 1996). This means that there may not be a definite endpoint that marks 'recovery' from grief or 'closure'. Successful mourning does not involve relinquishing attachment but in constructing new connections to the deceased over time. Important relationships continue to influence us whether the person is physically present or not. Constructing new connections may involve a search to find a narrative, or story, that provides a way of understanding the meaning of the loss and all that has happened (Parkes 1993b; Walter 1996; Niemayer 2000). Niemayer (2000) describes this as not merely a cognitive process but also as a 'tacit, passionate process that unfolds in a social field' (p. 552). In palliative care, an important theme in bereavement support may be enabling people to make sense of all that has happened to them on the roller coaster journey from diagnosis to the present reality of living without the deceased.

Stroebe and Schut (1999) conceptualize grief as a dual process. Bereaved people cope by oscillating between behaviour that is focused on their loss (e.g. thinking about the deceased, pining, holding onto memories, expressing feelings) and behaviour that is focused on managing everyday life (e.g. suppressing memories and taking 'time off' from grief, keeping busy, regulating emotions). Neither mode of coping is inferior and the degree of oscillation is influenced by such factors as time since bereavement, personality, gender and cultural background. This model, therefore, suggests that avoidance of affect may be functional rather than problematic. However, as in traditional models, coping behaviour that focuses exclusively on emotional expression (chronic grief) or on distraction (absent grief) is conceptualized as problematic.

Martin and Doka (2000) argue that personality has a major influence on ways of experiencing and expressing grief. People who are primarily in touch with their feelings experience 'intuitive' grief as described in the traditional models. However, people who are primarily thinkers experience grief as a cognitive process or 'instrumental' grief. They prefer to cope by seeking information, thinking through problems, taking action and seeking diversion. Most people will have one mode as dominant and the other as subordinate. Martin and Doka (2000) argue that 'instrumental' grief may be disenfranchised and be seen as problematic rather than as a way of managing grief. For example, controlling emotions may be seen as indicative of successful coping by some people but be judged as risky by professionals who rely on traditional models to inform their work. Martin and Doka (2000) suggest that helpers should seek to understand and validate individual ways of coping to enable people to build on their strengths while developing their range of coping strategies.

These developments in our understanding of bereavement demonstrate how views of 'risky' behaviour change over time. There may be discrepancies between how bereaved people and professionals conceptualize risk. Risk assessment, therefore, should be used as part of a process aiming to understand and respond to individual ways of coping rather than to predict outcome or to judge whether reactions are 'healthy' or not. This view is consistent with a 'naturalistic' rather than a positivist paradigm and reflects the real world of service delivery where the understanding of how best to support service users develops over time. Such a process is proposed in a set of Australian minimum standards for palliative care bereavement services (Centre for Grief Education 2001). These standards recommend that structured assessment tools should be used from admission to review the needs of care-givers as well as patients in order to plan care. After the death, a summary bereavement risk assessment should be discussed in multi-professional team meetings and, from this point, any subsequent action should be coordinated by the bereavement service. If assessment is unclear, it may be carried out by the bereavement service coordinator and include communicating with other professionals, such as general practitioners (GPs). Unfortunately, there has been no published audit of these standards. Kissane and Bloch (2002), drawing on family systems theory, describe an ongoing process focusing on whole family assessment and intervention.

In palliative care, the psychosocial needs of both care-givers and patients should be reviewed regularly by the multi-professional team, making it possible in many cases to make informed decisions about the need for ongoing bereavement support. Those who are likely to be vulnerable should be offered support by skilled people whose understanding of grief goes beyond a simplistic notion of 'grief work' and stage models. Risk factors should be used as indicators of what may influence grief rather than predictors, and people who do not want support should not be pressured into accepting. As assessment may be unreliable, access to support should be provided for those viewed as 'low' risk. Written information about grief and details of how to contact local and national services for both bereaved adults and children should be given routinely to all bereaved people. Where no bereavement service is available, providing such information should be a priority and a risk summary statement can be sent to GPs. Great care needs to be taken to avoid pathologizing grief while recognizing that many people want to talk about their experiences to someone who is prepared to listen and to understand.

How transferable are methods of risk assessment pioneered in palliative care to acute health care? Clearly, it will be more difficult to assess vulnerability in settings where psychosocial needs are a low priority and the patient is the focus of care rather than the family. However, understanding the factors that influence the course of grief, particularly the importance of the circumstances surrounding the death, can help to ensure that the needs of care-givers are taken into account. What happens at times of crisis is very important and poor communication, failures, frustration and suffering will be remembered and dwelt on after bereavement. Written information about common grief experiences and support services can always be provided to enable people to understand their reactions and to access support.

Conclusions

The health consequences of bereavement are well documented. Risk assessment and intervention have been conceptualized within a positivist paradigm that views the course of grief as predictable. Risk factors relating to lasting health problems after bereavement may be divided into three groups: situational, individual and environmental. Strong arguments have been made that these should be used to assess risk and to target resources on those who may be more vulnerable. This practice has been widely adopted by specialist palliative care. Decisions are made either by relying on clinical judgement or by using formal methods and risk assessment tools. The latter practice is associated with having a bereavement service to provide systematic ongoing support. A number of factors have been discussed that limit the reliability of current methods of risk assessment. Following this discussion, it is suggested that assessment may be reframed as an ongoing process of understanding, and responding to, individual ways of coping rather than predicting outcome. This recognizes that the experience of bereavement is multidimensional and that the expression of grief is contextual.

References

Averill, J.R. (1968) Grief: its nature and significance. *Psychological Bulletin*, 70: 721–48.

Bartrop, R.W., Lazarus, L., Luckhurst, E., Kiloh, L.G. and Penny, R. (1977) Depressed lymphocyte function after bereavement. *The Lancet*, 1: 834–6.

Beckwith, B.E., Beckwith, S.K., Gray, T.L. *et al.* (1990) Identification of spouses at high risk during bereavement: a preliminary assessment of Parkes and Weiss' risk index. *The Hospice Journal*, 6: 35–45.

Berardo, F.M. (1970) Survivorship and social isolation: the case of the aged widower. *Family Co-ordinator*, 19: 11–25.

Bowlby, J. (1961) Process of mourning. *International Journal of Psycho-Analysis*, 42: 317–40.

Bowlby, J. (1980) *Attachment and Loss, Vol. 3: Loss, Sadness and Depression.* London: The Hogarth Press.

Bowlby, J. and Parkes, C.M. (1970) Separation and loss within the family, in E.J. Anthony and C. Koupernik (eds) *The Child in His Family*. New York: Wiley.

Bunch, J. (1972) Recent bereavement in relation to suicide. *Journal of Psychosomatic Research*, 16: 361–6.

Centre for Grief Education (2001) *Minimum Standards for Bereavement Support Programs in Palliative Care Services in Victoria*. Victoria: Centre for Grief Education.

Cleiren, M.P.H.D. (1991) *Bereavement and Adaptation: A Comparative Study of the Aftermath of a Death*. Washington, DC: Hemisphere.

Cleiren, M.P.H.D., van der Wal, J. and Diekstra, R.F.W. (1988) Death after a long term disease: anticipation and outcome in the bereaved – Part II. *Pharos International*, 54(4): 136–9.

Doka, K.J. (1989) *Disenfranchised Grief*. Lexington, MA: Lexington Books.

Duke, S. (1996) An exploration of anticipatory grief. MA dissertation, Oxford Brookes University, Oxford.

Eve, A. and Jackson, A. (1994) Palliative care services – where are we now? *Palliative Care Today*, 2: 22–33.

Eve, A., Smith, A. and Tebbit, P. (1997) Hospice and palliative care in the UK 1994–5, including a summary of trends 1990–5. *Palliative Medicine*, 11: 31–43.

Field, D., Dand, P., Ahmedzai, S. and Biswas, B. (1992) Care and information received by lay carers of terminally ill patients at the Leicestershire Hospice. *Palliative Medicine*, 6: 237–45.

Gallagher-Thompson, D.E., Futterman, A., Farbarrow, N. and Peterson, J.A. (1993) The impact of spousal bereavement on older widows and widowers, in M.S. Stroebe, W. Stroebe and R.O. Hansson (eds) *Handbook of Bereavement*. Cambridge: Cambridge University Press.

Gibson, D.W. and Graham, D. (1991) *Bereavement Risk Assessment in Australian Hospice Care Centres: A Survey*, Ballarat University College, Ballarat, VIC.

Irwin, M. and Pike, J. (1993) Bereavement, depressive symptoms and immune function, in M.S. Stroebe, W. Stroebe and R.O. Hansson (eds) *Handbook of Bereavement*. Cambridge: Cambridge University Press.

Kim, K. and Jacobs, S. (1993) Bereavement and neuro-endocrine change, in M.S. Stroebe, W. Stroebe and R.O. Hansson (eds) *Handbook of Bereavement*. Cambridge: Cambridge University Press.

Kissane, D.W. and Bloch, S. (2002) *Family Focused Grief Therapy*. Buckingham: Open University Press.

Klass, D., Silverman, P.R. and Nickman, S.L. (1996) *Continuing Bonds*. Washington, DC: Taylor & Francis.

Lattanzi-Licht, M.E. (1989) Bereavement services: practice and problems. *The Hospice Journal*, 5: 1–28.

Lehman, D.R., Ellard, J.H. and Wortman, C.B. (1986) Social support for the bereaved: recipients' and providers' perspectives on what is helpful. *Journal of Consulting and Clinical Psychology*, 54: 438–46.

Levy, L.H., Derby, J.F. and Martinowski, K.S. (1992) The question of who participates in bereavement research and the bereavement risk index. *Omega: Journal of Death and Dying*, 25: 225–38.

Littlewood, J. (1987) Bereavement status: a neglected area of research. Paper presented to the *First International Conference on Multi-Disciplinary Aspects of Terminal Care*, Glasgow, September.

London Bereavement Network (2001) *Standards for Bereavement Care in the UK*. London: London Bereavement Network.

Lopata, H.Z. (1979) *Women as Widows: Support Systems*. New York: Elsevier.

Lowton, K. and Higginson, I.J. (2002) *Early Bereavement: What Factors Influence Children's Responses to Death?* London: King's College London/National Council for Hospice and Specialist Palliative Care Services.

Lund, D., Caserta, M.S. and Dimond, M.F. (1993) The course of spousal bereavement in later life, in M.S. Stroebe, W. Stroebe and R.O. Hansson (eds) *Handbook of Bereavement*. Cambridge: Cambridge University Press.

Machin, L. (1996) Living with loss: a survey of the bereavement response of 97 people, in L. Machin and G. Pierce (eds) *Research: A Route to Good Practice*. Keele: University of Keele, Centre for Counselling Studies.

Maddison, D. (1968) The relevance of conjugal bereavement for preventive psychiatry. *British Journal of Medical Psychology*, 42: 223–33.

Maddison, D. and Raphael, B. (1975) Conjugal bereavement and the social network, in B. Schoenberg, I. Gerber, A. Wiener *et al.* (eds) *Bereavement: Its Psychosocial Aspects*. New York: Columbia University Press.

Maddison, D. and Walker, W.L. (1967) Factors affecting the outcome of conjugal bereavement. *British Journal of Psychiatry*, 113: 1057–67.

Martin, T.L. and Doka, K.J. (2000) *Men Don't Cry . . . Women Do*. Philadelphia, PA: Taylor & Francis.

McCrae, R. and Costa, P.T. (1993) Psychological resilience among widowed men and women: a ten year follow-up of a national sample, in M.S. Stroebe, W. Stroebe and R.O. Hansson (eds) *Handbook of Bereavement*. Cambridge: Cambridge University Press.

Murphy, G.E. and Robins, E. (1967) Social factors in suicide. *Journal of the American Medical Association*, 199: 303–8.

Niemayer, R.A. (2000) Searching for the meaning of meaning: grief therapy and the process of reconstruction. *Death Studies*, 24: 541–58.

Parkes, C.M. (1975) Determinants of outcome following bereavement. *Omega: Journal of Death and Dying*, 6: 303–23.

Parkes, C.M. (1980) Bereavement counselling: does it work? *British Medical Journal*, 281: 3–6.

Parkes, C.M. (1981) Evaluation of a bereavement service. *Journal of Preventive Psychiatry*, 1: 179–88.

Parkes, C.M. (1990) Risk factors in bereavement: implications for the prevention and treatment of pathologic grief. *Psychiatric Annals*, 20: 308–13.

Parkes, C.M. (1993a) Bereavement, in D. Doyle, G.W.C. Hanks and N. Macdonald (eds) *Oxford Textbook of Palliative Medicine*. Oxford: Oxford University Press.

Parkes, C.M. (1993b) Bereavement as a psychosocial transition: processes of adaptation to change, in M.S. Stroebe, W. Stroebe and R.O. Hansson (eds) *Handbook of Bereavement*. Cambridge: Cambridge University Press.

Parkes, C.M. (1995) Attachment and bereavement, in *Proceedings of the Fourth International Conference on Grief and Bereavement in Contemporary Society*. Stockholm: Swedish National Association for Mental Health.

Parkes, C.M. (1996) *Bereavement. Studies of Grief in Adult Life*, 3rd edn. London: Penguin.

Parkes, C.M. and Weiss, R.S. (1983) *Recovery From Bereavement*. New York: Basic Books.

Parkes, C.M., Relf, M. and Couldrick, A. (1996) *Counselling in Terminal Care and Bereavement*. Leicester: BPS Books.

Parkes, C.M., Laungani, P. and Young, B. (1997) *Death and Bereavement Across Cultures*. London: Routledge.

Payne, S. and Relf, M. (1994) A survey of bereavement needs assessment and support services. *Palliative Medicine*, 8: 291–7.

Payne, S., Horn, S. and Relf, M. (1999) *Loss and Bereavement*. Buckingham: Open University Press.

Petersen, A. and Lupton, D. (1996) *The New Public Health: Health and Self in the Age of Risk*. London: Sage.

Pottinger, A.M. (1991) Grieving relatives' perception of their needs and adjustment in a continuing care unit. *Palliative Medicine*, 5: 117–21.

Raphael, B. (1977) Preventive intervention with the recently bereaved. *Archives of General Psychiatry*, 34: 1450–4.

Relf, M. (2000) The effectiveness of volunteer bereavement care: an evaluation of a palliative care bereavement service. Unpublished PhD thesis, University of London.

Riches, G. and Dawson, P. (1997) Shoring up the walls of heartache: parental responses to the death of a child, in N. Small and D. Field (eds) *Race, Gender and Death*. London: Routledge.

Sanders, C.M. (1981) Comparison of younger and older spouses in bereavement outcome. *Omega: Journal of Death and Dying*, 11: 217–32.

Sanders, C.M. (1983) Effects of sudden versus chronic illness death on bereavement outcome. *Omega: Journal of Death and Dying*, 11: 227–41.

Sanders, C.M. (1993) Risk factors in bereavement outcome, in M.S. Stroebe, W. Stroebe and R.O. Hansson (eds) *Handbook of Bereavement*. Cambridge: Cambridge University Press.

Schilling, R.F. (1987) Limitations of social support. *Social Services Review*, 61: 19–31.

Schleifer, S.J., Keller, S.E., Camerino, M., Thornton, J.C. and Stein, M. (1983) Suppression of lymphocyte stimulation following bereavement. *Journal of the American Medical Association*, 250: 374–7.

Shuchter, S.R. and Zisook, S. (1993) The course of normal grief, in M.S. Stroebe, W. Stroebe and R.O. Hansson (eds) *Handbook of Bereavement*. Cambridge: Cambridge University Press.

Silverman, P.R. (1986) *Widow to Widow*. New York: Springer.

Silverman, P.R. and Klass, D. (1996) Introduction: what's the problem?, in D. Klass, P.R. Silverman and S.L. Nickman (eds) *Continuing Bonds*. Washington, DC: Taylor & Francis.

Sobell House Annual Reports (yearly) Oxford: Sir Michael Sobell House.

Stroebe, M.S. (1992) Coping with bereavement: a review of the grief work hypothesis. *Omega: Journal of Death and Dying*, 26: 19–42.

Stroebe, M.S. and Schut, H. (1999) The dual process model of coping with bereavement: rationale and description. *Death Studies*, 23: 197–224.

Stroebe, M.S. and Stroebe, W. (1983) Who suffers more? Sex differences in health risks of the widowed. *Psychological Bulletin*, 93: 279–301.

Stroebe, W. and Stroebe, M.S. (1987) *Bereavement and Health*. Cambridge: Cambridge University Press.

Stroebe, W., Stroebe, M.S. and Domittner, G. (1988) Individual and situational differences in recovery from bereavement: a risk group identified. *Journal of Social Issues*, 44: 143–58.

Stylianos, S.K. and Vachon, M.L.S. (1993) The role of social support in bereavement, in M.S. Stroebe, W. Stroebe and R.O. Hansson (eds) *Handbook of Bereavement*. Cambridge: Cambridge University Press.

Vachon, M.L.S., Freedman, K., Formo, A., Rogers, J. and Freedman, S.J.J. (1977) The final illness in cancer: the widow's perspective. *Canadian Medical Association Journal*, 117: 1151–4.

Walter, T. (1996) A new model of grief: bereavement and biography. *Mortality*, 1: 7–25.

Walter, T. (1999) *On Bereavement: The Culture of Grief*. Buckingham: Open University Press.

Worden, J.W. (1983) *Grief Counselling and Grief Therapy*. London: Tavistock.

Wortman, C.B. and Silver, R.C. (1989) The myths of coping with loss. *Journal of Consulting and Clinical Psychology*, 57: 349–57.

Wortman, C.B., Silver, R.C. and Kessler, R.C. (1993) The meaning of loss and adjustment to bereavement, in M.S. Stroebe, W. Stroebe and R.O. Hansson (eds) *Handbook of Bereavement*. Cambridge: Cambridge University Press.

28

Bereavement support services

David Kissane

A natural continuity ought to exist between support for the grieving process among patients and their carers during palliative care and its maintenance for the bereaved after the death. Health care organizations caring for the dying have an invaluable opportunity to deliver such seamless continuity of care and thus minimize the rates of morbid consequence arising in the bereaved (Wilkes 1993). The configuration of bereavement support services is the practical manner in which this ideal is achieved.

Nurses at the coalface of clinical care are intimately involved with not only the dying but also their loved ones and carers – those family members and friends who subsequently become the bereaved. Moreover, knowledge of and familiarity with these people enables nurses to sustain a supportive role during that peak of emotional distress, the early phase of bereavement. Their contribution to any programme of bereavement support is crucial to its success (Foliart *et al.* 2001).

The nature of grief and the mourning process has been described (see Chapter 22) as has the care of the newly bereaved person present at the moment of death (see Chapter 23). The district nurse's perspective on bereavement support is also covered in Chapter 26. Here the focus is on the formal and informal support services provided by hospices and specialist palliative care services, with particular attention being paid to the nurse's role given the principles, stated above, of continuity of care and the nurse's intimate, prior connection with those who become bereaved.

Aims of bereavement support programmes

The goal of these programmes is to deliver relevant and effective support to the bereaved in a manner that is both clinically appropriate and cost-effective. A targeted response is necessary to reach certain groups whose needs might otherwise be neglected, while a preventive approach is worthwhile for its capacity to reduce costs significantly by assisting those at high risk of a pathological outcome before more serious difficulties arise. Three broad levels of care of the bereaved therefore emerge:

1 Generic support for all the bereaved provided by the whole treatment team and broad community.

2 Targeted support for those at high risk to prevent morbid grief.

3 Specific interventions for those experiencing complicated grief.

Such a multi-level approach helps to separate generic support from specialist bereavement services as well as ensure that programmes are indeed focused in a cost-effective manner.

Appropriate credentialling of staff holding special skills is required to competently deliver the highest or third level of bereavement care provision in which specific interventions are applied when complicated grief has intervened. In contrast, team education and in-service up-skilling about bereavement care underpins the generic delivery of support to all involved with a hospice or palliative care programme. The middle level of bereavement service provision is addressed by a mixed contribution from general and specialist staff.

Potential staff involved with bereavement support programmes include both generalist and specialist palliative care nurses, the general practitioner, the allied health team incorporating social worker, psychologist, psychiatrist, occupational therapist, pastoral care worker or chaplain and, finally, the team of trained community volunteers. The palliative care medical consultant, and for that matter others such as the medical oncologist, surgeon or consultant physician, are generally the least involved beyond ensuring that the members of the team are appropriately engaged in such relevant supportive work. An understanding of the operation of bereavement support services is highly pertinent to nurses working in hospice and palliative care.

Generic bereavement support programmes

These services are intended for all of the bereaved in a non-discriminatory manner. They form the bedrock of any bereavement support programme, and are the common starting point when a new palliative care service is established. Key components of such a generic programme include: (i) attendance at the funeral; (ii) expression of sympathy via cards or telephone calls; (iii) brochures about grief; (iv) follow-up visits to the home; and (v) commemorative services as the year unfolds (Wilkes 1993; Payne and Relf 1994; Foliart *et al.* 2001).

Attendance at the funeral

Not only is the funeral a key social ritual in which the life of the deceased is celebrated, but it also symbolizes continuity for the living, albeit without the family member that has died. Such rituals have great cultural relevance and personal meaning to the bereaved, who are usually therefore touched by the presence of representatives of the health care team (Vachon 1995). However, ethical, practical and time/cost constraints impact on decisions about such attendance, and they should be considered on a case-by-case basis.

By their very nature, funerals are time-consuming and necessarily costly in terms of the staff time involved in attendance. Does a single person represent the team, or do they feel the need for companionship as well? It quickly becomes burdensome to the palliative care service if two or more staff attend every funeral. Routine consideration of whether the service needs to be represented and who should be involved is therefore desirable.

First, where a series of health care teams have been involved in the patient's and family's care, identification of who was primarily involved seems sensible. For instance, sometimes an oncology service has had several years of intense involvement in contrast with the palliative care service's final week. Knowing that the oncology nursing staff intend to attend the funeral can free the palliative care team from unnecessary duplication. Similarly, a long period of time with the home care team might contrast with a short time as a hospice in-patient. In different circumstances, a patient dying from stroke or respiratory disorder may have had negligible contact with any service, in which case attendance may signify willingness to help in a manner that both inspires the family and connects staff with needy relatives.

What are the reasons for involvement in a funeral service? While the health care team hopes to benefit the bereaved through attendance, no harm should ever be caused by intrusiveness (Kissane and Bloch 2002). The latter might arise when the palliative care service has been viewed ambivalently by the relatives, sometimes associated with treatment complications or poor health outcome. From time to time, particular staff 'get offside' with relatives due to some attitudinal or personality clash. In any setting of conflict, the bereaved will want respect and privacy, which may lead to an active decision that the palliative care service will not be represented at the funeral.

How might attendance prove beneficial to the bereaved? Generally, it symbolizes connectedness with and concern for the bereaved, conveying considerable respect while also providing an opportunity for the attendee to invite continued contact: 'Please let me know if I can be of assistance.' Where the attendee has both known and cared for the deceased, their presence communicates powerfully a commitment to remain supportive of the bereaved. They may later be the logical choice for contact should the bereaved perceive difficulties to be developing.

The literature on clinician burnout also identifies attendance at funerals as a means of the health professional attending to their own grief (Vachon 1995). They may have lost a person they felt especially attached to. An ethical caution is needed here, however. When the actions of any professional are directed to their own rather than the patient's or family's needs, there is a potential danger of abuse through boundary transgression. Careful reflection about the motivations of the professional serves to guide this decision making. If personal gain was the primary reason for attendance at the funeral, some alternative approach to grieving with their professional colleagues is warranted, exemplified by a debriefing group for staff (Demmer 1999). The ethical rationale for nurses' attendance at funerals ought to be its potential benefit to the bereaved.

A common quandary is the level of involvement during the funeral service. Attendance at the church or funeral parlour for a commemorative service has different connotations to presence at the graveside, which, in turn, is different from returning home with the bereaved for a wake following the burial. What meaning does each level of involvement convey and what message does it give to the family? Differences exist here between the doctor or nurse providing physical health care and the chaplain or pastoral care worker dealing with the spiritual and religious aspects of the ritual. In general, it is sufficient for clinical staff to pay their respects in association with the commemorative service and then discreetly withdraw to allow the family to grieve with their own community and friends.

From time to time, conflict arises within palliative care teams about who should attend. On what basis does one select between a nurse who has had daily contact for several weeks and a social worker who has had a single, extended session? Generally, the greater the sense of connectedness, the more supportive that person's attendance will be perceived. However, consideration might be given to future support needs, and where greater risk prevails of morbid outcome, one professional could be of greater potential benefit than another. In such decisions, the focus is clearly ethically based on the needs of the bereaved rather than the staff members involved. Occasionally, joint attendance evolves, worthwhile when one is relatively inexperienced and likely to benefit from a colleague's support until greater experience is established.

In summary, then, palliative care teams do well to discuss the who and why of funeral attendance in every case of death, so that cogent reasons underpin any staff attendance, rather than having random, or worse, routinized patterns prevail.

The sympathy card or telephone call

Often, nurses will be off duty at a time when a patient with whom they have been considerably involved dies. In these circumstances, a telephone call to the bereaved from a key individual will be greatly appreciated over subsequent days. For a team, however, a sympathy card enables several to sign where multiple phone calls would be inappropriate. Furthermore, a message of continued availability for advice and support can be added helpfully. This not only serves as a source of reassurance but, not surprisingly, key nurses become the first point of contact when relatives are distressed, because these nurses have been prime sources of support during the final illness of the deceased. In this sense, the card or telephone call symbolizes an important link (Wilkes 1993).

Sometimes the final admission of a dying patient breaks continuity for nurses who may have been involved for months. They are not present at the time of death but learn about it over the next few days. Calls or correspondence are then a sensitive means of expressing sympathy to the bereaved once death has occurred. Hospices or home care services around the world employ a number of variations on this theme dependent on local conditions. When several deaths occur each week, staff may have a fortnightly or monthly card writing session. Attention to some systematic process ensures that families are not overlooked because of temporary circumstances. Some teams select the primary author of the correspondence from within their core group, based on who knew the relatives best or felt some affinity to the carer. Others see this as a duty of the nurse in charge.

Whatever the local method, documentation of this activity fosters compliance and ensures that the process is not postponed. All services discover that care of the current workload of patients takes precedence over those lost, and the bereaved are readily neglected by well-intentioned people (Lattanzi-Licht 1989). Implementation of a structured process with its own documentation protects against avoidance, delay or neglect, and later facilitates follow-up when periodic memorial services are being planned for these relatives and friends of the deceased.

The anniversary of the death is another occasion when a card offers support and may provide an opportunity for someone who is struggling to be directed to appropriate care (Gibson and Graham 1991). A systematic yet personalized method of generating such cards is essential.

Brochures and educational material

Information about what to expect emotionally and the normal course of mourning is greatly appreciated by the bereaved. A survey of Californian hospices identified that over 90 per cent offer educational material routinely (Foliart *et al.* 2001). Many hospices also permit library books to be borrowed by the bereaved.

Follow-up visits

Where community teams have supported a dying person and their family in the home, follow-up visits to the bereaved are greatly appreciated (Longman *et al.* 1989; Matsushima *et al.* 2002). The activities of the district nurse are considered from this perspective by Birtwistle in Chapter 26. From the point of view of the team, dialogue about such practice is worthwhile when allied health members have also been involved. Is there confidence about the resilience of the bereaved, or some concern about risk, which warrants consistent follow-up? Is a general practitioner involved? Does the team know the general practitioner's usual practice regarding follow-up of the bereaved? Has this been discussed or is it worth a call to clarify? Especially when a nurse has concern about the welfare of a recently bereaved carer, discussion with the general practitioner usefully engages that person in a plan of continued preventive care.

What is the ideal timing of follow-up visits to the home of a widow or widower? No single guideline will suffice as circumstances can be so varied. A visit 1–2 weeks after death is most common, but some of the bereaved will stay with other relatives for a time, making a visit 1–2 months later the practical option. Insight into family plans is clearly helpful here.

The content of conversation with the bereaved is worth special comment. Not only should the nurse ask about their welfare and coping, but questions that review the dying process are also valuable. Thus:

- How do you think X's death evolved?
- Were there difficult moments for you?
- Were you left with questions about what happened?
- Did you talk to the doctor about what would go on the death certificate?
- How did the funeral go?
- Are there family members you are concerned about?
- How are you coping now?

This conversation, typically occurring over a cup of tea or coffee, will precipitate active grieving, and the nurse should feel quite comfortable about the normality and appropriateness of this. Within appropriate cultural norms, tearfulness should be understood as natural, even desirable, and with time and patient listening, the nurse will generate a sense of valuable support. Beyond affirmation of the appropriateness of grief, accompaniment is the key therapeutic activity; solutions are generally not needed, as the context now exists that grief will unfold over many subsequent months. A new phase of life has been entered into which the bereaved will be required to effect considerable change and adaptation, but there is plenty of time in which to accomplish this (Parkes 1998). The nurse might conclude the visit by offering congratulations about the care and dedication given to the dying relative. An offer of availability in the future – 'simply call me if needed' – sustains the continuity of the preceding care. The nurse can thus be a genuine reference point of enquiry should problems develop.

Memorial services

As many societies have become less religious, a tradition of palliative care teams running memorial services has been established (Matsushima *et al.* 2002). The rationale is to both provide a multi-denominational ritual to facilitate normal grieving and to provide a contact point as time passes at which staff have the opportunity to meet the bereaved and check on their overall coping. Nurses are a pivotal part of this process because of their personal knowledge of the relatives involved. If the local culture has a very high level of involvement with religious ceremonies, exemplified by Buddhist ceremonies in Japan, the spirit of bereavement care may be embodied in the existing ceremonies (Matsushima *et al.* 2002). Nonetheless, palliative care staff can be actively involved.

Dependent of the size of any palliative care programme, these commemorative services are usually conducted every 6 months or yearly. Practical considerations such as the size of a chapel and what is manageable for the staff usually prevail. Planning may be designated to key staff members, but a team is generally needed to cope with the multiplicity of arrangements. Planning becomes systematized once a few have been conducted.

When the team meets, the list of potential invitees is reviewed for the relevant period, and invitations are issued on behalf of the programme. Some services select team members who will be remembered by the bereaved to sign the invitations, using linkages that foster attendance.

Chaplains usually assist with the content of the ceremonies, which can combine prayers, songs or hymns and readings from a variety of religious traditions. Families are often invited to write the name of their deceased relative in a commemorative book, these names being read out at an appropriate moment during the ritual. Family members can be invited to come forward and light a candle in memory of their loved one. Having medical, nursing or allied health staff read Scripture or other spiritual prayers and poetry during the ceremony is appreciated by the families and proves to be one way of ensuring that such staff attend. Once medical practitioners appreciate the benefits of the memorial to families and enjoy hearing how they are coping several months after their relative's death, they tend to return for subsequent memorials. The serving of refreshments following the ceremony is a *sine qua non* of the format, as it facilitates reunion.

Attendance by the bereaved at such memorial services tends to signify a reasonable adaptation to the loss. Non-attendance, when based on avoidant mechanisms, may be associated with the development of complicated grief. Hence a review of those who apologized or did not attend is as important a feature of the bereavement support programme as the memorial itself. What is known about the mourning of the non-attendees? Did any of them carry high risk factors for the development of complicated grief? A team member could make contact to review the coping of any who appear to be a concern.

The memorial programme has many covert benefits for the contributing staff through building cohesion, a spirit of generosity and a spiritual dimension to the team-as-a-whole. It is generally perceived to be a worthwhile extra-curricular activity for the multidisciplinary team.

Targeted support for those at high risk

Factors that increase the risk of complicated grief developing in the bereaved are described in Chapter 27 by Relf and are summarized here in Table 28.1. The goal of this aspect of a bereavement support programme is to select and apply a preventive model of care to counter and minimize the

Table 28.1   Classification of evidence-based risk factors for the development of complicated grief in the bereaved

1. Antedecedent factors

Nature of the carer's personality and individual vulnerabilities

- Their coping style and prior history in dealing with loss (e.g. anxious worrier or low self-esteem)
- Any past history of psychiatric disorder (e.g. depression)
- The build-up of cumulative experiences of loss

Nature of their relationship with the dying patient

- An ambivalent relationship (e.g. anger and hostility at alcoholism, gambling, infidelity, financial ruin)
- An overly dependent relationship (e.g. clinging and possessive from basic insecurities)
- An avoidant relationship (e.g. distant and awkward in an insecure manner)
- An unrecognized relationship (e.g. secret)

2. Decedent factors

Nature of the death

- One that is untimely in the life cycle (e.g. death of a child)
- Sudden or unexpected at that time (e.g. event-related, such as sepsis or pulmonary embolism)
- Traumatic (e.g. large bedsores with debility)
- Stigmatized or disenfranchising (e.g. AIDS or suicide)

3. Post-death factors

Nature of their family

- Dysfunctional (e.g. poor communicators, high conflict, poor cohesion)
- Reconstituted in a problematic manner (e.g. remarriage creating ambivalent step relationships; estate and legal conflicts)

Nature of their support network

- Isolated from extended family and friends (e.g. new migrant)
- Alienated from neighbours (e.g. perception of poor community support carried by the individual)

likelihood of morbidity in a proactive and cost-effective manner. To optimize compliance with such a programme, standardization of the risk assessment procedure is strongly recommended (Payne and Relf 1994). In the early 1990s, surveys of palliative care teams revealed that only between one-quarter and one-third utilized a standardized risk assessment procedure, and for 85 per cent of these it was done by a nurse (Gibson and Graham 1991; Payne and Relf 1994).

Such targeted support can be delivered individually, or via a group or family approach. Usually time-limited in design, the therapeutic approach is commonly supportive-expressive or psycho-educational in its application. The former utilizes the notion of encouraging active grieving through the sharing of thoughts and feelings with the counsellor; the latter offers information about the nature and course of the grief journey, a group environment being selected as a means of the bereaved sharing their experiences with others in a comparable predicament (Lieberman and Yalom 1992; Lund and Caserta 1992).

Credentialling processes require the choice of a therapist who has been formally trained in bereavement counselling for these models to be competently applied. Nurses, however, make a valuable contribution as co-facilitators of a bereavement group, particularly when they bring a sense of continuity through having known the deceased relative.

Preventive individual therapy with the bereaved

Where factors indicative of high risk for morbid outcome are present in the bereaved, a preventive approach in which a counsellor provides a limited number of sessions (for instance, six) over the next 6–12 months has been shown to reduce morbidity (Raphael 1977). There are certain risk factors that point to the appropriateness of an individual model of preventive support: (a) personal vulnerabilities, for instance a past history of depression or an anxious worrying style with limited coping reserves; (b) ambivalent relationships, including a lot of anger; (c) the disenfranchised, where the loss cannot be openly acknowledged and publicly mourned (Doka 1989); and (d) a degree of avoidance or shyness, suggesting they will be less willing to join a group environment.

The danger of an individual model is the development of dependence on the counsellor, for which reason this approach is often combined with a group or family approach for the added socialization the latter can provide. Sometimes two or three individual sessions will build up sufficient trust in the counsellor to allow movement into a group that this counsellor also facilitates.

The therapy model in individual preventive interventions is generally supportive-expressive, with the work of several theorists serving as a guide (Melges and Demaso 1980; Mawson *et al.* 1981; Raphael 1984; Worden 1991). Attention is given both to nurturing the expression of grief through remembering and sharing stories and, in parallel, adjustment to life without the deceased through active coping. Stroebe and Schut (1999) have termed this the dual process model of coping with loss.

Preventive group therapy with the bereaved

Group therapy is very cost-effective and serves to connect the bereaved with others caught up in the loneliness and isolation that often follows loss of a significant companion. Risk factors that point to the value of a group approach include: (a) a poorly supportive social network, where the individual is isolated or alienated from others; (b) an overly dependent relationship with the deceased, leaving the bereaved isolated and vulnerable as a result; and (c) an identifiable subgroup within society, who will profit from linking with others that share a comparable experience of loss. Examples of the latter include the spousally bereaved (Lieberman and Yalom 1992), adolescent or sibling groups (Stokes *et al.* 1997) and relatives of people who have committed suicide or died in a traumatic natural disaster (Schwab 1995–96; Goodkin *et al.* 1996–97). Strong satisfaction is generally reported with any group experience, but it varies with both the group's objectives and its setting (Hopmeyer and Werk 1994).

Group approaches can be facilitated by a trained counsellor or operate at a self-help level, incorporating the assistance of volunteers. The greater the risk of morbid complications for the bereaved, the more important that the former criterion operates; the latter approach can complement an individual supportive programme run by a trained counsellor (Thuen 1995; Foliart *et al.* 2001). High participant satisfaction with bereavement support groups is relatively strongly related to the quality of group leadership (Thuen 1995). Self-help groups need the wisdom of experience to draw the wary into a safe environment, avoid cliques, provide variety and foster socialization. Directed activities such as a walking group, which concludes with refreshments and discussion, appeal to some of the bereaved. Organizations such as Cruse, Solace and Compassionate Friends are very helpful to bereavement counsellors in running such group programmes (Kirschling and Osmont 1992–93; Wheeler 1993–94).

The models of therapy used when a trained counsellor leads groups include psycho-educational, supportive-expressive and psychodynamic (Yalom and Vinogradov 1988). Hospice programmes will typically adopt the psycho-educational approach because of its time-limited nature (six to eight sessions) and its ability to reassure the bereaved about normal grieving through some informational content. All groups deliver support and the opportunity for expression of feelings about the loss. Facilitators foster cohesion through the use of refreshments and active invitation to the members to exchange their contact details. A successful short-term bereavement group will have its members continue to support one another long beyond the formal life of the group.

Short-term groups are usually closed in that new members are not added once the group process has begun. Longer-term groups may be open, with new members (who are generally more recently bereaved) being added as some more senior members withdraw. In the latter setting, the relative improvement of older group members is used therapeutically to support the fragility of more recent members, while a psychodynamic approach may make use of patterns of relationship evident across a life span to provide insight into problems that repeatedly interfere with relationships in the present. Longer-term groups are generally conducted by regionally based bereavement counselling services rather than smaller hospice programmes and they seek to meet the needs of the especially high-risk bereaved (Foliart *et al.* 2001).

Group processes address unmet dependency needs in the lonely bereaved through connecting them to a network of people rather than a single therapist. The greater the homogeneity of membership in age and other social circumstances, the more easily connectedness will develop. Care needs to be taken whenever a group becomes unbalanced through a member being noticeably different in some characteristic and potentially challenging to integrate with others. Formal training in group therapy is invaluable to ensure that facilitators develop a healthy and nurturing environment.

Preventive family therapy with the bereaved

As the family is often the primary social network of the bereaved, identification of families at high risk of morbid bereavement outcome enables adoption of a family-centred model of care in keeping with the goals and rhetoric of the hospice movement. Risk factors that identify families suitable for a preventive family approach include: (a) a dysfunctional method of relating as a family unit through poor communication, cohesiveness or conflict resolution (Kissane *et al.* 1994, 1996); (b) a stage in the life cycle when the family especially matters to the health and development of its membership – for instance, the death of a child or adolescent (Davies *et al.* 1986); and (c) the cumulative experience of losses through multiple illnesses, disabilities or deaths in a family that is stretched to its limits, including a stigmatized or traumatic death – for instance, death from AIDS, suicide or homicide (Walsh and McGoldrick 1991).

The model of therapy is typically brief (four to eight sessions) and its focus can be supportive-expressive (Paul and Grosser 1965) or directed to the family's functioning (Kissane *et al.* 1998). The latter approach, termed family-focused grief therapy, makes use of a screening strategy that identifies families at greater risk of morbid outcome through the routine administration of the Family Relationships Index (FRI; Moos and Moos 1981), a 12-item pencil-and-paper questionnaire that informs about family functioning. The FRI is completed when the patient is first admitted to the palliative care or hospice unit. Continuity of family work is then established before the death of the ill family member, and the therapist's intimate knowledge and memory of this deceased person is hugely advantageous to later work during bereavement. Optimizing family functioning while promoting sharing of grief facilitates the development of a supportive environment with those most touched by the death – the immediate family (Kissane and Bloch 2002).

Therapists leading such family interventions need formal training in family therapy and typically come from such disciplines as social work or psychology. However, the co-therapy approach strengthens the overall application of family-focused grief therapy when it combines input from clinical staff with a detailed understanding of the care needs of the dying family member. The nurse plays a useful role here. Moreover, co-therapy deepens the involvement of the multidisciplinary team with the family in a therapeutically powerful manner.

Grieving families who have lost a child benefit clearly from a family-centred approach to support. Black and Urbanowicz (1985) in the UK and Davies *et al.* (1986) in the USA provide outstanding examples of such family-oriented approaches. A family approach to bereavement support is also remarkably suitable for many adult families who have lost a parent and seek to support more effectively their remaining parent.

Specific interventions for those experiencing complicated grief

Most specialist bereavement counselling is with the 20 per cent of the bereaved who develop some form of complicated grief (Middleton *et al.* 1993). No longer is the intervention preventive, as the morbidity associated with such distortion of normal grieving calls for specific interventions to alleviate the distress.

Chronic grief is well-suited to a cognitive-behavioural model of therapy where greater socialization is accomplished by activity scheduling and the bereaved person is drawn out of an entrenched pattern of retreat and avoidance. Depression as a complication of grief is appropriately treated with antidepressant medication alongside psychotherapies (see Chapter 14). Traumatic grief warrants desensitization to the cues that trigger recurrent distress. Special skills are needed in responding to these forms of complicated grief (Raphael *et al.* 2001).

An important nursing role is the recognition of poor coping and the sensitive referral of people with complicated grief to specialist bereavement counsellors – psychologists and psychiatrists – for appropriate interventions. Resistance to referral may be based on avoidance, fear, ignorance of the possible help available or a sense of stigma about needing help. Here the trust that the nurse has established as a sensible and caring advocate will help the bereaved accept guidance about appropriate referral.

Efficacy of bereavement support services

Since early descriptions of the possible profile of bereavement support services in hospice care (see, for example, Parkes 1981), few studies have evaluated their efficacy (Lattazi-Licht 1989; Longman *et al.* 1989; Rognlie 1989; Longman 1993; Hopmeyer and Werk 1994; Payne and Relf 1994; Thuen 1995; Bromberg and Higginson 1996; Payne 2001; Matsushima *et al.* 2002). Evaluations of bereavement support services tend to report high levels of satisfaction with the care provided (Longman *et al.* 1989; Hopmeyer and Werk 1994; Thuen 1995), but there are several methodological difficulties with such endeavours, particularly the social desirability of such a response.

The majority of palliative care or hospice programmes in the UK, the USA, Canada, Australia and New Zealand now accept bereavement support as integral to their services. The current challenge is to integrate this support to deliver continuity of care rather than have bereavement support added on as 'an extra' after death.

A survey by the Californian Hospice and Palliative Care Association identified that volunteers accounted for almost one-quarter of bereavement staff (Foliart *et al.* 2001). Payne (2001) explored this contribution of volunteers to bereavement support in New Zealand. While two-thirds had generic volunteer training, only one-third had specific training in bereavement and most (71 per cent) recognized previous personal bereavements. That half found their work emotionally distressing and one-quarter had problems with 'boundaries' points to the imperative for both training and supervision. Volunteers are a valuable asset, but sound training is an imperative.

In the USA, 55 per cent of a random sample of teaching hospitals reported some form of bereavement support, generally provided by a social worker or chaplain (Billings and Pantilat 2001). A comprehensive survey of hospice settings across Japan found that three-quarters provided some form of bereavement follow-up, most frequently using cards (84 per cent) and memorial services (59 per cent) (Matsushima *et al.* 2002). Nurses were actively involved. The prevalence of social groups was 35 per cent, telephone calls 32 per cent, home visits 22 per cent, individual counselling 22 per cent, self-help groups 11 per cent and family counselling 8 per cent.

Guidelines for setting up bereavement services

Where services are establishing bereavement support programmes, attention to published guidelines about their development can prove helpful. The then National Association of Bereavement Services in the UK published guidelines in 1994 (see Stewart 1994), the National Hospice Organization in the USA in 1997 and the Centre for Palliative Care in Australia in 1999.

Conclusions

In summary, the nurse makes a worthwhile contribution to bereavement support services through the following approaches:

1   Generic bereavement support provided by the whole treatment team:

   • attendance at the funeral;
   • expression of sympathy via cards or telephone calls;
   • availability of educational brochures about grief and bereavement;
   • follow-up visits to the home;
   • commemorative services.

2   Targeted preventive support for those at high risk:

- when factors predictive of high risk of pathological or complicated grief are present;
- individual grief counselling is suitable for the bereaved with (a) personal vulnerabilities, (b) ambivalent relationships, (c) the disenfranchised and (d) the avoidant;
- group approaches nurture socialization and reconnection when the bereaved person is isolated or belongs to a homogeneous subgroup – adolescent/siblings or the traumatically bereaved;
- preventive family approaches such as family-focused grief therapy optimize family functioning and mutual support.

3   Specific interventions for those with complicated grief:

- identification and referral of the bereaved with complicated grief is an important nursing role.

Evaluation of bereavement support services and demonstration of their utility and efficacy remains a relevant research agenda.

References

Billings, J.A. and Pantilat, S. (2001) Survey of palliative care programmes in United States teaching hospitals. *Journal of Palliative Medicine*, 4: 309–14.

Black, D. and Urbanowicz, M. (1985) Bereaved children – family intervention, in J. Stevenson (ed.) *Recent Research in Developmental Psychopathology*. Oxford: Pergamon Press.

Bromberg, M.H. and Higginson, I. (1996) Bereavement follow-up: what do palliative support teams actually do? *Journal of Palliative Care*, 12: 12–17.

Centre for Palliative Care (1999) *Bereavement Risk Assessment Guidelines*. Melbourne, VIC: Centre for Palliative Care, University of Melbourne.

Davies, B., Spinetta, J., Martinson, I., McClowry, S. and Kulenkamp, E. (1986) Manifestations of levels of functioning in grieving families. *Journal of Family Issues*, 7: 297–313.

Demmer, C. (1999) Death-related experience and professional support among nursing staff in AIDS care facilities. *Omega: Journal of Death and Dying*, 39: 123–32.

Doka, K.J. (1989) *Disenfranchised Grief: Recognizing Hidden Sorrow*. Lexington, MA: Lexington Books.

Foliart, D.E., Clausen, M. and Siljestrom, C. (2001) Bereavement practices among California hospices: results of a statewide survey. *Death Studies*, 25: 461–7.

Gibson, D.W. and Graham, D. (1991) Bereavement risk assessment in Australian hospice care centres: a survey. Unpublished dissertation, Ballarat University College, Ballarat, VIC.

Goodkin, K., Burkhalter, J.E., Tuttle, R.S. *et al.* (1996–97) A research derived bereavement support group technique for the HIV-1 infected. *Omega: Journal of Death and Dying*, 34: 279–300.

Hopmeyer, E. and Werk, A. (1994) A comparative study of family bereavement groups. *Death Studies*, 18: 243–56.

Kirschling, J.M. and Osmont, K. (1992–93) Bereavement network: a community based group. *Omega: Journal of Death and Dying*, 26: 119–27.

Kissane, D.W. and Bloch, S. (2002) *Family Focused Grief Therapy: A Model of Family-Centred Care During Palliative Care and Bereavement*. Buckingham: Open University Press.

Kissane, D.W., Bloch, S., Burns, W.I. *et al.* (1994) Perceptions of family functioning and cancer. *Psycho-Oncology*, 3: 259–69.

Kissane, D.W., Bloch, S., Dowe, D.L. *et al.* (1996) The Melbourne family grief study, I: perceptions of family functioning in bereavement. *American Journal of Psychiatry*, 153: 650–8.

Kissane, D.W., Bloch, S., McKenzie, M., McDowall, A.C. and Nitzan, R. (1998) Family grief therapy: a preliminary account of a new model to promote healthy family functioning during palliative care and bereavement. *Psycho-Oncology*, 7: 14–25.

Lattanzi-Licht, M.E. (1989) Bereavement services: practice and problems. *Hospice Journal*, 5: 1–28.

Lieberman, M.A. and Yalom, I. (1992) Brief group therapy for the spousally bereaved: a controlled study. *International Journal of Group Psychotherapy*, 42: 117–32.

Longman, A.J. (1993) Effectiveness of a hospice community bereavement programme. *Omega: Journal of Death and Dying*, 27: 165–75.

Longman, A.J., Lindstrom, B. and Clark, M. (1989) Preliminary evaluation of bereavement experiences in a hospice programme. *Hospice Journal*, 5: 25–37.

Lund, D.A. and Caserta, M.S. (1992) Older bereaved spouses' participation in self-help groups. *Omega: Journal of Death and Dying*, 25: 47–61.

Matsushima, T., Akabayashi, A. and Nishitateno, K. (2002) The current status of bereavement follow-up in hospice and palliative care in Japan. *Palliative Medicine*, 16: 151–8.

Mawson, D., Marks, I.M., Ramm, L. and Stern, R. (1981) Guided mourning for morbid grief: a controlled study. *British Journal of Psychiatry*, 138: 185–93.

Melges, F.T. and Demaso, D.R. (1980) Grief-resolution therapy: reliving, revising and revisiting. *American Journal of Psychotherapy*, 34: 51–61.

Middleton, W., Raphael, B., Martinek, N. and Misso, V. (1993) Pathological grief reactions, in M.S. Stroebe, W. Stroebe and R.O. Hansson (eds) *Handbook of Bereavement*. Cambridge: Cambridge University Press.

Moos, R.H. and Moos, B.S. (1981) *Family Environment Scale Manual*. Stanford, CA: Consulting Psychologists Press.

National Hospice Organization (1997) *A Pathway for Patients and Families Facing Terminal Illness: Self-determined Life Closure, Safe Comfortable Dying and Effective Grieving*. Alexandria, VA: NHO.

Parkes, C.M. (1981) Evaluation of a bereavement service. *Journal of Preventive Psychiatry*, 1: 179–88.

Parkes, C.M. (1998) *Bereavement: Studies of Grief in Adult Life*, 3rd edn. Madison, CT: International Universities Press.

Paul, N.L. and Grosser, G.H. (1965) Operational mourning and its role in conjoint family therapy. *Community Mental Health Journal*, 1: 339–45.

Payne, S. (2001) The role of volunteers in hospice bereavement support in New Zealand. *Palliative Medicine*, 15: 107–15.

Payne, S. and Relf, M. (1994) The assessment of need for bereavement follow-up in palliative and hospice care. *Palliative Medicine*, 8: 291–7.

Raphael, B. (1977) Preventive intervention with the recently bereaved. *Archives of General Psychiatry*, 34: 1450–4.

Raphael, B. (1984) *The Anatomy of Bereavement*. London: Hutchinson.

Raphael, B., Minkov, C. and Dobson, M. (2001) Psychotherapeutic and pharmacological interventions for bereaved persons, in M.S. Stroebe, R.O. Hansson, W. Stroebe and H. Schut (eds) *Handbook of Bereavement Research*. Washington, DC: American Psychological Association.

Rognlie, C. (1989) Perceived short- and long-term effects of bereavement support group participation at the Hospice of Petaluma. *Hospice Journal*, 5: 39–53.

Schwab, R. (1995–96) Bereaved parents and support group participation. *Omega: Journal of Death and Dying*, 32: 49–61.

Stewart, J. (1994) *Guidelines for Setting Up a Bereavement Service*. London: National Association of Bereavement Services.

Stokes, J., Wyer, S. and Crossley, D. (1997) The challenge of evaluating a child bereavement programmeme. *Palliative Medicine*, 11: 179–90.

Stroebe, M. and Schut, H. (1999) The dual process model of coping with bereavement: rationale and description. *Death Studies*, 23: 197–224.

Thuen, F. (1995) Satisfaction with bereavement support groups: evaluation of the Norwegian Bereavement Care Project. *Journal of Mental Health*, 4: 499–510.

Vachon, M. (1995) Staff stress in hospice/palliative care: a review. *Palliative Medicine*, 9: 91–122.

Walsh, F. and McGoldrick, M. (eds) (1991) *Living Beyond Loss: Death in the Family*. New York: Norton.

Wheeler, I. (1993–94) The role of meaning and purpose in life in bereaved parents associated with a self-help group: compassionate friends. *Omega: Journal of Death and Dying*, 28: 261–71.

Wilkes, E. (1993) Characteristics of hospice bereavement services. *Journal of Cancer Care*, 2: 183–9.

Worden, J.W. (1991) *Grief Counselling and Grief Therapy*, 2nd edn. New York: Springer.

Yalom, I.D. and Vinogradov, S. (1988) Bereavement groups: techniques and themes. *International Journal of Group Psychotherapy*, 38: 419–46.

Families and children facing loss and bereavement

Childhood bereavement services – a diversity of models and practices

Liz Rolls

This chapter is concerned with the services designed to help children and their families facing loss and bereavement. Although it is not known how many children and young people are bereaved each year, a number of estimates have been made. For example, Easton (2001) suggests that when the deaths of parents, siblings, grandparents and other significant people are taken into account, approximately 1.4 million children are bereaved annually. Winston's Wish (2002) provides a more conservative estimate, suggesting that 3 per cent of 5- to 15-year-olds have experienced the death of a parent or sibling, equating to 510,000 children in the UK. Despite the uncertainty about the number of children and young people affected by the death of a significant person, there was a marked increase, during the closing years of the twentieth century, in the number of services within the UK for children and their families who had been bereaved (Rolls and Payne 2003).

However, 'children' are not a homogeneous group, and understanding what is needed to support them is a complex enterprise. At the heart of the development of services are implicit assumptions about the development of children, that bereavement has an impact on them, and that supporting children and young people following bereavement will have a favourable influence on their present and/or future life. These assumptions provide the basis for the development of childhood bereavement services, the models and practices on which service provision is based, and for what is considered 'best' for helping bereaved children and young people.

Here, I use Bronfenbrenner's (1992) bioecological model of development to explore childhood bereavement services and their diversity of models and practices. I begin by describing this model within the broader context of theories of human development and their relationship to bereavement theories. I then use the model to consider briefly some of the ways in which loss and bereavement impact on children. Finally, I explore the ways in which childhood bereavement services contribute, through

Bronfenbrenner's 'ecological systems', to meeting the needs of bereaved children and their families facing loss and grief.

In this chapter, the terms 'child', 'children' and 'childhood' refer to children, young people and young adults between the ages of 0 and 18 years. The terms 'parent' and 'family' are problematic. Broadly, the term 'parent' is used to mean biological and adoptive parents, while the term 'family' is used to mean the 'network of people in the child's immediate psychosocial field' (Carr 1999: 3), including those who play a significant role. However, the broad use of these terms does not intend to ignore the variety of family compositions within the UK, nor foreclose on later consideration of the impact of the individual family constellation on a child who has been bereaved.

Theories of human development and their relationship to bereavement theories

The nature–nurture continuum of human development

Theories of socialization and development centre on a series of competing models. In the more biologically deterministic models, development is seen as a 'forward-looking' linear process, the outcome of which is adulthood. Furthermore, there is a view that human capacities are genetically endowed and immutable. In this model, the socialization of children involves training – sometimes viewed as 'taming' – them to *become* a competent adult member of society. Within this view, the focus is on children's futures not their present (Corsaro 1997). In contrast to viewing growth and development as passive and unilateral, the constructivist or interpretive model of development sees the child as an active, creative agent in their development, 'appropriating information from her environment to use in organising and constructing her own interpretations of the world' (Corsaro 1997: 11). Corsaro argues that theorists such as Piaget ([1937] 1954) believed 'that children from the first days of infancy interpret, organize, and use information from the environment, and that they come to construct conceptions (known as mental structures) of their physical and social worlds' (Corsaro 1997: 12). Vygotsky's (1978) socio-cultural view of children's social development is based on the idea that this is 'always the result of their collective actions and that these actions take place and are located in society' (Corsaro 1997: 14). Thus, rather than being appropriated by, and consumers of, adult society, children are themselves appropriators of society through their active, creative, social agency (Corsaro 1997).

Relationship of theories of human development to bereavement theories

Clark *et al.* (1994) has identified three models, or typologies, of bereavement theory:

1   The 'blunt trauma' models of early perspectives on bereavement that attempt to link adult psychopathology with the loss of a parent in childhood.

2   The 'shock–aftershock' models in which bereavement is seen not as a single event, but one that is mediated by determinants and the impact is carried forward into adult life.

3   The 'cascade' models of bereavement, involving an interaction of the specific meaning of the death, the child's characteristics of resilience and vulnerability, and the child's stage of development.

The linear approach to development is paralleled in the 'blunt trauma' models of bereavement, while the interpretive models of development underscore the 'shock–aftershock' and 'cascade' models. However, while death is a universal event, the subjective experience of bereavement is not only mediated through the interaction of the specific meaning of the death, the child's characteristics of resilience and vulnerability, and the child's stage of development. It is also embedded in the social, cultural and historical context in which it takes place. These models of development and bereavement are limited in their capacity to illuminate the *processes* by which individuals develop, and experience bereavement, in their immediate environment within a particular social and cultural context. Stroebe and Schut (1999) attempt to address this in their 'dual process' model of coping with bereavement, arguing that, in particular, it is 'useful to describe cultural differences along the loss–restoration dimension' (Stroebe and Schut 1999: 220).

Bronfenbrenner's bioecological model of development

Bronfenbrenner (1992) has proposed an empirically testable 'systems' or ecological model of development that does more than emphasize the importance of the interpersonal, social relationships in the development of the child, and their capacity to act on their social world. It outlines the set of *processes* 'through which the properties of the person and the environment interact to produce constancy and change in the characteristics *over the life course*' (Bronfenbrenner 1992: 191; my emphasis).

The model is based on three propositions:

1   Human development takes place through processes of progressively more complex reciprocal interaction, between an active, evolving biopsychological human organism and the persons, objects and symbols in its immediate environment.

2   The form, power, content and direction of these 'proximal processes' affecting development vary systematically as a joint function of the:

   • characteristics of the developing person;
   • environment; and
   • nature of the development outcomes under consideration.

3   Proximal processes serve as a mechanism for actualizing genetic potential for psychological development, but their power to do so depends also on the three factors stipulated in (2) (Bronfenbrenner and Ceci 1994: 572).

This notion of 'social ecology' – the mutual accommodation through the life span between the changing environment and unique individual – occurs in the context of four structures, or environments:

1   *Microsystems*: the immediate settings, of places and people, including the activities, roles and relationships of significant people, that contain the developing child.
2   *Mesosystems*: the processes between two settings each of which contain the child, for example home and school.
3   *Exosystems*: processes between two or more settings, only one of which contains the developing person, but which impacts on and influences the processes of the setting within which the child is developing, for example the parents' place of work.
4   *Macrosystems*: the broad overarching cultural and subcultural environment (Bronfenbrenner 1994).

These systems are outlined in Figure 29.1.

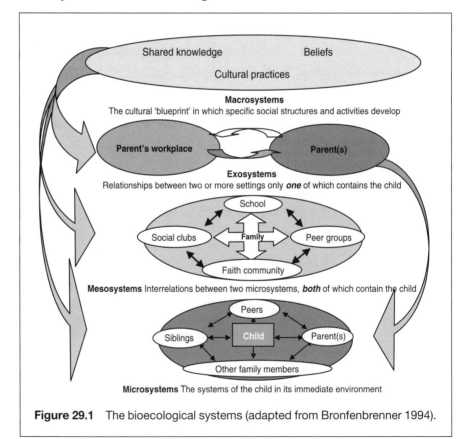

Figure 29.1   The bioecological systems (adapted from Bronfenbrenner 1994).

Bronfenbrenner's systems model of development outlines the dynamic process through which the genetic endowment of the child is actualized (Bronfenbrenner and Ceci 1994), and emphasizes the interrelated *dynamic* between the developing person, the processes or interactions and the context in which they occur, over and in time, and it is within this bioecological system that the death of a parent or sibling, the bereavement experience and childhood bereavement services are located.

The bereavement experience of a child

How a child experiences and responds to the death of a significant person, what happens afterwards and the accommodation or 'timely reconstitution' (Christ 2000) that a child is able to make, is the result of a complex set of processes or interactions between the significant relationships in, and features of, the microsystems and the mesosystems of which they are a part. Some of these include:

- who has died;
- the child's characteristics – age and stage of cognitive and emotional development;
- the circumstances surrounding the death, including how and what children are told, and what life is like afterwards; and
- relationships with peers and school.

These factors, often referred to as 'mediators', appear to be most powerfully associated with outcome (Christ 2000) and will be briefly explored here.

Who has died and who remains

Worden (1996) puts parents firmly in the role of the 'most significant other' for a child, suggesting that they are 'in effect their partners in negotiating the essential developmental tasks that will take them to adulthood' (p. 9). The death of a parent is, therefore, one of the most fundamental losses a child can face (Dyregrov 1991; Worden 1996). When the death of a sister or brother occurs, there will have been a history of a complex set of sibling relationships, and their death presents a different set of challenges for the bereaved child, who has been described as the 'forgotten mourner' (Hindmarch 1995). These include negotiating the ambivalent feelings often found in sibling relationships, as well as feelings of guilt and self-reproach (Dyregrov 1991). Furthermore, when a child has died of a life-limiting illness, the well siblings will have already been living in what Bertman (1991) calls 'houses of chronic sorrow' (p. 320; citing Bluebond-Langner 1989). There may be long-term implications for surviving siblings, who continue to report, 7–9 years after a child's death, various behaviours that they attribute to the death of their sibling (Davies 1991) and for whom there is a higher risk of psychiatric disorder in childhood (Rutter 1966) and in later life (Black 1996). However, there is some debate about the links between adult psychopathology and the bereavement of children in childhood (Harrington and Harrison 1999). Furthermore, the relationship with the parent prior to death may have been ambivalent and this will have an impact on the child's grieving (Dyregrov 1991)

As well as the relationship to the person who has died, the child continues in a relationship with those who remain. With the death of a partner, the remaining parent, in experiencing their own grief, presents a grave crisis to their child, in which

> never again will the world be as secure a place as it was before. The familiar design of family life is completely disrupted. The child suffers not only the loss of the parent, but is deprived of the attention he [*sic*] needs at a time when he craves that extra reassurance that he is cared for.
>
> (Grollman 1967: 15)

In the event of the death of a sibling, as well as experiencing the loss of that relationship, the bereaved child will be in the environment of parents who have lost a child, and on whom there are now 'conflicting demands both to let go of the parent role (in the case of the child who died) and, at the same time, to continue to be a parent to the remaining sibling' (Bertman 1991: 322). In grieving for their deceased child, Rubin (1993) suggests that 'parents' ability to maintain meaningful and balanced interaction with the surviving children is far from assured' (p. 285). Furthermore, they may put an intolerable emotional burden on their remaining children (Pettle and Britten 1995).

The active coping style of the surviving parent appears to affect outcome for the child (Christ 2000), and although the death of a sibling does not usually have the same developmental implications as the death of a parent (Nagara 1970), there may be increased parental anxiety and over-protection (Dyregrov 1991). Furthermore, while there were no significant differences between children who had lost a parent compared to those who had lost a sibling, there appear to be gender differences in the experience, with boys more affected by the loss of a parent and girls by the loss of a sibling (Worden *et al.* 1999).

The child's characteristics

The child's characteristics include their age, gender and cognitive and emotional development, each of which differentiates and affects the experience of bereavement. The characteristic of gender has been mentioned above, but what will be briefly discussed here is the effect of the child's cognitive and emotional development on their capacity to understand death and to mourn.

On their capacity to understand death

Wass (1991) suggests that individual differences in children's understanding of death are a function of 'maturation, life circumstances, experience, adult–child interactions, and a host of other factors' (p. 12). The capacity to understand death as permanent, irreversible, inevitable and universal comes with the child's cognitive maturation (Dyregrov 1991). According to Speece and Brent (1984), children under 7 years have a very limited understanding of the meaning of death, with children at 5 years conceiving of death as reversible (Nagy 1948) and meaning disappearance (Anthony 1940), although Black (1996) argues that even very young children have a concept of death. The idea of death as irreversible comes between the ages of 5 and 7 years (Speece and Brent 1984) and the sense of its inevitability as a natural biological process by 9–10 years (Nagy 1948). Noppe and Noppe (1997) suggest that the meaning of death evolves throughout adolescence. They link transformations in the death concept to the different developmental tasks across the early, middle and later years of adolescence, in particular to achieving emotional separation (younger adolescents), mastery and control (middle adolescents) and intimacy and commitment (later adolescents). However, Corr (1991) notes that while it is generally accepted that adolescents understand death as final, universal and inevitable, this capacity to conceptualize is different from understanding the significance of it.

Indeed, Wass (1991) argues that 'in a sense, the entire period of adolescence is about death and loss, the loss of childhood and of the protective warmth of the support coming with it' (p. 27). The death of a parent in adolescence, Abrams (1999) believes, 'interferes at every level with the business of being young and growing up . . . [and] . . . creates impossibly conflicting needs' (p. xiv). She argues that 'the struggle is not only how to cope with the bereavement itself, but also how to cope with it in the context of an unaccommodating world' (p. xiv).

On their capacity to mourn

There is uncertainty about the age at which a child has developed a capacity to mourn. Bowlby (1980) argues that grief reactions can be seen in children as young as 6 months, whereas others (e.g. Furman 1974) argue that this capacity comes later. Furman (1974) also argues that the expression of sadness does not require the child to have a concept of death. Christ (2000) has identified developmental differences in mourning, which in the younger age group (3–5 years) was related to their eventual acceptance of the finality of death. However, some would argue that it is an unproven assumption that children must grieve, and that a failure to mourn results in adult pathology (Harrington and Harrison 1999). Furthermore, grief may be differently expressed; for example, boys may have greater difficulty in showing and expressing their feelings than girls (Dyregrov 1991).

Circumstances around the death

The circumstances surrounding the death involve a number of aspects, including how the person dies, how and what children are told and how involved they are in the funeral, and what life is like afterwards.

How the person died

An anticipated death in which there is some warning helps lower anxieties (Black 1998). By contrast, a sudden death is 'a shock to the family system' (Handsley 2001), placing the family under great strain. These deaths often have a traumatic aspect resulting in a stronger impact on adults and the desire to protect children from too much detail (Dyregrov 1991). Indeed, children who have witnessed a violent death may develop post-traumatic stress disorder (Pynoos *et al.* 1987) and the children of murdered parents may well need specialized help (Black *et al.* 1992). The death of a parent or sibling by suicide presents particular difficulties for a child, not only because these are invariably violent deaths, but also because they challenge the child's notions of the world and what people can do (Dyregrov 1991). In addition, murder and suicide are often accompanied by stigma and notoriety, which have consequences for the bereaved person's future life, including fears for their own safety (Riches and Dawson 2000).

How and what children are told and how involved they are in the funeral

Learning of the death is a significant moment (Worden 1996) and parents are confronted with decisions about what, when and how to tell their children about the events surrounding the illness and death, and although children vary in their emotional and behavioural reactions, their responses are strongly influenced by those of the surviving parent and other adults (Worden 1996). Forewarning can help the child prepare (Black 1998), but for many reasons parents will deny their children information (Black 1996; Silverman 2000) or provide information at the time of diagnosis but not keep the child updated (Dyregrov 1991). Black (1998) argues that children benefit from attending funerals and other rituals, which are important mediators in the course and outcome of bereavement, helping children to acknowledge the death, honour the life of the deceased and provide support and comfort for the bereaved children (Worden 1996).

What life is like afterwards

Death has an impact on the practical aspects of everyday life (Melvin and Lukeman 2000), as well as on our 'internal working models' of the family (Riches and Dawson 2000: 5). According to Worden (1996), positive adjustment is associated with fewer daily life changes, but change is inevitable and may include changes in domestic arrangements such as who undertakes the chores and household duties, in sleeping arrangements and in arrangements for mealtimes and bedtimes (Worden 1996). Death may also involve more significant changes in the family's financial status, creating difficulties for the surviving members to manage (Corden *et al.* 2002). According to Worden (1996), the most frequent changes are experienced in the first 4 months, especially those related to chores, and there may be increased resentment at added responsibilities, especially following the death of a mother. However, this will depend on the quality of the pre-death relationship. With changing roles between partners and including children within the social economy of the household, this may not always be the case. When the parent(s) are unavailable, the child needs support from outside, and access to a replacement person can have positive effects on the child (Dyregrov 1991; Melvin and Lukeman 2000), although the surviving parent's new relationships may present the child with difficulty.

Significant changes in communication patterns also occur, including difficulty talking about the dead person or particular topics that may cause distress, the censoring of information and who talks to whom (Moos 1995). Balk (1990) argues that siblings, in trying to appear to cope, may not be given opportunities to talk, but children may also understand the burden under which the parent(s) struggle and adjust their behaviour accordingly (Silverman 2000). In addition, parents may be unwilling to discuss details of the death and their own feelings about it (Riches and Dawson 2000).

Child's relationship to peer and school

Relationships with peers and school are important microsystems of the child. Peers are a source of comfort, especially a friend who has had a similar experience, older friends and friends who knew the person who has died. But children may not talk to friends for a number of reasons, including their fear of crying, awkwardness on the part of friends, their not knowing or caring about the death, and it feeling too personal (Worden 1996). Late adolescents talk to peers more than to parents despite greater closeness to parents than in previous periods of adolescence (Noppe and Noppe 1997). The maintenance of contact with other children at school is important, especially if there is also parental grief (Walsh and McGoldrick 1991). However, many siblings feel peers and teachers do not understand their feelings (Hindmarch 1995), and school problems arise because of increased aggression, not being understood by peers and teachers, and poor concentration (Pettle and Britten 1995).

Childhood bereavement services: an ecological 'niche' for bereaved children and their families

Fundamental to Bronfenbrenner's (1992) thesis is not the fact that life events happen, but that our capacity to adapt and develop psychological health rests on successful adaptation to events that have occurred. This adaptation

– or its opposite, a failure to adapt – occurs in 'ecological niches', events that are 'favourable or unfavourable for the development of individuals with particular characteristics' (Bronfenbrenner 1992: 194). I now situate the work of childhood bereavement services, as an 'ecological niche', within the ecological systems of the bereaved child.

In this chapter, I use the term 'childhood bereavement services' in two conceptually different ways:

1   A childhood bereavement service is an *individual organization* comprising a number of paid and/or unpaid staff who provide some level of intervention for children and their families. There are similarities and differences between individual services in terms of what interventions they offer to children and their families, how they are organized and funded, and how they are staffed.

2   Childhood bereavement services are a *structural form* of health and social care provision for children arising in the specific cultural and historical context of the late twentieth-century 'developed' world.

Childhood bereavement services, as individual services and as a structural form, engage in a variety of practices that impact, directly and indirectly, on the environments of the child. In Bronfenbrenner's ecological systems model, childhood bereavement services, as a structural form, are *always* part of the exosystem, whether or not a child has been bereaved. Once a child has been bereaved, a childhood bereavement service *may* become part of the mesosystems, in that it becomes a setting containing the child and in which 'proximal processes' between the child and childhood bereavement service providers occur. This section will now consider some of the models and practices of childhood bereavement services from these two conceptually different positions. I draw on some of the data from the Clara Burgess Charity Research Study in which I was principal researcher. The aim of this qualitative research project was to identify and explore the key issues involved in providing UK-based bereavement support services for children. The three objectives were to:

•   identify the needs of the 'primary' (bereaved children and their care-givers) and 'secondary' (school and emergency service) users;

•   examine the procedures and processes that contribute to meeting the needs of the service users; and

•   identify the features that contribute to the development and maintenance of a childhood bereavement service within a community.

Childhood bereavement services in the mesosystems

Once a child 'uses' a childhood bereavement service, it becomes a setting in the mesosystems. Here, I broadly outline some of the differences between services as organizations, describe the variety of ways in which services are offered to children and, finally, identify some of the 'proximal processes' in which service providers engage.

The organization of childhood bereavement services

Childhood bereavement services, as individual service organizations, are structured in several different ways. For example, 85 per cent of services are provided through the non-statutory sector and 12 per cent of services are provided through the statutory sector, with a small group of services (2 per cent) being offered as joint initiatives between two organizations, within a sector or between the statutory and non-statutory sectors. Services are staffed by either paid or unpaid people, or a combination of both, with a diverse range of professional backgrounds, including counsellors (46 per cent), nurses (42 per cent), social workers (39 per cent), doctors (23 per cent), psychologists (10 per cent) and other professional groups (33 per cent), including occupational therapists, art and play therapists. The way in which services are organized is a feature of structural location, size and whether functional activities that support the organization, such as fund-raising and human resource management, are located within the childhood bereavement service or within the larger organization of which the service is a part. Service structures vary, with those that are located in a host structure, such as a hospice or as one part of the broader provision of a charity, being more informal, more fluid and less hierarchically structured than those that are organizations in their own right (Rolls and Payne 2002).

How services are offered

The majority of services (86 per cent) are offered to children between the ages of 0 and 18 years, with some services restricting their provision to a banded age group. Of the 16 services that offered support with respect to the death of a sibling only, 14 were hospices. The majority of services (71 per cent) worked with children who had been bereaved through any cause of death, including murder and suicide. Of the 26 services that restricted their work to children who are bereaved because of deaths from a life-limiting illness, including AIDS, cancer and motor neurone disease, 22 were hospices. In addition, 73 per cent offered a service to children irrespective of whether the death was sudden or anticipated, and of these 35 per cent were hospices. Some services (20 per cent), however, only worked with children whose bereavement had been anticipated, and the majority of these services (89 per cent) were located within hospices (Rolls and Payne 2002). Pre-bereavement support was offered by 64 per cent of services (Rolls and Payne 2003).

Services are offered in different modes: individually or in groups, with the child only or with families. Table 29.1 shows the matrix of activity and the percentage of services that offer each combination. Within this matrix of service provision, there is a further refinement of how services are organized: between the child and the parent, individual and group work, and the types of activities within them. This is illustrated in Figure 29.2.

Table 29.1   Percentages of services offering specific modes of intervention

Intervention	With the child	With the family
Individual work	62	86
Group work	45	64

Source: Rolls and Payne (2003).

Service focus is always on the child, but parents need to have their feelings recognized (Monroe 1995), and the extent to which the services focuses on the bereavement needs of parents varies between services. It may be undertaken in a parents' group, as part of family work, or parents may be referred to an adult service such as Cruse.

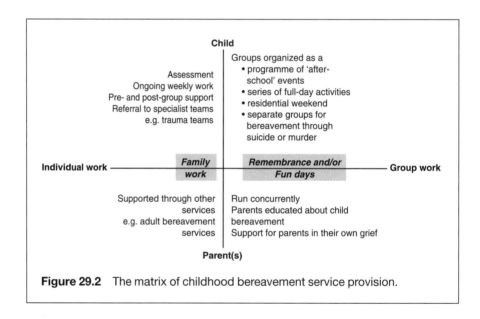

Figure 29.2   The matrix of childhood bereavement service provision.

The 'proximal processes' or interventions

As well as structuring service provision, service providers engage in a purposeful relationship with the child, and it is through these relationships, together with the associated objects and symbols that are generated in a range of activities, that the child's bereavement is 'processed'. The relationships and activities are not random, and while the specific activities may differ *between* services, and *within* services between service providers, they are purposeful. Three underlying objectives of the activities will be discussed here:

- remembering the person who has died;

- understanding and expressing feelings; and
- normalizing the experience and reducing isolation.

REMEMBERING THE PERSON WHO HAS DIED

Services help children remember through a number of activities, including creating a 'memory jar', making a special box into which important items can be placed or making and decorating a photograph frame. What is crucial to these activities is not just the making or collection of the artefacts, but helping the child talk about the meaning these have for them (Riches and Dawson 2000). This process supports the 'continuing bonds' (Potts *et al.* 1999), helps create a narrative, and also forms part of helping a child understand, give names to and express their feelings. Many services offer annual 'remembrance days', while others, such as hospices, keep a photograph album of all the children who have died.

UNDERSTANDING AND EXPRESSING FEELINGS

Riches and Dawson (2000) argue that opportunities for mentally processing the traumatic changes and unfamiliar feelings that the loss of a significant relationship brings are crucial. This includes both an opportunity for 'cognitive mastery' of the event, as well as stimulating emotional coping (Dyregrov 1991). There are many creative ways in which services help children understand and express their feelings, such as through the use of storytelling, puppets, 'anger walls' or other games, watching and talking about videos, and through other symbolic activities.

NORMALIZING THE EXPERIENCE AND REDUCING ISOLATION

Riches and Dawson (2000) suggest that there is a need to appreciate the normality of parental and sibling grieving, and both parents and children often feel isolated in such an extremely important event. Wright *et al.* (1996) argue that sibling groups can help overcome these feelings. Services usually run age-specific groups within their group activities and children can become supportive of each other both during the group sessions as well as afterwards.

Childhood bereavement services in the exosystems

Childhood bereavement services, as structural forms, are in the exosystem of all children. Exosystems are those environments which do not contain the child, but which have an impact on those that do. Services have relationships with others who have a relationship with the child. Some of the ways in which childhood bereavement services influence the systems surrounding the child include:

- *The mesosystems*: (1) offering advice and information to the *families* of children who have been bereaved; (2) supporting *schools* where either a member of staff or a child has died, or where a child has been bereaved.

- *The exosystems*: educating and training health, social care and other professionals, including teachers, police and other emergency service personnel.
- *The macrosystems*: influencing the social constructions, cultural assumptions and beliefs about childhood bereavement.

These influences are outlined diagrammatically in Figure 29.3.

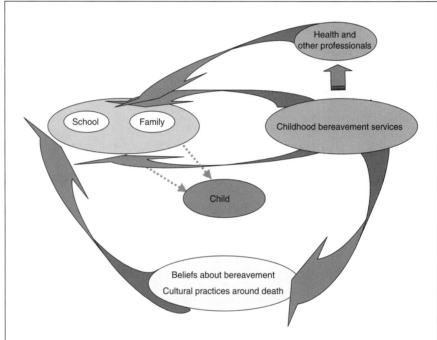

Figure 29.3   The influence of childhood bereavement services on the bioecological systems.

Advice and information to the families of children who have been bereaved

As we have seen, what and how children are told about events surrounding the death is important, and parents may need help in thinking about what to say to their child (Monroe 1995). Parents may also be confused about their child's response to the death, and uncertain how to help them understand both the events surrounding the death and the confusing set of feelings they are experiencing. Giving appropriate advice and information is, therefore, crucial in supporting parents to respond appropriately to their children's needs and in helping them anticipate difficulties. Services clearly feel this is an important aspect of their work, as 95 per cent of childhood bereavement services in the Clara Burgess study offered information and advice to families who have been bereaved, while 88 per cent of services provided resources, such as books and leaflets (Rolls and Payne 2003).

Supporting schools where either a member of staff or a child has died, or where a child has been bereaved

The school is an important setting for a bereaved child, either providing a potential haven of peace and normality (Pennells and Smith 1995) or being a source of increased distress and isolation (Hindmarch 1995). It is also a social environment that influences the meaning of loss (Rowling and Holland 2000). In some cases, the school community itself may be experiencing loss if one of its child or adult members has died. Schools that provide both open discussions about life and death for its pupils, as well as individual support if a death occurs, offer a protective moderating factor to the bereaved child (Dyregrov 1991). In the Clara Burgess Charity Research Study, 66 per cent of childhood bereavement services provided support to schools where there had been a death in the school community itself or where a child in the school had been bereaved. The level and type of support will range from advising teachers on how to support the bereaved child to supporting and assisting them in their own bereavement.

Educating and training health, social care and other professionals, including teachers, police and other emergency service personnel

While children may not have access to, or want to use, a specialized bereavement service, they are often in contact, in the course of their everyday life, with a range of professionals, such as teachers, doctors, school nurses and health visitors. Furthermore, groups of people, such as members of the emergency services or members of specialist groups such as hospice staff, will be in the environment in which the death had occurred. These groups are, therefore, important mediators of help and information about, as well as attitudes towards, bereavement. In the study, 32 per cent of services offered education and training opportunities to this group (Rolls and Payne 2003).

Influencing the social constructions, cultural assumptions and beliefs about childhood bereavement

According to Riches and Dawson (2000), there is now an ambivalent and contradictory attitude to death in modern society. On the one hand, death is very present, for example in the mass media, while at the same time serious discussion about our own deaths is still considered morbid. Mellor (1993) argues that the idea of death as a taboo subject, put forward by Gorer (1965) and Aries (1981), is no longer the case, and although death is very present in Western societies, there has been widespread 'sequestration' of it into the private space (Mellor 1993: 11). Death has been removed from public space and communal religious practices (Aries 1981) into hospitals (Illich 1976) and has become a technical matter (Glaser and Strauss 1968; Giddens, 1991). Funerals are now organized by specialists (Huntington and Metcalf 1979) and rituals have been deconstructed so people do not know how to act (Turner 1991). This privatization and subjectivization of the experience has consequences for individual experience, for as Mellor (1993) argues, 'the absence of death from the public space makes its presence in the private space an intense and potentially threatening one' (p. 21). Furthermore, it is not only death and bereavement that are sequestered into the private domain. Children themselves are subsumed within the privatized nuclear family and hidden statistically from significant events that affect them (for example, how many children are bereaved annually). Qvortrup (1997) argues that this is because 'they are not expected to have a stake in the present, social, economic or political arrangements' (p. 25).

Childhood bereavement services, individually and as structural forms, are increasingly playing an important role in influencing and defining cultural assumptions and beliefs about children and their experience of bereavement. They are taking children seriously, conferring dignity and importance to their experience and bringing children's experience out of the private into the public domain. They are increasingly advocating and campaigning on children's behalf at local and national levels, through the media and in government, as well as providing a vehicle through which children's own voices and experiences can be heard in their own right. The services in the study considered this an important aspect of their work, and all were able to engage in some way in changing attitudes and beliefs about children who have been bereaved.

However, there is a paradox. In influencing the shared knowledge, beliefs and attitudes about childhood bereavement, childhood bereavement services are increasingly *producers* of culture. But at the same time, childhood bereavement support is becoming increasingly specialized, bureaucratized and functionally differentiated (Rolls and Payne 2002) and part of the 'institutionalisation of bereavement support' (Winkel 2001), where 'expert discourse manipulates private experience' (Walter 1991: 39). In this capacity, they are *reproducers* of culture.

Conclusions

In thinking about loss and differential grief in families, Gilbert (1996) poses the question 'we've had the same loss, why don't we have the same grief?' She identifies the difficulty in understanding family dynamics in loss and grief, and that in paying attention to the family as a system can result in little attention being paid to the individual, intra-psychic processes. Locating this brief review of the impact of bereavement on a child in Bronfenbrenner's (1992) ecological systems model shows that the event occurs in, and is mediated by, a complex set of interrelationships within the microsystem and mesosystems of the child. Thus, children in any one family will experience the bereavement differently, not only because of the different qualitative relationship that they had to the person who died, but because of the proximal processes of the microsystems and mesosystems of which each of them is a part. For example, the high rates of divorce and remarriage may mean that a child will experience a number of family compositions.

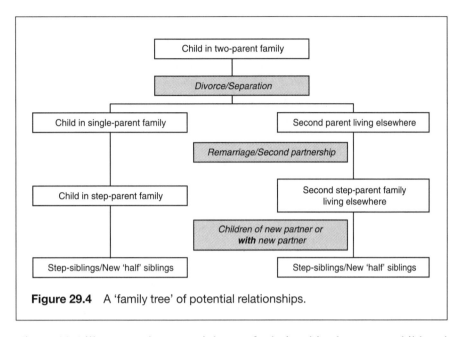

Figure 29.4 A 'family tree' of potential relationships.

Figure 29.4 illustrates the potential sets of relationships between a child and other family members when parents separate.

Bronfenbrenner's (1992) ecological systems model offers an opportunity to consider the child, and its respective systems and the relationships between these systems, simultaneously, rather than foregrounding one at the cost of another. It also identifies the primacy of relationship in mediating experiences. Service providers, while situated in an organizational structure, are a central group of people who can contribute to making order out of chaos and help provide a language for, and meaning to, a child's experience of grief and loss (Riches and Dawson 2000).

Childhood bereavement services, as a form of social provision, have the capacity to impact on the proximal processes within the mesosystems, exosystems and macrosystems surrounding a bereaved child. Bronfenbrenner's ecological systems theory provides a useful model to understand the set of 'intimate relations and the importance of social support' (Riches and Dawson 2000) as well as the dynamic of the processes by which these, together with the ever widening set of social relations and cultural context, can, over time, enable a bereaved child to accommodate and mature as a result of a death. It also helps identify the ways in which childhood bereavement services, as individual services and as structural forms of social provision, can provide favourable ecological niches for the bereaved child and their family. Finally, services are embedded in culture, but like the children with whom they work, they are active and creative agents influencing and shaping the world around them.

This chapter has linked some of the theory related to children and bereavement, and data from the Clara Burgess Charity Research Study, to a model of human development. Box 29.1 identifies several questions that you might like to use to help relate this to your practice.

Box 29.1   Relating the bioecological systems model to practice

1   Think about your own professional background and the work you do (or would like to do) with children who have been bereaved.

- Where would you situate this in the bioecological systems of the child?
- List the activities/interventions you use with children and their families. How do you think these will influence the bioecological systems of the child?
- In what ways could your work expand to influence other systems of the child?

2   Consider a child who has been bereaved. Using the bioecological systems model, what questions do you need to ask to assess the child's need for support and intervention?

Relevance to establishing a childhood bereavement service

Many factors need to be taken into account when establishing a childhood bereavement service, including those related to how the service will be staffed and funded. The bioecological systems model can help service providers and practitioners to:

- clarify the different terrain, or ecological 'field', that surrounds *each* bereaved child, even from within the same family;
- identify ways in which the respective ecological systems of the child can be made as favourable as possible for their future development.

In addition, the model can help services to:

- establish services and plan strategies that impact on the different systems;
- evaluate their service activity from the perspective of the different 'levels' at which they intervene.

Box 29.2 identifies a number of points to consider when establishing or developing a childhood bereavement service.

Box 29.2   Broad points to consider when establishing or developing a childhood bereavement service

- Where would you want to situate the work of your organization in the bioecological systems of the child?
- List the activities/interventions your organization could use or develop with children and their families. How do you think these will influence the bioecological systems of the child?
- What sources of support could your organization provide to these other systems?
- What do you need to have in place to do this?

References

Abrams, R. (1999) *When Parents Die: Learning to Live with the Loss of a Parent*, 2nd edn. London: Routledge.

Anthony, S. (1940) *The Children's Discovery of Death: A Study of Child Psychology*. London: Kegan Paul, Trench & Trubner.

Aries, P. (1981) *The Hour of Our Death*. London: Penguin.

Balk, D. (1990) The self-concepts of bereaved adolescents: sibling death and its aftermath. *Journal of Adolescent Research*, 5(1): 112–32.

Bertman, S. (1991) Children and death: insights, hindsights and illuminations, in D. Papadatou and C. Papadatou (eds) *Children and Death*. New York: Hemisphere.

Black, D. (1996) Childhood bereavement. *British Medical Journal*, 712(7045): 1496.

Black, D. (1998) Bereavement in childhood. *British Medical Journal*, 316: 931–3.

Black, D., Harris-Hendricks, J. and Kaplan, C. (1992) When father kills mother: post-traumatic stress disorder in the children. *Psychotherapy and Psychosomatics*, 57(4): 152–7.

Bluebond-Langner, M. (1989) Worlds of dying children and their well siblings. *Death Studies*, 13: 1–16.

Bowlby, J. (1980) *Attachment and Loss, Vol. 3: Loss, Sadness and Depression*. London: Hogarth Press.

Bronfenbrenner, U. (1992) Ecological systems theory, in R. Vasta (ed.) *Six Theories of Child Development*. London: Jessica Kingsley.

Bronfenbrenner, U. (1994) Ecological models of human development, in T. Husen and T.N. Postlethwaite (eds) *International Encyclodaedia of Education*, 2nd edn, Vol. 3. New York: Elsevier Science.

Bronfenbrenner, U. and Ceci, S.J. (1994) Nature–nurture reconceptualized in developmental perspective: a bioecological model. *Psychological Review*, 10(4): 568–86.

Carr, A. (1999) *The Handbook of Child and Adolescence Clinical Psychology*. London: Routledge.

Christ, G.H. (2000) *Healing Children's Grief: Surviving a Parent's Death from Cancer*. Oxford: Oxford University Press.

Clark, D., Pynoos, R. and Gobel, A. (1994) Mechanisms and processes of adolescent bereavement, in R. Haggerty, N. Garmezy, M. Rutter and L. Sherrod (eds) *Stress, Risk and Resilience in Children and Adolescents: Process Mechanisms and Interventions*. Cambridge: Cambridge University Press.

Corden, A., Sloper, P. and Sainsbury, R. (2002) Financial effects for families after the death of a disabled or chronically ill child: a neglected dimension of bereavement. *Child: Care, Health and Development*, 28(3): 199–204.

Corr, C.A. (1991) Understanding adolescents and death, in D. Papadatou and C. Papadatou (eds) *Children and Death*. New York: Hemisphere.

Corsaro, W.A. (1997) *The Sociology of Childhood*. London: Pine Forge Press.

Davies, B. (1991) Responses of children to the death of a sibling, in D. Papadatou and C. Papadatou (eds) *Children and Death*. New York: Hemisphere.

Dyregrov, A. (1991) *Grief in Children: A Handbook for Adults*. London: Jessica Kingsley.

Easton, C. (2001) Child bereavement and children's rights. *Childright*, 176: 15–16.

Furman, E. (1974) *A Child's Parent Dies: Studies in Childhood Bereavement*. London: Yale University Press.

Giddens, A. (1991) *Modernity and Self-Identity*. Cambridge: Polity Press.

Gilbert, K.R. (1996) 'We've had the same loss, why don't we have the same grief?' Loss and differential grief in families. *Death Studies*, 20: 269–83.

Glaser, B. and Strauss, A. (1968) *Time for Dying*. Chicago, IL: Aldine.

Gorer, G. (1965) *Death, Grief and Mourning in Contemporary Britain*. London: Cresset.

Grollman, E. (1967) Prologue, in E. Grollman (ed.) *Explaining Death to Children*. Boston, MA: Beacon Press.

Handsley, S. (2001) 'But what about us?' The residual effects of sudden death on self-identity and family relationships. *Mortality*, 6(1): 9–29.

Harrington, R. and Harrison, L. (1999) Unproven assumptions about the impact of bereavement on children. *Journal of the Royal Society of Medicine*, 92: 230–2.

Hindmarch, C. (1995) Secondary losses for siblings. *Child: Care, Health, and Development*, 21(6): 425–31.

Huntington, R. and Metcalf, P. (1979) *Celebrations of Death*. Cambridge: Cambridge University Press.

Illich, I. (1976) *Limits to Medicine*. London: Marion Boyars.

Mellor, P.A. (1993) Death in high modernity: the contemporary presence and absence of death, in D. Clark (ed.) *The Sociology of Death*. Oxford: Blackwell.

Melvin, D. and Lukeman, D. (2000) Bereavement: a framework for those working with children. *Clinical Child Psychology and Psychiatry*, 5(4): 521–39.

Monroe, B. (1995) Helping the grieving family, in S.C. Smith and M. Pennells (eds) *Interventions with Bereaved Children*. London: Jessica Kingsley.

Moos, N.L. (1995) An integrative model of grief. *Death Studies*, 19(4): 337–64.

Nagara, H. (1970) Children's reactions to the death of important objects: a developmental approach. *Psychoanalytic Studies of the Child*, 25: 360–400.

Nagy, M. (1948) The child's theories concerning death. *Journal of Genetic Psychology*, 73: 3–27.

Noppe, I.C. and Noppe, L.D. (1997) Evolving meanings of death during early, middle and later adolescence. *Death Studies*, 21(3): 253–76.

Pennells, M. and Smith, S.C. (1995) *The Forgotten Mourners: Guidelines for Working with Bereaved Children*. London: Jessica Kingsley.

Pettle, S.A. and Britten, C.M. (1995) Talking with children about death and dying. *Child: Care, Health and Development*, 21(6): 395–404.

Piaget, J. ([1937] 1954) *The Construction of Reality in the Child*. New York: Basic Books.

Potts, S., Farrell, M. and O'Toole, J. (1999) Treasure weekend: supporting bereaved siblings. *Palliative Medicine*, 13: 51–6.

Pynoos, R.S., Frederick, C., Nader, K. *et al.* (1987) Life threat and post-traumatic stress in school age children. *Archives of General Psychiatry*, 44: 1057–63.

Qvortrup, J. (1997) A voice for children in statistical and social accounting: a plea for children's right to be heard, in A. James and A. Prout (eds) *Constructing and Reconstructing Childhood*, 2nd edn. London: Falmer Press.

Riches, G. and Dawson, P. (2000) *An Intimate Loneliness: Supporting Bereaved Parents and Siblings*. Buckingham: Open University Press.

Rolls, L. and Payne, S. (2002) The social organisation of UK childhood bereavement services: a preliminary in-depth analysis of four UK childhood bereavement services. Paper presented to the *6th Annual Conference on the Social Context of Death, Dying and Disposal*, 5–8 September, York.

Rolls, L. and Payne, S. (2003) Childhood bereavement services: a survey of UK provision. *Palliative Medicine*, 17: 423–32.

Rowling, L. and Holland, J. (2000) Grief and school communities: the impact of social context, a comparison between Australia and England. *Death Studies*, 24: 35–50.

Rubin, S. (1993) The death of a child is forever: the life course impact of child loss, in M.S. Stroebe, W. Stroebe and R.O. Hansson (eds) *Handbook of Bereavement: Theory, Research and Intervention*. Cambridge: Cambridge University Press.

Rutter, M. (1966) *Children of Sick Parents*. Oxford: Oxford University Press.

Silverman, P.R. (2000) *Never Too Young to Know: Death in Children's Lives*. Oxford: Oxford University Press.

Speece, M.W. and Brent, S.B. (1984) Children's understanding of death: a review of three components of a death concept. *Child Development*, 55: 1671–86.

Stroebe, M. and Schut, H. (1999) The dual process model of coping with bereavement: rationale and description. *Death Studies*, 23: 197–224.

Turner, B.S. (1991) *Religion and Social Theory*. London: Sage.

Vygotsky, L.S. (1978). *Mind in Society*. Cambridge, MA: Harvard University Press.

Walsh, F. and McGoldrick, M. (1991) Loss and the family: a systemic perspective, in F. Walsh and M. McGoldrick (eds) *Living Beyond Loss: Death in the Family*. New York: Norton.

Walter, T. (1991) Modern death: taboo or not taboo? *Sociology*, 25: 293–310.

Wass, H. (1991) Helping children cope with death, in D. Papadatou and C. Papadatou (eds) *Children and Death*. New York: Hemisphere.

Winkel, H. (2001) A post-modern culture of grief? On individualization of mourning in Germany. *Mortality*, 6(1): 65–79.

Winston's Wish (2002) *Key facts – Children and Bereavement*. Handout at the Childhood Bereavement Network Conference, Birmingham, 28–29 June.

Worden, J.W. (1996) *Children and Grief: When a Parent Dies*, New York: Guilford Press.

Worden, J.W., Davies, B. and McCown, D. (1999) Comparing parent loss with sibling loss. *Death Studies*, 23: 1–15.

Wright, J.B., Aldridge, J., Gillance, H. and Tucker, A. (1996) Hospice-based groups for bereaved siblings. *European Journal of Palliative Care*, 3(1): 10–15.

PART FOUR

Contemporary issues

30

Overview

Christine Ingleton and Jane Seymour

Changes in population demographics, health needs and reforms in health-care delivery and work practices have had a major impact on the nursing profession in many developed countries. Moreover, the transfer of nurse education into higher education in the UK over the last decade and in North America over the past 20 years has heralded substantial changes in the way nurses are educated and prepared for practice. Nurse education in Australia has also experienced significant changes since the 1980s, including transfer of undergraduate preparation from hospital-based programmes to more formal learning in the tertiary sector and, more recently, growth in post-graduate degrees and clinical specialization (Lee *et al.* 2002).

In the UK, before the radical revision of the education strategy called Project 2000 (UKCC 1987), nurses were taught in training schools attached to hospitals. Two levels of qualification existed, enrolled and registered, and separate courses educated trainees for four areas of nursing: general (adult), sick children, mental health and mental handicap. Over 60 per cent of train-ees' time was spent in providing rostered service, during which time they were responsible to a service manager. Thus nurse training has moved from an apprenticeship model of preparation where trainees worked as 'pairs of hands' to an educationally driven model of preparation where students attend university-based courses.

The need for reform in nursing in the UK emerged from challenges in four main areas: education, service, recruitment and retention, and changes both in health needs and in the NHS. The reforms impacted both upon education and service provision. Educationally, diploma level education was introduced, replacing the previous two-tier system of enrolled and registered nurses. The four specialist routes to qualification were replaced by a Com-mon Foundation Programme (12–18 months) followed by a branch pro-gramme in a chosen specialism. Students are now provided with a bursary rather than a salary and are responsible to educationalists rather than service managers.

At the same time, increases in the age profile of populations, the rising incidence of cancer and the worldwide spread of HIV/AIDS, point to an increase in the need for palliative care in the coming years. As the need for palliative care increases, so the need for general and specialist palliative care education both pre- and post-registration continues to grow. However, meeting those needs is particularly challenging because the nature of palliative care means that teaching and learning about it can be complex and problematic (Macleod and James 1994, 1997). Box 30.1 shows the particular challenges facing nursing in palliative care education both pre- and post-registration. These will be discussed in turn.

Box 30.1   Educational challenges in palliative care education

- Changes in the initial preparation of nurses
- Changes in the continuing education of nurses
- The provision of general palliative care education programmes
- The scarcity of resources and teaching staff with skills in general palliative care
- The paucity of evidence to indicate the effect of education on practice
- The distance and access to effective programmes of education

---

Changes in the initial preparation of nurses

As noted above, palliative care education worldwide has undergone massive reforms in terms of where and how nurses are prepared in both pre-registration training and in subsequent continuing professional development. In the 1980s, Field and Kitson (1986) conducted a survey of UK schools of nursing to explore whether nurses are prepared educationally to deal with dying patients, death and bereaved relatives. The survey was repeated by Lloyd-Williams and Field (2002), the results of which are highlighted in Box 30.2.

It is difficult to make direct comparisons with other countries, since current data are not readily available. However, it is worth noting that the average amount of time spent on death education in general pre-registration nursing programmes has been estimated as 4.39 hours in Canada (Sellick *et al.* 1996) and 19.25 hours in Australia (Yates *et al.* 1996).

The recent Draft Plan from the National Council for Hospices and Specialist Palliative Care Services (NCHSPCS 2002) expresses concern about pre-registration education and training and suggests that a number of fundamental issues require attention: 'Pre-registration nurse training in palliative care consists of a core module in care of the dying which does not specifically identify the role of palliative care as either a speciality, nor as a "philosophical" approach to care. It is focused on the care of the patient dying with cancer' (p. 32). The NCHSPCS goes on to call for the following

> **Box 30.2** Results of surveys of UK schools of nursing examining palliative care education in pre-registration training
>
> The authors found that death education appeared to receive important attention in nursing schools and was provided at a level similar to that found in an earlier survey of British medical schools (Field 1984). The mean hours of teaching death and dying was 13.5 hours for students undertaking a nursing degree, 9.8 hours for students on traditional RGN courses and 6 hours for students on the then enrolled nurses' course. Medical students received 6.3 hours of formal instruction about death and dying. More recently, Lloyd-Williams and Field (2002) repeated the survey of nursing schools to explore the current provision of palliative care teaching to undergraduate nurses and the results paint a less positive picture some 18 years later. One hundred and eight questionnaires were sent out, of which 46 were returned, yielding a disappointing 40 per cent response rate. Diploma students received a mean of 7.8 hours (range 2–26; median 4) and degree students 12.2 hours (range 3–42; median 9) of teaching in palliative care during their undergraduate training. It was found that entry level student nurses received little generic teaching in palliative care and the teaching that did occur was mainly theoretical; palliative care knowledge was not formally assessed in 76 per cent of the degree programmes and 82 per cent of the diploma courses that responded to the questionnaire.

elements to be incorporated into the pre-registration curriculum, as a minimum requirement:

- a basic understanding of the role and function of the palliative care team and when to transfer to that service;
- a basic understanding of the psychological support needs of patients and their carers from pre-diagnosis onwards to ensure better arrangements and working practices in out-patients and other departments, as well as in the in-patient settings.

From the information that is currently available, it would appear that palliative care education has not been incorporated adequately within undergraduate training in the UK with any degree of uniformity. Given the growing volume of work in both the acute and community sectors in providing care for those patients with chronic, life-limiting diseases, palliative care education should take greater prominence than at present.

Changes in the continuing education of nurses

In the past, nursing has been viewed as a practice-based profession, with little expectation of education beyond that needed to inform and perform practical tasks. As the academic profile of nursing has developed, the number of post-registration practitioners seeking higher education courses to update their academic qualifications to first or higher degree level has increased markedly. Currently, a major issue facing registered nurses is the ongoing challenge of maintaining professional competence in the context of rapidly changing health care systems. In terms of continuing professional development for nurses, a significant policy development within the UK has been the introduction of what has come to be known as PREP (Post-Registration Education and Practice: UKCC 1994). Since this development, nurses have been required to undertake a minimum of 5 days study or equivalent every 3 years. At the same time, all programmes of specialist education for nurses have been required to meet the UK Central Council (the statutory body for nursing, later replaced by the Nursing and Midwifery Council) standards within the profession and, importantly, be linked to a higher education accreditation system. Credits for appropriate prior learning (APL) and appropriate prior experiential learning (APEL) were introduced, acknowledging and recognizing previous education, skills and experience. Furthermore, the development of AP(E)L[1] has greatly increased the ability of students to gain credit for professional achievement and to include this as part of their degree. The concept and principle of APEL was first developed in the USA in the 1970s and 1980s. It recognizes that learning has always taken place outside of education and training courses, and that APEL offers a process for quantifying this learning and giving it credit.

A hallmark of AP(E)L is modularization of courses and programmes of study. The modularization of programmes that have university approval has impacted upon all courses, including those relating to palliative care. While this mode of delivery does offer choice and flexibility for students, there is a danger that learning may be seen as a series of fragmented and unrelated chunks of content. To prevent this occurring, there is a need to consider educational approaches that pay attention to the educational *process* as well as the *outcome*, so that material from within modules is integrated into the whole experience and practice (Sheldon and Smith 1996). In the context of palliative care education, as with other educational programmes, there remains the concern that the requirements of educational institutions regarding course structure, credit levels and course validation may dominate and skew what is being offered to students.

Arguably (in the context of specialist palliative care), maintaining the balance between fostering growth 'in spontaneity and opportunities for charismatic individuals whose training has not followed a set path' (Sheldon and Smith 1996: 102) and applying a more systematic approach to education provision continues to be one of the most challenging aspects of specialist palliative care education. As the NCHSPCS draft paper points out:

> post registration courses in palliative care are in a state of flux with a plethora of different certificates, diplomas, and degree courses all accredited by differing institutions but with little or no common academic 'currency' or 'transferability'. Rather than a shortage of courses in palliative care there are too many, but with little or no central co-ordination. Identifying a clear training pathway for nurses is difficult

and there is an urgent need to develop the training pathway for nurses wishing to specialise in palliative care, with core training modules identified for nurses starting at D and E grade, and then moving on to the higher clinical grades.

(NCHSPCS 2002: 3)

The provision of general palliative care education

Historically, adult palliative care has been largely confined to those patients with cancer. Figures available for 1999–2000 in England suggest that 95 per cent of palliative care services are delivered to cancer patients.[2] While some patients require specialist palliative care, the vast majority need general palliative care focusing on holistic care provision and palliation of symptoms (Lloyd-Williams and Field 2002). A greater awareness that most patients with palliative care needs are cared for in general acute and community settings rather than specialist palliative care settings might improve nurses' impetus to access specialist training in palliative care.

The movement of the speciality away from patients with terminal cancer to encompass those with other life-threatening illnesses has caused confusion for those educators who have emphasized cancer-related palliative care in their teaching, at the expense of a more broad based multi-professional approach. Dowell (2002) suggests that education in palliative care should reflect the principles and practices of palliative care and, therefore, should be multi-professional in orientation, multi-modal in delivery and emphasize process *and* outcomes of care. However, the gaps in palliative care education discussed above, and assumptions that the knowledge base is wedded closely to cancer-related palliative care, may lead to inappropriate teaching and lack of multidisciplinarity.

Scarcity of resources and teaching staff with skills in general palliative care

In some palliative care units, there is a scarcity of resources to support learning, especially in the workplace. In many units, there are not the finances to establish a library and employ a librarian; nevertheless, a model of service provision could be considered before the purchase of costly resources such as journal subscriptions and books. Journal subscriptions are an annual, costly expense yet are essential in education, training and lifelong learning of staff. Furthermore, textbook material may be limited. For example, Ferrall *et al.* (1999) conducted a wide-ranging analysis of end-of-life content in nursing textbooks and revealed that there was little provision of information in undergraduate nursing textbooks on palliative care.

An additional constraint to the delivery of high-quality palliative care education appears to be lack of trained and experienced teachers to deliver educational programmes (Yates *et al.* 1996; Lloyd-Williams and Field 2002). In Lloyd-Williams and Field's (2002) survey, 82 per cent of respondents felt education about palliative care should be a core component of entry level diploma or degree education, but they recognized significant problems in providing such teaching: two-thirds indicated that they had difficulty in finding appropriately qualified staff to teach the subject. Moreover, this scarcity of teaching staff with skills in general palliative care, coupled with a lack of specialist palliative care units providing clinical placements, limits further educational provision in this area.

The paucity of evidence to indicate the effect on practice of education

In considering the availability of palliative care education for nurses and other health care professionals, studies have broadly focused upon two perspectives: first, examining whether nursing curricula incorporate teaching about death and dying and, second, exploring nurses' experience with dying patients (Copp 1994). In the USA, Quint's (1967) seminal work on the education of nurses to care for dying patients highlighted the considerable inadequacy of educational provision for nurses in this area. Quint's landmark study has gone on to profoundly influence the way in which these aspects of education have been incorporated and taught in schools of nursing throughout the developed world.

Although education is considered an integral part of the work of palliative care teams, there is little evidence to indicate the effect on practice of such education. Research examining the effectiveness of various education programmes on care of the dying has frequently revealed equivocal results. A recent review of the literature of studies related specifically to nurses' knowledge of palliative care (Proctor *et al.* 2000) found only three studies: one study conducted in Canada (Ross *et al.* 1996) and two studies conducted in Australia (Redman *et al.* 1995; Farrell 1998). Studies evaluating education often lack a theoretical basis, few employ controlled experimental designs and are predominantly concerned with participants' perceptions or assessment of their knowledge base. One of the reasons for this could be that, in common with research in palliative care generally, such research presents methodological challenges. Issues relating to research in palliative care are discussed in Chapter 35 by Ingleton and Davies. They highlight the methodological challenges researchers face in conducting studies in palliative care and the reasons for these difficulties. However, if we subscribe to the view that perceptions of increased knowledge, self-confidence and attitude change are more reliable (and meaningful) than measurable differences, there is substantial evidence to support the effectiveness of education in palliative care (Kenny 2001; Dowell 2002).

Distance, cost and access to effective programmes of education

Access to continuing education is a challenge for nurses who have work and family responsibilities, work shifts and may live a considerable distance from institutions of higher education (Canadian Nurses Association 1997). In a review of the evidence base for professional education for the cancer care nurse in England and Wales, it was found that at any one time, half the available places on English National Board specialist courses remain unfilled (Blunden and Langton 2001). Clearly, further work needs to be carried out to explain this lack of take up, which could relate to the difficulties nurses have in obtaining release from work to attend such programmes and/or lack of understanding of the need to undertake such specialist training if they work in non-specialist areas. However, it should be noted that attendance of staff members at educational courses and training does not necessarily ensure that palliative care practice will improve at an organizational level. If individual course members are to apply theory to practice, then certain organizational factors need to be in place: appropriate management and peer support, provision of financial resources and a collective commitment to developing practice (Froggatt 2000). In Chapter 36, Froggatt and Booth discuss the importance of the organizational context and organizational support needed in helping colleagues to improve palliative care practice.

Obstacles to accessing courses could be overcome with further development of more flexible modes of delivery, including providing work-based educational preparation, problem-based learning and through the promotion of inter-professional learning. These approaches are now discussed in turn.

Work-based learning

The type of courses available and mode of delivery must adapt to changing professional expectations; work-based learning in professional practice is one way of responding to these changes. Work-based learning, in valuing learning that takes place outside of an educational institution, and in integrating practice with theory, offers an interesting alternative to purely academic university-based courses (Hargreaves 1996). Work-based learning embraces a number of learning and teaching strategies that take place outside educational institutions and in students' workplaces. One of the primary modes of work-based learning is through the use of on-line materials, such as web-based resources. These are increasingly being employed to overcome the traditional barriers to continuing education. The potential role of the World Wide Web (see Chapter 34) in continuing nursing education is now attracting global interest (Billings and Rowles 2001; Washer 2001; Atack and Rankin 2002). A descriptive study of 57 registered Canadian nurses' experience with web-based learning found that while web-based learning can be an effective mode of delivery for nursing education, a number of challenges were faced when using this mode of delivery (Atack and Rankin 2002). For example, while access to the course from home was reported as very satisfactory for the majority, work users encountered a number of serious barriers, such as insufficient time and limited computer access. In addition, registered nurses made significant gains in their learning with email, internet, keyboard skills and word processing skills during the 16-week course. On the negative side, lack of computer skills, erroneous perceptions of course workload and inadequate preparation for web learning were largely responsible for most withdrawals. The authors conclude that teachers, peers, technology, course design and the learning environment are key variables that influence learners' experiences and success. Importantly, they suggest that advanced preparation and ongoing support from teachers and employers is required to make the learning experience a positive one for nurses. This shift away from viewing educational institutions as the principal places where learning takes place is discussed in Chapter 38 by Hopkins, who provides examples of how nurse managers can work to integrate learning into daily clinical practice in the palliative care setting.

Problem-based learning

Problem-based learning (PBL) is a method of group learning that uses true-to-life problems as a stimulus for students to learn problem-solving skills. More specifically, teachers facilitate learning in student-led group tutorials, but do not provide specific content information. In a synthesis of all available evaluative research from 1970 to 1992, comparing PBL with more traditional methods of medical education, Vernon and Blake (1993) concluded that the results generally supported the superiority of PBL, especially with regard to teacher attitudes, student mood, class attendance and academic process. Increasing numbers of nursing programmes have adopted PBL in various forms, because it is thought to promote higher-order thinking skills, and combines theory with practice. In analysing the strengths and weaknesses of PBL, for both teachers and students, Frost (1996) argues that PBL is more likely to bridge the gap between theory and practice, and equip nurses with the skills demanded by an ever-changing society. PBL used in a Canadian undergraduate programme nursing course was beneficial to students who learned community health nursing by analysing increasingly complex problems (Morales-Mann and Kaitell 2001). PBL in one Australian nursing programme produced a role change as students became active, self-directed learners with critical thinking and problem-solving skills (Little and Ryan 1998).

Inter-professional learning

There has been much written recently about how changes in patterns of health care delivery and structure of services have impacted upon the development of the health professions globally. These changes have included calls for collaboration between professions in health and social care. Inter-professional education is seen as one way forward in promoting professional and proficient teamworking. As this need for teamwork has been recognized, there is a need to change the way in which health care professionals are educated. The impetus for this has arisen, in part, from the belief that separate training encourages different health professional groups to hold onto their independence and autonomy, thereby detracting from effective teamwork. Cox and James explore the concept of boundaries and teamworking in palliative care in Chapter 31.

The need for change has also been accelerated in the developed world by the move towards shifting the balance from secondary to primary care and the need to use resources effectively and in a timely manner. Taken together, these changes have been instrumental in accelerating the growth and development of inter-professional learning in health care settings. Nevertheless, despite the growth and longevity of inter-professional learning, there is a lack of clarity surrounding the use of terms associated with 'shared learning'. Inter-professional, interdisciplinary, multi-professional, shared and collaborative (among others) are used interchangeably without any general agreement about their meaning (Hammick 1998). A recent systematic review by Cooper *et al.* (2001) on interdisciplinary education for undergraduate health care professionals revealed the literature to be diverse, including relatively small amounts of research data and much larger amounts of evaluation literature (Cooper *et al.* 2001). The researchers conducting the review used methodological rating schemes to test for confounding influences on the research studies. The number of studies found was 1421, but only 30 (21 per cent) were included in the analysis because of lack of methodological rigour in the research and poorly developed outcome measures. The review concluded that student health professionals were found to benefit from interdisciplinary education with outcome effects primarily relating to changes in knowledge, skills, attitudes and beliefs. Effects upon professional practice were not discernible and education and psychological theories were rarely used to guide the development of the education interventions.

As Sneddon points out in Chapter 33, in no other health care area is learning alongside different disciplines welcomed so readily as in the field of palliative care. In Lloyd-Williams and Field's (2002) survey of undergraduate teaching in palliative care, 22 per cent of respondents mentioned the desirability for palliative care to be taught as a multidisciplinary subject, though translating this into action is more problematic. It is postgraduate palliative care specialist education which has embraced the concept of inter-professional learning most enthusiastically, with many courses advertising themselves as having a multi-professional intake of students.

This appears to reflect the holistic and team approach mirrored in palliative care practice, although how this multi-professional group is engaged in the teaching and learning process is largely unknown. The wide variety of approaches and levels of study at different institutions can make application and integration difficult when applying learning to practice. Added to this, it is sometimes difficult to discern from the variety of course documents what the underlying educational philosophy is, whether it is being carried through in practice and whether there is any resonance of the educational philosophy with palliative care (Sheldon and Smith 1996).

The crucial question that remains unanswered is how inter-professional learning affects professional practice in palliative care. As yet there are no answers to this question. What is clear from the evidence available in the wider research literature is that a fundamental approach to inter-professional learning is required, one that integrates the best external evidence with educational expertise and students' choices. This highlights the need for greater discussion from an early stage between educators, practitioners and students to determine basic requirements (Cooper *et al.* 2001).

Inter-professional approaches to teaching and learning are increasingly being used in the context of research training in palliative care as attempts to strengthen the evidence base for the care and services provided to patients and their families continue. Although palliative care research is a growth activity with practitioners ever more involved in palliative care research as the field expands, this expanded contact with research is not without its pressures and problems, nor does this preclude the opportunity to build upon what has been already achieved. These problems and possible opportunities for advancing the contribution of nurses towards research activity in palliative care is the focus of the next section (see Box 30.3).

It is important to preface the following discussion by highlighting the difference in skills and knowledge which may be required by nurses, depending on their contribution towards research-based activity. The majority of clinical nurses are 'consumers of research'; they require appropriate access to research publications, libraries and sources of information to develop and implement evidence-based practice. Arguably, only a minority of nurses are 'research producers' and, as such, research methods skills, ethical knowledge and ability to disseminate findings are most relevant to their role. However, clearly research education should equip *all* nurses to assess critically those studies on which they plan to develop their practice.

Box 30.3 Problems and opportunities for advancing the contribution of nurses towards research-based activity

- Nurses' access to and use of research-based knowledge
- Developments in the acquisition of research skills
- Small-scale nature of studies conducted in palliative care
- Perceived dissonance between academic nursing and clinical practice
- Changes to ethical approval processes for research studies
- Expanding practitioner roles

Nurses' access to and use of research-based knowledge

Nurses' access to and use of research-based knowledge is considered an essential element of proposals to enhance the quality of health care (Department of Health 1999). Researchers at the Centre for Evidence Based Nursing at the University of York, UK (Thompson *et al.* 2001), conducted a study in which they hoped to identify the sources of information *actually* used by nurses, as well as those they *said* they used. Using a variety of data sources from 15 different clinical sites (none were specialist palliative care), three perspectives on information accessibility were identified. Human sources – that is, people – were perceived by nurses to be more accessible than text-based information. Clinical specialization was found to be associated with different approaches to information access and, in coronary care units, nurses were more likely to find local guidelines, protocols and on-line databases to be accessible than colleagues in general medical and surgical wards. Perhaps the most worrying finding was how little of the available text-based evidence had a research base, and how out of date the available textbooks were. In terms of what was *not* useful, no nurses viewed textbooks as a useful resource and equally the role of local information files was not found to be helpful. This was an important finding given that both of these resources were very much in evidence on the wards. More worryingly, perhaps, the internet, on-line databases and other library-based resources, such as the Cochrane Library, were not viewed as having much utility for practice. What emerged clearly from this study was that library skills and support to enable nurses to make the most of the often extensive resources available in each of the sites were seen as poorly developed. Physical access to research information is a significant barrier to research. There are parallels here with the findings relating to obstacles for nurses accessing continuing professional education for nurses, discussed above. Physical access to research information may present problems for specialist palliative care nurses who may not have the same facilities at their disposal as those offered to their counterparts employed in large acute units, attached to university departments.

Developments in the acquisition of research skills

Corner (1999) believes that professionals of all disciplines feel they lack the necessary skills to develop and execute robust research studies that are relevant to practice, and may find it difficult to compete for publication in top journals. In this way, nurses are not alone in finding the development of a research base for practice challenging.

Nurses arguably already possess many strengths and much of the expertise necessary to adopt the lead in practice. In particular, nurses possess the skills and temperament necessary to foster research collaboration, rather than competition (Corner 1999). This is crucial, as partnerships are essential to enable practice to develop (Bailey 1996; Corner 2001). Although the potential benefits of collaborative research partnerships are well established in palliative care, collaboration between health care professionals continues to be exceptional in the wider health care context where it is generally agreed that there needs to be an increase in interdisciplinary research projects.

Traynor and Rafferty (1997) sound a note of caution, however, at the wholesale adoption of a multidisciplinary approach to research, expressing their concern that in adopting a collaborative research framework nursing risked losing its unique identity. However, perhaps more important than the unique identity of nursing, is the contribution that nurses can make to the development of a wider body of health care knowledge through research. In 2003, Rafferty *et al.*, in an editorial in the *British Medical Journal*, reported that nursing receives only 20 per cent of the resources allocated to a national programme in teaching and learning of the Economic and Social Research Council. They observe starkly that without targeted investment, nurses 'will fail to deliver the benefits of evidence based practice' (Rafferty *et al.* 2003: 833).

Nurses have already made great strides in advancing palliative care knowledge in relation to the development of a number of key research approaches (see Chapter 35), but perhaps no more so than in their contribution to qualitative research studies. In a review of the nursing contribution to qualitative research in palliative care between 1990 and 1999, Bailey *et al.* (2002) reviewed critically 138 papers from 50 journals using a tool developed to assess both content and quality; in one part of this tool, reviewers recorded open-ended comments on the strengths and weaknesses of each paper. The authors presented a thematic analysis of reviewers' comments on a sub-group of 67 nursing papers from the main review. These were compared with an analysis of comments on 29 papers from a comparison group of papers from death studies, medical anthropology and sociology journals. Patterns of positive and negative evaluations were identified and used to generate an account of strengths and weaknesses in qualitative palliative care research in nursing. The authors found that nearly half the papers received were judged to be well written or to have a well-chosen topic. However, more than 40 per cent of papers generated negative comments about key methods-related issues. Overall, Bailey *et al.* concluded that over the last 40 years qualitative research in nursing has become an increasingly important focus in providing evidence for practice. It should be noted, however, that qualitative methods are not highly rated in Cochrane Reviews and thus studies employing these types of methodologies from this perspective do not count as 'evidence'. This seriously devalues a significant number of research studies conducted by nurses, which tend to draw heavily on qualitative methods of enquiry.

Arguably, the move of basic and post-basic nurse education into higher education institutions means that nurses are better equipped to conduct more advanced studies into areas of their practice. From an initial faltering start, the number of nurses undertaking doctoral level studies continues to grow (Corner 2001; Ingleton *et al.* 2001) and this is a positive move towards providing an international network of nurses in key positions in practice and academia, though much work remains to be done.

Small-scale nature of studies conducted by nurses in palliative care

Although the need for practice to be based on reliable evidence rather than anecdote has been recognized since the establishment of the modern hospice movement, much of the research undertaken to date has been limited and fragmented, with small-scale, single-centre studies being the norm. Ingleton and Davies delineate some of the explanations for this in Chapter 35. Similarly, much nursing research has been justly criticized as being small-scale, under-funded and locally based. Practitioners are exposed more to palliative care research as the field expands and larger numbers are now engaging in post-registration education, which often means that they undertake their own, small pieces of research (Daniels and Exley 2001). However, the extent to which findings from these small-scale local studies are applicable to policy development is unknown and many remain unpublished. Seymour *et al.* (2003) suggest that synthesizing data from studies with similar aims and designs highlights a methodological approach that may be valuable in palliative care research of this kind. They draw upon data on 37 patients' expectations and experiences of specialist palliative care services, as expressed in in-depth interviews across three evaluative studies of specialist palliative care services in the UK (Seymour *et al.* 2003). This approach provides an exemplar for synthesizing findings from small-scale qualitative studies and provides the possibility of demonstrating their applicability beyond local and specific contexts, while recognizing that caution must be shown in checking that methods of data collection and data analysis are comparable.

Perceived dissonance between academic nursing and clinical practice

A predominant theme in the nursing literature is the dissonance between academic nursing and clinical practice. Some writers have suggested that the gap between the two sectors arises primarily because of the '"idealised" views of nursing held by academic nurses, which seem incompatible with the "messy realities" of the practice world' (Dunn and Yates 2000: 166). The continuing tensions between academic and clinical nursing has resulted in calls to develop models for minimizing these tensions and to enhance links between academic and clinical settings. Establishing joint appointments is one means suggested for addressing the ambivalent relationship that has existed between academic and clinical nursing. The introduction of clinical chairs, which are joint appointments at the professorial level with links to both the academic and clinical settings, is one means by which more active cooperation between stakeholders can be achieved.

Dunn and Yates (2000) conducted a study to describe the roles of Chairs in clinical nursing in Australia. Eight clinical professors were interviewed using semi-structured telephone interviews. The participants highlighted the diversity of arrangements between university and health sector partners in establishing their respective roles. All roles included components of education, research and politics, but the relative contribution of each of these areas, and the viability of the posts, depended to a large extent on the ability of post holders to maintain sustainable income sources and to consolidate outcomes. Dunn and Yates conclude that although not a panacea, clinical professorial appointments do provide, perhaps, one of the best opportunities to bring together the major stakeholders in the nursing community: clinical, academic and professional.

There are others grappling with the same issues surrounding nursing scholarship and bridging the academic–practice divide in the USA (Brown 1995) and Australia (Roberts 1995). Possibilities in promoting scholarship within clinical practice relate not only to the establishment of clinical nursing professoriates as described above, but also the establishment of nursing-dedicated research wards and units, and maintaining the practice links of university-based nursing staff.

There are other models of scholarship emerging in the USA, such as the development of the National Center for Nursing Research, which emphasizes health care and promotion. In the light of continuing emphasis on evidence-based practice and clinical excellence, such a centre might provide an invaluable interface between evidence and practice.

Changes to ethical approval processes for research projects

In many parts of the developed world, policy changes to the ways in which ethical approval is sought are under review. In the UK, professional organizations involved in health care research have now established research ethics committees (first at local level and then at regional level) within the last decade. More recently, new governance frameworks for health and social care research and for research ethics committees (Department of Health 2002) have been developed in which it is made clear that attention to ethical issues are central to the whole research process from commissioning to dissemination (Seymour and Skilbeck 2002). These frameworks set out standards and mechanisms to protect and prioritize the well-being and safety of research participants, while at the same time creating an environment in which high-quality research is nurtured.

While this extra scrutiny can be seen as a positive move to academic excellence and rigorously conducted studies, it does present difficulties for some student projects or small-scale studies. The time-frames for these projects need to be scrutinized to take into consideration any comments or changes required by research ethics committees and research governance frameworks. This may make such projects difficult to complete. Already, additional aspects of research governance, such as the need for project research staff to hold honorary NHS contracts, even when working on projects involving minimal or no actual presence on NHS premises, have added to the difficulties of conducting research in the NHS.

Similar arrangements exist in Australia where the National Health and Medical Research Council (NHMRC) considers the ethical issues associated with research. Organizations in Australia that receive public funds administered by the NHMRC are required to establish another tier in the form of human research ethics committees to review research proposals involving humans. Lee and Kristjanson (2003), writing about human research ethics committees in Australia and the discomfort of the members of these committees who have no experience of palliative care, warn that committees may disallow access to palliative care patients and families as they perceive the notion of conducting research with this group as abhorrent. The authors, reflecting on 20 years' experience of presenting applications to human research ethics committees, call for a less adversarial approach to gaining ethics approval and an acknowledgement of the rights of palliative care patients, families and health care workers to choose to be involved in research.

Arguably, changes to research governance will have major implications for the type of research conducted in the future. Research projects involving staff members/professional groups have been the mainstay of undergraduate nursing and many postgraduate nursing projects. This has been a deliberate strategy to avoid the involvement of patients and to obviate the risk of their 'research fatigue' in research active environments (Watson and Manthorpe 2002). With the new difficulties envisaged in gaining ethical approval, this situation is likely to continue.

Expanding practitioner roles

Expanding practitioner roles to academic teaching and research has markedly changed the nature of nursing work roles and careers. Reflecting this, and writing from an Australian perspective, Roberts (1995) argues that, 'in an ideal world of nursing scholarship, the scholar would be a practitioner, researcher and teacher. The model of integrated scholarship ... [or] all-in-one scholar is a wonderful idea, but requires considerable amounts of support' (p. 218). For specialist nurses working in cancer and palliative care, the recommendation that research should be an integral aspect of their role has been outlined for some time. This may pose challenges and tensions within normal working practices. For example, Daniels and Exley (2001) conducted a small qualitative study with a group of specialist nurses at an independent hospice involved in palliative care research. From the interviews, the most important issue in ensuring the success of the research study were efforts to facilitate collaborative relationships between researchers and practitioners. Daniels and Exley reflect on their experiences and the difficulties they encountered, primarily with regard to obtaining informed consent from patients to take part in the research, and conclude by suggesting guidelines for conducting good quality research in palliative care.

The role of specialist nurses in palliative care

During the past 20 years, there has been a significant expansion in the number of specialist nurses practising in many areas of patient and family care. The designation of 'specialist nurse' is currently conferred on individuals with a wide range of knowledge and skills, with very different roles, remits and titles, and with diverse backgrounds in terms of education preparation. Accompanying this trend is a growing international literature concerned with the specialist nurses in palliative care (Colquhoun and Dougan 1997). As we have seen in Chapter 2, modern specialist palliative care services began earlier and have developed further in the UK than in other parts of Europe (Clark *et al.* 2000). One particular example of this is the number of palliative care clinical nurse specialists working in the UK, particularly those employed with initial support from the UK charity Macmillan Cancer Relief, normally referred to as 'Macmillan nurses' (see also Chapter 36). These posts have been influential in the models of specialist palliative care nursing adopted in other countries.

Macmillan nurse role

Macmillan nurse posts were first developed in the UK in the mid-1970s and have been established in both hospital and community settings. From being introduced as nurses with special responsibility for caring directly for terminally ill people and their families, the role of the Macmillan nurse has changed gradually to that of the clinical nurse specialist in which clinical, consultative, education, research and supportive functions are combined (Seymour *et al.* 2002). This evolution has, in part, occurred in response to the recognition that palliative care is a right for everyone with life-limiting illness. The parallel emergence of professional guidance on the development and definition of specialist nursing roles has been encouraged by wider policy initiatives emphasizing accountability and responsiveness to need.

Caddow (cited in NCHSPCS 1996) suggests a framework for the clinical nurse specialist role that has been widely accepted and adopted by Macmillan nurses. This involves considering the role as having four main elements:

- advice and information;
- consultative visit, preferably with the health care professional who has referred the patient – these are usually single visits unless otherwise requested;

- a short-term series of interventions with a patient or family – the intention is then to withdraw;
- ongoing multiple problem situations requiring continuing intervention and assessment.

Although the work of Macmillan clinical nurse specialists in palliative care is now well established, there has been little research into a number of key areas of the role.

Evaluation of the Macmillan nurse role

The extent to which Macmillan nurses can meet the ideals of specialist practice is little understood, although problems of role clarity and role overload have been linked to clinical nurse specialist posts more generally (Poole 1996; Bamford 2000). As Skilbeck and Seymour (2002) point out, there is little evidence about the character of Macmillan nurses' clinical work with patients; most work has concentrated on specific aspects of their duties, such as work patterns, referral trends, levels of support and stress, or have been small-scale evaluations. The extent to which generic Macmillan nurses are adapting to these new demands was addressed as part of a major evaluation study of UK Macmillan nursing in 12 sites in the Trent and Thames regions of the UK, commissioned by the UK charity Macmillan Cancer Relief. As part of this evaluation, Seymour *et al.* (2002) examined the extent to which Macmillan nurses are adapting to new working practices and procedures brought about by policy initiatives (Department of Health 1999, 2002).

Drawing on data from semi-structured interviews with 44 Macmillan nurses and 47 of their key colleagues, the study found differences of expectation between Macmillan nurses and their managers about the appropriate focus of their work, which led to problems of role ambiguity and role conflict. Moreover, Macmillan nurses were found to lack resources with which to develop an educative and consultative role and that problems existed in co-working with newly appointed cancer site-specific nurses and palliative medicine colleagues (Seymour *et al.* 2002). The authors conclude by pointing to a need to clarify the nature and scope of the Macmillan nurse role, to attend to issues of teamworking and to improve the skills of non-specialist staff in palliative care.

As part of this evaluation and acknowledging that there has been little research into the organizational context in which these nurses operate and the implications for the services they deliver, data were also collected about the Macmillan nursing care mix, nature of interventions and organization of workloads. The results showed a wide variation in the intensity of input into care of individual patients by Macmillan nurses. For the majority of patients, one or two contacts were undertaken with the purpose of resolving a particular problem or need. This variety of input was observed in the context of a caseload in which two-thirds of patients died within 200 days of referral to the services (Skilbeck *et al.* 2002). The evaluation also showed wide variation in organization and management of their practice (Clark *et al.* 2002). It would appear that there is a need to clarify the Macmillan nurse's role to ensure that their expertise is used effectively and efficiently. Other literature highlights the need for clarity over lines of responsibility, strategic planning and adequate resource allocation. These are all essential factors for nurses to accommodate change effectively. Overlaying these elements is the changing landscape of expanding roles and policy directives surrounding nurses' practice. For example, in recent years a range of risk management strategies has been introduced into health care settings in response to growing litigation and a transfer of the associated costs to health care providers. Within this context, nursing is being primed to play a more effective and central role in care delivery by developing new ways of working and promoting quality care through the use of clinical protocols, or care pathways, as a means of delivering evidence-based practice. The final section of this overview will explore the ways in which care pathways are being used and whether they offer the potential to improve palliative care delivery for patients and families.

Clinical protocols/integrated care pathways

The development and use of clinical protocols, or integrated care pathways (ICPs) as they have come to be known, has attracted substantial research interest. There appear to be three main reasons for the drive to develop these protocols: risk management, the speedier integration of research into practice and the standardization of practice to provide a more cost-effective and efficient health care system (Lawton and Parker 1999).

Widely accepted and used in the North American health care system, ICPs are increasingly being used in the UK. In the USA, advocates of pathways have placed them within an overall strategy for managed care, arguing that they result in resource efficiency while *maintaining* quality and managing costs. In the UK, rather than emphasizing the resource efficiency aspect, pathways are seen as a tool to implement clinical governance (see Chapters 37 and 38), which aim to *improve* the quality of care and ensure that clinical care is based on the latest research evidence (de Luc 2000).

Sometimes referred to as 'care maps', 'critical paths of care' or 'anticipated recovery paths', ICPs document any changes to the expected course of events through a variance sheet (Fowell *et al.* 2002). Riley describes the integrated care pathway as fulfilling the following functions:

> determines locally agreed multi-disciplinary practice, based on guidelines and evidence where available, for a specific patient client group. It forms all or part of the clinical record, documents the care given and facilitates the evaluation of outcomes of continuous quality monitoring.
> (Riley 1998: 2)

Lawton and Parker (1999) conducted a study to investigate the perceptions of doctors, nurses, midwives and health service managers towards the proposed development and implementation of clinical protocols. Twenty-four focus groups were convened across three hospitals in the UK. The effect of 'proceduralization' on professional autonomy and on the working relationships among professional groups emerged as an important theme. Importantly, the study revealed that successful implementation of protocols/guidelines depends on achieving the right balance between standardizing practice and allowing professionals to use clinical judgement.

De Luc (2000) reported on a quasi-experimental case study of two care pathways developed within one NHS Trust. In this study, de Luc makes a comparison of clinical care delivered before and after the introduction of the two pathways and the views of staff involved in the development and operation of the two pathways. Overall, the conclusions from this study are mixed. The findings suggest that the development aspects of pathways offer the easiest and most immediate route for change, including the development of multidisciplinary teamworking, design of clinical documentation and updating of clinical practice. The author points out that a considerable ongoing commitment of time and effort is required in the operation of pathways once implemented to engender a culture of continuous monitoring and comparing the standards of care provided. While these elements are ascribed to by many advocates of ICPs, they are rarely reflected in the increasing descriptive literature on pathways.

In the context of palliative care, Ellershaw *et al.* (1997) has piloted an ICP for the last 2 days of life and much of the developments since have been based on a variant of this influential work. Building on this work, Fowell *et al.* (2002) report on a pilot study to introduce a Wales-wide implementation of an ICP for the last 2 days of life. This occurred in four different care settings crossing the voluntary and statutory sectors. They found that initial analysis of 500 variance sheets generated by the ICP for the last 2 days of life indicate that the management of pain, agitation, excess respiratory secretions and mouth care may be problematic. However, while presenting an optimistic view of the use of ICPs, Fowell and colleagues acknowledge that further development work is needed on the variance sheet as a potential tool for the collection of data, as well as the need to establish inter-rater reliability across care settings.

In the USA, care pathways have been developed for hospice patients who die within one week of admission (Peterson and Hartman 2000). The problem here is that it is difficult to predict with any degree of accuracy when people are in their last week of life.

More generally, however, few evaluations have looked at either costs of development and implementation or, importantly, the efficacy of care pathways in changing practice and improving outcomes (Campbell *et al.* 1998). The need for systematic evaluations to measure the effectiveness of pathways has been cited by many writers in the international literature (e.g. Ebener *et al.* 1996).

In the context of palliative care, critics of ICPs suggest that, left unchecked, there is a danger that the 'process of dying' may be reduced to a number of flow diagrams (algorithms as they were called in some palliative care journals) and a series of boxes ticked by professional carers instead of recognizing the importance of spontaneity and creativity in palliative care (Kelly 2003). Importantly, the question still remains as to whether the introduction of pathways results in the benefits ascribed to them by their supporters and whether they warrant investment in time and resources to develop them.

Ultimately, though, for ICPs to be successfully introduced into palliative care settings, an integrated multi-professional approach and an open, flexible and participative culture is required. Otherwise, they may be viewed as a 'paper exercise' and merely another type of clinical audit tool; an approach to care that does not seem to resonate with philosophical statements about the individuality of patient needs.

In the remainder of this chapter, we introduce the eight chapters that form the final section of the book. The chapters are wide-ranging in character and set out contemporary issues in the fast-changing field of palliative care.

Overview of chapters in Part Four

Multi-professional working is said to be a key component of effective palliative care and it is generally recognized that the complex needs of patients and their families can best be met by a well-coordinated team of various professionals. In Chapter 31, Cox and James explore the concepts of boundaries, roles and teamworking within which palliative care is delivered. They detail how, over the last 30 years, the palliative care team has changed considerably in both its constitution and complexity. These changes have stemmed, in part, from patients' and families' increasingly high expectations of health care provision, in terms of power sharing, improved information giving, increased choice and better patient-centred care. However, the authors make the very salient point that these expectations will continue to be mediated by the fundamental need for human warmth and attention at times of vulnerability, when the needs for support and the potential desires to opt out by adopting a 'sick role' may be heightened.

As palliative care professionals are asked to respond to demands to extend their work beyond a focus on cancer, it follows that there is either a need to spread the effort further with few additional resources, or that there is a need to pay greater attention to the allocation of resources to those most in need, however these needs may be defined. Either way, this can add increasing pressure and stress to the daily work of palliative care professionals. While occupational stress and 'burnout' are common phenomena across health care settings, and are certainly not unique to palliative care, there are some characteristics of palliative care as a speciality that require specific attention. While acknowledging the significant work undertaken on occupational stress and burnout in palliative care, Aranda's chapter on occupational stress and coping strategies departs from influential work (most notably by Vachon) by exploring the relationship between the underlying philosophy of palliative care, what counts as 'stressful' and the meaning of this for nursing work in palliative care. Understanding how we perceive stress is critical to how the subject is approached. Aranda suggests that stress occurs at points of dissonance between the beliefs and values of the individual and their capacity to deliver care according to those values. The absence of a strong evidence base for preventing and managing the impact of this dissonance means that specialist palliative care services need to foster a flexible and varied approach to the provision of support in the workplace. Encouraging nurses to identify their personal approach to stress should be regarded as an overt part of professional development.

In Chapter 33, Sneddon focuses on education to prepare practitioners for a specialist role in palliative care, drawing on contemporary experience as a provider of multi-professional education in the UK and comparing experiences from other disciplines and contexts. She makes the point that palliative care has expanded greatly in the past 10 years, but not always in a coordinated way. In doing so, she suggests that it is timely to reflect on the future learning needs of professionals specializing in palliative care. However, Sneddon cautions educators to ensure that the education process mirrors the caring philosophy of palliative care. She calls for the skilful management of interpersonal learning opportunities, development of interpersonal skills and the use of creative learning and teaching strategies that reflect reality, in the delivery of specialist education in palliative care.

The use of creative learning and teaching strategies is the subject of Chapter 34 by Ahmedzai, who explores the current role and future scope of information and communications technology (ICT) in nursing as a vehicle for offering flexible education and professional development. Ahmedzai also looks at the role of information and communications technology in management, clinical practice and the nurse–patient interface. Ahmedzai quite rightly gives prominence to the use of ICT vehicles and their possible uses in specialist palliative care. The wide-ranging annotated description of current websites provided will be of relevance to a multi-professional palliative care audience. Ahmedzai concludes by reminding us of the speed at which communications technology is progressing, the massive impact it is having on all parts of health care and the concomitant challenges wrought by these developments, not least where the variability in quality ranks as the number one criticism.

The development of a wide-ranging and multidisciplinary programme of palliative care research is crucial to a more evidence-based approach to care. Within the broad field of palliative care, nursing is beginning to emerge as an important focus. In Chapter 35, Ingleton and Davies consider the relationship between scholarship, research and practice within palliative care. Although they concede there is still a long way to go, Ingleton and Davies conclude that nurses are making a growing contribution to the wider palliative care research community in terms of publications in international academic and professional journals and presentations at international conferences.

Looking to the future, joint ventures between clinical and academic centres and the establishment of designated research and practice units offer the opportunity to reduce the much discussed theory–practice gap. Such ventures are the focus of Chapter 36 by Froggatt and Booth. The authors present an account of expert nursing and its development through research and development in the context of palliative care. They draw on programmes of work undertaken when they were leaders of two national Macmillan Practice Development Units based in the UK. They illuminate practical examples of ways in which expert nurses in palliative care have been supported, drawing attention to a number of challenges to developing expert palliative care. While they do not dispute the need to have a sound basis for the decisions made about the treatment and care delivered within health care, they go on to suggest that an evidence-based practice approach can be constraining. Arguing that the evidence based-practice movement has narrowly defined the meaning of 'valid' evidence, they suggest it also places the highest confidence in only one type of evidence – that obtained through the conduct of randomized controlled trials.

Very few services escape the attention of resource management, clinical audit and clinical governance; specialist palliative care is no exception. The final two chapters of this part of the book deal with the interrelated issues of policy, audit and management within palliative care services. The authors of each of the two remaining chapters tackle these issues from the viewpoint of national policy and management. Barker and Hawkett outline contemporary UK government policy, making links to audit, evaluation and clinical governance. Drawing on her current work at the Department of Health, Hawkett considers the connections between policy and clinical practice and offers pragmatic suggestions about how clinical nurses might influence the policy-making process. Policy making is, of course, always an imprecise empirical process (Clark *et al.* 1997) and policy outcomes are necessarily complex, often difficult to forecast and subject to a plethora of influences, both predictable and unpredictable. As Barker and Hawkett show here, the extent to which palliative care providers can engage with, and influence, policy makers will be a crucial factor in shaping the future direction and form of palliative care. They delineate some of the difficulties in assessing quality in specialist palliative care and provide some clarity on how we variously define such potentially confusing terms as clinical governance, clinical audit and quality assurance and, importantly, what these mechanisms mean for specialist palliative care services. Inevitably, the need to adapt to an environment of greater scrutiny and performance review has driven palliative care providers to develop more robust and responsive strategies for effectively managing their teams.

In the final chapter, Hopkins picks up some of the themes introduced by Barker and Hawkett. He presents a model for leading and managing nursing teams, within the constraints of a changing policy environment. The model is derived from a review of nursing and human resource management literature, and from an empirical study undertaken by the author in a UK voluntary sector specialist hospice. The study, using a mixed-methods approach to data collection and a grounded theory approach to data analysis, produces aggregated themes that form the basis of a model of nursing leadership and management. Hopkins's model focuses on five components of nursing management as the key activities in improving the quality of nursing care delivered.

Notes

1 AP(E)L is the accepted way of referring to appropriate prior learning (APL) and appropriate prior experiential learning (APEL).
2 Hospice Information Service (2002) *Minimum Data Sets National Survey 1999–2000* (www.hospiceinformation.co.uk): accessed 16 October 2002.

References

Atack, L. and Rankin, J. (2002) A descriptive study of registered nurses: experiences with web-based learning. *Journal of Advanced Nursing*, 37(6): 506–11.

Bailey, C. (1996) Ethical issues in multi-centre collaborative research on breathlessness in lung cancer. *International Journal of Palliative Nursing*, 2(2): 95–101.

Bailey, C., Froggatt, K., Field, D. and Krishnasamy, M. (2002) The nursing contribution to qualitative research in palliative care 1990–1999: a critical evaluation. *Journal of Advanced Nursing*, 40(1): 48–60.

Bamford, J. (2000) The clinical nurse specialist: perceptions of practicing CNSs of their role and development needs. *Journal of Clinical Nursing*, 9: 282–92.

Billings, D.M. and Rowles, C.J. (2001) Development of continuing nursing education offering for the World Wide Web. *Journal of Continuing Education in Nursing*, 32: 107–12.

Blunden, G. and Langton, H. (2001) Professional education for the cancer care nurse in England and Wales: a review of the evidence base. *European Journal of Cancer Care*, 10: 179–82.

Brown, R. (1995) *Portfolio Development and Profiling for Nurses*. Salisbury: Quay Books.

Campbell, H., Hotchkiss, R., Bradshaw, N. and Porteous, M. (1998) Education and debate: integrated care pathways. *British Medical Journal*, 316: 133–7.

Canadian Nurses Association (1997) *The Future Supply of Nursing*. Toronto, ONT: Canadian Nurses Association.

Clark, D., Hockley, J. and Ahmedzai, S. (eds) (1997) *New Themes in Palliative Care*. Buckingham: Open University Press.

Clark, D., Ingleton, C. and Seymour, J. (2000) Support and supervision in palliative care research. *Palliative Medicine*, 14: 441–6.

Clark, D., Seymour, J., Douglas, H.R. *et al.* (2002) Clinical nurse specialist in palliative care. Part 2. Explaining diversity in the organisation and costs of Macmillan nursing services. *Palliative Medicine*, 16: 375–85.

Colquhoun, M. and Dougan, H. (1997) Performance standards: ensuring that the specialist nurse in palliative care is special. *Palliative Medicine*, 11: 381–7.

Cooper, H., Carlisle, C., Gibbs, T. and Watkins, C. (2001) Developing an evidence base for interdisciplinary learning: a systematic review. *Journal of Advanced Nursing*, 35(2): 228–37.

Copp, G. (1994) Palliative care nursing education: a review of research findings. *Journal of Advanced Nursing*, 19: 552–7.

Corner, J. (1999) Developing practice in palliative care. *International Journal of Palliative Nursing*, 5(4): 84–7.

Corner, J. (2001) Research and cancer care, in J. Corner and C. Bailey (eds) *Cancer Nursing Care in Context*. Oxford: Blackwell Science.

Daniels, L. and Exley, C. (2001) Preparation, information and liaison: conducting successful research in palliative care. *International Journal of Palliative Nursing*, 7(4): 192–7.

De Luc, K. (2000) Care pathways: an evaluation of their effectiveness. *Journal of Advanced Nursing*, 32(2): 485–96.

Department of Health (1999) *Making a Difference*. London: HMSO.

Department of Health (2002) *Research Governance Framework for Health and Social Care*. London: HMSO.

Dowell, L. (2002) Multiprofessional palliative care in a general hospital: education and training needs. *International Journal of Palliative Nursing*, 8(6): 294–303.

Dunn, S. and Yates, P. (2000) The role of Australian chairs in clinical nursing. *Journal of Advanced Nursing*, 31(1): 165–71.

Ebener, M., Baugh, K. and Formella, N. (1996) Proving that less is more: linking resources to outcomes. *Journal of Nursing Care Quality*, 10: 1–9.

Ellershaw, J., Foster, A., Murphy, D., Shea, T. and Overill, S. (1997) Developing an integrated care pathway for the dying patient. *European Journal of Palliative Care*, 4(6): 203–7.

Farrell, M.J. (1998) National palliative care education and training needs analysis. *Contemporary Nurse*, 7(2): 60–7.

Ferrall, B., Virani, R. and Grant, M. (1999) Analysis of end of life content in nursing textbooks. *Oncology Forum*, 26: 869–76.

Field, D. (1984) Formal instruction in United Kingdom medical schools about death and dying. *Medical Education*, 18: 429–34.

Field, D. and Kitson, A. (1986) Formal teaching about death and dying in UK nursing schools. *Nurse Education Today*, 6(6): 270–6.

Fowell, A., Finlay, I., Johnstone, R. and Minto, L. (2002) An integrated care pathway for the last two days of life: Wales-wide benchmarking in palliative care. *International Journal of Palliative Nursing*, 8(12): 566–73.

Froggatt, K.A. (2000) Evaluating a palliative care education project in nursing homes. *International Journal of Palliative Nursing*, 6(3): 140–6.

Frost, M. (1996) An analysis of the scope and value of problem-based learning in the education of health care professionals. *Journal of Advanced Nursing*, 24: 1047–53.

Hammick, M. (1998) Interprofessional education: concept, theory and application. *Journal of Interprofessional Care*, 12: 323–32.

Hargreaves, J. (1996) Credit where credit's due – work based learning in professional practice. *Journal of Clinical Nursing*, 5: 165–9.

Ingleton, C., Ramcharan, P., Ellis, L. and Schofield, P. (2001) Introducing a professional doctorate in nursing and midwifery. *British Journal of Nursing*, 10(22): 36–41.

Kelly, D. (2003) A commentary on 'An integrated care pathway for the last two days of life'. *International Journal of Palliative Nursing*, 9(1): 39.

Kenny, L. (2001) Education in palliative care: making a difference to practice. *International Journal of Palliative Care*, 7(8): 401–7.

Lawton, R. and Parker, D. (1999) Procedures and the professional: the case of the British NHS. *Social Science and Medicine*, 48: 353–61.

Lee, S. and Kristjanson, L. (2003) Human research ethics committees: issues in palliative care research. *International Journal of Palliative Nursing*, 9(1): 13–19.

Lee, W.S., Cholowski, K. and Williams, A.K. (2002) Nursing students' and clinical educators' perceptions of characteristics of effective clinical educators in an Australian university school of nursing. *Journal of Advanced Nursing*, 39(5): 412–20.

Little, P. and Ryan, G. (1998) Educational change through problem based learning. *Australian Journal of Advanced Nursing*, 5: 31–5.

Lloyd-Williams, M. and Field, D. (2002) Are undergraduate nurses taught palliative care during their training? *Nurse Education Today*, 22: 589–92.

Macleod, R.D. and James, C.R. (1994) *Teaching Palliative Care: Issues and Implications*. London: Cornwall Patten Press.

Macleod, R.D. and James, C.R. (1997) Improving the effectiveness of palliative care education. *Palliative Medicine*, 11: 375–80.

Morales-Mann, E. and Kaitell, C. (2001) Problem based learning in a new Canadian curriculum. *Journal of Advanced Nursing*, 33(1): 13–19.

National Council for Hospice and Specialist Palliative Care Services (1996) *Palliative Care in the Hospital Setting*. London: NCHSPCS.

National Council for Hospice and Specialist Palliative Care Services (2002) *Draft National Plan and Strategic Framework for Palliative Care: 2000–2005*. London: NCHSPCS.

Peterson, J. and Hartman, H. (2000) A pathway for patients who die within a week of hospice admission. *International Journal of Palliative Nursing*, 6(1): 39–45.

Poole, K. (1996) The evolving role of the clinical nurse specialist within the comprehensive breast care centre. *Journal of Clinical Nurse*, 5: 341–9.

Proctor, M., Grealish, L., Coats, M. and Sears, P. (2000) Nurses' knowledge of palliative care in the Australian Capital Territory. *International Journal of Palliative Nursing*, 6(9): 421–8.

Quint, J.C. (1967) *The Nurse and the Dying Patient*. New York: Macmillan.

Rafferty, A.M., Traynor, M., Thompson, D.R., Ilott, I. and White, E. (2003) Research in nursing, midwifery and the allied health professions. *British Medical Journal*, 326: 833–4.

Redman, S., White, K., Ryan, E. and Hennrikus, D. (1995) Professional needs of palliative care nurses in New South Wales. *Palliative Medicine*, 9: 36–44.

Riley, K. (1998) Definition of care pathways. *National Pathway Association Autumn Newsletter*, 2.

Roberts, K.L. (1995) Theoretical, clinical, research scholarship: connections and distinctions, in G. Gray and R. Pratt (eds) *Scholarship in the Discipline of Nursing*, Melbourne, VIC: Churchill Livingstone.

Ross, M., McDonald, B. and McGuiness, J. (1996) The palliative care quiz for nursing (PCQN): the development of an instrument to measure nurses' knowledge of palliative care. *Journal of Advanced Nursing*, 23: 126–37.

Sellick, S.M., Charles, K., Dagsvig, J. and Kelley, M.L. (1996) Palliative care providers' perspectives on service and education needs. *Journal of Palliative Care*, 12(2): 34–8.

Seymour, J. and Skilbeck, J. (2002) Ethical considerations in research user views. *European Journal of Cancer Care*, 11: 215–19.

Seymour, J., Clark, D., Hughes, P. *et al.* (2002) Clinical nurse specialists in palliative care, Part 3: issues for the Macmillan nurse role. *Palliative Medicine*, 16: 386–94.

Seymour, J., Ingleton, C., Payne, S. and Beddow, V. (2003) Specialist palliative care: Patients' experiences. *Journal of Advanced Nursing*, 44(1): 24–33.

Sheldon, F. and Smith, P. (1996) Life so short, the craft so hard to learn: a model for post-basic education in palliative care. *Palliative Medicine*, 10: 99–104.

Skilbeck, J. and Seymour, J. (2002) Meeting complex needs: an analysis of Macmillan nurses' work with patients. *International Journal of Palliative Nursing*, 8(12): 574–82.

Skilbeck, J., Corner, J., Bath, P. *et al.* (2002) Clinical nurse specialists in palliative care, Part 1: a description of the Macmillan case load. *Palliative Medicine*, 16: 285–96.

Thompson, C., McCaughan, D., Cullum, N. *et al.* (2001) Research information in nurses' clinical decision making: what is useful? *Journal of Advanced Nursing*, 36(3): 376–88.

Traynor, M. and Rafferty, A.M. (1997) *The NHS R&D Context of Nursing Research: A Working Paper*. London: Centre for Policy in Nursing Research, School of Hygiene and Tropical Medicine, University of London.

United Kingdom Central Council for Nursing, Midwifery and Health Visiting (1987) *The Scope of Professional Practice*. London: UKCC.

United Kingdom Central Council for Nursing, Midwifery and Health Visiting (1994) *The Future of Professional Practice: The Council's Standards for Education and Practice Following Registration*. London: UKCC.

Vernon, D. and Blake, R. (1993) Does problem-based learning work? A meta-analysis of evaluative research. *Academic Medicine*, 68: 550–63.

Washer, P. (2001) Barriers to the use of web-based learning in nurse education. *Nurse Education Today*, 21: 455–60.

Watson, R. and Manthorpe, J. (2002) Research governance: for whose benefit? (editorial). *Journal of Advanced Nursing*, 39(6): 515–16.

Yates, P., Clinton, M. and Hart, G. (1996) Improving psycho-social care: a professional development programme. *International Journal of Palliative Nursing*, 2(4): 212–16.

31

Professional boundaries in palliative care

Karen Cox and Veronica James

A boundary is a demarcation of some kind. Specialist palliative care is a small but important area in the growing complexity of bounded, community and acute care provision. It is an area which, with the patient and family seen as a whole unit, prides itself on the delivery of care through multidisciplinary teamwork. Thus, from the beginning, a tension arises. Patients and families want us to see them as a whole, and work in collaboration with them to meet a range of changing physical, psychological and domestic needs. They also want us to work with each other, seamlessly across the boundaries of general services and specialisms, acute and community, professions and organizations, without bands of fragmented specialists marching up the path. There is a danger that, despite a notion of teamwork, organizational fragmentation overrides the core purposes of palliative care – the central work with patients, or users, and families. Obviously, there must be considerable numbers of people, often working part-time, involved in running any 24-hour service efficiently and effectively. Yet the greater the number and types of professions and occupations, the greater the demarcations – and the greater the need for a team approach. So how should lay and professional expertise, community and in-patient organizations, and curative and palliative care intersect to focus on the family as the unit of care?

In this chapter, we explore the concepts of boundaries, roles and teamworking within which palliative care is delivered. We first consider the definitions of team and teamwork. Both these terms conjure up images of positive working relationships and a shared common goal. However, teams are complex and the work of the team in palliative care needs to be centrally concerned with the patient (or user) and family as key team players, albeit with a variable interest in decision making. Other members of the team, affected by funding, political and organizational agendas, contribute within the context of committed professional and occupational teams, intra- and inter-team boundaries, and external influences. We explore these issues further by considering the palliative care team within the overall perspective of patient and carer involvement in health and palliative care, taking account of new ideas of 'teams', their leadership and coordination.

Background

Over the last 30 years, the palliative care team has changed considerably. Traditionally, the focus of care delivery was within the setting of the hospice, which meant that the professionals involved worked in close proximity and were bounded by the physical space within which they worked. In addition, the nature of health care delivery at that time with its medical domination meant that the health care professionals involved, such as nurses and doctors, had fairly well-defined roles and responsibilities. This combination of a relatively clear demarcation between the contribution made by each of the team members and the physical boundary of the hospice meant that the palliative care team was relatively easily defined and understood. There are now, however, a multiplicity of palliative care settings and changing roles within the palliative care team. The relatively straightforward concept of health care provision (institution-based care led by medical staff) has shifted with the growth of broader-based public provision to a complex pattern of interrelated services (Payne 2000). Specialist teams for palliative care now do not simply reside in hospice settings. They can be found in acute and community settings, in public and private care. Teams work across disciplinary divides and institutional boundaries and need to be able to liaise effectively between a range of health and social care agencies (Clark and Seymour 1999). Similarly, shifts have occurred in relation to the roles and responsibilities of team members. Nursing in particular has undergone an enormous shift in terms of extended and advanced nursing roles and nurses are taking on tasks that were previously the preserve of their medical colleagues. Patients, users, consumers; family, lay and informal carers; inequality, difference; ethnic minorities, cultural diversity, cultural competence – these changes in terminology tell us something of the shifts that have occurred regarding role boundaries and the place of the patient as a team member since the modern hospice movement began in the 1960s. While variations in patient choice and involvement have always occurred as the result of different health insurance, funding and organizational systems, new movements to involve patients (Gillespie *et al.* 2002) mean that palliative care providers will want to look outward to broader health contexts, to see what patients and carers will be bringing with them to palliative care. The palliative care team of today is, therefore, a transformed and diverse entity.

The established view of teams and teamwork in palliative care

Palliative care teams are an interesting example of teamwork in the health care system. The National Council for Hospices and Specialist Palliative Care Services (NCHSPCS 1995) suggests that teamwork is a key element of specialist palliative care services. The current trend towards interdisciplinary teamworking and collaboration has been identified as a particular strength of specialist palliative care services, with hospice teams being described as good examples of inter-professional work (Ajemian 1993). Inter-professional work in this instance refers to people with distinct disciplinary training within the health service working together for a common purpose, as they make different, complementary contributions to patient-focused care (Leathard 1994). Furthermore, writers in this area also note that teamworking in palliative care is essential, as it provides mutual support in what can be emotionally draining work (in relation to caring for the dying) (Vachon 1987; Field 1989), as well as promoting enhanced clinical standards by facilitating exchange of knowledge, ideas and experience (Woof *et al.* 1998).

The established view of the palliative care team is invariably presented as a list of health and social care professionals from statutory and non-statutory services. Pick up any palliative care textbook and it will talk about team members and their roles, providing lists of professionals and their potential input to the team (Corr and Corr 1983; Hull *et al.* 1989; Dunlop and Hockley 1990; Saunders 1990; Clark *et al.* 1997; Faull 1998). Faull (1998), for example, provides a list of professionals and identifies 'who does what'. This description of roles includes health care-based services, such as medical roles (general practitioner, palliative care physician, hospital consultants), nursing roles (district nurse, specialist palliative care nurse, Marie Curie nurse, practice nurse, other nursing specialities), pharmacist, physiotherapist, occupational therapist, social worker, counsellor, clinical psychologist and dietician. Social services-based roles include home help, meals on wheels and voluntary organizations. Other services include private agencies, spiritual advisors and complementary therapists, in addition to the proliferation of services such as art, music and pets for health. Other authors (e.g. Hull *et al.* 1989; Ingham and Coyle 1997) use diagrammatic representations to convey the vast array of professionals involved in palliative care teams. These tend to be presented in a circular fashion, presumably to get away from the idea of any hierarchy, with the patient and family in the centre.

As can be seen from the *UK Hospice Information Directory 2002*,[1] not only are there national level teams of hospice leaders (for Africa, Australasia, Europe, North America) and hospice administration, fund-raising and management teams, but those delivering direct services have also divided into multiple, separate teams within the hospice system. These teams have drawn on an increasing range of medical and social care specialists from broader health and social care services with the effect that there is now no such thing as a 'standard' team.

While the lists and diagrams many textbook authors devise to represent these teams are useful for the reader who requires an insight into the variety of potential roles in palliative care and an outline of their area of expertise, they leave us asking a number of questions. There are two main ones that we will concentrate on in this chapter. First, these lists identify a huge number of people potentially involved and one has to question if the resulting combination actually amounts to a palliative care 'team' or simply denotes a loose grouping drawn from the multitude of specialist areas available within the NHS, social services and beyond, who may contribute to the care of any particular patient and their family. In addition, only limited reference is made to how professionals may or may not interact with each other or different agencies. Thus there is little attention given to issues such as ambiguity, overlap and conflict of roles, communication difficulties and leadership issues. Second, where is the patient in all this? The 'team', as presented in these texts, is invariably health care dominated, with little reference being made to the users of services playing a real part in the team even though they are now habitually claimed to be 'central' to the palliative care philosophy.

Limitations of the established view of palliative care teams

The absence of any critique of the development of palliative care teams could be attributed to what Dunlop (1998) refers to as a 'culture of niceness', which has been identified in particular with regard to voluntary hospices, as well as a natural reluctance on the part of the professionals within a team to expose their vulnerabilities. In effect, what we are left with is a limited understanding of the dynamics that are at play in specialist palliative care teams. This is not to criticize those who have attempted to outline the various roles involved in delivering palliative care services. Rather, it is an attempt to draw attention to the limitations of such analyses and identify the complexity of teams and the plethora of agencies and professionals involved in the delivery of this particular aspect of health care. It is to raise the question of what, in this context, does teamwork actually mean? To explore this question further, we need to refer to some of the theory on teams, team development and teamwork by social scientists and management theorists.

Theories of teams and teamwork

More people than ever will find themselves working in a team and health care workers are no exception (Dechant *et al.* 1993). Indeed, many health service providers have embraced team-based organization in an attempt to create new modes of delivery (Manion *et al.* 1996). It is important, then, that we understand how teams grow and develop and the contributions that are required from individual team members for this to happen (Dechant *et al.*

1993). However, defining 'teamwork' is not straightforward. The meanings of 'team' and 'teamwork' are controversial (Payne 2000) and there is little empirical evidence of what is effective teamwork (Opie 1997). A team is often defined as a group of people with diverse but related skills and knowledge who associate for the purpose of directing, coordinating and developing the separate parts as well as the sum total of their expertise (Pritchard and Pritchard 1994). In health care contexts, teamworking is often portrayed as a way to tackle the potential fragmentation of care, a means to widen skills and an essential part of the complexity of modern care (Firth-Cozens 1998). However, while the terms themselves may conjure up images of positive working relationships and a shared common goal, there is more to building an effective team than simply putting together a group of people (Zollo 1999).

Understanding teamwork and how it operates in health care delivery is complex. Health care teams have to contend with what Payne (2000) identifies as three paradoxes common to all types of teamwork. First, in the building of team relationships we may become more inward looking and yet, in care services, it is often also essential to build relationships with professionals in other agencies and teams. This is a common feature of many palliative care teams which have to look beyond their 'core' of staff to provide a comprehensive service for patients. Second, members of a team often value it for the mutual support it offers in the face of the institutional demands placed upon them, yet managers see teamwork as an instrument for carrying out the organization's objectives. Here again this can be seen as an issue grappled with by many palliative care teams who work in a stressful and demanding world and who often need to find support in like-minded colleagues. Finally, Payne (2000) suggests that teamwork forces us to think about our interactions with colleagues and yet, in the current health care climate, teams and the services they deliver should be responsive to users' needs. Again we can draw parallels with palliative care teams in that the focus on teams and writing about teams comes from a professional perspective, with professionals talking about other professionals in the team with limited reference to the users' perspective of the team and its workings. These three paradoxes mean that teamwork in health care settings is not straightforward, as teams are often struggling with the tensions between their own needs and the needs of the organizations and consumers whom they are supposed to serve.

Teams in health care have been predicated on a division of labour in terms of complex tasks. They are made up of individuals who have their own area of expertise, traditions, professional interests, working practices and professional regulatory requirements. Not only are teams made up of multiple professions, individuals with their own experiences, agendas and ambitions, but they also function within a global organizational culture, which demands more for the health dollar. This places increasing demands upon teams in terms of efficiency and effectiveness and, as it is politically driven, often operate on a short-term quick-paced agenda. Miller *et al.* (2001), in their study of inter-professional and occupational practice in health and social care, identify organizational issues that influence teamworking. These are: dependence on and response to recent government policies, the importance of team-orientated structures and processes, the diversity of patient populations, and the opportunities for the team to work closely. With the growth in the number of diseases being brought under the palliative care umbrella (HIV/AIDS, respiratory, renal, heart disease), it is little wonder that teams, while often being seen as a positive part of the work of health care delivery, can also be a source of angst and stress. Helping a team to develop and understand what is influencing it and how to overcome conflict is vital if a team is to survive. Palliative care teams need to be aware of the many pressures that have shaped the way they have developed and continue to shape the way they deliver services. Understanding how teams develop over time is crucial to this process.

In relation to clearly bounded teams, there are two main views about how teams develop: developmental and situational. Developmental views argue that teams go through a process of building up towards being a team. There are two versions of this view. The first, expressed by Brill (1976), holds that a group naturally develops and ends up as a team and that the team-builder's work is to speed it on its way. The second is that team development requires team-building to help overcome the barriers to effective teamworking (Shaw 1994). Probably the most cited and well-known developmental view is based on Tuckman's (1965) review of over 50 published papers on group development. He noted that groups go through four stages: forming (getting together), storming (rebellion and establishing roles), norming (agreement over the group work) and performing (getting on with the work) when they come together. Tuckman is careful to note that not all groups work through all of the stages, and not all of the stages the necessarily completed one after the other and in that order. Similarly, caution must be used when attempting to apply his findings in the real world of teamwork. The studies he reviewed were largely based on laboratory studies of small groups, as opposed to teams that had been together on a longer-term basis, had real tasks to deal with and were part of an organization with its own distinct imposed structures and responsibilities.

Situational views (in contrast to developmental views) suggest that different kinds of teams and teamwork are appropriate to different situations in which teams are placed. Team-building in this view requires an understanding of the factors that the team face and involves designing a plan of action, taking into account members' preferences, the type of work and the organization (Burrell and Lindström 1987). Situational views see team-building as responding to and improving work environments.

Building teams and teamwork in palliative care

In many respects, elements of both approaches are necessary if we are to build teams to work in health care settings because of the demands of service delivery and the range of different disciplines, backgrounds and organizations involved. Payne (2000) presents an interesting alternative to the models of team development and teamworking set out above but which contains elements of both. He argues for open teamwork, which combines the established view of teamwork with the concept of networking. Payne suggests that teams cannot just be about interpersonal relations between professionals working together, but require team members to reach out towards community, user and wider professional networks and to understand the contexts within which they are working. This concept of teamworking maps nicely onto palliative care where a core team may be required to interact with other teams, individuals and organizations in the course of its work. We will return to this later.

Teamwork is also affected by members' roles and the way in which members interact with each other (interpersonal relations). Early research in this area typically concerned the role of individual team members as opposed to how they interacted with each other. For example, Benne and Skeats (1948) refer to three types of group member: those who help the group to achieve its task, those who develop group cohesion and those concerned with personal needs. Later work focused on the effect of different personality types or behaviours on the functioning of the team (Brill 1976).

A major advance in the understanding of member roles within a team came in the early 1980s. Based on research among management teams, Belbin (1981) identified eight roles that were necessary for a successful team (company worker, chair, shaper, plant, resource investigator, monitor evaluator, teamworker, completer-finisher). Belbin suggested that a successful team will have all or most of these eight roles within it and that, if significant roles are missing, the team will not function well. Most people, however, have both main and secondary roles and, therefore, can contribute in multiple ways. Which roles they take on depends on other skills in the team (Payne 2000). Although Belbin's work has been highly influential, there are a number of cautions which must be applied. First, people are not always consistent and the roles they take on may change. Second, Belbin's model suggests that only changing team membership achieves the desired roles, and thus does not offer an intervention that can help an existing team make progress (Clark 1994). More recent work has focused on skills and competencies as the primary issues affecting the functioning of the team and refers to styles of the team members, such as contributors, collaborators, communicators and challengers (Parker 1990; Spencer and Pruss 1992; Margerison and McCann 1995). These kinds of role preferences are possibly more helpful than Belbin's team roles when considering the issue of teamwork in palliative care, where the team may be made up not only of individuals who work and meet together on a daily basis, but may also contain elements of distant working across organizational and professional boundaries. It may be useful for readers to consider their own teams in this way and note which role preferences they take on as well as considering their colleagues. Understanding where one another is coming from and how to use the strengths of individual team members in particular circumstances can make for a more effective and responsive team.

Another issue facing palliative care teams is the changing nature of health care professional roles. Contributions within a team are often shaped by how people see themselves within the team and where they locate the team's and their own boundary. For those involved in palliative care, the changing place and pace of care delivery, the increasingly vast array of individuals involved, and the changing roles and boundaries of health care professionals, mean that roles within the team are constantly changing. The place of the physician as the leader of the team is shifting and the rise of consumerism has secured the place of the patient and family at the centre of the team. Nurses are increasingly seen as the leader or coordinator of care in the palliative care setting, primarily because of their close proximity to the patient and family (Ingham and Coyle 1997). Indeed, nurses are now pioneering new approaches to care delivery and organization in palliative care, including nurse-led clinics for patients with breathlessness (Corner *et al.* 1995), managing ascites (Preston 1995) and the prescribing of medications. This shift in professional boundaries – that is, nurses taking over from the traditionally medically led service – is likely to have an impact on the team dynamics in terms of its development and functioning.

Teamwork in palliative care (as in any area of health care) is multilayered, delivered by a range of professionals, in a range of settings and from a variety of perspectives. Different individuals will be more or less important at a particular point in time according to the needs of the patient and their family. The palliative care team may be better viewed as a kaleidoscope of roles and skills, of teams within teams and of blurred boundaries, that will look different according to the needs and place of the individual and family they are caring for. This description does not fit neatly with the earlier descriptions of teams and teamwork, which present teams as fairly static entities. In contrast to the view that we have presented and Payne's (2000) concept of open teams, the older established view of teams took no account of the moving array of roles suggested here. Our kaleidoscope approach to viewing teams can, however, be disconcerting, as it raises questions about overall responsibility and issues of coordination. As such, it requires excellent communication skills and a clear understanding of each others' skills and abilities, collaborative practice – including conjoint problem solving, shared record keeping and shared accountability (Kedziera and Levy 1994) – an ability to cross organizational and professionals boundaries and to give up ownership of 'the patient'. This kind of teamwork requires members of the team to be more reflexive (Opie 1997). Being reflexive in this sense requires teams to review and critique their performance and move beyond familiar ways of working with each other (Opie 1997). Opie (1997) suggests that reflexive practice may be particularly important in complex cases or when the team believes that its work with the client is not progressing as well as it might.

Patients and the palliative care team

We now turn to the second of our concerns about teams and teamwork as traditionally described in the literature, which relates to the place of the patient and family in the health care team. It is natural that health care practitioners and researchers consistently conceptualize their own work in terms that position 'the patient' at the 'centre' of their approach, and this can be seen in a number of the familiar models of the palliative care team referred to earlier in this chapter (Corr and Corr 1983; Hull *et al.* 1989; Dunlop and Hockley 1990; Saunders 1990; Clark *et al.* 1997; Faull 1998). However, if we wish to deliver the best possible palliative care services, it is surely crucial to ask whether in reality patients are so consistently at the 'centre' of palliative care teams in practice, and the best way to do so is to explore patients' own experiences of the team and their place in it.

As previously stated, palliative teams consist of a range of health and social care professionals who deliver care in a variety of different settings. In practice, however, individual patients and their families may not see the complete cast of characters that health care professionals regard as the 'team' or, indeed, perceive that they are in fact also part of this 'team'. In the course of their dying trajectory, they may come across only one or two leading players, with other individuals only having bit parts. Professionals may be aware of all the others in the team and what is available, however the patient is likely not to have any idea about the characters 'backstage' and the alternatives available to them. The patient's perspective of the team is therefore likely to be very different to that of the professionals. Patients' and families' perspectives, as the users of palliative care services, are likely to throw a very different light onto our professional constructs of the palliative care team. It is important, then, for us to consider what the team looks like from the patient's perspective if the team is to have any meaning at all.

In a systematic review of the impact of specialist palliative care provision on consumer satisfaction, opinion and preference, Wilkinson *et al.* (1999) identified 83 studies relating to work undertaken in North America and Europe. The team noted that consumers were more satisfied with all types of palliative care, whether provided by in-patient units or in the community, than provided by general hospitals. However, the majority of the studies they reviewed were based on small-scale local studies that mainly focused on a single hospice. There was little research in relation to home care or other forms of palliative community-based services. In addition, there was little reference to patients' and families' perceptions of the palliative care team, rather the focus was on comparing place of care (i.e. hospice versus hospital), the satisfaction with specialist community services and preference for place of death.

The review concluded that there were few consistent trends in consumer opinion on and satisfaction with specialist models of palliative care. This lack of a consumer perspective may be related to some of the methodological difficulties of collecting information at a vulnerable time in patients' and families' lives (Fakhoury 1998). However, this kind of information is invaluable to providers of palliative care services, as it can present a unique perspective on the quality of the service, access to care provision, problem areas and service successes (Wilkinson *et al.* 1999). In examining consumer perceptions of teamwork, more consumer-oriented, qualitative approaches that take a longitudinal perspective may be one way to begin to uncover some of the experiences of being cared for by a palliative care team. This would allow for exploration of the concept of a team approach to care as perceived by the patient as well as exploring who they perceive to be responsible for which aspects of their care at different points in their illness trajectory. This kind of information can be used to develop more successful models of palliative care teams and team practices.

The effectiveness of palliative care teams

We noted earlier that various writers on interdisciplinary teams in palliative care suggest that such teamworking impacts positively on the quality of care received by dying patients and their carers, and that it is beneficial for staff (Vachon 1987; Hull *et al.* 1989; Hockley 1992; Opie 1997; Woof *et al.* 1998). There is little empirical evidence, however, to suggest that interdisciplinary teams improve patient outcomes (Opie 1997; Zwarenstein and Reeves 2000). The bulk of the literature presented earlier in relation to palliative care teams tends to be descriptive, focusing on team composition, teamworking and changing working practices, but with little reference to whether these teams are effective or not. In addition, the growth of palliative care services has in the main been unplanned and un-evaluated. Developments have largely been in response to local pressure, public demand and fund-raising activities and, while they are becoming an increasing part of mainstream provision, are often still situated in the voluntary and independent sectors (Faull 1998). As a result, there are now a wide variety of models and approaches to delivering palliative care. However, because of the haphazard approach to service development, there has been limited evaluation of the effectiveness of this kind of service provision. In the current health care climate, it is no longer sufficient to simply claim that the service you are delivering is effective. Services now have to provide clear evidence to this effect. For palliative care teams, this means being able to demonstrate clinical effectiveness, quality services, service-user involvement, collaborative working and cost-effectiveness. Questions on these issues are increasingly being asked of palliative care services and are a subject of debate among the palliative care community (NCHSPCS 2001).

Service level evaluations have not been able to demonstrate the superiority of specialist services over non-specialist services in palliative care (Robbins 1997). Indeed, many of the basic comparative studies, taking into account outcomes, measures of performance and cost, have not been carried out for palliative care services (Robbins 1997). A systematic review undertaken by Hearn and Higginson (1998), focusing on specific palliative care interventions, demonstrated improved outcomes for those cared for by specialist teams rather than standard care. In the 18 studies that they reviewed, they noted that effectiveness of the team was evidenced by an increased satisfaction on the part of patients and carers, better symptom control, a reduction in the number of days per hospital stay, more time spent at home and an increased likelihood of patients dying in the place of their choice. On this basis, Hearn and Higginson (1998) concluded that the palliative care approach does have an impact on the quality of care delivered. However, whether this was attributable to the fact that it was a team providing such interventions is debatable. It is notoriously difficult to identify which particular elements of the team or its approach are most effective. Similar work that has attempted to evaluate the impact of teamwork in specialist stroke services or breast care teams has identified analogous problems.

Measuring the effectiveness of health services is not straightforward. 'Effectiveness' itself is a multi-layered concept that can be approached from numerous perspectives, although 'value for money' and 'health gain' often emerge as two of its essential elements. Evidence of what might constitute 'effectiveness' is also a matter of debate, since the significance of one patient's experience, as compared with evidence produced by a large-scale, multi-centre randomized controlled trial of a large population, may be more or less appropriate and valuable to health care practitioners, depending upon the purpose and nature of the particular study. Health service research suggests that the complex and multi-faceted nature of health care means that traditional experimental approaches may be inappropriate for certain kinds of enquiry (Fitzpatrick and Boulton 1994; Klein 1996). Alternative approaches grounded in more naturalistic methods, such as pluralistic evaluation (Smith and Cantley 1985), may be more appropriate when outputs are less quantifiable and the process is also of importance. In addition, there is a real need to consider the user perspective in relation to the effectiveness of services. How do patients and families perceive the care they receive? What worked for them, what did not work as well? These how, what and why questions are important if we are to understand anything about the processes that are underway as palliative care is delivered and received. Simply relying on quantitative measurable outputs is not enough if we wish to be able to answer these more complicated in-depth questions. It appears that if we are to achieve any meaningful evaluation of palliative care teams, there is a need for a multi-method approach that embraces both quantitative and qualitative research data to help us identify how and why something is – or is not – effective.

Specialist palliative care teams pose another challenge for researchers. Specialist input in palliative care is invariably provided in addition to mainstream care. In some instances, they work alongside the mainstream caregivers or may simply provide additional resource in terms of information, advice or equipment. The point is that it is very difficult to identify a 'pure effect' – that is, make any comparison between the specialist service and the routine services as the two are often so intertwined. In addition, patients who do not receive any input from the specialist team may receive care of the same standard from mainstream services provided by numerous practitioners who have received additional education and training in palliative care. Hospices, for example, are no longer providing care that is radically different to mainstream health services (Seale 1989). This dispersal of palliative care knowledge has caused an interesting dilemma for palliative care teams. If professionals outside the specialist team are capable of providing the care and support traditionally within that team's domain, what is to become of the specialist team? In addition, if these same teams cannot provide evidence of their effectiveness, how can they defend the need for their existence?

Evaluating the effectiveness of specialist palliative care teams might appear, then, to be an impossible task. Yet palliative care teams, like all other branches of health service provision, need to be able to demonstrate their effectiveness to survive. They cannot continue simply on the basis of what has gone on in the past. What appears to be vitally important is that, first and foremost, there needs to be a clear definition of specialist palliative care teams (and this, as noted earlier, is notoriously difficult to achieve in the palliative care setting because of the plethora of professionals involved). Second, it is important to identify which elements of the team can be meaningfully assessed in relation to concepts of 'effectiveness'. Only with a clear definition and an identification of the assessable elements can any progress be made towards examining the effectiveness or otherwise of the specialist team in palliative care.

▌Conclusions

Patients and families have increasingly high expectations of health care provision and what services should offer. These include higher expectations of power sharing, improved information giving, increased patient choice and better patient-centred care (Gillespie *et al.* 2002). These will continue to be mediated by the fundamental need for human warmth and attention at times of vulnerability, the family support and tension created by illness, and a desire to adopt the 'sick role', with its version of opting out. Underpinning these changes is the challenge to the idea of 'professional/expert' and 'lay' boundaries, which, in turn, cause us to think anew about 'team' inputs. As palliative care continues to face the call for broader delivery of palliative care started in the mid-1980s, beyond the traditional cancer focus a wider range of teams will face the challenge of collaborative working. While users and families may welcome the different professionals who offer support, there is also the danger of intrusiveness as well as fragmentation. One thing remains certain, however – palliative care teams need to develop new models of practice and evaluations of that practice if the successes of their past are to be mirrored in their future. In summary:

- There are now a multiplicity of palliative care settings and changing roles within the palliative care team.
- Teams need to reach out towards community, user and wider professional networks and to understand the contexts within which they are working.
- Teams need to become reflexive in their practice and regularly review their functions and processes.
- Evaluations of teams are required that consider its effectiveness as well as the user perspective in order to develop future successful models of teams.

▎Note

1 See Help the Hospices and St Christopher's Hospice (2002) *Hospice Information Directory* (www.hospiceinformation.info).

▎References

Ajemian, I. (1993) Interdisciplinary teamwork, In D. Doyle, G. Hanks and N. Macdonald (eds) *Oxford Textbook of Palliative Medicine*. Oxford: Oxford Medical.

Belbin, R.M. (1981) *Management Teams: Why They Succeed or Fail*. Oxford: Heinemann.

Benne, K.D. and Skeats, P. (1948) Functional roles of group members. *Journal of Social Issues*, 4(2): 41–9.

Brill, N.I. (1976) *Teamwork: Working Together in the Human Services*. Philadelphia, PA: Lippincott.

Burrell, K. and Lindström, K. (1987) *Teamview: A Teambuilding Programme* (original Swedish edition, 1985). Hove: Pavilion.

Clark, D. and Seymour, J. (1999) *Reflections on Palliative Care*. Buckingham: Open University Press.

Clark, D., Hockley, J. and Ahmedzai, S. (1997) *New Themes in Palliative Care*. Buckingham: Open University Press.

Clark, N. (1994) *Teambuilding: A Practical Guide for Trainers*. London: McGraw-Hill.

Corner, J., Plant, H. and Warner, L. (1995) Developing a nursing approach to the management of dyspnoea in lung cancer. *International Journal of Palliative Nursing*, 1(1): 5–11.

Corr, C.A. and Corr, D.M. (1983) *Hospice Care: Principles and Practice*. London: Faber & Faber.

Dechant, K., Marsick, V.J. and Kasl, E. (1993) Towards a model of team learning. *Studies in Continuing Education*, 15(1): 1–14.

Dunlop, R.J. (1998) *Cancer: Palliative Care*. London: Springer.

Dunlop, R.J. and Hockley, J.M. (1990) *Terminal Care Support Teams: The Hospital–Hospice Interface*. Oxford: Oxford University Press.

Fakhoury, W.K.H. (1998) Satisfaction with palliative care: what should we be aware of? *International Journal of Nursing Studies*, 35: 171–6.

Faull, C. (1998) The history and principles of palliative care, in C. Faull, Y. Carter and R. Woof, *Handbook of Palliative Care*. Oxford: Blackwell Science.

Field, D. (1989) *Nursing the Dying*. London: Routledge.

Firth-Cozens, K.J. (1998) Celebrating teamwork. *Quality in Health Care*, 7 (suppl.): S3–S7.

Fitzpatrick, R. and Boulton, M. (1994) Qualitative methods for assessing health care. *Quality in Health Care*, 3: 107–13.

Gillespie, R., Florin, D. and Gillam, S. (2002) *Changing Relationships: Findings from the Patient Involvement Project*. London: King's Fund.

Hearn, J.H. and Higginson, J. (1998) Do specialist palliative care teams improve outcomes for cancer patients? A systematic review. *Palliative Medicine*, 12: 317–32.

Hockley, J. (1992) Role of the hospital support team. *British Journal of Hospital Medicine*, 48(3): 250–3.

Hull, R., Ellis, M. and Sargent, V. (1989) *Teamwork in Palliative Care*. Oxford: Radcliffe Medical.

Ingham, J.M. and Coyle, N. (1997) Teamwork in end of life care: a nurse–physician perspective introducing physicians to palliative care concepts, in D. Clark, J. Hockley and S. Ahmedzai (eds) *New Themes in Palliative Care*. Buckingham: Open University Press.

Kedziera, P. and Levy, M. (1994) Collaborative practice in oncology. *Seminars in Oncology*, 21(6): 705–11.

Klein, R. (1996) The NHS and the new scientism: solution or delusion? *Quarterly Journal of Medicine*, 89: 85–7.

Leathard, A. (1994) *Going Interprofessional*. London: Routledge.

Manion, J., Lorimer, W. and Leander, W.J. (1996) *Team-based Health Care Organisations: Blueprint for Success*. Gaithersburg, MD: Aspen.

Margerison, C.J. and McCann, D. (1995) *Team Management: Practical New Approaches*, 2nd edn. Oxford: Management Books.

Miller, C., Freeman, M. and Ross, N. (2001) *Interprofessional Practice in Health and Social Care: Challenging the Shared Learning Agenda*. London: Arnold.

National Council for Hospice and Specialist Palliative Care Services (1995) *Information Exchange*, No. 13. London: NCHSPCS.

National Council for Hospice and Specialist Palliative Care Services (2001) *What Do We Mean by Palliative Care? A Discussion Paper*. London: NCHSPCS.

Opie, A. (1997) Thinking teams, thinking clients: issues of discourse and representation in the work of health care teams. *Sociology of Health and Illness*, 19(3): 259–80.

Parker, G.M. (1990) *Team Players and Teamwork: The New Competitive Business Strategy*. San Fransisco, CA: Jossey-Bass.

Payne, M. (2000) *Teamwork in Multi-professional Care*. London: Macmillan.

Preston, N. (1995) New strategies for the management of malignant ascites. *European Journal of Cancer Care*, 4(4): 178–83.

Pritchard, P. and Pritchard, J. (1994) *Teamwork for Primary and Shared Care: A Practical Workbook*, 2nd edn. Oxford: Oxford University Press.

Robbins, M. (1997) Assessing needs and effectiveness: is palliative care a special case?, in D. Clark, J. Hockley and S. Ahmedzai (eds) *New Themes in Palliative Care*. Buckingham: Open University Press.

Saunders, C. (1990) *Hospice and Palliative Care: An Interdisciplinary Approach*. London: Edward Arnold.

Seale, C.F. (1989) What happens in hospices: a review of research evidence. *Social Science and Medicine*, 28(6): 551–9.

Shaw, I. (1994) *Evaluating International Training*. Aldershot: Avebury.

Smith, G. and Cantley, C. (1985) *Assessing Health Care: A Study in Organisational Evaluation*. Milton Keynes: Open University Press.

Spencer, J. and Pruss, A. (1992) *Managing Your Team: How to Organise People for Maximum Results*. London: Piatkus.

Tuckman, B. (1965) Developmental sequences in small groups. *Psychological Bulletin*, 63: 384–99.

Vachon, M.C.S. (1987) *Occupational Stress in Caring for the Critically Ill, the Dying and the Bereaved*. Washington, DC: Hemisphere.

Wilkinson, E.K., Salisbury, C., Bosanquat, N. *et al.* (1999) Patient and carer preference for, and satisfaction with, specialist models of palliative care: a systematic literature review. *Palliative Medicine*, 13: 197–216.

Woof, R., Carter, Y. and Faull, C. (1998) Palliative care: the team, the services and the need for care, in C. Faull, Y. Carter and R. Woof, *Handbook of Palliative Care*. Oxford: Blackwell Science.

Zollo, J. (1999) The interdisciplinary palliative care team: problems and possibilities, in S. Aranda and M. O'Connor (eds) *Palliative Care Nursing: A Guide to Practice*. Melbourne, Ausmed.

Zwarenstein, M. and Reeves, S. (2000) What's so great about collaboration? We need more evidence and less rhetoric. *British Medical Journal*, 320(7241): 1022–3.

32

The cost of caring

Surviving the culture of niceness, occupational stress and coping strategies

Sanchia Aranda

Palliative care nursing occurs in a context of significant human suffering, suffering in which nurses are both witness and participant. As palliative care nurses, every day we deal with people facing one of life's greatest challenges – people who are often distressed, in pain and struggling with questions of meaning. We are not immune to this suffering and, for most of us, our reason for working in this field is a desire to make a positive difference in the lives of dying people and their families.

We work in a setting that for the rest of health care is associated with the failure of modern medicine to hold death at bay. Our work is also often hidden from view in a social context where there is both a fascination with death and an avoidance of its proximity. We are lauded for the work we do because others see it as distasteful, yet the skill of our work is seen as hidden (Aranda 2001), innate rather than learned. Nursing in palliative care is even described as the quintessential spirit of nursing (Bradshaw 1996) – potentially little more than attention to the basics. For me, such beliefs minimize the complexity of our work and undermine the skill – a skill that is a combination of disease knowledge, clinical expertise and human compassion.

Believing that palliative nursing is natural rather than learned leads to what I consider to be a clear paradox in the self-perception of palliative care nurses – on the one hand, this is something everyone with a bit of humanity can do and, on the other, it is hard work and skilled practice. This paradox means we work in a constant balance between emphasizing the ordinariness of what we do and having to defend the need for skilled nurses in the delivery of palliative care. If nurses are to survive and even thrive in this context, attention must be paid to the skills and supports required to do this.

While occupational stress and burnout are common phenomena across health care and certainly not unique to palliative care, there are some characteristics of palliative care as a specialty that require specific attention. In this chapter, while acknowledging the significant work undertaken on occupational stress in palliative care (e.g. Vachon 1987, 1995, 1999), I seek to depart from this work through an exploration of the relationship between the underlying philosophy of palliative care, what counts as stressful and the meaning of this for nursing work in palliative care. It is from an understanding of this relationship that I argue for greater emphasis on self-knowledge and reflective capacity, both within individuals and teams, as the key mechanism for surviving and thriving as a palliative care nurse.

Stress in palliative care nursing

Stress in palliative care workers has received ongoing attention in the literature since the seminal work of Mary Vachon (1987). Terms associated with stress in health workers include compassion fatigue (Welsh 1999), burnout (Payne 2001) and chronic grief (Saunders and Valente 1994; Feldstein and Gemma 1995). Much of the descriptive work on stress in palliative care has focused on the identification of specific stressors and a summary of such stressors is presented in Box 32.1. While there is some evidence that levels of burnout are low in palliative care nurses and that stressors contribute to the burnout that does occur (Payne 2001), how we understand stress is critical to how the subject is approached.

Theoretical understandings of occupational stress and coping

Vachon, the leading author on occupational stress in palliative care, utilizes the person–environment fit framework to understand work stress in palliative care. This framework works from the principle 'that adaptation is a function of the "goodness of fit" between the characteristics of the person and the work environment' (Vachon 1999: 93). This framework requires an exploration of the needs of the person and the resources available to meet these within the environment and also a comparison between the abilities of the individual and the demands of the work environment. Essentially, stress occurs when the demands of the environment exceed the abilities of the person or when the environment cannot meet the needs of the individual. This framework makes intuitive sense in considering occupational stress in palliative care because it acknowledges that this field is built on a set of values and beliefs, about the care of people who are dying, which must at some level be shared by individuals who choose this work. These beliefs and values include a valuing of each individual, a belief that dying can be a time of personal growth and that quality of life in dying is a central goal of care.

However, the person–environment fit framework is limited when attempting to understand the nature of stress in palliative care more specifically. While it is sometimes said that working with the terminally ill is stress-

Box 32.1   Sources of stress

Environmental factors

- Working conditions
  - high workloads
  - staff shortages
- Inadequate preparation for work situation
- Inadequate preparation for care demands
- Lack of time to relax or grieve
- Poor or negative interrelationships between staff
- High levels of organizational change
- Lack of management support or appreciation
- Role conflict or lack of role clarity
- Role change
- High levels of uncertainty

Patient factors

- Role overlap with family members
- Nature of the patient's illness
- Patient's emotional state
- Family's emotional state
- Nature of the death

Personal factors

- Demographic variables often listed but relationship unclear
- Gaps between ideals
- Feelings of inadequacy
- Personality disorders
- Identification with the patient
- Provision of care that was not optimal
- Accumulated grief

ful (McNamara *et al.* 1995), it is not necessarily more so than in other specialist areas of health care. Why do some situations cause stress for one individual and not another? Why is a certain type of situation more stressful for the same individual at one time than at another? Lazarus and Folkman (1984) developed the transactional model of stress and coping that can help to answer such questions. They argue that individuals constantly appraise events in their environment in relation to the potential impact these events have for them. Stressful events are those that are appraised as indicating a threat, challenge or harm for the individual, thus it is the appraisal of the situation by the individual rather than an inherent characteristic of the situation that leads to stress as an outcome. Coping is anything the individual does 'to regulate the distress (emotion-focused coping) or manage the problem causing distress (problem-focused coping)' (Folkman 1997: 1216).

Benner and Wrubel (1989), in their book *The Primacy of Caring*, draw on Lazarus and Folkman's (1984) transactional model of stress and coping, arguing that stress occurs when things matter to the individual. Essentially, when the things that you hold to be important are threatened or challenged, stress is the result. If we apply this to stress in palliative nursing, we begin to see some of the daily stress facing nurses in this field. If what matters to you draws from palliative care philosophy, such as the ability to spend time with patients and families, the ability to alleviate symptoms, having the time to bring closure to a relationship with a patient by attending a funeral, then anything that reduces your capacity to do this is a potential cause of stress. While this may appear obvious, it is rarely brought out in work on stress in palliative care.

McNamara *et al.* (1995) offer a sociological perspective on stress that is consistent with both the person–environment and transactional models but which allows a closer examination of how the philosophical basis of palliative care both sets up what counts as stressful and frames the mechanisms through which nurses and others deal with stress. Essentially, their work draws from Saunders and Baines's (1983) contention that 'if we are to remain for long near the suffering of dependence and parting we need also to develop a basic philosophy and search, often painfully, for meaning even in the most adverse situations' (pp. 65–6). Thus the ability to work in palliative care in the long term is understood by McNamara *et al.* (1995) as residing in 'the development of a value system that supplies meaning and direction' (p. 223). This shared value system becomes the group's work driver and is closely related to their sense of efficacy and of having done a good job. For McNamara *et al.* (1995), '(p)erceptions of stress and strategies for coping, therefore, are not entirely idiosyncratic, but are grounded in a learned logic that is systematically shared' (p. 224). From this perspective, stress relates to threats to the practitioner's ability to deliver care according to these shared values and perhaps also to challenges to the shared strategies for dealing with such threats.

The values-based perspective on stress offered by McNamara *et al.* is afforded more theoretical strength by the recent work of Folkman (1997) on meaning-focused coping. Drawing on research with partners of men with HIV, Folkman argues that even in the event of an unfavourable resolution of a stressful event, such as a diagnosis of a terminal disease, individuals can modify the stress response through meaning-focused coping efforts. These efforts include positive reappraisal, revisited goals, spiritual beliefs and positive events. Significant similarities can be drawn here between the global way in which palliative care philosophy is an attempt to reappraise the negative outcome of death through emphasizing the growth possible in the face of death or acceptance of death and reconciliation of a life well lived (positive reappraisal), focusing on short- rather than long-term goals such as living day to day to the maximum (revisited goals), belief in an afterlife or having made a contribution that will be remembered (spiritual beliefs), or making opportunities for positive events in an otherwise distressing situation such as developing a memory book for a loved one (positive events). Thus stress in palliative care can be understood as intimately linked to the practitioner's capacity to personally engage in meaning-focused coping. I would argue also that the practitioner's experience of stress may be related to the degree to which their clients engage in meaning-focused coping, as it is through such coping efforts that patients can be understood to directly assume the values inherent in the delivery of palliative care.

The importance of understanding the relationship between palliative care values and stress becomes critical if one accepts my previously argued view that the philosophical basis of palliative care suffers from a lack of critique and in many respects is ideological rather than rooted in reality (Aranda 1998a). I have argued that values such as acceptance of the inevitability of death, the family as unit of care and excellence in pain and symptom management are often used in the language of palliative care but that little evidence exists to support the achievement of these values in practice (Aranda 1998a). More recently, I have argued that indeed several tyrannies of palliative care act to reduce open critique and thus leave the field in danger of further ideological stagnation (Aranda 2001). What is important from this for a discussion of stress is that without this critique palliative care nurses are more at risk of stress as care systems develop increasingly in ways that threaten their value system, but these systems are unable to be openly challenged. Much of this lack of open challenge relates to what I have previously referred to as the 'tyranny of niceness' (Aranda 2001).

The 'tyranny of niceness'

The 'tyranny of niceness' is referred to by Street (1995) as a culture that involves 'being nice; not making a fuss; smiling a lot; speaking in a sympathetic voice even if you go away and complain about the person afterwards; not letting on that you think the other person is being unfair; and always putting the other person first even when you know they are a "user" ' (p. 30). Street argued that for nurses in units where the tyranny of niceness operated, there was a blurring between being nice and being caring such that to be genuinely caring meant always being nice and fitting in with the unit/service expectations. What she found in her research was that although everyone on the study unit described the environment and people within it as nice, very few nurses felt as if they were good enough to be a part of the team and did not see themselves as fitting in. Importantly, she described how the expectation of always being nice prevented constructive critique and debate with others.

Being nice or good is a central value in palliative care. This is in part linked to the strong historical links between palliative care and religion, but also to the highly moral nature of palliative care philosophy. Thus one of the central, but perhaps unwritten, values of palliative care is being nice. Indeed, people who work in palliative care often make a distinction between the good of their world and the bad of mainstream health care. For example, in the study of McNamara *et al.* (1995), one of the nurses said: 'sometimes we live in a false world, everybody in hospice is so "nice". When you get outside of it, you find it's all a bit of a shock' (pp. 229–30). Added to this is the voice of believing palliative care to be work that is somehow unable to be understood by others or would be a burden to them. As another nurse from the above study said: 'You know it's not arrogance that we don't confide in our families. What we do is special and only we can understand really what it's like. We don't want to burden them with something they don't need to know' (pp. 232–3).

Thus the pre-existing drive towards being nice in palliative care has the potential to exacerbate the tyranny of niceness in ways that cover over or even silence critical thought about organizational and practice issues. The increasing gap between what we value and what we do as a result of health care reforms, such as mainstreaming and increased economic pressures, increases the potential dissonance between our capacity to deliver care according to our core values and the reality of our practice world, a dissonance that is difficult to fight against while the tyranny of niceness is operant.

The value of being nice or good is lived out in palliative care through the central value of the good death and understanding the challenges to our ability to deliver the good death is critical to understanding stress in palliative care nursing.

The good death

The good death is an ideal commonly associated with the efforts of palliative care practitioners to achieve positive outcomes in the lives of people who are dying and has received significant commentary in the palliative care literature (e.g. McNamara *et al.* 1994; Payne *et al.* 1996). Elements of a good death vary, but include open awareness of impending death, acceptance or adjustment to this, engaging in preparation for death, talking with others about death and making final farewells. Good death in this palliative care sense is in contrast to the use of the term within the euthanasia debate, where the emphasis is on a quick, painless exit.

McNamara *et al.* (1995) present an excellent account of the relationship between stress in palliative care nursing and ideas about the good death. In the context of their study, a good death referred to one where there was 'an awareness, acceptance and a preparation for death' undertaken by the person who was dying, characteristics I would argue are centrally linked to Folkman's ideas about meaning-focused coping. Many of the nurses in their study recalled stories of deaths that reinforced their belief that 'there must be a better way to die' and precipitated a decision to become a palliative care nurse. Thus an inherent part of becoming a palliative care nurse appears to be a commitment to achieving a good death for patients, often contrasted against previously encountered bad deaths. However, notions of a good death are largely ideological and it is common for patients to die deaths that may be in keeping with how they have lived their lives but might not fit with images of a good death. Patients may also not engage with attempts to portray their situation in a more positive light, becoming depressed and demoralized rather than actively embracing the growth palliative care portrays as possible at the end of life.

McNamara *et al.* (1995) articulated five threats to a good death that act as sources of stress for palliative care nurses. The five threats related to societal values and reactions, organization of the work environment, exchanges between nurses and patients and their families, exchanges between nurses and their families, friends and colleagues and personally facing death. Drawing on these threats I suggest that understanding the oppositions at the heart of these threats helps us to understand stress in palliative nursing as it relates to the good death. Centring on a simplistic binary split between good and bad, these oppositions are:

- dissonance between social reactions to death and the values of palliative care; and

- dissonance between the organization of the work environment and the values of care delivery.

While clearly binary oppositions overly simplify reality, they can be a helpful way of understanding the tensions that exist in practice.

Dissonance between social reactions to death and the values of palliative care

The first and fourth threats articulated by McNamara *et al.* (1995) concern a dissonance between the values of palliative care and the values of society and social reactions to what palliative care nurses do, both in terms of the nurses' relationship to society as a whole and to individuals within their family and friendship group. The binary opposition is that society generally sees death as a negative experience, while palliative care nurses have adopted a value system that reappraises the meaning of death in a more positive light, a natural part of life and not inherently negative. This then leads to a perception of isolation within the field of palliative care and a sense of not being understood. McNamara *et al.* report that some nurses felt unable to speak openly about their work in situations outside of palliative care because people did not want to be confronted by death in social situations. They suggest that nurses 'perceive stress, in this context, to be related to "the general society's" non-acceptance of death and, implicitly, to the ensuing disregard for their system of values' (p. 229). These feelings extended for some nurses into not feeling able to confide in family and friends, turning instead for support to fellow workers.

Essentially, these threats see the 'good' palliative care workers happily embracing death while bad society seeks to push it from view. Additionally, individuals within society are seen as lacking the capacity to understand or would be burdened by what palliative care nurses see and do. Indeed, the anthropologist Julia Lawton produced a powerful thesis arguing that society's inability to cope with the realities of dying is an important driver of the hospice movement. In her work (Lawton 1998, 2000), she argues that bodily disintegration resulting in incontinence and other forms of boundary loss are unacceptable to society, resulting in the sequestration of dying people within hospices. Palliative care nurses, particularly those who work in the hospice setting, can thus be understood as dealing with those aspects of death that society shuns. Obviously social attitudes to death and dying are not this simplistic. What is important though is that when palliative care nurses perceive themselves to be isolated from society, family and friends through differences in values about dying and death, through their different life experience or through fears about not being understood, they become isolated from the very social environments that provide them with necessary time out from this potentially draining work.

Spending more and more time in the company of other palliative care nurses because of a shared value system may be counterproductive in other ways. McNamara *et al.* (1995) reveal that some nurses identify a 'level of dishonesty' or a 'conspiracy of silence' around admitting to feeling personal pain or struggles with their work. The meaning-focused coping inherent in palliative care approaches to death portray a positive reappraisal of a negative situation that is not always easy to sustain and workers are likely to feel pain as bonds with patients and families are broken through death or when they cannot achieve a 'good' death for the patient. Taking the moral high ground in relation to palliative care values may also mean a reluctance to admit that this work involves personal struggle. In my work with Mary (see Box 32.2), she felt unable to talk about her struggles in caring for Lucy within the nursing team. While discussion sessions were held within this team to allow nurses to talk about their work, there was a perception that the team leader was holding back. This senior nurse was a nun and appeared to Mary to be trapped in a missionary approach to her work that meant her own needs were always secondary. In the team, this resulted in role expectations that meant personal needs were always subsumed to the needs of the patient. Thus on the surface and in the rhetoric of the group, team members understood themselves to be supportive of each other; in reality, much of each nurse's personal struggle was silenced.

Nurses in a study of nurse–patient friendships in cancer and palliative care were asked to consider this issue of team openness to personal struggle and the provision of support when it was raised by Mary (Aranda 1998b). At the group meeting where this was first discussed, Tessa suggested that her team was safe and allowed everyone to discuss personal feelings. However, at the following meeting Tessa expressed a modified view. Her discussions with one of her nursing colleagues over the ensuing weeks revealed that this nurse felt censored in the team and this had led to her hiding her feelings from the group. Tessa identified that safety and support were conditional within their nursing team with conditions set around behaving in certain ways and

---

Box 32.2 Case study

Mary was an experienced home-based palliative care nurse who, at the time of her participation in a research project on nurse–patient friendship, had just re-entered nursing after an experience of professional burnout. During our first interview she recounted the story of her work with Lucy, a young woman with terminal cancer that had led to significant weight gain and quadriplegia. Lucy had been a model and found these alterations to her body very distressing. Her husband, David, also found the changes distressing and this led to less and less contact between them and little involvement in Lucy's physical care. Mary described how in caring for Lucy her efforts focused on maintaining feelings of worth and personhood in the face of such degrading tasks as enemas and faecal disimpaction. In addition, Mary recognized Lucy's loss of physical contact with David and tried to meet some of these needs through massage and touch. She found herself spending more and more time delivering care to Lucy, making her late for other clients and often providing less than her usual care to them in order to fill the enormous care needs of Lucy, even past the time when it would perhaps have been appropriate for Lucy to be in the hospice. When Mary raised her concerns over Lucy within the nursing team, the response was usually one of giving her a break from the care, which served to silence Mary's concerns as she did not wish to be replaced or to stop caring for Lucy. Mary's reflections on her situation were in contrast to another nurse from this team who also participated in the study. Jane's reflections showed a concerned team willing to assist Mary; however, the nurse lacked the skills to know how to openly critique what was happening. The first interview for this study occurred many months after Lucy's death but resulted in a significant delayed grief response for Mary, requiring several sessions of grief counselling to work through the many issues that had resulted in Mary's burnout experience. Mary's resolution of her experience was also aided by her continued participation in the research project, providing extended opportunities for her to reflect on this and other experiences with patients who were dying. At the end of the study, Mary said that prior to this she probably had an in-built desire to rescue patients from their experiences (to provide a good death) and that she no longer felt this level of responsibility and was able to work to make a difference in their lives but understood that she could not make this happen always (Aranda 1998b).

   This is a real case but the names are pseudonyms and the identity of the setting is not revealed in keeping with the ethical requirements of the study. All participants signed a consent form acknowledging that the work would be used in subsequent publications and that their identity would not be revealed.

---

premised on length of time in the team. While palliative care teams may indeed be supportive in general and aim for a degree of openness and support not usual in team settings, achievement of this is hard work. The tyranny of niceness prevented this nurse disclosing her feelings because admitting them and thus criticizing the team for its lack of support for her would not be nice behaviour and would place her outside of the group. When we assume our teams to be supportive and fail to acknowledge the level of work required to create a supportive environment, the end result can be a significant dissonance between what we say, do and feel, generating potential for individual and team stress.

Dissonance between the organization of the work environment and the values of care delivery

Vachon (1987) argues that patients are not the major source of stress in palliative care and that the real problems are the work environment and the nurse's occupational role. The desire to assist the patient to achieve a good death is often thwarted by the work environment and role factors. Work environment factors include the involvement in care of individuals who appear not to share the values of palliative care, such as medical specialists who continue to treat the cancer beyond what the nurse considers reasonable. Indeed, attempts to avoid this source of stress are present in arguments that cancer treatments have no place in hospice settings, an argument that seeks to separate palliative care from mainstream health care, perhaps because of conflicting values (Biswas 1993).

Such arguments are based on a simplistic division between, for example, the 'bad' oncologist using yet more chemotherapy and the 'good' palliative care nurse wanting to protect the patient from harm. The patient is passive in the argument, ignoring both the patient's role in the decision and the complexity of balancing the side-effects of cancer treatments against the benefits that might be gained in terms of pain and symptom relief. All too often there is no attempt to openly discuss the apparent conflict between the various practitioners involved, a discussion that could lead to mutual understanding and hopefully improved sharing of patient care. The absence of conflict resolution in such situations leaves the palliative care nurse to deliver care in ways that are not consistent with his or her value system as the patient's acceptance of ongoing treatment is understood as indicating a lack of acceptance of death. While clearly patients can still be accepting of the inevitability of death while continuing to seek treatments that will either lengthen life or reduce symptoms, such choices are not always well accepted in palliative care.

Similarly, the work environment in palliative care is becoming increasingly mainstreamed, adding new pressures of workload that threaten the provision of time – a highly valued aspect of the palliative approach to care and a key factor in ensuring a good death. Palliative care is asked to respond to criticisms about being a form of deluxe dying for the few (Johnston and Abraham 1995) and to demands to extend their work beyond a focus on cancer (Clark and Seymour 1999). This means either spreading the effort further with few additional resources or greater attention to the allocation of resources to those most in need however this is defined. Ultimately, either outcome can add increasing pressure to the daily work of palliative care nurses. In Australia in the 1980s, a community palliative care nurse undertook a direct care role providing holistic care to about four patients a day, leaving sufficient time for prolonged visits with patients who needed this. Today, this same nurse is more likely to be sharing care with a generalist community nurse, have a role that is more case management than direct care and will visit six to eight patients in one day. The case management role also reduces the level of direct physical care that is provided and on observation this significantly reduces delivery of many of the comfort elements of palliative care, such as extended touch through massage (Brown *et al.* 2002).

Similarly, acute palliative care units focusing more on acute symptom management than care of the dying are gradually replacing in-patient hospices. Length of stay is reducing, patients may be receiving treatments such as intravenous antibiotics and patients who are not immediately dying may be transferred to nursing homes or go home when this might not be considered ideal. This reality threatens ideas about a good death by reducing the time spent with the patient, fracturing holistic care and reducing the palliative nursing role to monitoring of outcomes of acute treatments, such as intensive pain management. The result is greater dissonance between the shared values of palliative care and the daily reality of nursing work, a dissonance that threatens the meaning of our work and is thus likely to result in greater stress.

A further area of dissonance between the work environment and the values of palliative care is an increasing social acceptance of euthanasia as an end-of-life option. The modern hospice movement is significantly influenced by Christian values and the field's public position is thus overtly anti-euthanasia. Nurses want to see patients achieve a good death, yet the palliative definition of a good death rules out both euthanasia and physician-assisted suicide. Opting for a quick exit through euthanasia is seen to portray a life without meaning, while a significant part of palliative care work is about helping patients to obtain meaning in the face of death. Work stress can result when caring for patients with differing values about end-of-life decisions, when caring for patients who refuse to engage in a search for meaning in their death or when the nurse is not personally opposed to euthanasia.

Our earlier work around palliative care nurses' attitudes to euthanasia showed that not all were opposed to hastening death (Aranda and O'Connor 1995), demonstrating a potential dissonance between the nurse and the value system operating in the organization. In addition, at least three nurses in this study believed that they had been involved in euthanasia in the workplace. Leaving aside the more complex legal concerns this raises, from a stress perspective there are palliative care nurses who believe they have contributed to a patient's death but work in an environment where these issues are rarely discussed in open and frank ways.

The philosophy of palliative care and its anti-euthanasia position makes it very difficult for palliative nurses to hold views even moderately supportive of attempts to hasten death, let alone to discuss these in the workplace. However, it is possible for people with a desire for assisted death to be cared for within a palliative care environment (Aranda *et al.* 1999) by encouraging an open dialogue with patients that is respectful of their wishes and desires but reinforces the legal constraints and value position of the palliative care system.

The 'good nurse'

The nurse's role in a good death is one of involvement, provision of effective symptom control to allow the person to live as fully as possible until death, death that is pain-free and provision of an environment that allows death that is peaceful and dignified (McNamara *et al.* 1995: 234). A significant part of achieving this involves assisting patients to gain meaning in their lives at this time. Good palliative care nurses are skilled in symptom management because a patient with few symptoms can live their remaining life more fully. Good palliative care nurses are also willing to help patients talk about their deaths, helping them to resolve issues in their lives and thus find meaning in their deaths. Good palliative care nurses are also those who assist the patient to find meaning through their relationships with others, facilitating family discussions, helping patients create legacies such as letters for those they will leave behind, and bringing in others who can assist with issues like spiritual conflict and psychological distress.

Living up to this image is not always easy and a significant component of stress in palliative care nursing can be linked to not achieving a good death *vis-à-vis* not being a good palliative care nurse.

Reducing stress in palliative care

Strategies for dealing with stress in palliative care nursing are frequently discussed (e.g. Pearce 1998; Barnes 2001; Payne 2001). Box 32.3 provides an overview of some of the strategies mentioned in the literature; however, it is important to note that the evidence base for these strategies is poorly developed and there is a critical need to research the impact of various stress-reduction strategies. Significantly, coping efforts in palliative care are understood in the literature as a shared responsibility between the individual and the work setting. Nurses describe palliative care environments as being more supportive than those in which they had worked previously (Newton and Waters 2001).

While strategies such as 'developing realistic perspectives' about the work (Byrne and McMurray 1997) and seeing the bigger picture (Vachon 1998) are recommended and appear intuitively appropriate, few mechanisms to achieve such outcomes have been systematically evaluated. There is a significant emphasis now being placed on self-awareness and reflective capacity as critical tools in mastery over stress experienced in palliative care.

Box 32.3 Strategies for managing stress

Within the palliative care unit

- Teamwork and team cohesiveness
- Selecting staff to ensure environment–person fit
- Professional development/education programme
- Clinical supervision made available

By the individual

- Seek counselling
- Attend a support group
- Attend regular clinical supervision
- Change roles or take time out from role
- Undertake more education
- Establish outside interests
- Balance work and home life
- Exercise
- Religious beliefs
- Understand personal boundaries
- Having a sense of mastery
- Finding meaning in work

Mary's story is a clear example of the personal benefits that can be gained through opportunities to safely reflect on how we work as nurses in palliative care. Unfortunately for Mary, this did not occur until after a period of significant distress and burnout, which was hardly ideal.

Some significant attempts to investigate structured approaches to reducing stress in the care of people who are terminally are beginning to appear in the literature. For example, von Klitzing (1999) compared the development of reflective learning in a psychodynamic group with that of a group of general nurses, although the reflections predominantly focused on the care of people who were terminally ill. The study found that nurses could develop reflective capacity in this supported process, with these reflections becoming increasingly more high level when about the patient. Of concern was that the level of reflection about the nurse herself decreased over time, suggesting perhaps that this level of self-work may require specific emphasis over time.

A popular self-awareness strategy employed by disciplines such as social work and psychology is clinical supervision (see Chapter 38). In Chapter 38, Hopkins deals with clinical supervision from a management perspective. Use of clinical supervision in nursing was, until recently, largely confined to the psychiatric setting. One of the possible reasons for this is that nursing was largely understood as a collective profession, while clinical supervision was seen to focus on the issues arising from dyadic relationships between an individual practitioner and an individual patient. An interesting study from

Sweden (Palsson *et al.* 1994) examined the use of group clinical supervision in cancer care in terms of its effect in handling difficult situations. While caution must be exercised in interpreting the generalizability of the results of this qualitative study, they suggest an enhanced capacity to gain relief from distressing situations through the clinical supervision process. In addition, the nurses felt their professional roles and self-perceptions were confirmed through the group, with signs of increased knowledge, a greater sense of well-being and enhanced self-confidence.

Critical to the perspective taken in this chapter, the study of Palsson *et al.* (1994) was theoretically linked to Antonovsky's theory of sense of coherence. The components of this theory are comprehensibility, manageability and meaningfulness. I would argue that a strong sense of coherence can equate to a nurse whose values and beliefs about his or her work are consistent with the daily reality of practice, where he or she feels able to manage the work demands in making a difference for the dying person and family and where overall a sense of meaningfulness in this work is retained as a motivation to continue.

Conclusions

The overriding premise of this chapter is that stress occurs at points of dissonance between the values and beliefs of the individual and their capacity to deliver care according to these values. The absence of a strong evidence base to preventing and managing the impact of this dissonance on work stress means that palliative care services need to foster a flexible and varied approach to the provision of support in the workplace and to encourage nurses to identify their personal approach to stress as an overt part of professional development.

However, it is clear from the literature that in palliative care a sense of meaning in the work, of making a contribution and of helping the person to die a good death, when not idealized, are fundamental to professional well-being. The capacity to maintain a balance between making a difference and accepting the limitations of what can be achieved requires a significant level of self- and team-awareness. There is some evidence that this awareness can be promoted through processes such as clinical supervision and structured reflection. However, this reflection requires moving beyond the tyranny of niceness to an open and penetrating critique of what we do, how we do it and the effects of our work on both our patients and ourselves.

References

 Aranda, S. (1998a) Palliative care principles: masking the complexity of practice, in J. Parker and S. Aranda (eds) *Palliative Care: Explorations and Challenges.* Rosebery: MacLennan and Petty.

Aranda, S. (1998b) A critical praxis study of nurse–patient friendship. Unpublished doctoral thesis, La Trobe University, Melbourne, VIC.

Aranda, S. (2001) Guest editorial: the tyrannies of palliative care. *International Journal of Palliative Nursing*, 7(12): 572–3.

Aranda, S. and O'Connor, M. (1995) Euthanasia, nursing and care of the dying: rethinking Kuhse and Singer. *Australian Nursing Journal*, 3(2): 18–21.

Aranda, S., Bence, G. and O'Connor, M. (1999) Euthanasia: a perspective from Australia. *International Journal of Palliative Nursing*, 5(6): 298–304.

Barnes, K. (2001) Staff stress in the children's hospice: causes, effects and coping strategies. *International Journal of Palliative Nursing*, 7(5): 248–54.

Benner, P. and Wrubel, J. (1989) *The Primacy of Caring*. Menlo Park, CA: Addison-Wesley.

Biswas, B. (1993) The medicalization of dying: a nurse's view, in D. Clark (ed.) *The Future for Palliative Care: Issues of Policy and Practice*. Buckingham: Open University Press.

Bradshaw, A. (1996) The spiritual dimension of hospice: the secularisation of an ideal. *Social Science and Medicine*, 43: 409–20.

Brown, R., Aranda, S., Parker, J. and Wiltshire, J. (2002) Exploring nurses' work with people experiencing bodily decay at the end-of-life. Unpublished research data and work in progress. Melbourne, VIC: Melbourne University.

Byrne, D. and McMurray, A. (1997) Caring for the dying: nurses' experiences in hospice care. *Australian Journal of Advanced Nursing*, 15(1): 4–11.

Clark, D. and Seymour, J. (1999) *Reflections on Palliative Care*. Buckingham: Open University Press.

Feldstein, M.A. and Gemma, P.B. (1995) Oncology nurses and chronic compounded grief. *Cancer Nursing*, 18(3): 228–36.

Folkman, S. (1997) Positive psychological states and coping with severe illness. *Social Science and Medicine*, 45(8): 1207–21.

Johnston, G. and Abraham, C. (1995) The WHO objectives for palliative care: to what extent are we achieving them? *Palliative Medicine*, 9: 123–37.

Lawton, J. (1998) Contemporary hospice care: the sequestration of the unbounded body and 'dirty dying'. *Sociology of Health and Illness*, 20(2): 121–43.

Lawton, J. (2000) *The Dying Process: Patients' Experiences of Palliative Care*. London: Routledge.

Lazarus, R.S. and Folkman, S. (1984) *Stress, Appraisal, and Coping*. New York: Springer.

McNamara, B., Waddell, C. and Colvin, M. (1994) The institutionalization of the good death. *Social Science and Medicine*, 39(11): 1501–8.

McNamara, B., Waddell, C. and Colvin, M. (1995) Threats to the good death: the cultural context of stress and coping among hospice nurses. *Sociology of Health and Illness*, 17(2): 222–44.

Newton, J. and Waters, V. (2001) Community palliative care clinical nurse specialists' descriptions of stress in their work. *International Journal of Palliative Nursing*, 7(11): 531–40.

Palsson, M.E., Hallberg, I.R. and Norberg, A. (1994) Systematic clinical supervision and its effects for nurses handling demanding care situations. *Cancer Nursing*, 17(5): 385–94.

Payne, N. (2001) Occupational stressors and coping as determinants of burnout in female hospice nurses. *Journal of Advanced Nursing*, 33(3): 396–405.

Payne, S., Langley-Evans, A. and Hillier, R. (1996) Perceptions of a 'good' death: a comparative study of the views of hospice staff and patients. *Palliative Medicine*, 10: 307–12.

Pearce, S. (1998) The experience of stress for cancer nurses: a Heideggerian phenomenological approach. *European Journal of Oncology Nursing*, 2(4): 235–7.

Saunders, C. and Baines, M. (1983) *Living with Dying: The Management of Terminal Disease*. Oxford: Oxford University Press.

Saunders, J.M. and Valente, S.M. (1994) Nurses' grief. *Cancer Nursing*, 17(4): 318–25.

Street, A. (1995) *Nursing Replay: Researching Nursing Culture Together*. Melbourne, VIC: Churchill Livingstone.

Vachon, M. (1987) *Occupational Stress in the Care of the Critically Ill, the Dying, and the Bereaved*. New York: Hemisphere.

Vachon, M. (1995) Reflections on the history of occupational stress in hospice/ palliative care. *The Hospice Journal*, 14(3/4): 229–46.

Vachon, M. (1998) Caring for the caregiver in oncology and palliative care. *Seminars in Oncology Nursing*, 14(2): 152–7.

Vachon, M. (1999) Staff stress in hospice/palliative care: a review. *Palliative Medicine*, 9: 91–122.

von Klitzing, W (1999) Evaluation of reflective learning in a psychodynamic group of nurses caring for terminally ill patients. *Journal of Advanced Nursing*, 30(5): 1213–21.

Welsh, D.J. (1999) Care for the caregiver: strategies for avoiding 'compassion fatigue'. *Clinical Journal of Oncology Nursing*, 3(4): 183–4.

33

Specialist professional education in palliative care

How did we get here and where are we going?

Margaret Sneddon

In this chapter, I focus on education to prepare practitioners for a specialist role in palliative care. I focus mainly, but not exclusively, on post-basic nurse education in the UK. However, experiences from other disciplines and contexts, particularly medical education, will be used to draw comparisons or to explore different ideas. Basic professional training programmes or short courses aimed at generalists will only be discussed in as much as they have influenced the development of more advanced education programmes. The philosophy and principles of specialist professional education generally are discussed briefly with fuller consideration given to key elements of palliative care education and what constitutes best practice. The development of palliative care education is then outlined. It is not my intention to provide a historical account, but to consider the factors that have influenced, and will continue to influence, how specialist education develops. This will give rise to an exploration of the challenges to be faced in the future. In relation to the provision of specialist education, recent experience as a provider of multi-professional palliative care education is cited as an example, supported by comments from current and recent students to provide the consumer's perspective (permission was granted by the students concerned). Therefore, what participants of specialist professional education programmes might want or need from their experience is considered.

Specialist professional education

Education

Education is a complex concept that is difficult to define. It is not a discrete event but a process with a humanistic basis intended to enhance the participant's learning and understanding (Jarvis 1983). A humanist approach is concerned with 'human growth, individual fulfilment and self-actualization'

(Quinn 1995: 100) underpinned by the work of theories such as Maslow's hierarchy of needs and Roger's student-centred learning. Theorists argue that the intrinsic value of education enables the individual 'to travel with a different view' (Peters 1979: p. 8) on a journey to a destination where we never arrive. Implicit to this concept is the notion that the person is changed by the experience of education: they perceive and respond to subsequent experiences in a different way. The change that occurs can arise from many life experiences other than planned programmes of education. So when embarking on a planned educational experience, our perceptions and needs will be influenced by all of our past experiences. Recognition and affirmation of prior learning and individual needs is a key principle of adult education (Knowles 1984). Education, therefore, becomes an enabling process for personal growth and learning for the individual.

Professional education

By necessity, professional education tends to be more focused on outcome and professional growth, rather than process, individual needs or personal growth, to ensure the professional develops the knowledge, skills and attitudes that render them fit to practise in their particular field. For example, in nursing we have progressed from a 'training' mentality where the aim was to teach students to undertake specific tasks or procedures unquestioningly, to one that more readily appreciates the need to learn how to learn, to develop an enquiring mind, and to learn concepts and principles that can be applied flexibly in different situations.

Over the years, there has also been a growing recognition of the need for ongoing training and education to maintain satisfactory levels of practice to such an extent that it is now underpinned by legislation. Ongoing or continuing professional education (CPE) seeks in part to maintain the currency of existing knowledge, the half life of which is suggested to be 2–5 years in nursing (Ferrell 1988). It is also a means of extending knowledge and skills by meeting identified needs in relation to the professional's role or preparing them for a new role. There has been increasing specialization in every branch of health care as the knowledge base extends, making education beyond a basic professional qualification a necessity. CPE generally involves mature individuals with personal and professional life experience on which to 'hang' new learning. Usually, but not always, they have chosen to enter a particular programme of learning because it is of relevance to them professionally and so they are motivated to learn. They may have identified specific gaps in their knowledge or expertise. All these characteristics pertain to the 'adult learner' as described by Knowles (1984).

From a manager's perspective, there is little point in investing time, effort and money in CPE if it does not have an impact on practice, preferably beyond that of the individual. The subsequent ability to cascade knowledge and influence the practice of colleagues provides added value to any education programme. The focus on outcome, particularly achieving an impact on practice, may appear contrary to the humanistic philosophy of education that focuses on the student's needs. However, there is generally something to be gained on both sides.

Specialist professional education

Specialist professional education may involve those working in a specialist field of practice or those in the role, or preparing for the role, of specialist practitioner. Whether catering for specialist practitioners or those working in specialist fields, specialist professional education should seek to enable participants to deliver best clinical practice. The outcome should be practitioners who are able to assess comprehensively an individual's needs, implement interventions and, based on sound evidence, evaluate the outcome. Implicit in this is the ability to critically appraise research evidence and learn from the outcomes, so that practice continues to develop. In addition, specialist practitioners should also be able to influence practice through teaching, dissemination of research and implementation of change. Yet a recent study reported clinical nurse specialists in palliative care to be 'poorly prepared in terms of their educational background and information technology skills' (Seymour *et al.* 2002: 390) in order to fulfil the teaching part of their role. In nursing, specialist posts first appeared in the 1970s. There was no clear pathway or training to specialism, with most acquiring their knowledge and skills on the job, through self-learning and often with little support from others. The roles of clinical nurse specialists just 'kept growing without any direction or control' (Castledine 2002: 507). Their role is now much more clearly defined and there are expectations that they will be involved in teaching, advising, acting as a change agent, developing practice, providing a voice for the specialty and being familiar with, if not actively involved in, research activities. Such expectations are reinforced by standards for education of specialist practitioners in nursing that have been set out by professional bodies in the UK (now the Nursing and Midwifery Council). Specialist posts for allied health professionals have also been developed within the past 10 years. However, these are rare outside specialist palliative care units.

| Palliative care education

Several writers have drawn parallels between the philosophy of education and palliative care provision. Sheldon and Smith (1996) suggest that palliative care education should mirror that of the philosophy of palliative care provision in that it is a 'process that is *with* and *for* people rather than *on* people' (p. 100). Comparisons are drawn between students embarking on a programme of study and patients with advancing illness, who are each facing uncertainty with a potential for personal growth. This resonates with Peters's (1979) statement, that the analogy of a journey is often used in relation to the illness experience. Both the student and the patient need support and companionship along the way. However, it is their journey; they choose how they respond to the experience. Respect for their choices and feeling valued as an individual is important for each within their own context.

The holistic nature of palliative care should also be reflected in education provision. James and Macleod (1993) suggest that the interpersonal aspects of palliative care are more important to the patient than the more easily addressed physical aspects. The value placed on positive human interaction means that the most important tools practitioners have are themselves. Therefore, palliative care programmes must equip them with the interpersonal skills to meet the needs of patients and their carers, in addition to knowledge of particular problems and how these might be addressed. So, too, palliative care education must seek to enable students to achieve their personal potential, as their effectiveness lies not only in learning the application of strategies and techniques, but in responding intuitively as a fellow human being. Knowledge and skills are insufficient without the appropriate attitude, giving some credence to the saying 'palliative care is caught, not taught' (Anon.). That is not to say that these abilities are innate and cannot be learned – effectiveness lies in developing self-knowledge of their strengths and limitations and developing confidence in using themselves and their intuitive abilities. Such skills require an openness and willingness to explore personal values, attitudes and fears. The 'teacher' must ensure time, opportunity, a safe environment and trusting relationship to enable the abilities to be cultivated. Clearly, this is difficult to achieve in short didactic sessions with large groups of students. However, cultivating a safe environment is an important consideration when developing programmes that are more comprehensive. In relation to nurse education, Jodrell (1998) highlights the need to address issues of clinical excellence, research, management and leadership in education programmes to develop advanced levels of practice. In the UK, these elements are mandatory for the award of the Specialist Practitioner Qualification for nurses, recordable by the governing body of the Nursing and Midwifery Council. Similar requirements are stipulated for doctors preparing for consultant posts. Although there is no such equivalent qualification for other professions, the need to develop skills wider than the area of specialty is well recognized.

Multi-professional working is said to be a key component of effective palliative care (World Health Organization 1990). It is well recognized and supported by a small number of studies that the complex needs of patients and their families can best be met by a well coordinated team drawing on various professional skills (Jones 1993). In no other aspect of health care is learning alongside different disciplines so enthusiastically welcomed, despite the absence of strong evidence that it facilitates more collaborative teamworking. Indeed, Ford (1998) suggests that multi-professional education was moving from 'an accepted principle to a necessary practice' (p. 1167). However, multi-professional education is a term often used when all that has been done is the drawing together of a disparate group of professionals in one location (see Chapter 31). There may be minimal interaction of those involved.

Inter-professional education is perhaps a more apt term for the more desirable process that provides an opportunity for shared learning experiences with a potential for breaking down professional barriers, enhancing understanding of the role and strengths of others, enhanced communication and collaboration through a more interactive process (Barr and Waterton 1996). These benefits are not achieved without careful planning and social engineering. General principles of adult learning apply in relation to ensuring relevancy and meaningfulness, but can present a challenge when different professions are involved. Effort, creativity and consultation with others with different professional backgrounds will help to ensure that each participant is able to make a positive contribution and be valued within the group. Problem-based learning with scenarios that reflect the real world of practice and the complex needs of patients can be particularly effective in multi-professional groups.

Box 33.1 Example of creative use of real situations (Wee *et al.* 2001)

Multi-professional groups of undergraduate students (medical, nursing, social work, physiotherapy and occupational therapy students who are at least in the second year of their training) are joined by an individual who is currently involved in caring for a family member who is dying or someone who has recently been bereaved. Facilitators include a palliative nurse lecturer, palliative medicine consultant and lecturer in psychosocial palliative care. A senior physiotherapist or occupational therapist also assists. Certain tasks are set to encourage interaction and listening to the carer's story, after which the students reflect on key issues about the care provided. They then prepare a joint presentation. Although involving undergraduate students, this approach has considerable potential with more experienced professionals. However, this approach involving carers or patients must be well planned and sensitively handled by experienced teachers and practitioners.

Growth of palliative care education

Although the birth of the modern hospice movement in 1967 was heralded by the opening of St Christopher's Hospice in London, the term palliative care did not come into common usage until 1987 when it was recognized as a medical subspecialty by the Royal College of Physicians in the UK (Scott *et al.* 1998).

For many years, the main focus in palliative care education seemed to be in spreading the word, achieving a measure of credibility and convincing professionals in general health care settings that palliative care was more than good basic nursing care of dying patients, an approach that was often seen as criticism of their core skills. However, it was commonly believed that staffing levels that enabled extra time to be spent with the

> **Box 33.2** An example of acquiring professional specialty status for palliative medicine in the UK
>
> The Association of Palliative Medicine (APM), established in 1985 (Scott *et al.* 1998), lobbied for the specialty status of palliative medicine, developed a core curriculum for medical training and a programme for trainee consultants, making palliative medicine an appropriate career path for doctors. Although nurses may take the credit for stimulating recognition for the need for improvement in this area of care, the advances made would not have been possible without the change of name and the recognition by the Royal College of Physicians. Having a programme of medical training of specialists added credence to palliative care and recognition that it was more than good basic nursing care. The Association's success in having palliative medicine included in the undergraduate curriculum has ensured that the doctors of tomorrow will be better equipped.
>
> Specialty status required that the specialty be based on a sound body of evidence, giving rise to research and many improvements in pain and symptom control. This became a very useful hook with which to gain medical interest in terms of education. However, this trend has given rise to concern that palliative care is becoming too focused on symptom management and interventions and risks losing sight of the whole patient and the philosophy of palliative care (Dush 1990).
>
> Despite the fact that one of the criteria for recognition as a medical specialty is a sound body of knowledge and skills, this was fairly weak in 1987 when palliative medicine was given such recognition by the Royal College of Physicians. Little of what was practised was based on sound evidence and it became necessary to address this urgently.

patient and pleasant surroundings were all that was needed; these were considered luxuries unrealistic in busy hospital wards. Hospices were perceived to be the only institutions that could offer the appropriate environment in which to die and the quantity of staff to spend a lot of time with the patient and their family. The ability to facilitate care at home by specialist nurses such as Macmillan nurses was acknowledged, but only because they had a much smaller case load and could spend more time with the patients! It was clearly perceived as nothing to do with having particular knowledge, skills or attitudes. Based on work such as that of Mills and co-workers' (1994) observational study of terminal care in the acute setting, professionals began to acknowledge that there were many inadequacies in care provision. This qualitative study recorded the care provided to patients during the last week of life in several acute medical and surgical wards in a busy general hospital. It highlighted a tendency in some wards to follow the 'medical model' in that when cure was no longer deemed possible and medical interest waned, so too did the nursing attention. Many examples of failure to address basic care needs, such as prevention of thirst, were observed. It is interesting that although this study was carried out in the mid-1980s, the results were not published until 1994, partly because of resistance to the findings. It can be difficult for any professional to accept that they may share responsibility for the delivery of care that is less than optimal and this sometimes results in an attempt to shift blame to the institution or other professional groups. This was also seen in an earlier study in Canada by Mount (1976) that highlighted the views of various professional groups, including doctors, nurses, social workers and clergy. Each blamed the other for failure to provide good palliative care.

Despite an apparent reluctance to be overtly critical of their own practice, nurses were the first to become enthusiastic about palliative care education. Their interest gave rise to many short courses, study days and, later, professionally validated courses. Education for other professionals was *ad hoc* until the first multi-professional university-accredited programmes came into being in the UK in 1994. One of these courses focused on psychosocial palliative care and was geared in particular towards social workers and nurses. The growth in academically accredited specialist palliative care programmes has been substantial. No other branch of health care has spawned so many specialist courses. Within 7 years of becoming a medical specialty, Sheldon and Smith (1996) reported that there were seven specialist postgraduate diploma or master's programmes in the UK and many others related to social work or nursing that included at least one palliative care module. In addition, there were numerous professionally validated courses for nurses. In 2002, the Hospice Information Service records 13 degree level programmes in palliative care, several other degree courses with opportunities to specialize in palliative care and many diploma programmes and modules. Master's specialist programmes have remained static at seven (two by distance learning), probably reflecting a relatively limited need at this level. However, there are more general programmes with significant palliative care components. Most are multi-professional, although some specify they are for nurses and professions allied to medicine, but not doctors. There is one postgraduate diploma/master's for doctors alone. At the time of writing, five institutions in Scotland and considerably more in England and Wales offer professionally validated courses with specialist practitioner qualifications for nurses in palliative care. In addition, most hospices have an education department to cater for the needs of their own staff and other professionals in the locality. They continue to 'spread the word' and generate further interest in education.

Many other countries have developed palliative care programmes. Distance learning courses are available in Uganda, Kenya, Argentina and South Australia. The USA has two master's programmes, both for nurses, and a multi-professional programme is currently being developed. Australia has three multi-professional master's courses. France has one diploma course, but the rest of Europe is not very well served in terms of academically accredited programmes.

Influencing factors

Several inter-related factors have stimulated expansion of palliative care education, partly through awakening health service managers to the need to equip health professionals in many areas of care with core palliative care skills.

Political

The UK has a state-funded health care system, the National Health Service (NHS), so there is a single employer who can determine educational requirements. Reorganization of the NHS and initiatives driven by a need to develop more cost-effective services, such as the Calman-Hine recommendations for cancer services (Expert Advisory Group on Cancer 1995), have helped to shape the role of specialist nurses, requiring the development of new skills in service and policy development (Seymour *et al.* 2002). In addition, a clinical governance framework (discussed in Chapters 37 & 38) for health and social care workers requires employers and individual professionals to ensure that practitioners are appropriately skilled to deliver quality care. Although most hospices are run independently of the NHS, most seek to achieve the standards set nationally. To ensure staff are adequately skilled, a number of strategies have been introduced. Individual professionals have been encouraged to undertake critical reflection on their practice, a strategy that inevitably leads to identification of learning needs. Statutory requirements for continuing professional development, such as the Post Registration Education and Practice initiative for nurses (UKCC 1994), have been introduced for most health professionals, stimulating an expectation of continual learning throughout an individual's professional career. Evidence-based care is another requirement of clinical governance and is also necessary for credibility, status as a medical specialty and for funding reasons. Therefore, in addition to maintaining knowledge of new research, skills in research appraisal and activity have been needed for all disciplines.

Economic

Charitable funding is one key reason why the UK has been able to develop so many educational programmes. Macmillan Cancer Relief and Marie Curie Cancer Care have supported many educational initiatives in support of their aims to improve patient care. Although some short programmes may generate income for an institution, longer award-bearing programmes rarely do. Without charitable funding, or the free provision of teaching from hospices, few of the existing programmes would have developed. Charities have also played a key role in funding research, which, in turn, is constantly raising new issues for professionals. The introduction of specialist Macmillan nurses and Marie Curie home care nurses in the early 1970s and later palliative care consultants into community and hospital settings were another significant influence in that general health care professionals gained first-hand experience of the specialist skills. The nature of Macmillan Cancer Relief funding meant that posts were pump-primed for an agreed period and then taken over by the institution, mostly in the NHS. In this way, more and more specialist posts were able to be integrated into the health care system. The potential for improved symptom management, particularly pain control and early discharge, could not be denied and led to demands for education in these areas.

Another factor relates to insufficient resources to enable all individuals with palliative care needs to be cared for in specialist units. More and more responsibility for providing palliative care is being devolved to other settings. So there has been a move towards employing more specialists in acute and community settings as a resource for generalist colleagues. As generalists have also been keen participants of palliative care education, specialists perceive a need to further their own education to remain confident in their specialty and maintain credibility.

Social

The growing elderly population, increase in chronic life-limiting illnesses and improved treatment for cancer has stimulated public demand for improved palliative care provision. This is partly due to the example provided by hospices, but also reflects a growing awareness and interest in all topics related to dying and death by the public and the media. The public are also better informed about health issues generally through the internet and more demanding of information and support. Recognition that palliative care is appropriate in many disease trajectories other than just cancer has added to the demand. Additionally, there is a desire to increase the choices available to patients, including where they are cared for and where they may die. The generally accepted belief is that most patients wish to stay at home as long as possible, and also to die at home with adequate support, although there is limited evidence to support this.

Limited charitable resources have curtailed significant expansion of hospices. However, there is also a realization that palliative care should not be the icing on the cake, but a core part of statutory provision, for which resources are limited.

Expansion of knowledge base

Expansion of the knowledge base, which has in part resulted from education, has also fuelled the need for more education. In learning more, knowledge gaps become more evident; more research is stimulated and knowledge expands. The much needed development of research has necessitated constant updating of professionals in addition to the acquisition of skills to determine the quality of the research. This has changed the nature of palliative care education from a 'recipe' approach to managing symptoms and problems on a more solid research base. It has also spawned several specialist journals in which research can be disseminated. Published in the UK, but with international representation on the editorial boards, are *Palliative Medicine, Progress in Palliative Care, International Journal of Palliative Nursing* and *Mortality and the European Journal of Palliative Care*. Outside the UK, we find the *Journal of Pain and Symptom Control* (USA), *Journal of Palliative Medicine* (USA), *American Journal of Hospice and Palliative Care* (USA) and *Journal of Palliative Care* (Canada). The growing educational provision not only utilizes such journals as a learning resource, but also feeds new knowledge into them as skills in writing and research are developed.

Box 33.3   What's in a name?

Prior to 1987 when palliative medicine was a recognized medical specialty, this branch of health care was generally referred to as terminal care and was considered the province of nursing. I well remember as a young nurse considering anyone with cancer, especially recurrent cancer, being considered 'terminal' and of little interest to the medical profession. However, a change of terminology enabled it not only to be an acceptable area of interest for doctors, but also broadened the scope of involvement and reflected the emphasis on living rather than dying. The result was that practitioners were required to adopt a much more active role in enhancing quality of life rather than simply the quality of death. Care was required over a much longer period, particularly as symptoms became more effectively controlled. In short, it was no longer enough to care about dying people and their families, many diverse skills had to be developed in addition to the resilience required to cope with such demanding work.

What does the specialist or aspiring specialist want and need from an education programme?

It is important to consider that whatever educationalists think should be included in a programme of study may be at odds with what either participants or managers want. The tension between what students wanted and what was required for master's level study was apparent when the author was developing and directing a multi-professional palliative care programme at higher degree level, which began in the early 1990s. The programme could be taken full-time over 1 year or part-time over 2 or 3 years for the Postgraduate Diploma or Master's of Science, respectively. This section highlights key observations gained through that experience.

A needs assessment identified that research skills were not especially highly valued by potential participants, including nurses, doctors, clergy and allied health professionals. The main interest lay in pain and symptom management, communication skills, emotional and spiritual care and bereavement. Initially, these aspects provided the main content of the programme. Generic skills such as critical appraisal and teaching were integrated to some extent throughout and, it could be argued, covertly.

Since the programme began, participants have come from a variety of professional backgrounds but fall into three broad categories:

- those already in a specialist role or specialist setting;
- those aspiring to be in a specialist role or setting;
- those generalists whose remit involves them substantially in caring for people with palliative care needs.

The most common reasons for applying are:

- awareness that they could care more effectively, particularly in managing pain and other symptoms;
- validation of their existing expertise and enhanced credibility through gaining a qualification;
- to learn alongside members of other professions and enhance understanding of roles;
- to gain confidence in communicating with patients and relatives and responding to emotional and spiritual distress;
- to gain understanding of disease processes and treatment strategies (non-clinical professions, e.g. social work or clergy);
- to gain confidence in their knowledge base to enable them to teach others; and
- to develop research or teaching skills (expressed by more recent students).

It quickly became apparent that the generic component was insufficient if the education was to have the desired impact on patient care. After 2 years, a reconfiguration of the programme introduced a specific module on teaching skills and more substantial input on communication skills, particularly inter-professional communication, research, critical appraisal and professional issues such as quality, ethics and implementation of change.

Rigorous evaluation of each module, and the overall programme, by students and teachers and a reflexive approach by the programme director sought to ensure that it was a positive learning experience for the students in addition to meeting their educational needs and contributing to course development. The impact on practice has been demonstrated through course work. Examination of programme evaluations frequently identifies the multi-professional nature of the programme as being most valuable. Opportunities to work in groups has never been perceived as enough, indicating the value placed on learning derived from fellow students. Students state that they were attracted by the specific palliative care content of the programme, particularly pain and symptom management. However, they perceive ultimately that the communication skills and the professional issues content has been more influential in changing their practice. The communication skills module is experiential. Assessment of practical skills is undertaken alongside that of their abilities to critically appraise their own practice through a scoring system developed for the programme and through critical analysis of their strengths, limitations and consideration of alternative strategies. The perceived impact of the professional issues component relates to three aspects. First, their enhanced understanding of ethical issues and decision making in relation to this. Second, their confidence and ability to seek out and make judgements on published work and research, which they frequently admit to accepting blindly prior to the programme. Third, how they relate to other professionals and their understanding of differing perspectives.

Despite the perceived value of the multi-professional approach, there are limitations in respect of meeting the needs of some professional groups. The uptake by some professional groups, such as clergy, social work, occupational therapy, physiotherapy or other therapies is variable and, on occasions, there has been only one member of a particular profession represented. Moreover, the evidence base for palliative care is dominated by medicine and nursing. It can be very challenging for the isolated professional and for the programme teachers to ensure their particular needs are met.

Recent changes to the course have resulted in a programme with considerably more of a generic component, although all course work must be focused on palliative care. The intention is that the programme should better prepare students with the principles and strategies to enable them to take responsibility for further learning and practice development. The change has also been influenced by a need to rationalize existing education and utilize resources more effectively, a strategy advocated by Koffman (2001) to help encourage more learning from other disciplines and those outside the specialist field.

How effective is specialist professional education in palliative care?

In the second edition of the *Oxford Textbook of Palliative Medicine* (1998: 1205), Jodrell was critical of the fact that 'the paucity of systematic evaluations of educational programmes in palliative care has not improved since the first edition of this Textbook'. This remains the situation. There is fairly weak published scientific evidence to support a positive impact of education on clinical practice, with most evaluations focusing on participant perceptions. However, Fuhrmann and Weissberg (1978) assert that perceptions of increased knowledge, self-confidence, performance achievements and attitude changes are more reliable than actual measurable differences and, therefore, are valid predictors of behaviour. If this is accepted, then there is substantial evidence in support of the effectiveness of education, particularly if the evaluation is undertaken at some point after the education to avoid the bias of 'happiness indexes' (Gosnell 1984). Just as it is difficult to

---

Box 33.4 Portfolios as a learning and assessment strategy

A portfolio is a collection of evidence of learning and achievement. In the context of the MSc/Postgraduate Diploma in Palliative Care run in Glasgow, it is used to identify learning needs and to record the process of learning that ensues. With much resistance from colleagues, portfolios were introduced as a learning and assessment strategy at the outset. In view of the diversity of the participants' educational and professional backgrounds, portfolio learning was considered a way of ensuring each individual's learning needs could be identified and met. With support, each student was encouraged to reflect on existing knowledge, skills and attitudes and identify priorities for learning that would be meaningful to their own professional practice and then to plan strategies to achieve their stated outcomes. Developing a portfolio was a new and daunting concept for most and initially many were unable to see the point of it all. By the end of the programme, with very few exceptions, students leave feeling very proud of their achievements and delighted that they are documented in the portfolio. The portfolios also provide evidence of a positive impact in practice as a result of education. As the programme continues over 2 years, how understanding, attitudes and practice have changed is clearly demonstrated. There is also little doubt that many practice initiatives would not have been implemented had it not have been for the need to produce evidence of application of learning to practice. Therefore, the portfolio acts as a prompt for practice development. Despite their value as evidence, the portfolios are personal, no copies are retained and for ethical reasons they have never been used to systematically gather such evidence.

Using portfolios as an assessment strategy remains somewhat controversial because of their subjectivity. However, the whole concept encourages self-appraisal and, with clear guidelines on what is required, the standard is generally very good. Educators are enthusiastic about the concept and it has been used widely in nursing and medical education (Snadden and Thomas 1998) and very successfully in other palliative care programmes (Finlay *et al.* 1993). However, there has been little formal evaluation. One exception is preliminary work by Challis *et al.* (1997), who reported that participants perceived portfolio learning to be effective in meeting pre-determined objectives and those arising from critical incidents in practice. It also appeared to stimulate a more collaborative approach to learning. However, there was subjective and objective evidence that maintaining the portfolio was more time-consuming than more traditional methods of learning.

---

measure many aspects of palliative care in a quantitative way, so it is with education. Sheldon and Smith (1996) suggest that a positivist approach to measuring the impact of palliative care education is pointless, as it is denies the whole philosophy of promoting personal growth alongside safe practice. It could be argued that the best evidence of personal growth and altered attitudes and values must come from individuals themselves. Examples of evaluations focusing on perceived impact after completion of the programme include those of Sneddon (1992), Kenny (2001) and MacDougall *et al.* (2001). All involved evaluation a few months after the education ended and all reported changes in practice as a consequence of the education by most of the participants, with specific examples provided. However, the studies by MacDougall *et al.* (2001) and Keogh *et al.* (1999) had a low completion rate for the final evaluation.

Sneddon's (1992) study also highlighted the importance of factors other than the education provided in determining if learning was applied to practice. Of the 36 nurses on the education programme, 64 per cent reported changes in practice or ability to influence colleagues, giving specific examples of doing so. Increased knowledge, skills and confidence were the main facilitating factors; shortage of staff and lack of support were the main inhibiting factors. Presence or absence of support from nurse managers was a key factor. Other inhibiting factors included:

- having no clear or effective strategy with which to instigate change (sometimes giving rise to conflict);

- lack of credibility and authority in junior staff (staff nurses had more difficulties than ward managers);

- negative or disinterested attitudes of colleagues (only some perceived it as an opportunity to learn).

Sneddon's (1992) results supported other findings that education is only part of the equation (Keiser and Bickle 1980). Knowledge and skills gained are not necessarily put into practice (Sanzaro 1983) and the individual must be motivated to improve practice and be adequately supported to do so (Lawler 1987). Sneddon also highlighted the need to prepare students to negotiate and plan appropriate strategies for change. The need for support in the work environment has also been demonstrated by Wilkinson (1991) and Booth *et al.* (1996) in relation to the impact of communication skills courses. Similarly, in a study of clinical nurse specialists in palliative care, Seymour *et al.* (2002) identified a need for formalized support such as clinical supervision to enable specialists to fully develop their roles. Therefore, to reflect the

---

Box 33.5 Examples of manager support

Example of positive manager support
One manager who appeared really interested to hear the nurse's views of the course asked her to share her experience with colleagues and negotiated that she spend time in a variety of wards to disseminate her new knowledge and skills. There was no indication that the manager devoted a lot of time to staff development, but the attitude and ability to convey a sense of support and value was significant.

Example of negative manager support
Another nurse was bitterly disappointed to be told that there was no place for what she had learned in the unit (care of elderly). For others, there was no mention of the course on their return: 'It's as if I had never gone.'

true impact of education, evaluation processes must take into account factors other than the educational experience. Moreover, in programme development, ways of overcoming the barriers need to be explored.

How planned education is delivered is another aspect that lacks rigorous evaluation. It is accepted that effective palliative care depends on various disciplines working collaboratively and communicating well, but there is little more than anecdotal evidence that multi-professional education facilitates this. In addition, various distance learning initiatives have developed with scope to develop more electronic means of learning. While these meet the need of practitioners who are unable to access face-to-face teaching, formal evaluation of outcomes of the various approaches would be useful as they are not necessarily less expensive to provide.

What are the challenges for the future?

There is little doubt that the increasing prevalence of chronic life-limiting illnesses will result in more people requiring palliative care and so demand will continue to grow in the foreseeable future. So, too, will the need for education. In view of the number of existing programmes, it is questionable as to whether more are needed. However, palliative care programmes have developed in an *ad hoc* fashion, not always driven by need in terms of the various levels of provision. Therefore, rationalization and consideration regarding the best way forward is essential. In view of the success of the strategy of the Association of Palliative Medicine, perhaps some national standardization of educational outcomes, programme components and levels might overcome the inconsistency and *ad hoc* development of additional programmes. This could be linked with career paths for the various professions. Developing standards and employing benchmarking could also be a way of encouraging greater collaboration between education providers. The core curriculum identified by the International Society of Nurses in Cancer Care (1991) and endorsed by the World Health Organization would be a useful starting point. However, this could now be informed by the considerable experience of palliative care education gained in the past 10 years.

There remains a relatively weak evidence base for some aspects of palliative care, providing an insecure footing for education. It is essential that professionals have opportunities to develop the appropriate skills to further develop the specialty and become more active in research to enhance the knowledge base. While more generic components would help to develop these skills, there is concern that it may result in more dilute programmes, which, in turn, may result in what Scott *et al.* (1998) warn are 'anaemic models of palliative care' (p. 1187).

Specialist practitioners must have a sound knowledge of the specialty and so any specialist education programme should include a strong palliative care component that is underpinned by the philosophy to maximize quality

> **Box 33.6**   Core curriculum for palliative care suggested by the International Society of Nurses in Cancer Care
>
> - The politics of health care: death, society and palliative care
> - Nursing theory: the nurse in palliative care
> - Counselling theory and practice
> - Interdisciplinary teamwork
> - Pain and symptom management
> - Loss and grief
> - Spirituality
> - Legal and ethical issues

of life of the individual patient and their family. Particular emphasis should be placed on the interpersonal aspects of practice, to enable practitioners to use themselves to maximum therapeutic benefit. Practitioners must also be equipped to appraise the growing body of literature, evaluate practice and implement change if they are to influence practice. Therefore, more general managerial and professional skills should be developed in a specialist education programme. The 'cook book' approach is inappropriate for this level of education, as it is essential that specialist practitioners can apply their knowledge and skills flexibly in diverse situations and appropriate to the unique needs of the individual. Because of its wide scope, there are particular challenges for palliative care in terms of:

- time – potentially from diagnosis to the bereavement period;

- diagnosis – any chronic life-limiting illness;

- recipient – patient, family and support network;

- remit – physical, psychological, social and spiritual;

- philosophy of teamwork and support for colleagues.

The palliative care needs of people with diseases other than cancer (e.g. dementia) are increasingly being recognized, and is likely to give rise to demands for education relevant to these conditions. Education must embrace this wider focus.

Finally, education is only part of the picture. Educators must work with managers and practitioners with the aim of maximizing impact on practice. This would involve continuing support during and following formal education programmes. Creative approaches to programme evaluation need to be developed, for example to utilize the available student-generated evidence of impact on practice. Only by demonstrating effectiveness will comprehensive programmes be selected by managers over short, sharp and much cheaper courses.

Conclusions

Palliative care education has expanded greatly in the past 10 years in particular, but not always in a coordinated way. It is time to reflect on the future learning needs of professionals specializing in palliative care, planning new education or modifying existing education accordingly. Needs assessments, involving practitioners, managers and service users, together with more creative approaches to evaluation of education should inform future development. However, careful balance of generic and specialist components will best equip students to maximize the impact of learning on practice and enable further development of the specialty. Educators must be careful not to lose the elements that distinguish palliative care in their programmes, ensuring that the education process mirrors the caring philosophy of palliative care. Skilful management of inter-professional learning opportunities, development of interpersonal skills and creative strategies that reflect reality are necessary components of specialist education. Key learning points include:

- The expectation of specialist palliative care education is that it will result in a positive impact on practice, preferably beyond the individual participant. Therefore, participants also need to be equipped with skills of negotiation, change implementation, teaching and leadership.

- Learning in relation to psychosocial, spiritual and interpersonal elements of palliative care is not only the most difficult, but also the most vital and valued by patients.

- Inter-professional education that is effective in facilitating collaborative working requires careful planning and use of strategies to enable all participants to make a positive contribution. Problem-based learning reflecting practice is a useful learning strategy.

- Support in the workplace is critical to the implementation of learning.

- Development of educational standards nationally would aid the development of a more coordinated approach to education.

Further reading

Harden, R.M. (1998) AMEE guide No. 12: Multiprofessional education: Part 1 – effective multiprofessional education: a three-dimensional perspective. *Medical Teacher*, 20(5): 402–16.

Jeffrey, D. (ed.) (2002) *Teaching Palliative Care: A Practical Guide*. Oxford: Radcliffe Medical Press.

Kaye, P. (ed.) (1997) *Tutorials in Palliative Medicine*. Northampton: EPL Publications.

Leininger, M. and Watson, J. (1990) *The Caring Imperative in Education*. New York: National League for Nursing.

McGill, I. and Weill, S. (eds) (1993) *Making Sense of Experiential Learning: Diversity in Theory and Practice.* Milton Keynes: Open University Press.

Parsell, G. and Bligh, J. (1998) Educational principles underpinning successful shared learning. *Medical Teacher*, 20(6): 522–9.

References

Barr, H. and Waterton, S. (1996) *Interprofessional Education in Health and Social Care in the United Kingdom.* London: CAIPE.

Booth, K., Maguire, P.M., Butterworth, T. and Hillier, V.F. (1996) Perceived professional support and the use of blocking behaviours by hospice nurses. *Journal of Advanced Nursing*, 24: 522–7.

Castledine, G. (2002) The development of the role of the clinical nurse specialist in the UK. *British Journal of Nursing*, 11(7): 506–8.

Challis, M., Mathers, N.J., Howe, A.C. and Field, N.J. (1997) Portfolio-based learning: continuing medical education for general practitioners – a mid-point evaluation. *Medical Education*, 31: 22–6.

Dush, D.M. (1990) High-tech, aggressive palliative care: in the service of quality of life. *Journal of Palliative Care*, 9(1): 37–41.

Expert Advisory Group on Cancer (The Calman Hine Report) (1995) *A Policy Framework for Commissioning Cancer Services: A Report by the Expert Advisory Group on Cancer to the Chief Medical Officers of England and Wales.* London: Department of Health and the Welsh Office.

Ferrell, M.J. (1988) The relationship of continuing education offerings to self-reported change in behaviour. *Journal of Continuing Education*, 19(1): 21–4.

Finlay, I.G., Stott, N.C.H. and Marsh, H.M. (1993) Portfolio learning in palliative medicine. *European Journal of Cancer Care*, 2: 41–3.

Ford, G. (1998) Multiprofessional education, in D. Doyle, G.W.C. Hanks and N. MacDonald (eds) *Oxford Textbook of Palliative Medicine*, 2nd edn. Oxford: Oxford Medical Publications.

Furhmann, B.S. and Weissburg, M.J. (1978) Self-assessment, in M. Morgan and D. Irby (eds) *Evaluating Clinical Competence in the Health Professions.* St Louis: Mosby.

Gosnell, D.J. (1984) Evaluating continuing nursing education. *The Journal of Continuing Education in Nursing*, 15(1): 9–11.

International Society of Nurses in Cancer Care (1991) *A Core Curriculum for a Post-basic Course in Palliative Nursing.* Manchester: Haigh & Hochland.

James, C.R. and Macleod, R. (1993) The problematic nature of education in palliative care. *Journal of Palliative Care*, 9(4): 5–10.

Jarvis, P. (1983) The concept of education, in P.J. Hills (ed.) *Professional Education.* London: Croome Helme.

Jodrell, N. (1998) Nurse education, in D. Doyle, G.W.C. Hanks and N. MacDonald (eds) *Oxford Textbook of Palliative Medicine*, 2nd edn. Oxford: Oxford Medical Publications.

Jones, R.V.H. (1993) Teams and terminal cancer care at home: do patients and carers benefit? *Journal of Interprofessional Care*, 7(3): 239–45.

Keiser, G.J. and Bickle, I.M. (1980) Attitude change as a motivational factor in producing behaviour change related to implementing primary nursing. *Nursing Research*, 29(5): 290–4.

Kenny, L.J. (2001) Education in palliative care: making a difference to practice. *International Journal of Palliative Nursing*, 7(8): 401–7.

Keogh, K., Jeffrey, D. and Flanagan, S. (1999) The Palliative Care Education Group for Gloucestershire (PEGG): an integrated model of multidisciplinary education in palliative care. *European Journal of Cancer Care*, 8: 44–7.

Knowles, M. (1984) *The Adult Learner: A Neglected Species*, 3rd edn. Houston: Gulf Publishing.

Koffman, J. (2001) Multiprofessional palliative care education: past challenges, future issues. *Journal of Palliative Care*, 17(2): 86–92.

Lawler, T.F. (1987) Effecting change in a community hospital: implications for staff development. *Journal of Continuing Education in Nursing*, 18(2): 59–63.

MacDougall, G., Mathew, A., Broadhurst, V. and Chamberlain, S. (2001) An evaluation of an interprofessional palliative care education programme. *International Journal of Palliative Nursing*, 7(1): 24–9.

Mills, M., Davies, H.T.O. and Macrae, W.A. (1994) Care of dying patients in hospital. *British Medical Journal*, 309: 583–6.

Mount, B.M. (1976) The problem of caring for the dying in a general hospital: the palliative care unit as a possible solution. *Canadian Medical Association Journal*, 11(2): 119–21.

Peters, R.S. (1979) *The Concept of Education.* London: Routledge and Kegan Paul.

Quinn, F.M. (1995) *The Principles and Practice of Nurse Education*, 3rd edn. London: Chapman & Hall.

Sanzaro, P.J. (1983) Determining physicians' performance: continuing medical education and other interacting variables. *Evaluation and the Health Professions*, 6(2): 197–210.

Scott, J.F., MacDonald, N. and Mount, B. (1998) Palliative medicine education, in D. Doyle, G.W.C. Hanks and N. MacDonald (eds) *Oxford Textbook of Palliative Medicine*, 2nd edn. Oxford: Oxford Medical Publications.

Seymour, J., Clark, D., Hughes, P. *et al.* (2002) Clinical nurse specialists in palliative care. Part 3. Issues for the Macmillan nurse role. *Palliative Medicine*, 16(5): 386–94.

Sheldon, F. and Smith, P. (1996) The life so short, the craft so hard to learn: a model for post-basic education in palliative care. *Palliative Medicine*, 10: 99–104.

Snadden, D and Thomas, M. (1998) The use of portfolio learning in medical education. *Medical Teacher*, 20(3): 192–9.

Sneddon, M.C. (1992) Continuing education in palliative care nursing: an exploration of perceived outcome and factors influencing application of learning, Unpublished thesis, University of Glasgow.

United Kingdom Central Council for Nursing, Midwifery and Health Visiting (1994) *The Future of Professional Practice: The Council's Standards for Education and Practice Following Registration*. London: UKCC.

Wee, B., Hillier, R., Coles, C. *et al.* (2001) Palliative care: a suitable setting for undergraduate interprofessional education. *Palliative Medicine*, 15: 487–92.

Wilkinson, S. (1991) Factors which influence how nurses communicate with cancer patients. *Journal of Advanced Nursing*, 16: 677–88.

World Health Organization Expert Committee (1990) *Cancer Pain Relief and Palliative Care*. Technical Report Series 804. Geneva: WHO.

34

Information and communication technology in nursing

Current role and future scope

Hilde Ahmedzai

In this chapter, I offer a basic introduction to concepts in information and communication technology and some practical applications for nurses in terms of relevant web materials and how to access them. I do not mean to provide a critique of the specialist field of information and communications technology in nursing. I begin by clarifying and defining some of the most common terms used in this field. I then go on to describe and exemplify the relevance of these technologies within various aspects of palliative care nursing. I also refer to research where this is applicable. A paper by Ada Spitzer (1998) raised the following question: 'Moving into the information era: does the current nursing paradigm still hold?' A few years have passed since this publication, but it is likely that the question relating to nursing and the transition into the information era is still valid in most industrialized countries today. The rapid growth of the information society and the closely related information and communication technologies has had an enormous impact on all areas of health care, including nursing. It is imperative that all disciplines involved in delivering, managing or researching health care assess their existing framework with the view of embracing and adapting innovative developments to make further progress in the care of patients.

Information and communications technology in nursing

The UK Council for Health Informatics Professions define health informatics as: 'The knowledge, skills and tools which enable information to be collected, managed, used and shared to support the delivery of healthcare and promote health'. Norris and Brittain discuss the confusion that exists between various terms like 'medical informatics', 'health care information management', 'health care informatics' and 'medical librarianship'. They argue that the term health care informatics comprises (a) information for clinical purposes and (b) information for the management of health care. As health informatics is becoming an increasingly important part of health care, it is important that the nursing profession develop and take forward these elements of health informatics which are applicable to nursing (see Table 34.1).

Each health discipline operates within its own defined framework and it is therefore important that the information and communication technologies employed to support nursing interventions are developed and studied within the arena of the nursing profession. Although it is useful and necessary to build upon the knowledge base of health informatics, it is equally important for the nursing profession to relate, adapt and further develop these theories to support nursing interventions. This requirement does imply – both good and bad – a further splitting and sub-specialization both within the field of nursing as well as the field of health informatics. As a result, we have seen the growth of nursing informatics becoming a recognized specialty in many parts of the developed world.

Table 34.1   Stakeholders' main areas of interaction with information and communication technology (ICT)

Stakeholder group	ICT vehicle	Potential value	Considerations
Nurse practitioners	Emails, websites, discussion lists, newsgroups, electronic patient record, care pathway systems, videoconferencing	Information on request, information sharing – integrated care across multiple providers, procedures and guidelines, professional development	Privacy concerns, incomplete data, unregulated use of ICTs, lack of standards for vocabulary
Nurse researchers/ academics and students	Websites, evidence-based databases, e-learning	Convenience, improved out-reach	Quality of data, confidentiality of data storage, unethical collection and use of health care information
Nurse managers	Patient admission, discharges and management, financial systems, executive information systems, on-line databases and statistics, on-line policies	Public health agenda, report generation, care planning, resource planning and costing, automated collection, structuring and codification of data	Training for staff in ICT, investment in equipment, errors due to failed or unavailable technology, performance testing
Patients	Email consultations, information portals, discussion lists, videoconferencing	Convenience, patient empowerment, increased patient choice and involvement in care	Patient acceptance, access, privacy concerns, quality of internet resources, incorrect self-diagnosis and treatment, inequity

Nursing informatics

Although this book is aimed specifically at nurses with an interest in palliative care, it would still be worthwhile taking a glimpse at another area of nursing, namely that of nursing informatics. The term 'nursing informatics' originated from work by Scholes and Barber in 1980 and was approved by the American Nurses Association as a nursing specialty in 1992 (Saba 2001). Nursing informatics emerged as a result of the integration of information science and computer science with nursing science. Saba and McCormick define it as:

> The use of technology and/or computer system to . . . process . . . and communicate timely data and information in and across health care facilities that administer nursing services and resources, manage the delivery of nursing care, link research resources and findings to nursing practice, and apply educational resources to nursing education.
>
> (Saba and McCormick 2001: 226)

This definition suggests that, in spite of being a distinctive specialist field that many might feel is distant from hands-on palliative care, nursing informatics is highly relevant for palliative care nursing and it is important that both fields are open to collaboration across the specialist boundaries. To a certain extent, all nurses are regularly utilizing aspects of information and communication technologies in the ways described above and, as such, are taking part in the growing field of nursing informatics, often without having any conscious notion about the connection. Before we investigate some of the specific applications information and communication technology can have for palliative care nursing, it is helpful to briefly describe the most common vehicles that we currently use for these purposes. 'Vehicles', in this context, refers to the various mediums or technical methods in which information and communications are being processed.

Information and communication technology vehicles

Of all the various elements of information and communication technologies, the *internet* is crucial in linking it all together. The internet is basically one vast worldwide network that links all other smaller networks together. For us to get access to this big network, our personal computer has to be connected to one of the smaller networks, which are provided by organizations like universities and national health services or by a variety of commercial companies who act as internet access providers or internet service providers.

Within a period of no more than 10 years, the internet has developed from being a novelty for a few people to an increasingly pervasive part of our lives and has vastly increased the rate at which information is obtained

---

Box 34.1   Section key points

Nursing informatics

- Computer science
- Information science
- Nursing science

Vehicles for information and communication technology

- The internet
- World Wide Web
- Electronic mail
- Mailing lists
- Newsgroups
- Internet relay chat
- Videoconferencing

---

and disseminated, certainly in the environments of work and education, and increasingly also in people's own homes. However, estimated figures for internet usage vary enormously throughout the world, with a total of 605.6 million people (about 10 per cent) linking up to the internet worldwide as of September 2002. Looking at a few of the English-speaking countries with high numbers of users, we find the following figures: for the UK in September 2002 it was 34.3 million (57 per cent of the population), for Australia in February 2002 it was 10.63 million (54 per cent), for the USA in April 2002 the figure was 165.75 million (59 per cent) and for Canada in March 2002 it was 16.84 million (52 per cent). On the other hand, the situation is very different in other countries and examples of countries with low numbers of users include Turkey in December 2001 (2.5 million users, 3 per cent), Vietnam in December 2001 (400,000 users, 0.49 per cent) and India in December 2001 (7 million users, 0.67 per cent) (Nua.com 2002).

The *World Wide Web* is often thought of as being the same as the internet, although this is not the case. More specifically, the internet is the infrastructure or the framework in which the World Wide Web functions as only one of several vehicles used to exchange information between computers that are connected to this internet system. The World Wide Web is the interface, or the medium, we use to access text, graphics, moving images and sound via documents called websites, which again consist of individual web pages (Kiley 1999). Although the World Wide Web is making the information available to us, we still need a so-called *web browser* to enable us to access the various documents or web pages that have been submitted to the World Wide Web part of the internet. A web browser, like Microsoft Explorer or Netscape, enables us to make sense of all the coded information hidden behind the web pages, so that we can navigate, or find our way around, the various sections within individual websites and

> **Box 34.2** Some basic terms explained
>
> - The internet is the overall system connecting millions of computers around the world
> - The World Wide Web (www) is the part of this system allowing us to access web pages
> - Web pages are like chapters or paragraphs in a website
> - A website is the total collection of all web pages belonging together
> - The homepage or landing page of a website is the front page or introduction page of a website
> - A web browser is the technical computer program used to search for and access individual web pages

enables us to jump from one piece of information to another in exploring the huge range of resources available. A popular term for this is 'surfing the net', as we seem to effortlessly glide around different information resources with one resource leading us onto the next one. We are, of course, not dependent upon finding one website by the help of another one, usually presented as 'links' on a website. The same way as a piece of printed information can be identified by a title, an ISBN code and so on, each web page is equipped with a specific code or address so that it can be found directly. The term for this is *URL* (uniform resource locator), as it is unique for each individual web page on the internet. For example, the URL (website address) http://www.hpna.org/ has the following messages embedded in it:

- 'http' (hypertext transfer protocol) tells the computer how it should communicate with the internet, as http is a method of codes for writing content for the internet.

- 'www' indicates that the information you are looking for is placed on the World Wide Web.

- 'hpna' is the acronym for Hospice and Palliative Nurses Association and relates specifically to that website.

- Finally, 'org' indicates that you are looking for a website belonging to an organization and not a commercial site, as that would usually have 'com' at the end. Neither 'org' nor 'com' tell you which country the website originates from, whereas for instance 'ac.uk' tells you that you are looking for an academic (ac) institution in the UK.

Electronic mail (email) is another vehicle that has revolutionized the way we communicate with each other. The BBC's (British Broadcasting Corporation) on-line internet guide (WebWise 2002) at http://www.bbc.co.uk/webwise refers to email as 'the internet's killer application', because even if you never surf the World Wide Web, you will still probably end up using email at some point. Email is a particular method of using the internet for communicating with each other and is not part of the World Wide Web. However, it should be pointed out that one can use the World Wide Web system for email communications as well.

Mailing lists, discussion lists or *listservs* is a facility whereby emails are automatically distributed to names on a list. Such lists are usually organized for topic-related discussions so that people with a common interest can easily share information and otherwise communicate with each other. One will have to subscribe to a particular mailing list(s) of one's choice and members of the list can read emails from others without responding or can reply or write their own email message that will be distributed to all members of that particular mailing list. Many find a mailing list more convenient than a newsgroup, as the user does not have to access any website on the World Wide Web to read or post messages.

Newsgroups, also called *usenet, message board* or *note board*, is another system enabling electronic communication between people either working within the same field or who are otherwise share a common interest. As opposed to a mailing list, this kind of communication takes place via the World Wide Web and participants will not receive messages directly to their email. Nor is it necessary to formally subscribe to a newsgroup. Newsgroups are established for any imaginable topic and they can either be moderated (monitored and screened so that a moderator decides which messages will be published) or messages can be posted directly to be shared with the group. Newsgroups will usually provide an archive of previous messages, giving a flavour of the type of discussions taking place within each particular group.

Internet relay chat refers to the way in which one can communicate with other people in real time via the internet. The communication occurs by participants in a so-called *chat room* typing their own messages, submitting them to the communal chat room on the internet and thereby making them readable by other participants, who, in turn, can instantly type and make available their own message to everyone participating in the chat. It is also possible for individuals in a chat to break out of the group discussion and enter a so-called private area of communication, where the other participants in the initial chat are excluded. This is perhaps the most intimate and at the same time the most vulnerable and often unsafe manner of communication taking place via the internet. Most chat rooms are unmoderated, although the potential for abuse has led to an increasing number of moderated chat rooms. This is particularly important with regard to protecting vulnerable users like children, but it does necessarily require substantial resources with regard to manpower.

The internet began as a way of exchanging text-based information in various formats as described above, but developments in telecommunications have brought about advances far beyond that, with *videoconferencing* having particular relevance for health care disciplines. This enables people to talk to each other at the same time as seeing each other live on the computer screen.

Applications for palliative care nursing

Increasingly, providers of clinical information and educational materials are taking advantage of the recent developments in information and communication technology, resulting in multiple choices of accessing such resources at one's own convenience via the internet. As such, the internet provides an unparalleled opportunity to utilize modern technologies for enhancing nursing care. In this section, I look at how the vehicles described above can be applied to support various aspect of palliative care nursing.

Nursing documentation is an important part of overall clinical documentation and is a crucial element of palliative care nursing. It is essential for good patient care and for effective communication within the team of health care professionals. A variety of computer-based nursing documentation systems have been in use for many years and have enjoyed a rather mixed reception among nurses. The overall aim is to achieve best possible documentation quality with the minimum effort in operating the documentation system. It also serves as an important tool for nursing management and for nursing research, and it is an important vehicle for the storage and retrieval of data. One of the main criticisms of these systems has been that they fail to reveal the true complexity of the nursing process. Also, the lack of a standardized nursing language and the many different documentation formats make the systems more difficult to operate and the documentation less transferable than paper versions. Computer-based nursing documentation systems aim to ease the input of patient data and improve the standardization of nursing documentation, but there are strong limitations of such systems. They do, however, provide a structured documentation system within an individual organization and between organizations using the same software. Compared with traditional paper documentation, which is often incomplete and even illegible, computerized nursing documentation is regarded as a superior system, in spite of its need for improvements. Electronic nursing care protocols, cover all areas, from referrals, care planning and outcome ratings through to discharge planning.

While some services are in their infancy in terms of information and communication technology, others are pioneering new systems like wireless technology, enabling efficient point-of-care access to their computer-based patient record. At Southmead Hospital in Bristol, UK (Duffin 2003), nurses successfully piloted a wireless portable screen for accessing information on medication rounds, thereby reducing the potential for errors. They carried a small screen from bed to bed and accessed their patients' details with a special pen instead of referring to paper records. Information was automatically updated on screen when doctors amended the records on their computers.

Electronic networks will increasingly play a crucial role in communicating clinical information within and between services. An important element of communication in networks and closely linked to computerized nursing documentation are the various applications of electronic patient records, also called computerized patient records. This is an electronic record that contains all the health information of a patient, from a single episode of care to life-long health care information. Electronic patient records are being developed and implemented worldwide and they are the subject of much attention from clinicians, nurses, researchers, health care managers, consumers and government bodies alike. They are specifically raising questions about such issues as ownership of the records and who should be eligible for sharing the information held in the records.

The role of the World Wide Web in clinical nursing practice

Beyond local documentation systems and electronic networks for restricted areas, lie the phenomenal opportunities of the World Wide Web as a vehicle for enhancing clinical nursing practice. A study of nurses' use of the internet (Estabrook *et al.* 2003) showed that although the number of nurses using the internet is rising – particularly internet use at home – nurses' internet use at work and particularly for the purpose of practice information was low compared with that of other groups, such as physicians and the general public. There is little data on how information and communication technology is being used in the field of palliative care in general and with regard to palliative care nursing in particular. Pereira *et al.* (2001) conducted a survey in which they explored internet use by palliative care health professionals. The survey was placed on the World Wide Web and palliative care health care professionals were invited to participate via a palliative-care-related website, listserv and newsletter. A total of 417 completed responses were received over a 4-month period. Of these, 36 per cent were from physicians and 30 per cent were from nurses; one-third of respondents were practising palliative care full time. Although 63 per cent of respondents were from North America, countries from all over the world were represented. Eighty-eight per cent of respondents were searching the internet for clinical information, 80 per cent were using email, 69 per cent were accessing on-line medical journals and 59 per cent were subscribers to a palliative-care-related listserv or newsgroup. One such newsgroup specifically targeting palliative care professionals can be found at http://www.mailbase.org.uk/lists/palliative-medicine/. This allows for discussion on all aspects of palliative medicine and palliative care and aims to facilitate communication between practitioners involved in research or educational initiatives, as well as allowing the exchange of information or advice relating to clinical matters.

Integrated care pathways are playing an increasingly important role in clinical practice (see Chapter 30) and, as such, is a topic lending itself very well to dissemination to the wider nursing audience through the internet. The website for the National electronic Library for Health in the UK incorporates a database named the National electronic Library for Protocols and Care Pathways (NeLPCP), accessed at http://www.nelh.nhs.uk/carepathways/. This database was launched in 2001 and provides detailed information for over 2000 care pathways currently in use or in preparation in various areas, including palliative care and care of the dying. The information includes details on the organizations involved, the nature of and the stage of development of the pathway, together with contact details for further information.

The Department of Pain Medicine and Palliative Care at Beth Israel Medical Center in New York also provides access to a pathway for Palliative Care for Advanced Disease (PCAD), which can be downloaded from their website at http://www.stoppain.org/. Furthermore, this website is an excellent educational resource for various topics in palliative care, particularly in dealing with symptom control. Also in the area of clinical resources, the Canadian website for the Edmonton Regional Palliative Care Program (http://www.palliative.org/index.htm) offers a section called 'Clinical Information'. This is a high-quality resource for health care professionals, aimed at helping them reflect on their practice. The section is split into eight subsections, including assessment tools and guidelines, palliative care tips with 'how-to' suggestions for common problems and 'Nursing Notes' with articles written by palliative care nurses.

Another recommended site for clinical issues is one by the Palliative Care and Rehabilitation Medicine Department at the MD Anderson Cancer Center, University of Texas (http://www.mdanderson.org/departments/palliative/). As a highly innovative feature of a palliative care website, it is worth mentioning the section called 'Palm files'. This provides access to files that can be easily downloaded to a hand-held computing device such as the Palm Pilot (R), using the software (computer program) AvantGo(R), which allows users to synchronize the Palm Pilot with selected web pages. The website provides instruction on how to download and use these files and this is clearly an excellent option for more technologically minded practitioners on the move and by the bedside.

As nurses become increasingly involved in drug administration and drug prescribing, it is paramount to have access to up-to-date knowledge in the field. Palliativedrugs.com Ltd. provides such information (http://www.palliativedrugs.com/). Here nurses can find essential information on this topic, with relevance worldwide, and a separate section is included for UK professionals addressing the issues of using licensed drugs for unlicensed purposes.

As these examples illustrate, the most common role of the internet in health care is to act as a medium for transferring and making available existing information to a wider audience. In this sense, it is merely acting as a vehicle for information delivery and does not have any impact on the nature of the information it disseminates. At other times, however, the internet as the medium becomes a crucial element of the process taking place, enabling new innovative procedures for patient care. This is clearly illustrated by Kuebler and Bruera (2000), who describe how the specialized field of end-of-life care can greatly benefit by utilizing the internet to ensure comprehensive palliative care for remote rural areas or areas that otherwise have limited access to specialist palliative care. The authors developed a standardized communication format titled the Collaborative Consultative Model. This model provides the collaborating practitioners with a standardized communication form containing various valid and reliable psychometric assessment instruments. It is designed to be accessed from any computer via the internet and, in this study, the model was demonstrated as a collaborative tool between a rural palliative care nurse practitioner in the USA and an urban medical research physician in Canada. By using this system, they were able to provide expert consultation for individual patients through the internet.

Videoconferencing

Another application that is subject to increasing attention from palliative care relates to the use of videoconferencing. Advances in technology and reductions in the costs of equipment have resulted in renewed interest in this particular medium. Research and developments in this area are often categorized by the terms of telemedicine and telecare. The Telemedicine Information Service (http://www.tis.port.ac.uk/index.htm), run by the University of Portsmouth in the UK, describes telemedicine as a new way of delivering health care, from a centralized service to one which is patient-centred, recource-efficient and where decisions are made at a local level close to the patient. The term is used when referring to a number of applications of information and communication technology to medicine. Similarly, they define telecare as 'the use of information and communication systems to give patients with or without their healthcare professional or informal carer access to information sources wherever they are located'.

Regnard and colleagues have carried out extensive work on using videoconferencing in palliative care (Regnard 2000). Through the IMPaCT (Interactive Multimedia Palliative Care Training) project, they assessed the practicalities and educational effectiveness of videoconferencing in palliative care. Regnard (2000) describes how 946 people were linked during 88 videoconferencing sessions, covering a wide range of different purpose, with 136 professionals at distant sites for palliative care education. According to an update on the Telemedicine Information Service website (http://www.tis.port.ac.uk/index.htm), in July 2003 it was reported from the project that videoconferencing was still used on a regular basis and that 14 hospices in the UK had videoconferencing equipment. The uptake remained very low but there was a discernible shift in cancer and palliative care to using videoconferencing to save time and costs. As part of the IMPaCT project, it was intended to test out 'patient-to-professional links', but although this was not feasible in the first part of the study, it is planned to assess the feasibility of remote patient consultations in the future.

Ahmedzai and colleagues addressed this issue in a small study in the UK, in which they examined the acceptability of using videoconferencing between cancer patients or carers and health care professionals. A web camera was installed on several computers, allowing cancer patients from a hospital, a hospice and a research centre access to consultations with a dietician, radiographer or social worker from the cancer centre. A total of 12 people took part in the testing, of whom five patients and two carers were from the local hospice. The evaluation showed that, not surprisingly, none of the participants definitely preferred the use of a video telephone to a face-to-face consultation (Figure 34.1). However, two patients/carers replied that they might possibly prefer a video telephone to face-to-face consultation. They argued that such a system offered an element of distance that was not possible in a face-to-face setting. They also valued the potential flexibility of the system and thought it to be an efficient use of the professional's time. Recordings of the time spent on the videoconferencing link showed an average consultation time of about 25 minutes, which does not imply that the consultation itself occupied less time than a traditional face-to-face consultation. However, it was an advantage that neither the patient nor the professional had to travel to take part in the consultation. Comparing video telephone to ordinary telephone consultation, the majority replied that they would definitely prefer using the video telephone (Figure 34.2).

Positive aspects highlighted included the ability to see the face as well as the voice of the health professional and how this increased the confidence that patients/carers had in the person they were seeking advice from. They thought this especially important if they were talking to a professional who they did not know prior to the consultation. It is generally thought that telecare would have the greatest impact in countries where people are living in remote areas or where the specialist services available cannot adequately meet the demand for face-to-face consultations. Although this may be the

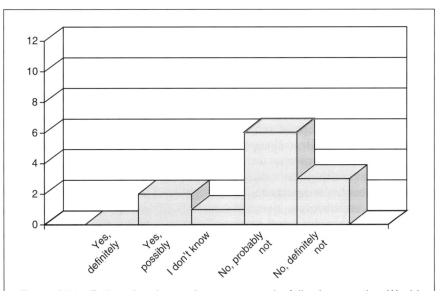

Figure 34.1   Patients' and carers' responses to the following question: Would you prefer video telephone to a face-to-face consultation? (*n* = 12)

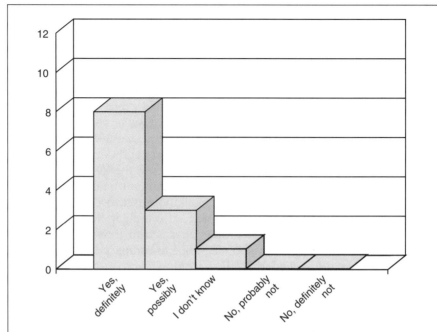

Figure 34.2 Patients' and carers' responses to the following question: Would you prefer video telephone to an ordinary telephone consultation? (*n* = 12)

most obvious arena for its use, all 12 people in our study said that they would definitely use such a service if it existed. In particular, it seems a good option for patients living at home, who may be too weak to travel for consultations with specialist services.

The future success of telemedicine and telecare will depend on patient and provider acceptance of such technologies. It is, therefore, imperative that the views and experiences of the users and providers of health care services are sought to enable problems to be resolved and issues to be addressed before these techniques are further developed and implemented.

Information and communication technology in nurse management is in many areas closely related to, and dependent upon, the previously mentioned computerized clinical information systems. These systems are important sources of information for nurse managers about patient demographic statistics and they can provide an overall picture of the complexity of the nursing care involved. Information and communication technology systems are also widely used in managing staffing and scheduling of nurses. Equally, they can provide essential information relating to accessibility of health care services, which have particular relevance for the field of palliative care. Furthermore, as the information society rapidly develops, it opens up insights into a wealth of information on government policies and guidelines that can be accessed via the internet. This is of great value, but at the same time presents the common challenge when locating information on the internet: with the magnitude and diversity available, it can be difficult to make the optimal selections. In the past, one could rely on getting relevant publications, plans and guidelines in the post, whereas the internet provides access to a whole range of additional information, including some that may only marginally relate to one's own field. However, there is no doubt that the internet facilitates easy access to crucial documents and as an added bonus enables insight into policy documents and developments within other countries as well. Among the growing number of electronic databases, the National electronic Library for Health provides a 'guidelines finder' at http://www.nelh.nhs.uk/guidelinesfinder/. As of April 2003, it holds information and links to various guidelines for the UK, the USA, New Zealand, Australia and Canada.

Nurse–patient interface

The exchange of information between the patient and members of the health care team is crucial for high-quality patient care. As previously mentioned, a shared electronic record is an important tool for facilitating storage and viewing of all patient data. In a review by Sitting (2002), 27 personal health records of various complexity and stage of development were identified as available in some form for public viewing. In his review, Sitting defined internet-based personal health records very broadly. This included something as simple as a form that the patient can print and fill in to an application that would enable patients to view and annotate (via a secure internet connection) their electronic medical record held by their doctor in his office. In Sitting's review, only commercially created personal health records were included, but he did refer to systems created by academic clinical departments that have available internet-based personal health records through their local health care system's website. The use of internet-based personal health records is still in the very early days of development and testing, but this important tool is likely to be of benefit to both patients and all the health care professionals involved in their care and treatment. It must be noted that internet-based personal health records raise additional concerns regarding data ownership, patient confidentiality and patient rights and these issues must be addressed responsibly in the creation and use of these systems.

An essential part of patient empowerment is helping people understand more about their illness and potential related problems. They also need to know about treatment options and ways of supporting them in their illness. A poll conducted for the British Medical Journal Publishing Group (2002) found that 88 per cent of general practitioners (GPs) surveyed reported that they had experienced patients bringing health information obtained from the internet when attending consultations. Although 60 per cent of the GPs were in favour of patients exploring on-line health information, less than half provided any advice to their patients about which on-line sources to access. Ullrich and Vaccaro (2002) quote a figure as low as 4 per cent of patients who were recommended a health care website for their condition, although 70 per cent of all patients would like their physicians to do so. Similar results have been shown in several other surveys and it is very reasonable that patient information and education is an area where nurses should play an important role.

Ahmedzai and colleagues have addressed this issue with the development of a website acting as a gateway to high-quality resources for cancer patients and carers. The initiative is called PIES – Personalized Information, Education and Support – and is for cancer patients and their carers, and is located at www.piesforcancer.info. PIES is based on an overwhelming amount of existing English information resources for cancer patients, but at the same time the recognition of inconsistencies in quality of such resources and the difficulties many consumers have in finding relevant and high-quality information. Responding to these issues, PIES assists consumers in pulling together existing information resources of high quality, categorized according to cancer type and other topics relating to living with cancer, and providing links to applicable information resources according to individual needs. As well as providing a service, we also need to explore patients' and carers' views on using information technologies for obtaining information and support in relation to cancer. To answer some of these questions, PIES is undergoing an evaluation to establish its benefits and limitations.

A further area where nurses could play an important role is as facilitators or monitors of email discussion groups and chat rooms for patients. This was well illustrated in a study by Cudney and Weinert (2000), who investigated the role of the nurse monitor in a project using telecommunication technology for providing information and support to middle-aged rural women living with chronic illness. Cudney and Weinert describe the nurse monitor's role as covering four main areas of computer-based support for women. The *Conversation* area is intended to be primarily an exchange between the women and the nurse monitor stimulates this exchange initially and encourages it throughout the duration of the computer sessions. Through *Mailbox*, she responds appropriately to any woman who chooses to have a private conversation via email. In *HealthChat*, she takes a lead role in selecting topics for discussion and also provides new information, prepares printed materials, shares resources on topics, answers questions and arranges for participation of guest consultants. The nurse monitor also scans current literature and works directly with the voluntary health agencies to obtain current information to be shared in the section called *Resource Rack*.

Furthermore, there is an increasing amount of literature on doctors' interaction with patients via email correspondence and web-based consultations (Ball and Lillis 2001; Sitting *et al.* 2001). There is little evidence of nurses' contribution in this field, but the potential is clearly there and the survey by Sitting *et al.* (2001) showed that a large number of patients with access to email would like to have a dialogue with their health care provider.

Education and professional development

Education and professional development is an area with potential for utilizing the contributions of information and communication technology. Resources range from on-line discussion groups to comprehensive e-learning, which allows students to study for postgraduate degrees and other forms of continuing professional development via the World Wide Web. Distance learning programmes are becoming increasingly popular and also increasingly more feasible as information and communication technology improves and widens the possibilities for course delivery. As the demographic characteristics of students see them becoming older, part-time, non-residential, performing paid work alongside their studies and increasingly computer literate, they will desire convenient education that is available anyplace and anytime. Taking traditional distance learning a step further and fully exploiting the potentials of information and communication technologies is demonstrated by the growth of web-based courses.

The use of videoconferencing has been investigated by Anderson *et al.* (2003), who compared the effectiveness of palliative care education delivered by videoconferencing with face-to-face delivery. They found that given the choice, community nurses prefer face-to-face teaching, but they learn just as effectively when a session is delivered over the videoconferencing link. It was also clear that establishing videoconferencing education requires early training, regular support and an organizational commitment that takes up to a year to develop. Furthermore, although individual enthusiasm is important, this does not guarantee success. Documenting the important factor of costs, they found that cost savings in travel time recouped the cost of the equipment in one year.

For e-learning initiatives to be functional and effective options, nurses must be equipped for the challenge. Accordingly, health information management and information technology will increasingly play a central role in the curriculum for nurses. As well as serving as the medium for undertaking courses, the internet also serves as an excellent platform for sharing information and experiences within that field. An example is the Center to Advance Palliative Care (CAPC), http://www.capcmssm.org, a resource to hospitals and other health care settings interested in developing palliative care programmes. It is based in New York and the key aim of the website is to assist developing palliative care programmes. There is extensive content on that topic and one of the sections is called 'building a program'. There is also a 'CAPC How To Manual', offering advice on how to establish a palliative care programme with links to case studies describing the development of various programmes.

Through an email survey of nursing programmes, Wells *et al.* (2003) assessed the type of technological infrastructure available to educators in US nursing programmes, the programme's end-of-life content and the needs and preference for end-of-life care teaching materials. The final sample represented 25 per cent of all US nursing programmes, of which only 3 per cent reported having a dedicated course for end-of-life issues, whereas 40 per cent wanted to increase this content in their curricula. The findings of this survey provided the basis for the development of the Toolkit for Nurturing Excellence at the End-of-Life Transition (TNEEL), which was created by the Cancer Pain and Symptom Management Nursing Research Group at the University of Washington School of Nursing. On the basis of the survey, the developers were able to tailor the toolkit to its users, taking into consideration the computer technologies available to nursing faculties, their skills, needs and preferences. The toolkit has been distributed at no charge to all US undergraduate nursing programmes and is seen as a valuable contribution in helping to standardize end-of-life curricula for nursing and also as an important potential of adding end-of-life content to all nursing programmes in the USA.

The internet offers a wealth of educational resources of a less formalized nature by disseminating information on courses, conferences and other events for specialist nursing groups. It provides access to professional associations and interest group organizations like the International Association for Hospice and Palliative Care (http://www.hospicecare.com), the European Association for Palliative Care (http://eapcnet.columbusnet.it/), the Australian and New Zealand Society of Palliative Medicine (http://www.anzspm.org.au/), Palliative Care Australia (http://www.pallcare.org.au/), the American Academy of Hospice and Palliative Medicine (http://aahpm.org/), the British Columbia Hospice Palliative Care Association (http://www.hospicebc.org/), and the National Council for Hospice and Specialist Palliative Care Services (http://www.hospice-spc-council.org.uk/). Increasingly, palliative care organizations offer electronic newsletters delivered directly to the end user's email account and, as such, benefits greatly both information providers and consumers by fast and convenient up-to-date information delivery. Among the many search tools available on the internet is Growthhouse.org, specially tailored to palliative care resources. It is run by the Inter-Institutional Collaborating Network on End of Life Care (IICN), which links major organizations internationally in a shared on-line community. The IICN includes palliative care organizations in the USA, Canada, the UK, Spain, Hong Kong and Malaysia and can be found at http://www.growthhouse.org/iicn.html.

The ability to exchange information and experiences on an informal basis is potentially valuable to nurses. Traditionally, this has taken place within small groups of nurses who already have established a relationship, whether it is a group of colleagues in a workplace or nurses with affiliations to a specific organization. A fast growing tool for expansion in this area is the use of on-line discussion lists and newsgroups. These allow participants the opportunity to communicate with colleagues worldwide, regardless of whether they know each other or not. One example of a widely used discussion forum within palliative care is the bulletin board provided by PalliativeDrugs.com. One must register via the website at http://www.palliativedrugs.com. Once a member of the group, one can receive a continuous update of current discussions by having all messages that are submitted to the group forwarded to one's email. Participation in the discussion is facilitated by using the bulletin board section on the website.

Research

One of the most important functions of modern information and communication technology in health care is the role it plays in the area of research and scholarly activity, as the growth of evidence-based practice is influencing all areas of health care. Most adults grew up with the library being the all-important source of knowledge and one had to physically go there to identify and retrieve any wanted information. This is changing and we now have a host of options for gathering information, with the internet taking the leading role. Via electronic journals and medical databases like Medline and the Cochrane databases of systematic reviews, we have immediate access to up-to-date information and evidence. The Cochrane Collaboration (http://www.cochrane.org./) is an international, non-profit-making organization that aims to assist well-informed decisions about health care by preparing and presenting systematic reviews of the effects of treatments. The Cochrane Library is the main output of the Collaboration, updated quarterly and distributed on an annual subscription basis on disk, CD-ROM and via the internet. The Cochrane Library contains several different databases and 50 Cochrane 'review groups', each preparing systematic reviews for a specific area of health care. With specific relevance for palliative care, the Cochrane Pain, Palliative Care and Supportive Care Group (PaPaS), http://www.jr2.ox.ac.uk/cochrane/, focuses on reviews for the prevention and treatment of pain, the treatment of symptoms at the end of life, and supporting patients, carers and their families through the disease process.

Future scope

The development of information and communication technology is progressing faster than in any other area of modern life. It is hard to find other fields where the changes are so radical within such short time spans. It is very likely that by the time this chapter has reached its audience, many areas addressed here will have changed and new innovative developments will have taken place.

It is not possible to provide a comprehensive and reliable prediction of what is in store for us in this field, although some likely scenarios present themselves. Most certainly, the technical specifications of the equipment we are using will improve and we will be operating from computers that will have better technical specifications, allowing more data to be stored as well as retrieved at a higher speed, when at the same time being much smaller in size.

Wireless connection to the internet is already starting to make an impact on health care services and is a very promising development that is likely to improve access to information and support for both nurses and patients in palliative care. In connection with the evaluation of the previously mentioned PIES project, a wireless computer is being installed in an in-patient unit at a hospice in Barnsley, UK. This allows a laptop computer to be transported wireless around the unit, facilitating internet access for patients and carers at the bedside or in a private room anywhere within the unit, or in areas of the garden if needed. This kind of mobile access is likely to have an enormous impact on future nursing care. Not only will we use more wireless desktops and laptops, but hand-held and wearable computers will become increasingly common, providing nurses convenient access to relevant information at the point of care.

A further area utilizing the advances in information and communication technology relates to consumer involvement (see Chapter 4). Consumers now have the ability to obtain and disseminate information of a kind and in a way that was previously reserved for the health care professions. This will increasingly influence the way consumers and health care providers interact with each other and will no doubt have an impact on the traditional balance of power. In particular, it presents a challenge for health care professionals in that they are forced to examine and maybe redefine their role in a world where information that was previously only accessible to them is now also widely available to the consumers.

Conclusions

It is beyond doubt that the recent developments in information and communication technology have had and will continue to have an enormous impact on all parts of society, including health care. As this chapter has demonstrated, the internet has currently the most prominent role in this field and, as such, is frequently the subject of attention. As a tool for disseminating information, the internet has many advantages – flexibility, speed and the potential for reaching a wide audience. Against this, it also has a concomitant set of challenges, where the variability of quality ranks as the number one criticism. Of additional concern is the way in which information is organized – or rather not organized – on the internet and the implications this has for identifying information that is relevant for one's needs.

Furthermore, as Norris (2002) points out, there is much concern about the divisive nature of information and communication technologies – referred to as the 'digital divide' – creating a class of people disadvantaged by their lack of knowledge and/or inability to access information and services offered through modern technologies. This concern is also discussed by MacPherson and Wilkinson (2001), who looked at the issue of culture with regard to access and participation in the information society. They argue that the emphasis on cultural and ethnic categorization only further divides people and fails to reduce inequalities and suggest transculturalism as a more useful way of approaching cultural differences.

Clearly, for the many people who are not as deft with the internet, today's information-intensive health care system can be both confusing and frustrating. This relates equally to patients as well as health care professionals and lack of training and basic familiarity with information tools does still represent an important factor in professional resistance to the so-called 'information revolution'.

These are among the many challenges we face when travelling at high speed on the information highway. It is important that nurses in palliative care do not take the back seat as passengers on this journey, but rather take a leading role in the driving seat to ensure that they and patients alike will benefit from what is on offer along the way.

Useful websites

- American Academy of Hospice and Palliative Medicine: http://aahpm.org
- Australian and New Zealand Society of Palliative Medicine: http://www.anzspm.org.au
- BBC, London, UK: http://www.bbc.co.uk/webwise
- British Columbia Hospice Palliative Care Association: http://www.hospicebc.org
- Center to Advance Palliative Care (CAPC), New York, NY: http://www.capcmssm.org
- Cochrane Collaboration: http://www.cochrane.org
- Cochrane Pain, Palliative Care and Supportive Care Group (PaPaS): http://www.jr2.ox.Ac.uk/cochrane/
- Department of Pain Medicine and Palliative Care at Beth Israel Medical Center, New York: http://www.stoppain.org/
- Department of Palliative Care and Rehabilitation, MD Anderson Cancer Center, University of Texas, Dallas, TX: http://www.mdanderson.org/departments/palliative
- Edmonton Regional Palliative Care Program, Edmonton, Alberta, Canada: http://www. palliative.org/index.htm
- European Association for Palliative Care: http://eapcnet.columbusnet.it
- Inter-Institutional Collaborating Network on End of Life Care: http://www.growthhouse.org/iicn.html
- International Association for Hospice and Palliative Care: http://www.hospicecare.com
- Mailbase newsgroup: http://www.mailbase.org.uk/lists/palliative-medicine/
- MSc's in Clinical Oncology and Palliative Care: http://www.ncl.ac.uk/cancereducationonline/index.htm
- National Council for Hospice and Specialist Palliative Care Services: http://www. hospice-spc-council.org.uk/
- National electronic Library for Health (NeLH) Guidelines Finder: http://www.nelh.nhs.uk/guidelinesfinder/

- National electronic Library for Protocols and Care Pathways (NeLPCP): http://www. nelh.nhs.uk/carepathways/
- Nua.com 2002: http://www.nua.ie/surveys/
- Palliative Care Australia: http://www.pallcare.org.au
- Palliativedrugs.com Ltd.: http://www.palliativedrugs.com
- PIES, Personalized Information, Education and Support: www.piesforcancer.info
- Telemedicine Information Service, University of Portsmouth, Portsmouth, UK: http://www.tis.port.ac.uk/index.htm

References

Anderson, K., Regnard, C. and van Boxel, P. (2003) The effectiveness of palliative care education delivered by videoconferencing compared with face-to-face delivery. *Palliative Medicine*, 17: 344–58.

Ball, M.J. and Lillis, J. (2001) E-health: transforming the physician/patient relationship. *International Journal of Medical Informatics*, 61: 1–10.

Cudney, S.A. and Weinert, C. (2000) Computer-based support groups: nursing in cyberspace. *Computers in Nursing*, 18(1): 35–43.

Duffin, C. (2003) Portable screen proves a success after ward trials. *Nursing Standard*, 17(18): 8.

Estabrook, C.A., O'Leary, K.A., Ricker, K.L. and Humphrey, C.K. (2003) The Internet and access to evidence: how are nurses positioned? *Journal of Advanced Nursing*, 42(1): 73–81.

Kiley, R. (1999) *Medical Information on the Internet – A Guide for Health Professionals*, 2nd edn. Glasgow: Churchill Livingstone, Bell & Bain Ltd.

Kuebler, K.K. and Bruera, E. (2000) Interactive collaborative consultation model in end-of-life care. *Journal of Pain and Symptom Management*, 20(3): 202–9.

MacPherson, S. and Wilkinson, M. (2001) Health informatics and the cultural divide: a UK perspective: *Health Informatics Journal*, 7(2): 62–5.

Norris, A.C. (2002) Current trends and challenges in health informatics. *Health Informatics Journal*, 8: 205–13.

Pereira, J., Bruera, E. and Quan, H.J. (2001) Palliative care on the net: an online survey of health care professionals *Palliative Care*, 17(1): 41–5.

Regnard, C. (2000) Using videoconferencing in palliative care. *Palliative Medicine*, 14: 519–28.

Saba, V.K. (2001) Nursing informatics: yesterday, today and tomorrow. *International Nursing Review*, 48(3): 177–87.

Saba, V.K. and McCormick, K.A. (2001) *Essentials of Computers for Nurses: Informatics in the Next Millennium*. New York: McGraw-Hill.

Sitting, D.F. (2002) Personal health records on the internet: a snapshot of the pioneers at the end of the 20th century. *International Journal of Medical Informatics*, 65: 1–6.

Sitting, D.F., King, S. and Hazlehurst, B.L. (2001) A survey of patient–provider e-mail communication: what do patients think? *International Journal of Medical Informatics*, 45: 71–81.

Spitzer, A. (1998) Moving into the information era: does the current nursing paradigm still hold? *Journal of Advanced Nursing*, 28(4): 786–93.

Ullrich, P.F., Jr. and Vaccaro, A.R. (2002) Patient education on the internet: opportunities and pitfalls. *Spine*, 27(7): E185–E188.

Wells, M.J., Wilkie, D.J., Brown, M.A. *et al.* (2003) Technology survey of nursing programs: implications for electronic end-of-life teaching tool development. *Computers, Informatics, Nursing*, 21(1): 29–36.

35

Research and scholarship in palliative care nursing

Christine Ingleton and Sue Davies

Introduction

There has been a remarkable growth in the extent of research activity in palliative care in recent years, much of it driven by attempts to strengthen the evidence base of the specialty. Research in palliative care has come a long way from the isolated endeavours of its founders in the early 1960s and we now have the prospect of both national and international communities of interdisciplinary research interest. Collaboration between centres, inter-professional and multi-professional working, as well as diverse interests and approaches, all are features of the contemporary scene.

Within the broad field of palliative care research, nursing is beginning to emerge as an important focus. Palliative care is a challenging and expanding area of nursing, with major developments in service organization and the creation of new nursing roles (Shewan and Read 1999; Seymour *et al.* 2002). Such initiatives require ongoing systematic evaluation, demanding research skills and capacity in the form of dedicated research posts, access to funding and a supportive infrastructure. Developments in the organization and provision of palliative care nursing services have been paralleled by changes in the education and preparation of nurses for palliative care nursing practice, which, in turn, reflect a more general transformation in nurse education. Throughout the industrialized world, there has been a gradual but comprehensive integration of nursing education into higher education. This has resulted in increased emphasis on the need to develop the evidence base for practice, and has placed pressure on both nurse educators and practitioners to actively engage in research and scholarly activities (Humphreys *et al.* 2000; Royal College of Nursing 2001).

In this chapter, we explore some of the challenges and opportunities offered by research and scholarship in palliative care nursing. We begin with a consideration of the relationship between scholarship, research and practice with particular reference to nursing in palliative care settings. We follow this with a brief overview of the current context and status of palliative care nursing research, including a summary of substantive themes and issues within the palliative nursing research literature, and areas yet to be explored. We then consider a range of challenges and opportunities in conducting and participating in palliative care nursing research and scholarship, particularly in relation to:

- creating an infrastructure to support research and scholarly activity in palliative care nursing;
- identifying factors shaping research agendas and research priorities;
- selecting appropriate and ethically sensitive methods for conducting palliative care nursing research;
- working collaboratively to ensure that research in palliative care is relevant to service users and practitioners;
- getting research findings into the public domain to influence practice and service development.

We conclude with suggestions for meeting these challenges and ensuring that research and scholarship continue to provide the foundation for palliative care nursing practice.

The relationship between research and scholarship in palliative care nursing

Internationally, scholarship has been identified as a priority for nursing and nursing education (Department of Health 2000; Pullen *et al.* 2001; Ramcharan *et al.* 2001). Scholarship has been described as a professional value and intellectual process, grounded in curiosity about why patients respond in the way they do and why we, as nurses, do the things we do (Pullen *et al.* 2001: 81).

Kitson (1999: 773) proposes that the skills of scholarship coalesce around:

- being able to find and understand what has gone before (literature searching, comprehension, critical appraisal, interpretation);
- reviewing the published literature in a fair and unbiased way, accurately reflecting the state of the field, showing judgement and the ability to integrate and synthesize a diverse body of work;
- the ability to communicate ideas effectively, cogently, coherently and concisely through the written word and orally;
- the ability to think logically and clearly and knowing how to present the pros and cons of an argument in a balanced way.

However, Ramcharan *et al.* (2001) argue that the value and relevance of scholarship to nursing practice and education has been undermined by a pre-occupation with research products and outputs such as peer-reviewed publications. They suggest that systems of recognition and reward should be equitably distributed between the wide areas of potential scholarship. In the context of higher education, this will mean universities accommodating different models of scholarship and nurses recognizing their responsibility to contribute to scholarly activity. In a practice-based profession, a number of authors have identified the need to reconceptualize what constitutes scholarship (Burgener 2001; Ramcharan *et al.* 2001). Burgener (2001), for example, suggests that there is a need to delineate scholarship of practice and differentiate between the characteristics of scholarship of practice and traditional research approaches. For example, a practice-based profession needs timely information about practice and service development in addition to what may be termed 'pure' knowledge. Researchers and practitioners are increasingly exploring the concept of 'practice development' and how this can best be achieved in a range of care settings [see, for example, the work of Unsworth (2000) for an exploration of the concept of practice development].

There is little doubt that the complex problems and challenges faced by palliative care nurses deserve a scholarly approach. However, in common with nurses in other fields of practice, palliative care nurses and researchers face a number of challenges in attempting to engage in and sustain scholarly activity. First, intellectual isolation may be a problem, since most palliative care is provided in community and hospice settings where access to wider resources and networks for supporting scholarly activities may be lacking or limited. Second, few would disagree that meeting the needs of patients and carers takes precedence over establishing a sound knowledge base for practice (Richards *et al.* 1998; Field *et al.* 2001). Third, only recently has the development of skills in the critical evaluation and conduct of research become a significant focus within nurse preparation (Scott 1998). Furthermore, specific training for research in palliative care has been largely absent from within postgraduate programmes. Practitioners may therefore lack the confidence to draw upon the knowledge base to influence and shape practice, particularly within the context of a multidisciplinary arena.

In common with research activity, scholarship requires a supportive infrastructure. Pullen *et al.* (2001), for example, suggest that scholarship is likely to flourish where creativity, questioning and innovation are promoted and valued, and where senior scholars and expert practitioners serve as role models and mentors. Moreover, scholarship, in whatever discipline, reflects a 'transdisciplinarity, both in methodology and in dialogue' (Kitson 1999). Consequently, nurse scholars need to be able to engage in debate with scholars of other disciplines and appreciate a range of methodological perspectives. In this context, there is a need for more mentorship and supervision for nurses, accompanied by opportunities for international exchange and multidisciplinary collaboration (Kitson 1999). This is essential if nurses are to continue to make an important contribution to palliative care research and scholarship.

What contribution is nursing making to palliative care research and scholarship?

Research in palliative care has been influenced by a number of traditions and disciplines. Historically, early research in pain management was influential in establishing the specialty of palliative medicine (Saunders 1958; Twycross and Lack 1983; Hanks and Justins 1992) and involved clinical studies of the effectiveness of treatment, particularly the treatment of pain. Alongside these clinical studies, research adopting sociological and psycho-social perspectives has explored experiences of death and dying (Glaser and Strauss 1965; Quint 1967; Field 1989), with bereavement and communication studies emerging as important and influential themes (Kubler-Ross 1969; Murray Parkes 1970; Faulkner 1992). These early studies were crucial in establishing the speciality of palliative care and provided important data on care of the dying person. In her review of research in palliative care published in the period 1966–82, Corner (1996) found that pain and symptom control accounted for 21 per cent of the work, studies of health carers accounted for 17 per cent and studies evaluating patient care covered 9 per cent. These studies were characteristically descriptive, employing survey methods, retrospective views of patients' case notes and reviews of admissions to hospices and palliative care. Although nurses were contributing studies to the body of work, numbers were small and the rather embryonic nature of the research as a whole was a feature of the work reviewed.

In the current climate of health care, practitioners have become accustomed to working within a constantly changing environment, and palliative care is no exception. Changes in government health policy within industrialized countries are generally aimed at raising standards of care and service delivery within a cost-constrained environment. For example, within the UK National Health Service, initiatives have included the introduction of clinical governance, the National Institute for Clinical Excellence and the Commission for Health Improvements (Department of Health 1998). All these initiatives are aimed at ensuring that health care practice is based upon research evidence wherever possible. Consequently, the need for a research base in palliative care nursing is imperative and this has been well recognized by UK authors (Payne 2000; Wilkinson 2001) and others (Chang and Daly 1998; Wilkes 1998).

This leads us to consider the contribution that nursing is making to the body of palliative care research. In a recent selective review of the literature, Corner and Bailey (2002) explored the contribution nursing is making to palliative care research by identifying the character of nursing research and the unique ways that nurses as researchers, and nursing as the subject of research, have – and are – contributing to palliative care (Corner and Bailey 2002). They identified several areas where progress has been made and where nurses have made a key contribution towards the overall research effort in palliative care research (see Box 35.1).

> **Box 35.1**   Nurses' contribution to research in palliative care
>
> - Prevalence of symptoms
> - Pain control
> - Control of other symptoms
> - Needs/experiences of patients
> - Studies of carers
> - Conventional care
> - Place of death
> - Bereavement care
> - Specialist palliative care services
> - Assessment tools
> - Policy issues
> - Communication skills

On the basis of their analysis of this selective review, Corner and Bailey (2002) made the following observations about the contribution of nursing research to palliative care. First, much of the research undertaken by nurses in palliative care is characterized by a deep interest in the personal and interpersonal aspects of care for people who are dying. More specifically, several studies have involved observation of nurses in their work with dying patients (e.g. Quint 1967; Melia 1987; Payne *et al.* 1996; Copp 1999). Second, much of the research to date has focused on the nurse's role in palliative care (e.g. James 1989; McNamara *et al.* 1994; Froggatt 1998). Third, a number of seminal studies of palliative care nursing have been undertaken by researchers from other disciplines, particularly sociologists and anthropologists (e.g. Field 1989; Lawton 1998). Finally, a more recent theme to emerge is the concept of palliative care nursing as a therapeutic activity (e.g. Corner 1996; Bredin *et al.* 1999). Several studies have provided the opportunity to elucidate the nature of nurses' therapeutic work with patients experiencing breathlessness (O'Driscoll *et al.* 1999), fatigue (Richardson and Ream 1998) and lymphoedema (Badger 1997), as well as evaluating training and communication skills (Faulkner 1992).

Wilkes *et al.* (2000) reviewed 59 published and unpublished projects relating to nursing research on palliative care in Australia between 1990 and 1996. There are interesting parallels between this review and that of Corner and Bailey (2002). For example, Wilkes *et al.* found that the majority of studies focused on professional issues and management of the patient's pain. However, in common with UK studies, little research on families and carers of palliative care patients was evident. Wilkes *et al.* (2000) called for further research to focus on projects that evaluate the nurse's role in the palliative care team, determine the effectiveness of interventions for symptom control and explore the nurse's contribution to meeting the psychosocial needs of patients and families.

In relation to the process and context of palliative care nursing research, many of the studies have been small in scale, fragmented and locally based.

Few well-designed intervention studies have been published and there is a lack of rigorous evaluation. This is perhaps unsurprising, since much of the knowledge base for nursing practice in general has been generated through small-scale research projects, often undertaken by nurses as part of their continuing professional development. These projects are most useful if the information derived from them forms part of a continuing research agenda and this can be best achieved if the results are published. These small research projects may also function as preliminary and pilot studies where they play a useful role in assessing whether the method is feasible and whether it is possible to recruit an appropriate sample within a certain time-frame.

As with other fields of health care, there is a need for greater synthesis of research in palliative care and integration of research findings into clear indicators for practice development. One way of achieving this is through the conduct and dissemination of systematic reviews. Well-conducted systematic reviews can assist practitioners to evaluate and interpret otherwise unmanageable volumes of research. They are particularly useful when there is uncertainty regarding the potential benefits or harm of an intervention and when there are variations in practice – situations that are both common in the rapidly expanding field of palliative care (Hearn *et al.* 1999). In addition to providing a better basis for clinical practice, systematic reviews identify gaps in research, enabling future research priorities to be set in a more organized and objective way (Hearn *et al.* 1999). A number of good examples of systematic reviews are emerging within palliative care (see, for example, Wilkinson *et al.* 1999; Luddington *et al.* 2001; Hotopf *et al.* 2002).

Within the UK, several organizations have been established with a specific remit to conduct systematic reviews in health care, including the Cochrane Collaboration in Oxford and the NHS Centre for Reviews and Dissemination at the University of York. A Pain, Palliative Care and Supportive Care Collaborative Review Group has recently registered as part of the Cochrane Collaboration with the aim of producing and maintaining reviews in these areas, though no guideline have yet been published from this group.

Having considered the current 'state of the art' in palliative care nursing research, we will now explore ways of sustaining the progress that has already been made.

Challenges and opportunities in conducting and participating in palliative care nursing research and scholarship

In many respects, palliative care nursing research is still in its infancy and requires a sustained programme of investment if nursing practice in palliative care is to be underpinned by a sound and well-constructed knowledge base. In the UK context, a recent report for the Higher Education Funding Council (CPNR/CHEMS 2001) suggested that the nursing profession's failure to make a optimal contribution in relation to research and scholarship was due to a combination of a lack of professional confidence and coordination as well as institutional barriers. Some of these challenges will now be described.

Creating an infrastructure to support research and scholarly activity in palliative care nursing

Three criteria must be met to create an organizational culture that is supportive of research and scholarship: staff with the requisite research skills and practice, access to funding, and effective support and supervision. Each of these will now be considered in turn.

Staff with research skills and experience

Academic departments, provider units and commissioning agencies all require individuals with research skills and expertise. A small proportion of health care practitioners will have research activities as a major part of their job description. For these individuals, an explicit career structure that affords access to professional development opportunities and guidance in career planning is crucial. However, in contrast to medicine, nursing offers little opportunity to build research into a continuing clinical career. Funded posts in nursing research are usually fixed-term in nature and permanent posts are rare. Even nurses employed in new nursing roles, which have research as an integral element of their job description (such as the nurse consultant posts in the UK), are often unable to make the conduct of research a priority (Guest *et al.* 2001).

Within academic settings, the employment of researchers on fixed-term contracts is a major barrier to the development of expertise and a programmatic approach to research: 'Universities attachment to hire and fire practices with research staff is more to do with the antiquated way in which so much of their research is managed. Too often it is individual rather than team work. Each project stands alone (Solesbury 2001: 17).

Practices such as pooling staff between projects and rolling contracts can alleviate some of the difficulties associated with the short-term nature of much funded research. However, the deficit in research skills is not simply a function of the way that funded research in nursing is organized: training and preparation for research are also crucial in both clinical and academic environments. Although graduate degrees in nursing have become more common, doctorally prepared nursing professionals are not being produced in sufficient numbers to meet the growing need (Ingleton *et al.* 2001). Certainly, a lower proportion of nurse lecturers hold a PhD than in most other academic disciplines (Clifford 1997). There are also barriers to clinical nurses developing research skills. These include a lack of dedicated time to undertake research in clinical settings, limited access to formal research training and isolation from academic departments. One solution is to focus resources on enabling nurses to undertake higher degrees in order to build research capacity. However, there is also a need for post-doctoral support, in the form of access to funding and academic role models to enable career researchers to develop programmes of research (CPNR/CHEMS 2001). There are now several well-established university-based or linked centres for palliative care in the UK and in other countries, where clinicians and academics can share ideas and expertise.

Access to funding for palliative care nursing research

Most research projects require financial support, for equipment, personnel to assist in data collection and management, or for dissemination and publication costs. Because internal sources of support within higher education worldwide have declined while research costs have escalated, acquiring external funding has become the essential first step for almost all studies. In fact, learning to write proposals for research funding has become an important component of masters and doctoral education in many nursing programmes (Ingleton *et al.* 2001). The first step in preparing a successful proposal is knowing where to apply for funding. There are many types of potential funders for palliative care research (see Box 35.2) and many types of grant opportunities available for would-be researchers to access. These range from explicit invitations to tender to undertake a clearly specified project, to a more flexible and open agenda in which funding agencies invite researchers to develop their own ideas within broad parameters. However, funding for palliative care has, at least until recently, been scarce (Richards *et al.* 1998), though increasingly many of the current opportunities arising from research priorities are particularly relevant to the area of palliative care (Box 35.3).

Developing funding proposals and accessing sources of funding are skilled and time-consuming activities. It may be beneficial for a novice researcher to collaborate with a senior researcher on several studies before attempting a proposal on his or her own, although not all neophyte

---

Box 35.2 Types of potential funder with UK examples

- Government- and state-funded health and social care research agencies, e.g. NHS and Department of Health National and Regional programmes
- Research Councils, e.g. Medical Research Council/Engineering and Physical Sciences Research Council (EPSRC) and Economic and Social Research Council (ESRC)
- Health care and disease-specific charities, e.g. Macmillan Cancer Relief, Marie Curie Cancer Care, Nuffield Small Grants, Cancer Research UK
- Professional organizations, e.g. Royal College of Nursing, International Council of Nurses
- Pan National Organizations, e.g. European Union
- Institutional funding, e.g. university and hospital sources
- Partnerships with industry, e.g. drug companies

Box 35.3 Opportunities arising from British NHS priorities

- Consumer involvement
- Inter-agency working
- Interdisciplinary
- Move to applied research/problem-based
- Use of quantitative and qualitative methods
- Primary care or research at primary–secondary interface
- Clear funding streams

---

researchers are in the fortunate position of having an obvious association with a senior researcher with a proven 'track record' in grant capture. A good way to build a track record is to begin with limited aspirations and seek small-scale funding from local sources, particularly from the institution in which the researcher works. Using a programmatic approach, a research project can build on the previous one, providing evidence that further studies are worthy of major funding.

Effective support and supervision for researchers

Much attention has rightly been given to the well-being of research participants in the conduct of palliative care research (Seymour and Ingleton 1999). However, one group often neglected in any consideration of the demands of palliative care research is the researchers themselves. Researchers in health care face numerous challenges that extend beyond individual research conduct (Sque 2000). Research is, increasingly, a team activity that may require high levels of collaboration between different professional groups and disciplinary perspectives. In this context, the research team is required to engage with both political and personal issues, some of which pose particular challenges in the area of palliative care research and scholarship.

Repeated exposure to the distress of others may raise other considerations. For example, palliative care research may require extended contact with patients who have complex, intractable and life-limiting clinical problems, which may result in an 'unhealthy' pre-occupation with death and dying. For example, the researcher may self-monitor for signs of disease, or may experience a sense of identification with, and injustice for, those affected. Thus, prolonged contact with individuals suffering from life-limiting illnesses can raise personal fears and anxieties about one's own mortality, or for that of family and friends (Clark *et al.* 2000).

This can be exacerbated when the research participants nonetheless give their time willingly, without complaint and in the belief that it may help others in the future, if not themselves. Researchers may feel unsure how to respond to such altruism, or experience stress as they try to fulfil research participants' expectations of the outcomes of the research. Moreover, considerable 'emotional labour' (James 1989) may be required to mask feelings elicited by the close interpersonal involvement with very ill people.

Clinical and non-clinical researchers may experience these difficulties differently (Kenyon and Hawker 1999). The clinical researchers may feel frustrated at wanting to intervene to ameliorate care-giving, to relieve suffering or take on the role of therapist directly. Non-clinical researchers may, in turn, feel frustrated at an inability to assist. Moreover, both groups may develop a sense that the research is less important than trying to improve the immediate situation.

Research projects or departments may develop mechanisms to support researchers faced with these dilemmas. One approach is to make available access to an independent counsellor. This approach is advocated by Payne and Westwell (1994), who suggest that allowance for this type of 'outside' support be budgeted for in grant applications. This person would usually be outside the organizational structures of project management but would be skilled in dealing with personal issues identified by researchers. This is a form of support that may be given to individual or teams of researchers and which is carried out on a confidential basis.

An alternative model is a concept of research supervision that tackles *both* task and process. Within this framework researchers may address with their supervisors both the personal and emotional consequences of their work, as well as matters of reaching milestones and maintaining targets. This calls for a particular commitment on the part of all concerned. Supervisors must learn to provide space to the non-intellectual and non-mechanistic aspects of the research process. Researchers must be willing to share vulnerabilities, doubts, concerns and errors with a senior colleague. Both will have to be willing to set aside regular, protected time without interruptions and to prepare appropriately in advance for supervision sessions. This may mean a change in organizational culture in those settings where research targets are detached from their personal consequences and where even to acknowledge such issues may be construed as a sign of weakness or unsuitability for the work.

An additional component of effective supervision is to address researchers' goals for professional development. Supervisors should be aware of the need to engage with issues around career advancement and in particular the need to publish work and present it at conferences.

Identifying factors shaping research agendas and priorities

Engaging effectively in palliative care nursing research requires an awareness of the range of influences that stimulate and shape the agenda for research and development, and determine which areas are considered as priorities. Within any health care system, these factors are likely to include:

- demographic factors;
- global policy;
- government policy;
- service users' views;

- the views of professional organizations; and
- the views of funding bodies.

Examples of ways in which these factors may impact upon priorities for palliative care research are shown in Table 35.1. It is understandable that practitioners engrossed in clinical work and academics engulfed in teaching responsibilities might imagine that they do not have a role in influencing these agendas. However, it is essential that priorities for research are grounded in the challenges of practice and the needs of service users and their families. Practitioners have access to this information and should seek opportunities to help identify research questions. This could be achieved through membership of special interest groups within professional organizations, publishing work that identifies problem areas arising from practice and making contributions at conferences and networking groups.

Table 35.1   Factors influencing agendas and priorities for palliative care research

Influences	Examples relevant to the UK
Demographic factors	Ageing population, patterns of cohabitation
Global policy	World Health Organization definitions of palliative care (WHO 2002)
Government policy	NHS Cancer Plan (Department of Health 2000): increased funding for cancer research with palliative care identified as an area of priority. National Service Framework for Older People (Department of Health 2001): end-of-life care identified as a priority within research programme to support the objectives of the framework
Service user views	Alzheimer's Society: consumer panel for identifying research priorities identified the effect of care standards and carer support as two priority areas in 2002–2003
Views of professional organizations	Palliative Care Research Society of the UK and Ireland: aim is to promote the interest of palliative care research locally, nationally and internationally. National Cancer Research Institute: purpose is to improve the number of patients entering clinical trials of cancer treatment and to improve the level of research activity within each of the 34 cancer networks within the UK
Views of independent charities	National Council for Hospice and Specialist Palliative Care Services: purpose is to promote the extension and improvement of palliative care services, in part through encouraging improved professional education and research

In addition to identifying and shaping priorities for research in palliative care, the factors and organizations presented in Table 35.1 also exert an influence on how the research is undertaken. This is the focus of the next sub-section.

Selecting appropriate and ethically sensitive methods for conducting palliative care nursing research

The growing literature on palliative care reflects a range of philosophical and methodological persuasions, suggesting that a variety of methods are appropriate for research in this area. Furthermore, the willingness of researchers in the field of palliative care to work across disciplines has facilitated an eclectic approach to the selection and use of research methods. However, individuals in need of palliative care services and their carers (both formal and informal) have particular needs and vulnerabilities and it is essential that these are borne in mind when research approaches and methods are selected.

The specific challenges posed by any research study in palliative care will be dependent upon the particular methodological approach adopted. In quantitative studies, practical challenges include the need to recruit a sample of people who are representative of palliative care patients and the difficulty of attrition due to progression of disease and death. Problems also arise in relation to instrumentation. Few outcome measures have been designed specifically for use with this group of patients, raising questions about the validity and reliability of measures. There may also be particular problems in using some methods; for example, self-completion measures may be inappropriate as many patients are too ill to complete them. In some cases, a questionnaire may be completed by a proxy, such as a professional or family member, on behalf of the patient. However, this has the potential to introduce bias (Hearn and Higginson 2001).

As a result of concerns about making demands on people who are terminally ill, many studies have been based on the retrospective accounts of family members as a proxy measure for the dying person's experiences. However, this also introduces the potential for bias. Hinton (1996), for example, noted that relatives' retrospective accounts of terminally ill patients' experiences were unreliable in several important respects.

Small numbers of patients available within local settings means that it may not be possible to study some questions, for example those requiring a randomized controlled trial design. Few palliative care services have sufficiently large numbers of patients to enable recruitment of samples necessary to detect statistically significant findings. Other issues affecting sample size include:

- high rates of attrition;
- complexity of treatment regimes; and
- low percentage of recruitment into trials.

Collectively, these challenges indicate that prospective, multi-centre studies over a long period may be required. However, multi-centre studies are complex to manage and require good collaborative relationships and sufficient resources.

The generally more interactive methods of qualitative research may be particularly appropriate to study people's views on their end-of-life needs. Biographical and narrative methods can be helpful in providing a framework for addressing past and present experiences, together with anxieties about the future (Clarke and Hanson 2000). Typically, research paradigms in palliative care nursing have allocated a mainly passive role to patients and carers, involving them in responding to questionnaires and structured measures of quality of life (Payne 2002). Qualitative, participatory and action research approaches provide an opportunity to create a more active role for research participants; in this way, the users are empowered and the research is more likely to be directed to their real needs (Gott *et al.* 2000). However, whatever methodological approach is selected, research in palliative care raises a number of ethical issues that will now be considered.

Ethical challenges

The study of ethics in health care research stresses the balance between the desire of researchers to extend knowledge with the rights of the research participants (Robbins 1998). Such tensions are exacerbated when research involves people who are particularly vulnerable, such as people who are terminally ill and their families. Concerns about the ethics of involving people who are dying in research have been widely expressed and debated (de Raeve 1994; Wilkie 1997; Field *et al.* 2001). Field *et al.* (2001), for example, highlight two views about the appropriateness of research in palliative care. One is that research in palliative care settings places too great a demand on people who are very ill. The other view is that research is an ethical imperative to ensure that quality of care is enhanced. These authors make it clear that they subscribe to the latter view, but suggest that researchers must ensure that research questions are relevant and that the research design is rigorous: 'there is an absolute requirement to ensure that such studies are carefully designed to reduce burden [on research participants] to a minimum and to make optimal use of data collected. These data are very precious' (Field *et al.* 2001: 78).

Again the particular ethical challenges posed by a research study in palliative care will be dependent upon the research design. Wilkie (1997) describes the main ethical issues in qualitative research in palliative care as intrusion, the raising of false hopes and prompting painful and difficult emotions. She also discusses the possibility that some research participants may find their involvement therapeutic, raising the question of what happens when the study finishes. Conversely, quantitative studies may hold little obvious benefit for participants, particularly when their involvement requires the completion of lengthy and time-consuming research instruments. Longitudinal studies, which require participants to complete the same questionnaire on a number of occasions, may provide valuable information about the progression of a person's illness, but are likely to be particularly onerous at a point when time has become a precious commodity. Experimental designs are also important in determining the effectiveness of interventions but usually require random allocation of participants to intervention or control groups. These designs raise particular challenges in palliative care research, where potential recruits to a study are likely to prefer to try any intervention, even an unproven one, rather than consent to the possibility of receiving no treatment at all.

Robbins (1998) suggests several safeguards for protecting the interests of patients participating in palliative care research. These include:

- monitoring procedures for gaining consent, including renegotiating consent at intervals during the research;
- careful piloting of research methods to determine the impact of the research on participants;
- submitting all palliative care research to a research ethics committee;
- being flexible – particularly in relation to the completeness and timing of observations to ensure that the privacy of terminally ill patients is not invaded unnecessarily.

Some of the methodological and ethical challenges discussed here can be ameliorated through effective multidisciplinary teamwork, which is the focus of the next sub-section.

Working collaboratively to ensure that research in palliative care is relevant to service users and practitioners

Whereas multidisciplinary collaboration may be perceived as a challenge, it also provides many opportunities in the context of palliative care research. Collaboration can take various forms across the span of a research project. Beattie *et al.* (1996) refer to a 'matrix' of collaboration that occurs at any one instant in time and on multiple levels during the conduct of the research. There may, for example, be collaboration between various professionals within and outside the team (Beattie *et al.* 1996), different organizations (Clark *et al.* 2000) and between research commissioners, participants and researchers (Clark *et al.* 2002). This may call for a sharing of information and expertise among disciplines that have historically worked independently. Furthermore, it requires that practitioners (often from a range of different professions) and academics come together. To achieve a successful collaborative partnership, a readiness for individuals to work together is required, as well as recognition of the demands of each other's roles. However, personal readiness needs to be complemented by a supportive culture within the various clinical areas, departments and institutions within which individuals work.

Developing and nurturing a sense of security about one's own discipline requires that members of the team have respect and trust for each other.

Both respect and trust develop over time; yet when undertaking commissioned work, deadlines are sometimes tight, perhaps affording less opportunity to develop trust with colleagues. As Clark *et al.* point out:

> In order to realize the full potential of multi-disciplinary, collaborative research, an open and flexible attitude, and a willingness to respect (and accept) the differences between and within disciplines are required. Professional jealousies need to be relinquished . . . The risk of cultural hegemony in which one set of values is regarded as more valid than any other, may unwittingly exclude some parties from contributing to the research enterprise.
>
> (Clark *et al.* 2000: 445)

In spite of these challenges, it might be argued that the constructive development of collaborative relationships now frequently underpins the whole research enterprise. Viewed in this light, it is little different from the clinical practice of palliative care. The successful negotiations of these relationships should mean that all members of the team should have access to professional, personal and administrative support. Moreover, successful collaboration can resolve problems of professional conflicts, contrasting organizational agendas and varying career concerns, all of which may disrupt an otherwise sound project.

Getting research findings into the public domain to influence practice and service development

General and specialist practitioners have repeatedly articulated the need for better dissemination of research (Le May *et al.* 1998; Mulhall 2001). Practitioners and researchers are often working with different agendas and within differing organizational constraints. For practitioners working within a multidisciplinary team, there may be conflict about the usefulness and application of different types of research evidence (Mulhall 2001).

For researchers working within academic departments, other factors may come into play. There may be a number of conflicting pressures that have to be reconciled at the dissemination stage of the research project. For example, projects that relate to new products and treatment interventions may be tentative about reporting findings due to constraints by commercial sponsors. Commissioned research, in particular evaluation studies, undertaken for government departments, health authorities and trusts, or major evaluations may be subject to contractual clauses that restrict or control the process of dissemination. In academic departments within the UK, the pressure of the research assessment exercise may create imperatives to publish findings in particular journals and within specific time-frames (see Box 35.4).

Although publication in peer-reviewed journals is often advocated by academic departments to ensure positive research assessment exercise ratings, such journals may not be those to which nurses working in palliative care and cancer care subscribe, and so the impact of evidence upon practice may be limited (Richardson *et al.* 2001). There is also the question of how

Box 35.4   Identifying audiences for research reports

For colleagues, peers and editorial boards of refereed journals, the theoretical framework and how findings relate to the discovery of knowledge in the discipline are important. For practitioners, the descriptive elements in portraying some real-life situation, as well as the implications for action, may be the most salient features. For the commissioners of the research, the significance of the findings and recommendations, whether cast in academic or practical terms, is perhaps more important than the details of how the research was undertaken. Finally, for a higher degree, mastery of the methodology, understanding of the theoretical issues and evidence that the researcher has successfully negotiated all phases of the research process are imperative.

others will react to the work itself. The mechanisms of peer review, external examination of research degrees and conference presentations act as quality control mechanisms to some extent. Citation indexes provide some evidence of whether the research appears to have contributed to knowledge, changed attitudes or influenced policy or practice.

Unfortunately, dissemination of findings is something that is usually thought about at the conclusion of the project rather than at the outset. It is incumbent upon researchers, when agreeing the brief for any particular project, to encourage thinking about how the findings will be disseminated once they are available. This is part of the research process that is frequently allowed little or no time; it must somehow be fitted alongside other commitments. As a consequence, the potential impact of a piece of work may be eroded. Imaginative approaches to dissemination are called for, making appropriate use of new technologies, but also incorporating ideas from community development, action research and partnership projects.

Practitioners, service providers and research commissioners usually cannot wait years for some research evidence about a problem. In short, they require instant knowledge for purposes of immediate action. That is where the difficulties between academic researchers and practitioners begin, because the demand for instant solutions appears incompatible with the long and painstaking processes of scholarly research, where what may be seen as quite insignificant from the perspective of a practitioner can capture the imagination of the researcher for years. One way in which this is manifest is in the different ways in which scholarly research and report material are presented, and the emphasis placed on the various components, depending on the audience. There is a diversity of audiences, each with different needs and no single report or paper will serve all audiences simultaneously. An essential task in designing the overall study report is to identify the specific audiences of the report (see Box 35.5).

In summary, ensuring that the findings of palliative care nursing research are accessible to a range of stakeholders requires an imaginative dissemination strategy which produces timely, meaningful and relevant outputs in a range of formats.

Box 35.5   The UK Research Assessment Exercise

Within the UK, the quality of university-based nursing and health care research is assessed at intervals within the context of the Research Assessment Exercise (RAE). The purpose of the RAE is to produce ratings of research quality for the higher education funding bodies to determine research funding allocations to universities. Assessment of quality is based on peer review by subject panels whose members are appointed on the basis of nomination. Service user representatives are included in the nursing panel in addition to established academics and service provider representatives. The most recent exercise was conducted in 2001 and demonstrated an overall improvement in the quality and international standing of research across all disciplines within UK universities. In relation to nursing research, the assessment demonstrated an overall improvement since the previous exercise in 1996, although nursing remains at the bottom of the league table of all subjects.

The nursing panel identified some important strengths in the work submitted, including that on palliative care. There were also some strong examples of interdisciplinary research, links with service providers and involvement of users of health services. However, the panel also noted a lack of depth in some of the work submitted and reported that programmatic approaches were rare. The Report of the RAE Nursing Panel suggests that, while nursing research within UK universities is undoubtedly contributing to the knowledge base for nursing practice, substantial investment and development is required if the ultimate goal of ensuring that research in nursing enhances the care and well-being of patients, their families and communities is to be achieved.

Conclusions

Research and scholarship in palliative care nursing has come a long way in the last 30 years. Nurses are making a growing contribution to the wider palliative care research community in terms of publications in international academic and professional journals and presentations at interdisciplinary conferences. Designated research and practice units now exist and greater resources and effort are being put into both synthesizing the evidence in the form of systematic reviews and producing evidence relevant to practice. Nurses already possess the many strengths and skills necessary to foster research collaboration and find a clear and distinct position within the mainstream of interdisciplinary effort. Looking to the future, joint initiatives between clinical and academic centres may enhance the relevance and timeliness of research and so reduce the much discussed theory–practice gap (Richardson *et al.* 2001). Similarly, the development of collaborative research groups within and between academic and service organizations, and web-based special interest groups, are further mechanisms for creating working partnerships.

In summary, the future holds huge potential for palliative care nursing research to make a difference to the experiences of the users of palliative care services, their families and staff working with them. However, this potential will only be fully realized if a supportive infrastructure is created and maintained, which will ensure access to resources and enable effective partnerships to develop.

References

Badger, C. (1997) A study of the efficacy of multi-layer bandaging and elastic hosiery in the treatment of lymphoedema, and their effects on the swollen limb. Unpublished PhD thesis, King's College London.

Beattie, J., Cheek, J. and Gibson, T. (1996) The politics of collaboration as viewed through the lens of a collaborative nursing research project. *Journal of Advanced Nursing*, 26: 682–8.

Bredin, M., Corner, J., Krishnasamy, M. *et al.* (1999) Multi-centre randomized controlled trial of nursing intervention for breathlessness in patients with lung cancer. *British Medical Journal*, 381: 901–4.

Burgener, S.C. (2001) Scholarship of practice for a practice profession. *Journal of Professional Nursing*, 17(1): 46–54.

Chang, E. and Daly, J. (1998) Priority areas for clinical research in palliative care nursing. *International Journal of Nursing Practice*, 4(4): 247–53.

Clark, D., Ingleton, C. and Seymour, J. (2000) Support and supervision in palliative care research. *Palliative Medicine*, 14: 441–6.

Clark, D., Hughes, P., Ingleton, C. and Noble, B. (2002) *Evaluation of Powys Macmillan GP Clinical Facilitator Project*. Sheffield: The University of Sheffield.

Clarke, A. and Hanson, E. (2000) Death and dying: changing the culture of care, in T. Warnes, L. Warren and M. Nolan (eds) *Care Services for Later Life: Transformations and Critiques*. London: Jessica Kingsley.

Clifford, C. (1997) Nurse teachers and research. *Nurse Education Today*, 17: 115–20.

Copp, G. (1999) *Facing Impending Death: Experiences of Patients and Their Nurses*. London: Nursing Times Books.

Corner, J. (1996) Is there a research paradigm for palliative care? *Palliative Medicine*, 10: 201–8.

Corner, J. and Bailey, C. (2002) Nursing research in palliative care. Paper delivered to the *Royal Society of Medicine Conference*. London, November.

CPNR/CHEMS (2001) *Promoting Research in Nursing and the Allied Health Professions*. Report to Task Group 3 by the Centre for Policy in Nursing Research, CHEMS Consulting, the Higher Education Consultancy Group and the Research Forum for Allied Health Professions. London: HEFCE.

Department of Health (1998) *A First Class Service: Quality in the New NHS*. London: Department of Health.

Department of Health (2000) *The NHS Plan: A Plan for Investment, a Plan for Reform*. London: HMSO.

Department of Health (2001) *The National Service Framework for Older People*. London: HMSO.

De Raeve, L. (1994) Ethical issues in palliative care research. *Palliative Medicine*, 8: 298–305.

Faulkner, A. (1992) The evaluation of training programmes for communicating skills in palliative care. *Journal of Cancer Care*, 4: 175–8.

Field, D. (1989) *Nursing the Dying*. London: Routledge/Tavistock.

Field, D., Clark, D., Corner, J. and Davis, C. (eds) (2001) *Researching Palliative Care*. Buckingham: Open University Press.

Froggatt, K. (1998) The place of metaphor and language in exploring nurses' emotional work. *Journal of Advanced Nursing*, 28(2): 332–8.

Glaser, B. and Strauss, A. (1965) *Awareness of Dying*. Chicago, IL: Aldine.

Gott, M., Stevens, T., Small, N. and Ahmedzai, S. (2000) *User Involvement in Cancer Care: Exclusion and Empowerment*. Bristol: Policy Press.

Guest, D., Redfern, S., Wilson-Barnett, J. *et al.* (2001) *A Preliminary Evaluation of the Establishment of Nurse, Midwife and Health Visitor Consultants*. Report to the Department of Health. London: King's College.

Hanks, G.W. and Justins, D.M. (1992) Cancer pain: management. *The Lancet*, 339: 1031–6.

Hearn, J. and Higginson, I. (2001) Outcome measures in palliative care for advanced cancer: a review. In D. Field, D. Clark, J. Corner and C. Davis (eds) *Researching Palliative Care*. Buckingham: Open University Press.

Hearn, J., Feuer, D., Higginson, I. and Sheldon, T. (1999) Systematic reviews. *Palliative Medicine*, 13: 75–80.

Hinton, J. (1996) How reliable are relatives' retrospective accounts of terminal illness? Patients' and relatives' accounts compared. *Social Science and Medicine*, 43: 1229–36.

Hotopf, M., Chidgley, J., Addington-Hall, J. and Lan, L.K. (2002) Depression in advanced disease: a systematic review. Prevalence and case finding. *Palliative Medicine*, 16: 81–97.

Humphreys, A., Gidman, J. and Andrews, M. (2000) The nature and purpose of the role of the nurse lecturer in practice settings. *Nurse Education Today*, 20(4): 311–17.

Ingleton, C., Ramcharan, P., Ellis, L. and Schofield, P. (2001) Introducing a professional doctorate in nursing and midwifery. *British Journal of Nursing*, 10(22): 1469–76.

James, N. (1989) Emotional labour. *Sociological Review* 37: 15–42.

Kenyon, E. and Hawker, S. (1999) Once would be enough: some reflections on the issues of safety for lone researchers. *International Journal of Social Research Methodology: Theory and Practice*, 2(4): 313–27.

Kitson, A. (1999) The relevance of scholarship for nursing research and practice. *Journal of Advanced Nursing*, 29(4): 773–5.

Kubler-Ross, E. (1969) *On Death and Dying*. London: Tavistock.

Lawton, J. (1998) Contemporary hospice care: the sequestration of the unbounded body and 'dirty dying'. *Sociology of Health and Illness*, 20(2): 121–43.

Le May, A., Mulhall, A. and Alexander, C. (1998) Bridging the research–practice gap: exploring the research cultures of practitioners and managers. *Journal of Advanced Nursing*, 28(2): 428–37.

Luddington, L., Cox, S., Higginson, I. and Liversey, B. (2001) The need for palliative care for patients with non-cancer diseases: a review of the evidence. *International Journal of Palliative Nursing*, 7(5): 221–6.

McNamara, B., Waddell, C. and Calvin, M. (1994) The institutionalization of the good death. *Social Science and Medicine*, 39(11): 1501–8.

Melia, K. (1987) *Learning and Working: The Occupational Socialization of Nurses*. London: Tavistock.

Mulhall, A. (2001) Bridging the research–practice gap: breaking new ground in health care. *International Journal of Palliative Nursing*, 7(8): 389–94.

Murray Parkes, C. (1970) Seeking and finding a lost object: evidence from recent studies of reaction to bereavement. *Social Science and Medicine*, 4: 187–201.

O'Driscoll, M., Corner, J. and Bailey, C. (1999) The experience of breathlessness in lung cancer. *European Journal of Cancer Care*, 8: 37–43.

Payne, S. (2000) Research involves small steps not giant leaps (editorial). *International Journal of Palliative Nursing*, 6(2): 56.

Payne, S. (2002) Are we using the users? (guest editorial). *International Journal of Palliative Nursing*, 8(5): 212.

Payne, S. and Westwell, P. (1994) Issues for researchers using qualitative methods. *Health Psychology Update*, 16: 7–9.

Payne, S., Hillier, R., Langley-Evans, A. and Roberts, T. (1996) Impact of witnessing death on hospice patients. *Social Science and Medicine*, 43(12): 1758–94.

Pullen, R.L., Jr., Reed, K.E. and Oslar, K.S. (2001) Promoting clinical scholarship through scholarly writing. *Nurse Educator*, 26(2): 81–3.

Quint, J.C. (1967) Institutional practices of information control. *Psychiatry*, 28: 119–32.

Ramcharan, P., Ashmore, R., Nicklin, L. and Drew, J. (2001) Nursing scholarship within the British university system. *British Journal of Nursing*, 10(3): 196–201.

Richards, M.A., Corner, J. and Clark, D. (1998) Developing a research culture for palliative care. *Palliative Medicine*, 12: 399–403.

Richardson, A. and Ream, E. (1998) Recent progress in understanding cancer-related fatigue. *International Journal of Palliative Nursing*, 4(4): 192–8.

Richardson, A., Miller, M. and Potter, H. (2001) Developing, delivering and evaluating cancer nursing services: building the evidence base. *Nursing Times Research*, 6(4): 726–35.

Robbins, M. (1998) *Evaluating Palliative Care: Establishing the Evidence Base*. Oxford: Oxford University Press.

Royal College of Nursing (2001) *Charting the Challenge for Nurse Lecturers in Higher Education*. London: RCN.

Saunders, C. (1958) Dying of cancer. *St Thomas's Hospital Gazette*, 56(2): 37–47.

Scott, C. (1998) Specialist practice: advancing the profession? *Journal of Advanced Nursing*, 28(3): 554–62.

Seymour, J. and Ingleton, C. (1999) Ethical issues in qualitative research at the end of life. *International Journal of Palliative Nursing*, 5(2): 65–74.

Seymour, J., Clark, D., Hughes, P. *et al.* (2002) Clinical nurse specialists in palliative care: Part 3. Issues for the Macmillan nurse's role. *Palliative Medicine*, 16: 386–94.

Shewan, J. and Read, S. (1999) Changing roles in nursing: a literature review of influences and innovations. *Clinical Effectiveness in Nursing*, 2: 75–82.

Solesbury, W. (2001) Fixed-term contracts and other worrying symptoms *Research Fortnight*, 25 April, p. 17.

Sque, M. (2000) Researching the bereaved: an investigator's experience. *Nursing Ethics*, 7(1): 23–34.

Twycross, R.G. and Lack, S.A. (1983) *Symptom Control in Far-Advanced Cancer: Pain Relief*. London: Pitman.

Unsworth, J. (2000) Practice development: a concept analysis. *Journal of Nursing Management*, 8(6): 317–26.

Wilkes, L. (1998) Palliative care nursing research trends from 1987–1996. *International Journal of Palliative Nursing*, 4(3): 128–34.

Wilkes, L., Tracy, S. and White, K. (2000) The future of palliative care nursing research in Australia. *International Journal of Nursing Practice*, 6(1): 32–8.

Wilkie, P. (1997) Ethical issues in qualitative research in palliative care. *Palliative Medicine*, 11: 321–4.

Wilkinson, E., Salisbury, C., Bosanquet, N. *et al.* (1999) Patient and carer preference for, and satisfaction with, specialist models of palliative care: a systematic review. *Palliative Medicine*, 13: 197–216.

Wilkinson, S. (2001) Nurses must seize the opportunity (guest editorial). *International Journal of Palliative Nursing*, 7(1): 4.

World Health Organization (2002) *National Cancer Control Programmes: Policies and Managerial Guidelines*, 2nd edn. Geneva: WHO.

36

Developing expert palliative care nursing through research and practice development

Katherine Froggatt and Katie Booth

In this chapter, we present an account of expert nursing and its development through research and practice development in the context of palliative care. The meaning of expertness in the current climate of evidence-based practice is explored for individual practitioners in the context of organizational constraints and macro-policy initiatives. Our own expertise is based in the two national Macmillan Practice Development Units, funded by a leading UK cancer charity (Macmillan Cancer Relief). The units are involved in the production, dissemination and utilization of knowledge for and about practitioners working at an advanced level as clinical nurse specialists in cancer and palliative care.

We draw on different aspects of the programmes of work undertaken over the last 8 years in these two units to illuminate practical examples of ways in which expert nurses in palliative care have been supported. To do this, we will initially present an overview of the nature of expertness within health care in general, and within nursing in particular, and outline factors and pressures that currently shape the development of expert nursing. In conclusion, a number of challenges to developing expert palliative care nursing are presented.

Expertise and expertness: definitions and dimensions

Professional expertise is described by Higgs and Andresen (2001) as being grounded in three types of knowledge: research and theory, professional craft knowledge and personal experience. Expertness has many dimensions and, importantly, does not have absolute properties, as it is an individual attribute that is socially constructed (Higgs and Bithell 2001). Higgs and Bithell (2001) utilize two perspectives to understand professional expertise – historicism and the dimensions of expertise. In this way, they have contextually located expertise as well as discussed its manifestations in the current climate.

Historicism, as used by Higgs and Bithell (2001), is concerned with understanding a phenomenon in its historical and cultural contexts. Higgs and Bithell (2001) propose that a number of historical and cultural contexts can be used to explore professional expertise, including the origins of expertise in experience, professionalization, models of practice, ethics, consumerism and social responsibility. The main focus of our discussion is professionalization – that is, expertise for the collective of a profession, the professional socialization of individuals into their particular professional group and models of practice. It is a collective process that describes the historical and political emergence of occupational groups or professions (Higgs and Bithell 2001).

Expertise in this context is concerned with the holding of an exclusive body of knowledge and high levels of skill that are not for sharing with other professional groups, or with patients when considering the domain of health care. Professions are established through the identification and up-keeping of formal entry qualifications. Regulatory bodies are created to administer the entry gates and to discipline members who are deemed no longer to be a part of the profession. Some professions such as nursing are considered to be emerging, and for them there is an aspiration to become like the established professions such as medicine or law. In this context, expertise is seen as the key to the status and privilege accorded to the 'professional' and the rationale for the professional's judgements to be respected. Regulation for nursing in the UK has therefore been widely seen as a cornerstone to nursing developing as a profession.

In contrast, the process of professional socialization is about the development of individuals. Higgs and Bithell (2001) identify a number of different models of professional socialization within health care. Each model places a different emphasis upon the meaning of expertise. Some are concerned with the nature of knowledge, others with how knowledge is used and others with the context for which knowledge is generated and used. One of the earliest models of professional socialization is that of apprenticeship, where the learner acquires their knowledge on the job. Expertise is, therefore, a product of the master's competence and the experience obtained within the work. Within health care, other models of socialization place a greater emphasis upon the attainment of knowledge that is deemed to be more scientific, for example the health professional model and the scientist practitioner model. The latter model clearly links expertise with scientific rigour and evidence-based practice and is seen as a result of the need to demonstrate credibility among practitioners. Therefore, overt measures of competence are sought within the scientific domain. In contrast, in other models of socialization expertise is framed as the processual skills of practitioners, their ability to work with information and knowledge, for example the clinical problem-solver model, the reflective practitioner model and the interactional professional model. Lastly, the competent clinician model is framed within an efficiency domain where expertise is concerned with cost-efficiency and cost-effectiveness.

Socialization of individuals into professional groups can be thought of as being shaped by the models outlined above. However, the model of health care current within a particular health care system or an organizational unit is also important, as this creates another frame within which the expertise is used. Different frameworks for health care can include a medical model, a wellness model, a social responsibility model or a rehabilitative model. Much thought within nursing has been directed towards making clear distinctions between models relevant for nursing and medical models of care, but it can be argued that such debates, if divorced from the day-to-day realities of understanding and delivering expert care in clinical settings, can diminish professional dialogue and become sterile (Booth *et al.* 1997).

Although expertise cannot be easily defined or objectified, the dimensions of expertise can be explicated to build up a picture of the complex concept that is expertise. Within the nursing context, discussion about expertness frequently refers back to the work of Benner and her work about the practice of expert nurses (Benner 1984). Based on the work of Dreyfus, who studied chess players and airline pilots, Benner has applied a model of skill acquisition within nursing. The Dreyfus model proposes that there are five levels of proficiency that a student has to pass through before they are deemed an expert. These levels of proficiency are: novice, advanced beginner, competent, proficient and expert. Benner's framework is linked closely to this skills acquisition model and there is a strong emphasis placed on experience and its role in obtaining knowledge and, ultimately, expertise.

Although seminal in terms of its influence in nursing education and curriculum development, this model has been criticized for its lack of definition of the concept 'expert' (Jasper 1994) or the characteristics of expert nursing (Conway 1996). Benner instead describes its application in clinical practice, placing an emphasis upon the context-specific nature of expertness. However, it is possible to identify key features of expert practice within Benner's work; these include perceptual and intuitive abilities and pattern recognition. To clarify the ambiguity present within the thinking around the notion of an 'expert' within nursing, Jasper (1994) undertook a concept analysis of the term 'expert' and proposed that the defining attributes of an expert are: possession of a specialized body of knowledge and skills, great experience in a particular field of practice, well-developed levels of pattern recognition and the expert being acknowledged as such by others around them.

With respect to knowledge, an expert is not just concerned with knowing about, but also with know-how. It is hard to define what constitutes the specific content of an expert's knowledge, as this is context-dependent. For example, within palliative care nursing challenges are currently being made to the expertness of palliative care nurses to address the needs of other disease groups. This is explored further (see Box 36.3). As well as possessing specialized knowledge, experts are in a position to create it. Knowledge is also more than having educational qualifications, as experience is also crucial. Through experience, knowing-about is shaped into knowing-how. Experience is often assumed to refer to the amount of time spent working within a clinical speciality, in this instance palliative care. However, as already indicated, a number of years spent working in a discipline does not necessarily ensure that an individual nurse is an expert, as it is possible to work but not engage with the work. Pattern recognition within complex situations is an attribute that an expert is able to engage with, as Benner (1984) describes in the example of the flight instructors who were able to identify errors on numerous screens and dials faster than their students. This was not because they could look more quickly, but rather that they did not follow the rules they themselves had taught their pupils.

Jasper also identifies recognition by others as defining an expert. However, without externally validated criteria of what is an expert, this may be a self-referring system. Identified 'experts' identify other 'experts'. Ascription is a subjective and relative process and may say as much about the values and experiences of the people doing the ascribing of the expertness as is does about the person so described. It is worth noting that Conway (1996), for example, has raised questions about robustness, particularly in terms of the ways in which 'expert' participants are identified (Manley and Garbett 2000). There is a great reliance on the identification of experts by peers as means of identifying the 'expert' population. Without an articulation of how the identifiers of the expertise have themselves been chosen and an understanding of their own concepts of expertise, there is a lack of rigour to these processes.

Despite this limitation, the framework for understanding expertise from an individual's perspective as proposed by Conway (1996) is useful, in that it recognizes both fluidity and the context-dependent nature of expertise. Conway suggests that the worldview of practitioners directly shapes their understanding and utilization of expertise. In addition, several attributes influencing expert nurses can be related to the nurses themselves and the organizational context they work in. Each nurse holds particular values and goals, has his or her own ability to reflect, personal authority to exert, educational attainments and ability to make relationships. However, the organization in which nurses work will also hold values and have goals that may or may not be in concord with that of the nurse. There are also resource issues that may act as a constraint on the nurse and his or her practice. Conway (1996) identifies four types of expert (technologists, traditionalists, specialists and humanistic existentialists) that draw upon different worldviews – that is, they value different types of knowledge, hold varying values and have particular goals.

Technologists demonstrate a wide range of knowledge, specifically anticipatory knowledge, diagnosis knowledge, 'know-how' knowledge and monitoring knowledge, about junior medical staff and patients. Transmission of this knowledge usually occurs in a didactic fashion. Traditionalists, in contrast, are concerned with survival and 'getting the work done'. Their focus with respect to care is task-allocated and they operate as medical assistants overseeing medical work. These practitioners feel powerless to change the wider context. Specialists, meanwhile, visibly extend their roles, bringing about change, although the way they do this reflects the other three types of expert, for example some specialists operate within the technologist domain. Specialists have distinctive roles, for example in palliative care or breast cancer; they value their extended knowledge base, have a consultative role for other nurses, develop autonomy and innovation in their work and use protocols to extend their role. Humanistic existentialists are dynamic with a strong nursing focus to the care they offer. As well as feeling passionate about their work, they are able to change the context they work in to support the development of their care and, consequently, are influential in terms of nursing.

It is possible to identify three features across these four dimensions of expertise. One feature of these dimensions concerns what is known, be it knowledge or skills. Second, there are processual features pertaining to how what is known is used and, finally, there is reference to the context within which it is used.

Across the different health care contexts within which expertise is located and in the dimensions of expertise identified, it is apparent that expertise is a complex and interactive attribute, whether it is considered for an individual practitioner or for the collective of the nursing profession. However, expertise in palliative care nursing is more than a conceptual dialogue – it is grounded within the speciality of palliative care, which is itself located in the wider health care system.

Expertise in context: policy and organizational demands

At a macro level, policy makers and the government of the day work together to shape the decisions made about health care and nursing delivery. Within the UK, expertise is seen as central to the drive over the past few years to improve the quality of health services and refers to both the collective nursing profession and individual nurses. For instance, in 1998 the Department of Health stated that 'Driving up standards will rely on the commitment and expertise of all those who work in the health service' (p. 11). In this climate, there are evident pressures on those delivering services to provide care of a suitable expert quality. For example, 'From the time of diagnosis, each patient should have access to a named nurse who has been trained in counselling patients, who has specialist knowledge of cancer and who can offer continuity of care' (Department of Health 1997: 21). In this case, policy guidance about colorectal cancer has implications for nurse training in counselling skills, in specialist knowledge and in the way service is delivered (so enabling the nurse to offer continuity of care).

Potentially, collective nursing expertise can be built through contributions to policy and service development. However, in cancer and palliative care, this expertise may well be overlooked by policy makers. For instance, a recent textual analysis of cancer guidance documents demonstrated that although nurses were integral to implementing service improvements, the majority of references to the essential nursing roles were indirect or implied (Booth *et al.* 2001a). This suggests that collective nursing expertise is relatively invisible and that despite their knowledge and experience, nurses can find themselves powerless in policy terms. The question is why? For one thing, the explicit nursing role in implementing guidelines seems to have been hidden within the term 'team'. This perhaps serves to hide the tension of power relationships and masks a general expectation that it is the doctor who is in charge. However, in terms of UK health care, there is a growing acceptance that a meaningful contribution from all members of the health care professionals is essential. For example, the Department of Health (1998) has called for 'Total involvement of staff in shaping services and planning change, with open communication and collaboration' (p. 75).

It must be remembered that there is evidence that being a member of a nominated team does not automatically bring with it smooth working. Medical team members may find expert help from nurses somewhat undermining (Field 1998) and nurses may not insist on bringing their expertise to the fore to protect working relationships (Griffiths and Luker 1997). So it would appear that expert knowledge needs to be explicitly acknowledged by those who implement policy before it can be fully utilized for service development. Building this expertise into decision-making structures is a sensible way forward. However, another example of research conducted by one of the Macmillan Practice Development Units underlines the importance of organizational culture in the utilization of nursing expertise in cancer and palliative care (see Box 36.1).

Collective nursing expertise can be facilitated through the work of specialist nurses (Closs and Cheater 1994) and, in relation to cancer care, *The Nursing Contribution to Cancer Care* (Department of Health 2000) stipulates the need for specialist nurses to take the lead in ensuring that patient care is not only of a high standard, but also that interventions are based on sound evidence. However, the ability of the specialist nurse to pass on their expertise is shaped by the organizational context they work in (Conway 1996). For example, a large study using questionnaire and focus group data, undertaken by the Manchester Practice Development Unit, demonstrated that organizational support and guidance were essential if specialist nurses in cancer and palliative care were to feel adequately prepared to help colleagues improve their practice (Booth *et al.* 2003).

Several themes are present within the policies presented: these concern increasing advice and regulation and the type and nature of knowledge that is valued within health care. First, with respect to regulation, there is a need to demonstrate professional competence. Recent UK government policy publications (e.g. Department of Health 1999a,b) have led to an increasing emphasis on expertise being seen in terms of competency and competency assessment (Manley and Garbett 2000). The nursing profession is also measuring and assessing expertise and competence through accreditation as public protection is deemed to be required.

Box 36.1   Expert nurses' influence in developing service

As a result of the influential Calman-Hine Report in England and Wales, con-sultant grade clinician posts were created to facilitate, organize and coordinate high-quality, comprehensive cancer services. In addition, although they were not explicitly called for, lead cancer nurse posts began to emerge. These post were designed to complement the work of the lead cancer clinician by facilitating the necessary strategic planning to ensure nursing aspects of the transformed cancer and palliative care services were identified and nurtured.

By 1998, Macmillan Cancer Relief had entered into funding arrangements to support a number of lead cancer nurse posts in England, Scotland and Wales, and considered a structured evaluation of these innovative posts was important and timely.

A study of 12 lead cancer nurses conducted over a 2-year period as they developed their posts was illuminating in this respect (Booth *et al.* 2001b). It was found that despite considerable variation between the 12 sites in terms of length of time in post, the person's previous experience and current job description, all the lead nurses had made notable contributions within their organizations and had implemented a wide range of service developments. Three factors were identified as being particularly important in assisting the lead nurse to achieve their goals:

1   Developing advantageous alliances with those closely associated with the delivery of cancer services.
2   The ability to recognize and harness the help of powerful colleagues.
3   Accommodating to the climate of change which was current throughout the duration of the investigation.

Most lead nurses experienced some difficulties in the following three areas:

1   Frequent developments and changes in NHS policy, in addition to Trust mergers and service restructuring.
2   Restricted resources.
3   Cancer care is organized in a site-specific way, which is problematic when trying to bring a unifying approach to cancer services.

Overall, this study indicates that success in the lead role was not simply about ideal characteristics pertaining to the person occupying the lead nurse post; instead, success was concerned with a working partnership between the lead nurse and the organization. In addition, it is important for lead nurses to be supported in dealing with difficult situations that arise both within the organization and as a consequence of external influences.

Note: This example is adapted from an Executive Summary of the Lead Nurse Project distributed by Macmillan Cancer Relief.

Second, there are aspirations that, in the UK, the National Health Service (NHS) will increasingly use evidence as a foundation, as exemplified by systems to manage and monitor the use of evidence – for example, the National Institute of Clinical Excellence and the Commission for Health

Improvement. These institutions reflect the broader underlying movement of evidence-based practice that is very influential in the UK. The drive for evidence-based health care provision is an illustration of 'technical rationality' and mirrors the scientist practitioner model of professional practice, outlined earlier. This approach to developing practice, through the identification of 'valid' sources of knowledge to evaluate their credibility to support rational decision making (Sackett *et al.* 1997), sits within the dominant paradigm within Western thinking of positivist logical empiricism, exemplified in the medical model of health care. Arising from a contemporary response to the control of risk in a culture of increasing managerialism and audit (Trinder 2000), evidence-based practice is a product of its time, which is being challenged by other voices such as the user movement (see Chapter 4) and a recognition that certainly within nursing other types of knowledge are present and valued (Blomfield and Hardy 2000).

Against this complex background of differing priorities and voices, it is possible to identify ways in which expert palliative care nursing and nurses are being developed within the UK. Education, research, quality initiatives and practice development are variously used to develop practitioners to become more expert. The nature and impact of education and research and scholarship on the development of palliative care nursing is explored elsewhere (see Chapters 33 and 35). Here we describe the work of two sister national research and practice development units and consider their impact upon the development of expert palliative care nursing and what issues this has raised.

Macmillan Practice Development Units: a strategy for development

Charities have been important players in the development of palliative care nursing in the UK, together with higher educational focused on the delivery of palliative care education and research. We focus here upon the work that has been undertaken by one of the main cancer charities in the UK, Macmillan Cancer Relief, to ensure that practitioners are appropriately prepared to deliver expert care to patients and their families.[1]

As well as supporting people with cancer with information, financial grants and support, Macmillan Cancer Relief also invests in the funding of posts in nursing, medicine and other allied health professions. Nurses comprise the largest group of health care professionals supported by Macmillan Cancer Relief. As of December 2002, there were 2029 clinical nurse specialists out of a total of 2510 funded posts. The postholders are funded by Macmillan but are predominantly employed by the acute hospital Trusts and primary care Trusts within which they work; however, Macmillan offers ongoing support to these postholders. This support is overseen by the Department of Education, Development and Support at Macmillan Cancer Relief through education, provision of resources and research and practice development. The Macmillan National Institute of Education has lecturers located in seven regions of the UK, and these lecturers offer professional development and support to postholders. Professional resources, including research reports, syntheses of evidence, other resources and information, are developed and disseminated to all postholders and beyond.

Macmillan also fund two Practice Development Units (PDUs), currently located in Manchester and Southampton. The first unit was funded in 1994 at the Institute of Cancer Research in London (moving to the School of Nursing and Midwifery at the University of Southampton in 2002), and the second was established in 1997 at the School of Nursing and Midwifery at the University of Manchester. The units have core funding, which has enabled substantial programmes of work to be established and has allowed for the development of ideas and effective dissemination.

The two units hold common values about practice development and research. The overarching aim of the work is to improve the care received by people living and dying with cancer. The ultimate objectives are to support the provision of practical, realistic and desirable improvements in clinical practice and to ensure that these improvements have theoretical credibility (see Kitson *et al.* 1996). The units are not just concerned with the development of knowledge. They also find ways based upon the evidence to promote the implementation of knowledge into practice. The focus on practice development is significant, because in addition to the development of new knowledge (through the undertaking of research), the units are concerned with understanding how knowledge is (or is not) used in practice. Looking back on the work since 1994, it is possible to identify several strategies that have been adopted that facilitate the development of expert practice among clinical nurse specialists in palliative care and cancer:

1 *Production of knowledge* to support practitioners and improve the care for patients. This may be new knowledge obtained through the undertaking of empirical research, or it may be the synthesis of knowledge elsewhere in areas of relevance to practitioners in this speciality. The two units have focused on different areas, for example the unit now based in Southampton has had a strand of work focused upon the management of difficult symptoms. Examples of this work include developing an intervention to manage breathlessness (Bredin *et al.* 1999), understanding the experience of fatigue (Krishnasamy 1996) and exploring the significance of weight loss to patients, their carers and professionals (Poole and Froggatt 2002). In Manchester, the work has had a psycho-social focus concerned with information needs and decision making and the psychological impact of a cancer diagnosis (Chalmers *et al.* 2001; Foy and Rose 2001). The endeavour is to understand how to provide and sustain effective nurse-led interventions for these issues. Understanding nursing delivery and nurses' work has been important in several pieces of work, including the practice development role of clinical nurse specialists (Booth *et al.* 2003), the work of lead nurses (Booth *et al.* 2001b) and the development of the provision of palliative care in nursing

homes through education and clinical nurse specialist work (Froggatt 2000; Froggatt and Hoult 2002, Froggatt *et al.* 2002b).

2 *Capacity building for clinical practice and research* occurs through the links made between the units and clinical areas. Strengthening the research base of cancer care and investment in staff through education and development are both essential elements of the NHS Cancer Plan (Department of Health 2000). This reflects the increasing recognition at policy level that development of capability in research is fundamentally important to the wider development of high-quality health care. It is therefore considered vital to extend and enhance research capability within the Macmillan workforce. Two models of working have been used to date to undertake this aspect of the unit's work. In the first, several posts have been established that allow clinical practitioners to spend time working in the units. Individuals are either seconded to work in the unit for a specified period of time, or joint posts are established so that individuals work part-time in the unit and part-time in practice. Based on this model, the connection between research and practice is located within particular individuals, who have to bridge these two worlds. There are costs to this model, not only in terms of finance because of the higher proportion of part-time staff in any one location, but also in terms of the time, as senior unit staff have to supervise the work of these staff members.

In the second model, the research practitioners employed to work full-time in the unit base their research within the relevant clinical area so that they are actively present as researchers in clinical practice. The advantage to the practitioners working in this model is that they are integrated into the research unit and the whole unit can support individuals. The transition from practice to research can be a hard one. For some individuals, working full-time in a research unit, even one that is committed to the development of practice and using research methods that are participative, this change is too great and they may return to practice relatively quickly. Other individuals thrive on an opportunity to step back and be more critical about issues that relate to practice.

Through both these approaches, the units and the clinical areas are strengthened. Heightened research awareness and critical skills are present in the clinical area and the research foci and research approaches adopted within the units are grounded in the priorities of clinical practice. More experienced unit staff are also involved in the supervision of master's and doctoral students. The project topics can usually complement the unit's core programme of work and add to our understanding of expertise in clinical practice. The units also offer reactive support, usually by telephone, to a wide range of health care professionals regarding research and clinical practice projects. This is more usually signposting to the most appropriate source of information and more local support, but is an important feature of the work as a resource across the UK.

3 *Support of evidence-based practice* has been developed within the units in several ways. The outcomes of the empirical research already outlined are being integrated into the activity of Macmillan Cancer Relief more cen-

trally, as their relevance and importance are recognized. A quarterly bulletin *Evidence Update* is produced from the Manchester Unit in conjunction with the University Library and the Christie Hospital Library. This publication provides accessible, up-to-date information about relevant published evidence in the area of cancer and palliative care nursing. All Macmillan post-holders have received this directly. In the future, the *Update* will be available on the Macmillan website, making it accessible to a wider audience. Library support services have also been developed.

The following cases (Boxes 36.2 and 36.3) illustrate in more detail the ways in which the research and practice development undertaken by the units has helped facilitate the development of expert practitioners within palliative care and also promoted the expertness of palliative care nursing as a consequence. In Box 36.2, some of the challenges to the development of expertness are highlighted arising from a programme of work into the management of breathlessness. In Box 36.3, the context in which expertise is used is challenged in a different way, and translation is required across specialities. This example clearly illustrates that expertise is not static and to be an expert requires individuals to be able to adapt their knowledge base to suit the contexts in which they are working.

The challenges of developing expertise in an evidence-based health care system

Several challenges to the development of expert palliative care nursing can be identified. While not disputing the need to have a sound basis for the decisions made about the treatments and care delivered within health care, an evidence-based practice approach can be very constraining. The evidence-based practice movement has narrowly defined the meaning of 'valid' evidence, placing the highest confidence in only one type of evidence – that obtained through the conduct of randomized controlled trials. There are practical and ethical difficulties that exist in generating evidence through randomized controlled trials in the palliative care population (Hardy 2001). Other forms of evidence need to be acknowledged and there is a wide spectrum that can potentially contribute to the nature of knowledge and expertise. Within palliative care nursing, the nature of evidence will need to reflect the philosophy that underpins the care of people within this discipline. For palliative care, the key ideals of holism, multidisciplinary working and the needs of the patients and their wider carers all impact upon the knowledge that is required to be an expert palliative care nurse. The user voice (both from patients and their family carers) also needs to be heard and allowed to contribute to the nature of the knowledge that is valued (see Chapter 4).

It can also be seen that the promotion of evidence-based care does little to address how this evidence can be used and what shapes its use. Although it is assumed that the presence of evidence from systematic reviews is

---

Box 36.2   Dissemination and utilization of a non-pharmacological intervention to manage breathlessness: expertise and pragmatics

Over the last 8 years, Macmillan has funded a programme of work in the management of breathlessness within the Practice Development Unit, formerly based in London at the Institute of Cancer Research. As is described elsewhere (Bredin *et al.* 1999), a non-pharmacological intervention to manage breathlessness in advanced lung cancer was developed by practitioners at the unit. This work is currently being disseminated, a number of resources have been developed (e.g. information booklets and a CD-ROM) and educational courses have been established (Connelly and O'Neill 1999), including a new Master's module in collaboration with the Macmillan National Institute of Education. A number of issues have been raised about the dissemination and utilization of this intervention that pertain to the development of expert nurses.

Froggatt *et al.* (2002a) have explored some of the issues raised for the unit as it began to facilitate the dissemination of the intervention and tried to establish networks and resource centres to support the work. It was interesting to note that despite attendance at training and educational initiatives that have been developed in the UK, the practitioners concerned still reported feeling inadequate and lacking confidence to use aspects of the intervention in their own practice (Froggatt *et al.* 2002a; Johnson and Moore 2003). Practitioners – clinical nurse specialists in lung cancer and palliative care as well as other disciplines (physiotherapists and occupational therapists) – perceive the original researchers involved in the research project as being the experts and continue to look to them for their expertise and support. Why is this? The evidence for the intervention is readily available in the form of published papers, resources (e.g. a CD-ROM) and study days.

Johnson and Moore (2003), two practitioners who have used the intervention in their own practice and who have been involved in teaching others, have explored some reasons for the difficulties in taking this 'evidence' and using it in practice. These relate to the differences between doing research focused on this one study and being a practitioner with competing demands from a number of people with differing clinical needs. There are organizational issues of how to establish a clinic and even the appropriateness of this form of service provision for people with breathlessness. They consider the issue of confidence and propose that this may arise from the demands within the intervention to work in a therapeutic way with patients (Bailey 1995), which can be threatening to practitioners if they are not adequately prepared and supported once in practice.

Some practitioners have begun to address these issues for themselves. Early findings from an evaluation of the Master's module mentioned earlier indicate that those practitioners who have attended the module courses have moved on in their practice. For example, where they regarded the original researchers as experts, as a consequence of attending the module they find themselves being perceived as the experts in their locality. This duality of inexpertness and expertness held within one practitioner is an indication of the complexity of the issue. The practitioners were also addressing issues of translation of knowledge from one setting to another. The empirical research work was undertaken in an out-patient setting, whereas practitioners wishing to use this intervention worked in a variety of settings, including hospital wards and people's homes in the community. Consequently, expertise in one context has begun to be translated to fit the needs of other settings.

---

sufficient to ensure it is used, wider individual and organizational issues shape to what extent expert evidence is utilized in practice. Interestingly, the National Institute of Clinical Excellence, which commissions evidence and then prescribes its use, is doing this not only on the basis of the scientific evidence, but also on economic grounds. Best practice is not only about rigorous clinical evidence, but is also linked to the financial implications and

---

Box 36.3 The provision of palliative care in nursing homes: expertise in context

There is increasing interest from specialist palliative care practitioners and educators in the provision of palliative care in nursing homes. The ways in which palliative care practices in nursing homes are being currently developed raise a number of questions about the methods of development and assumptions about expertise that may be held within palliative care and the nursing home sector (Froggatt 2001). Clinical nurse specialists have a role to play in the provision of palliative care in nursing homes, as well as supporting the development of palliative care practices within this setting (Froggatt *et al.* 2002b).

In this situation, there is an interplay of two dimensions of expertise outlined earlier – the knowledge base and the recognition by others of being an expert. Clinical nurse specialists in palliative care do have expertise in specialist palliative care, but they are also ascribed expertise by nursing home staff who perceive them to be experts about palliative care. An important question arises from this ascription of expertise in this context. To what extent can an expert in one area of palliative care (e.g. specialist palliative care for people with cancer) be an expert in another speciality (e.g. gerontological care)? In nursing home care, cancer is not the dominant cause of death, and nursing home residents live and die with a complexity of chronic conditions that interplay to create a different dying trajectory that is likely to be longer and marked by more uncertainty (Komaromy 2002).

What should be recognized is that a new expertise needs to be articulated that draws upon the expertise of specialist palliative care as well as gerontology to provide end-of-life palliative care for residents in nursing homes that is diverse enough to encompass the varying needs of this population.

---

costs of implementing such knowledge. Kitson *et al.* (1996) propose that if the successful implementation of a new initiative is to be achieved – that is, evidence is utilized in practice – not only is evidence required, but issues of context (McCormack *et al.* 2002) and facilitation (Harvey *et al.* 2002) also need to be addressed.

In summary, challenges to the development of palliative care nursing expertise include:

- Valuing the range of evidence that exists within nursing, including intuitive and non-rational sources.
- Learning from others in other professions and health care disciplines.
- Maintaining expertness and the ability to be creative in the midst of increasing regulation and prescription from the centre, based on economic markers.
- Incorporating the user perspective, patients and their carers.

Being an expert is about knowledge, skills to utilize this knowledge and working in a situated context.

Conclusions

The development of expert nursing in palliative care is a complex matter and draws upon a variety of sources for its energy and momentum. We have outlined here some of the conceptual issues about the nature of expertise and being an expert nurse, indicating the various factors that shape how expert nurses and practice can be developed in the contemporary culture of the UK health care system.

Promoting the development of nurses to ensure that nursing is developed is too simplistic a strategy. A multi-pronged strategy is required that addresses the professional developmental needs of nurses, while at the same time challenging and changing the organizational contexts within which they work. We have drawn upon concrete examples of work *in situ* in the Macmillan Practice Development Units, which has its roots in research and practice development. As described in other chapters in this book, education, research and scholarship, and audit are also important for the development of expertise among palliative care nurses, which will ultimately benefit individuals who are dying and members of their families.

Note

1   Marie Curie Cancer Care, another large nationwide cancer charity in the UK, has also been involved in supporting the educational, research and development needs of its staff.

References

Bailey, C. (1995) Nursing as therapy in the management of lung cancer. *European Journal of Cancer Care*, 4: 184–90.

Benner, P. (1984) *From Novice to Expert: Excellence and Power in Clinical Nursing Practice*. Menlo Park, CA: Addison-Wesley.

Blomfield, R. and Hardy, S. (2000) Evidence-based nursing practice, in L. Trinder and S. Reynolds (eds) *Evidence-Based Practice: A Critical Appraisal*. Oxford: Blackwell Science.

Booth, K., Kenrick, M. and Woods, S. (1997) Nursing knowledge, theory and method re-visited. *Journal of Advanced Nursing*, 26: 804–11.

Booth, K., Kirshbaum, M., Eastwood, L. and Luker, K.A. (2001a) Guidance on commissioning cancer services: an investigation of the implications for nursing. *Clinical Effectiveness in Nursing*, 5: 73–80.

Booth, K., Kirshbaum, M. and Luker, K.A. (2001b) *Evaluation of the Macmillan Lead Nurse Initiative*. Project report submitted to Macmillan Cancer Relief.

Booth, K., Luker, K.A., Costello, J. and Dows, K. (2003) Macmillan cancer and palliative care specialists: their practice development support needs. *International Journal of Palliative Nursing*, 9(2): 73–9.

Bredin, M., Corner, J., Krishnasamy, M. *et al.* (1999) Multi-centre randomised controlled trial of nursing intervention for breathlessness in patients with lung cancer. *British Medical Journal*, 318: 901–4.

Chalmers, K., Luker, K.A., Leinster, S., Ellis, I. and Booth, K. (2001) Information and support needs of women with primary relatives with breast cancer: development of information and support needs questionnaire. *Journal of Advanced Nursing*, 35(4): 497–508.

Closs, J.S. and Cheater, F.M. (1994) Utilization of nursing research: culture, interest and support. *Journal of Advanced Nursing*, 19: 762–73.

Connelly, M. and O'Neill, J. (1999) Teaching a research-based approach to the management of breathlessness in patients with lung cancer. *European Journal of Cancer Care*, 8: 30–6.

Conway, J. (1996) *Nursing Expertise and Advanced Practice*. Salisbury: Mark Allen.

Department of Health (1997) *Guidance on Commissioning Cancer Services: Improving Outcomes in Colorectal Cancer. (The Manual)*. London: HMSO.

Department of Health (1998) *A First Class Service: Quality in the New NHS*. London: HMSO.

Department of Health (1999a) *Agenda for Change: Modernising the NHS Pay-system*. London: Department of Health.

Department of Health (1999b) *Making a Difference: Strengthening the Nursing, Midwifery and Health Visiting Contribution to Health and Healthcare*. London: Department of Health.

Department of Health (2000) *The Nursing Contribution to Cancer Care*. London: Department of Health.

Field, D. (1998) Special not different: general practitioners' accounts of their care of dying people. *Social Science and Medicine*, 46(9): 1110–20.

Foy, S. and Rose, K. (2001) Men's experiences of their partner's primary and recurrent breast cancer. *European Journal of Oncology Nursing*, 5(1): 42–8.

Froggatt, K.A. (2000) Evaluating a palliative care education project in nursing homes. *International Journal of Palliative Nursing*, 6(3): 140–6.

Froggatt, K. (2001) Palliative care and nursing homes: where next? *Palliative Medicine*, 15: 42–8.

Froggatt, K.A. and Hoult, L. (2002). Developing palliative care practice in nursing and residential care homes: the role of the clinical nurse specialist. *Journal of Clinical Nursing*, 11: 802–8.

Froggatt, K.A., Corner, J. and Bredin, M. (2002a) Dissemination and utilisation of an intervention to manage breathlessness: letting go or letting down? *NT Research*, 7(3): 2–10.

Froggatt, K.A., Poole, K. and Hoult, L. (2002b) The provision of palliative care in nursing homes and residential care homes: a survey of clinical nurse specialist work. *Palliative Medicine*, 16: 481–7.

Griffiths, J.M. and Luker, K.A. (1997) A barrier to clinical effectiveness: the etiquette of district nursing. *Clinical Effectiveness in Nursing*, 1: 121–30.

Hardy, J. (2001) Placebo controlled trials in palliative care: the argument for, in D. Field, D. Clark, J. Corner and C. Davies (eds) *Researching Palliative Care*. Buckingham: Open University Press.

Harvey, G., Loftus-Hills, A., Rycroft-Malone, J. *et al.* (2002) Getting evidence into practice: the role and function of facilitation. *Journal of Advanced Nursing*, 37(6): 577–88.

Higgs, J. and Andresen, L. (2001) The knower, the knowing and the known: the threads in the woven tapestry of knowledge, in J. Higgs and A. Titchen (eds)

Practice Knowledge and Expertise in the Health Professions. Oxford: Butterworth Heinemann.

Higgs, J. and Bithell, C. (2001) Professional expertise, in J. Higgs and A. Titchen (eds) *Practice Knowledge and Expertise in the Health Professions*. Oxford: Butterworth Heinemann.

Jasper, M.A. (1994) Expert: a discussion of the implications of the concept as used in nursing. *Journal of Advanced Nursing*, 20: 769–76.

Johnson, M. and Moore, S. (2003) Research into practice: the reality of implementing a non-pharmacological breathlessness intervention into clinical practice. *European Journal of Oncology Nursing*, 7(1): 33–8.

Kitson, A., Ahmed, L.B., Harvey, G. and Seers, K. (1996) From research to practice: one model for promoting research-based practice. *Journal of Advanced Nursing*, 23: 430–40.

Komaromy, C. (2002) The performance of the hour of death, in J. Hockley and D. Clark (eds) *Palliative Care for Older People in Care Homes*. Buckingham: Open University Press.

Krishnasamy, M. (1996) *An Exploration of the Nature and Impact of Fatigue in Advanced Cancer: A Case Study*. London: Macmillan Practice Development Unit, Centre for Cancer and Palliative Care Studies.

Manley, K. and Garbett, R. (2000) Paying Peter and Paul: reconciling concepts of expertise with competency for a clinical career structure. *Journal of Clinical Nursing*, 9: 347–59.

McCormack, B., Kitson, A., Harvey, G. *et al.* (2002) Getting evidence into practice: the meaning of 'context'. *Journal of Advanced Nursing*, 38(1): 94–104.

Poole, K.A. and Froggatt, K.A. (2002) Loss of weight and loss of appetite in advanced cancer: a problem for the patient, the carer or the health professional? *Palliative Medicine*, 16: 499–506.

Sackett, D.L., Richardson, W.S., Rosenberg, W. and Haynes, R.B. (1997) *Evidence-Based Medicine: How to Practice and Teach EBM*. New York: Churchill Livingstone.

Trinder, L. (2000) Introduction: the context of evidence-based practice, in L. Trinder and S. Reynolds (eds) *Evidence-Based Practice: A Critical Appraisal*. Oxford: Blackwell Science.

37

Policy, audit, evaluation and clinical governance

Liz Barker and Sue Hawkett

Introduction

In this chapter, we outline recent UK government policy linking audit, evaluation and clinical governance. We demonstrate how this has shaped specialist palliative care services and the implications for professional practice. Most of the material is drawn from the *NHS Plan* (Department of Health 2000d), the *NHS Cancer Plan* (Department of Health 2000c) and subsequent documents. Although these deal with services in England, there are similar policy directions in other UK countries. European developments have not been addressed.

Where do we begin? What are the connections between policy and clinical practice? Does policy make any difference? And how can clinical nurses influence the process? These are some of the questions we should consider. It is important to see how clinical practice is informed and directed by policy *and* how practice influences policy. The National Health Service (NHS) for the UK established some 50 years ago was, and continues to be, founded on the principle of health care provision for all irrespective of condition or ability to pay. In 1997, the incoming government signalled a new direction for health care. The *New NHS: Modern Dependable* (Department of Health 1997) set out a 10-year plan focusing on improving the quality of care, proposing a new model which brought together responsibility for quality at local level with clear national standards. The aim was to reduce variations in outcomes of, and access to, services, as well as to ensure that clinical decisions were made based on the most up-to-date evidence and were known to be effective. There are three main elements to the 10-year plan.

- Setting clear national quality standards through national service frameworks (NSFs) and the establishment of an independent National Institute for Clinical Excellence (NICE).
- Mechanisms for ensuring local delivery of quality clinical services

through clinical governance supported by programmes of lifelong learning and local delivery of professional self-regulation.

- Systems for monitoring delivery of quality standards in the form of a statutory Commission for Health Improvement (CHI), a NHS performance assessment framework together with national patient surveys.

The policy scene was set, therefore, to provide a framework of national standards (NSFs) to ensure consistent quality services, based on evidence (NICE), informed by patients' views which are monitored (CHI).

Building on the *New NHS: Modern and Dependable* (Department of Health 1997), the *NHS Plan* (Department of Health 2000d) was published, setting out a vision and investment for a health service for the twenty-first century designed around the patient. Although major improvements in health had been delivered, they fell short of the standards patients expected and staff wanted to provide. The emphasis was to ensure the NHS provided a service that patients wanted and needed.

It was clear that patients wished to be treated with dignity and respect, to have clear information about their condition, good communication from health care professionals and to receive the best possible symptom control and psychological support. To address these issues, there needed to be major changes in the way health care was funded and staff worked. This theme was emphasized again in the *NHS Cancer Plan* (Department of Health 2000c) published later in the same year.

How these major shifts in culture would be achieved and what it meant for professional practice and accountability were set out in the following subsequent documents:

- *Shifting the Balance of Power Within the NHS: Securing Delivery* (Department of Health 2001b);
- *Shifting the Balance of Power Within the NHS: The Next Steps* (Department of Health 2002a);
- *Delivering the NHS Plan: Next Steps on Investment, Next Steps on Reform* (Department of Health 2002b).

These described how the *NHS Plan* (Department of Health 2000d) would be implemented.

Shifting the balance of power

In *Shifting the Balance of Power Within the NHS: The Next Steps* (Department of Health 2002a), the Department of Health outlined the vision for achieving both organizational and cultural change:

- empowering frontline staff to have a say in the way in which services were delivered and resources allocated;

- empowering patients to be informed and active partners in their care and, most importantly, involving them in the design, delivery and development of local services;

- changing the current culture by devolving decision-making power to frontline staff and primary care trusts (primary care trusts) led by clinicians and local people, and by building clinical networks across organizations.

What did this mean for how the NHS was run? A major and radical reorganization was taking place. The most significant change was devolving 75 per cent of NHS budgets to PCTs, with the aim of putting power at the frontline of clinical care. Health authorities, which had in the past been responsible for commissioning services, were replaced with fewer strategic health authorities. These authorities had responsibility for developing strategy and performance managing PCTs, NHS Trusts and Workforce Development Confederations in order to secure delivery and ensure a consistent approach. In effect, they managed the NHS on behalf of the Department of Health. Four Directors of Health replaced the regional offices to become Directorates of Health and Social Care. Their role was to support and develop the NHS, provide local contact and performance manage the strategic health authorities.

The development of clinical networks across organizations and sectors was a key element in changing the culture and devolving decision making to frontline staff and local people. The concept of networks as an effective way of delivering services had been developed in the *NHS Cancer Plan* (Department of Health 2000c). Thirty-four cancer networks, each serving a population of between 500,000 and 3 million, are organizational models bringing together health service commissioners, primary care trusts, providers (primary and community and hospitals), the voluntary sector and local authorities. Central to the role of a network is the development of strategic service delivery plans for all aspects of cancer care, including palliative care. These plans are fully integrated within the wider planning process through health improvement programmes, which target health priorities for the total population and service and financial frameworks matching resources to priorities.

The success of the cancer networks was acknowledged and provided an example of how services could be delivered (Department of Health 2002a). Managed cancer networks were seen to facilitate integrated care, improve clinical outcomes, develop cost-effective services and to improve patient experience and equity of service provision. Primary care trusts and strategic health authorities would be responsible for commissioning services but would achieve this through cancer networks, which would provide an established route for care delivery across the care pathway. It was seen that NHS Trusts and PCTs would be accountable for the delivery of the cancer targets and implementing the *NHS Cancer Plan* (Department of Health 2000c), working together within cancer networks.

Improvements in commissioning health care would ensure that (Department of Health 2002b):

- Patients would be provided with timely, comparable information on practices and hospitals, which would be updated regularly.
- Patients would be offered a choice of general practitioners (GPs), hospitals and consultants.
- Where choice was exercised, cash for treatment would follow the patient irrespective of health care provider.
- Price for units of activity would be set, allowing PCTs to focus on volume, appropriateness and quality. For this to function, an 'open book' relationship was required between PCTs and NHS Trusts.
- Significantly, health resource groups – a system by which a process of care is costed – and benchmarks would be used to establish a standard tariff for the same treatment regardless of provider.
- Local commissioning would focus on volume, appropriateness and quality not price, as this would be fixed using regional tariffs to reflect unavoidable differences in costs in different parts of the country.

In describing changes for patients, it was stated that 'Hospitals will no longer choose patients. Patients will choose hospitals' (Department of Health 2002b: 22, para. 5.4). This is one of the fundamental principles of delivering an effective health service.

The most significant policy development for specialist palliative care is the *NHS Cancer Plan* (Department of Health 2000c), which sets out four main aims.

- to save more lives;
- to ensure people with cancer get the right professional support and care as well as the best treatments;
- to tackle inequalities in health; and
- to build for the future through investing in the workforce, through strong research and preparation for the genetics revolution.

The plan set out a strategy to bring cancer services up to the level of the best in Europe and to improve the experience of care for those affected by cancer. To achieve this, the *NHS Cancer Plan* outlined a supportive and palliative care strategy. This would mean that for the first time a comprehensive service to support patients, families and carers, from the time that cancer was first suspected through to death and into bereavement, would be established.

Why was such a strategy needed? We know that when the diagnosis of cancer is first made, it can have a devastating impact on the quality of patients' lives. Patients need to have access to information, communication, emotional, social and spiritual support and good symptom control. Carers may also need information and support throughout the care pathway and into bereavement. For this to be achieved, equitable provision of supportive and palliative care needs to be established in each cancer network and in line with other national service frameworks, supported by evidence-based service guidance and national standards. The provision should reflect partnership agreements between the NHS, social services and the voluntary sector. One of the main elements of the supportive and palliative care strategy is the development of evidence-based guidance developed by the National Institute for Clinical Excellence (2002). The supportive and palliative care guidance, being developed in two parts, will provide service delivery recommendations on: the overall organization of service delivery, information, communication, psychological support services, general palliative care, specialist palliative care, social, emotional and spiritual support, complementary therapies, bereavement and carer support. The first part of the guidance will include a chapter on specialist palliative care and can be found at www.nice.org.uk. The completed guidance will be available in late 2003.

The direction has been set by national policy on how to deliver a service that meets the needs of the patient and carers and ensures a quality service that is continually improving. This is the goal; how will it be delivered? Specialist palliative care services must be delivered within the context of evidence-based services, delivered against nationally agreed standards and monitored both locally and nationally. So what does this mean for specialist palliative care? By specialist palliative care, we mean care provided by those specialists who have received additional training and qualifications in palliative care and acquired considerable practical experience (NCHSPCS 2002b).

All health care delivery must have clear standards, which are evidence-based, and encompass the concepts of equity, access, effectiveness and efficiency. Specialist palliative care services are no different. Translating policy into practice means providing evidence of high-quality care, looking across the whole patient journey, regardless of setting. In specialist palliative care, as in health care generally, there are failures of coordination and communication between professionals and services that must be addressed.

In delivering a specialist palliative care service, all the departments must work seamlessly to create a quality service. We must look critically at the service we provide, at each part which makes up the whole and how the parts interlink to provide a seamless service. The quality of service provision delivered to patients depends on how the organization operates as a whole (Klein 1998).

Assessing quality in specialist palliative care creates challenges. Quality improvement is about change and change involves changing practices and behaviours, the burden of gathering data, additional reporting and external review, all of which bring added pressures. For change to succeed, it must be both managed and led (Garside 1998). However, if the culture of the organization values the contributions of individuals, is open, does not apportion blame (Department of Health 2000b) and has decentralized decision making, this can help facilitate change (Ferguson and Lim 2001; Rycroft-Malone *et al.* 2002). The critical role of top management and their leadership in quality management is emphasized by Thiagarajan and Zairi (1997), who believe 'Leadership in fostering an environment where quality is a way of life sets the foundation for the implementation of quality assurance in an organisation' (p. 270).

Introducing a quality and change culture to staff requires the ability to demonstrate how the quality approach links with their values and motivation (Ovretveit 1992). Ownership of quality initiatives and any changes that arise are vital, as change is successful only when the entire organization participates (Kanter *et al.*, cited in Garside 1998).

Definitions

Terms associated with quality can be confusing, not least when we look at definitions. Many alternative quality terms are used interchangeably. Shaw (1980) illustrates this terminological confusion of titles by identifying 96 possible alternative terms for the activity of measurement and improvement of the quality of care. The following are several commonly used definitions:

- *Policy*: a set of ideas or a plan of what to do in particular situations that has been agreed officially by a group of people, a business organization, a government or a political party (*Cambridge International Dictionary of English* 2002).

- *Clinical governance*: a framework through which NHS organizations are accountable for continuously improving the quality of their services and safe-guarding high standards of care by creating an environment in which excellence in clinical care will flourish (Department of Health 1998).

- *Clinical audit*: the systematic and critical analysis of the quality of clinical care, including the procedures used for diagnosis, treatment and care, the associated use of resources and the resulting outcome and quality of life for the patient (Department of Health 1989).

- *Patient satisfaction*: the ultimate validator of quality of care (Donabedian 1966). The degree to which the clients' experience of the service exceeds their expectations, at a particular time (Ovretveit 1992).

- *Standards*: a means of applying qualitative or quantitative measures to which values can be assigned (Williamson 1992).

- *Quality assurance*: initiatives designed to ensure minimum standards of (existing) care, and the mechanisms created to identify and deal with those whose performance does not meet those standards (Buetow and Roland 1999).

- *Quality improvement*: approaches that seek to improve care and prevent poor care on a continuous basis as part of everyday routine (Buetow and Roland 1999).

Clinical governance places equal attention on accountability for existing care and improving future care – that is, a combination of quality assurance and quality improvement. It encompasses national standards and guidelines and systems for monitoring quality and performance.

What does this mean for specialist palliative care services?

Quality, partnership and performance are key issues in the provision of hospice and specialist palliative care services; getting the care right is essential when time is limited and there is no second chance to improve the quality of the care. It is important to choose a suitable measure, one that reflects the goals of care, to reduce pain, discomfort and anxiety (NCHSPCS 1995; Hearn and Higginson 1997).

But how can this be measured? The National Council for Hospice and Specialist Palliative Care Services (NCHSPCS 1999) produced a briefing bulletin that looked at the definition and measurement of quality in palliative care. The NCHSPCS suggested that the quality framework shown in Figure 37.1 may be useful when examining the quality of specialist palliative care.

Policy objectives can be summarized as:

- All people with life-threatening illness and their families should have access to palliative care appropriate to their needs.

- Access should be when and for as long as they need it.

- The care provided should produce the intended benefits of that care.

- Care should be provided in a way and in a place that is acceptable to those receiving it.

- The cost of providing care should be the least, which is appropriate to the service being provided.

National Policy Objectives
Generate
National standards
Generate
High-level Performance Indicators
Generate
Data Requirements

Figure 37.1 Quality framework.

Current national standards applicable to specialist palliative care services

Currently, there are three main sets of national standards that apply to specialist palliative care services:

- the draft national specialist palliative care standards issued to cancer network in September 2001 (NCHSPCS 2001);

- the *Manual of Cancer Standards* (Department of Health 2001a); and
- the National Care Standards.[1]

It should be noted that not all of these standards apply to all settings. The draft national standards and performance indicators for specialist palliative care will be reviewed following the publication of the NICE guidance on supportive and palliative care and become part of the *Manual of Cancer Service Standards*. These national standards will apply to all specialist palliative care services regardless of setting. Standards for individual providers such as those developed by Trent Hospice Audit Group (1998), Health Quality Service (1999) and Quality by Peer Review (2001) need to demonstrate compatibility with the national standards.

An assessment of how far palliative care services are meeting these standards and providing care that satisfies patient and family need, requires the development of performance indicators. Performance indicators can be both proxy and direct. *Proxy* performance indicators may be the presence or absence of a multi-professional specialist palliative care team, since evidence suggests that such a team does improve the quality of care, or the use of evidence-based guidelines. *Direct* performance indicators measure how far pain control has been effective for individual patients, with results aggregated to provide an overall indicator.

In addition to the development of national standards, health resource groups and health benefit groups will be established. Health resource groups will establish standard tariffs for specific treatments and costs per case within specialist palliative care services and are being developed by the NHS Information Authority. This work links with the developing Cancer Data Sets, which will include palliative care. The NCHSPCS, supported by the Department of Health, currently collect data for the Minimum Data Set. The aim of this work is to ensure that a database is available that will inform national policy and assist networks in developing network-wide strategies and service delivery plans in conjunction with PCTs.

Manual of Cancer Service Standards

The *Manual of Cancer Services Standards* (Department of Health 2001a) was developed from the series 'Improving Outcomes in Cancer Care' on breast, colorectal and lung cancer. The manual sets out arrangements for cancer networks. Currently, the standards apply to cancer and palliative care services provided in secondary care. These standards provide the basis for the Cancer Peer Review visits and assessment.

The National Care Standards Commission

The National Care Standards Act (Department of Health 2000a) estab-lished the National Care Standards Commission (NCSC), which is a non-governmental, independent organization, and in April 2002 replaced the Registered Homes Act 1984 (under which hospices were previously inspected). This Act applies to all independent health care providers – that is, those not part of the NHS, which includes hospices and a total of 38,000 private health care establishments.

The NCSC was established to provide a means of regulating private and voluntary health care. Eighteen days after being established, a press release announced that all inspections of health care would fall under a new body, the Commission for Health Audit and Inspection. This will be a combination of the Commission for Health Improvement, the Audit Commission and the NCSC. This new body will require new legislation, but will ultimately be responsible for regulating the quality of *all* health services provided by both the National Health Service and the private sector.

Clinical governance

As mentioned earlier, in 1997 the British government introduced a statutory duty of quality on the NHS, that of clinical governance (Department of Health 1997). All NHS providers are bound by this duty of quality. Although there is no legal obligation for voluntary hospices to be bound by clinical governance, hospices care for NHS patients under service level agreements and are in receipt of NHS funding. Acknowledging their independence, the NCHSPCS defined clinical governance for voluntary hospices as:

> An internal framework through which voluntary sector providers of hospice and SPC [specialist palliative care] demonstrate accountability for and ensure continuous improvement in the quality of their services for patients and those who care for them and the safeguarding of high standards of care by creating an environment in which clinical care will flourish.
>
> (NCHSPCS 2000: 9)

This definition recognizes the independence of voluntary hospices, which are responsible for their own affairs and are accountable to the general public. The expectation for voluntary hospices is that the NHS will want to see evidence that arrangements are in place to ensure quality of care similar to that in the NHS.

Clinical governance gives us a framework which encompasses many elements of quality improvement. Assessing quality involves measurements in several domains (see Figure 37.2). However, many questions about quality

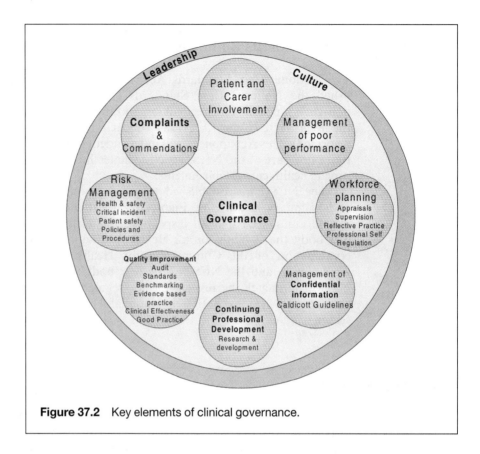

Figure 37.2   Key elements of clinical governance.

converge on one central theme: what does it mean to provide quality care, how can quality be measured and what information do we need to assess quality? Currently in specialist palliative care there is no single system available that incorporates all these elements, but examining quality in any of the dimensions requires collection of data and then analysis of that data.

Quality of what, perceived by whom?

Quality improvement and the evaluation of palliative care are important to improve the quality of that care, to increase client satisfaction, to assess the costs of palliative care and to allow comparisons between interventions (Normand 1996). But whose quality? Ovretveit (1992) proposes that quality should be viewed from three perspectives – client, professional and management – to ensure integrated, comprehensive and appropriate standards are developed. Much has been written about the different perceptions of quality and the fact that professionals view quality from a different perspective than patients. Professionals view technical expertise designed to make us better (i.e. outcomes of care) as being a marker for quality, whereas patients view the quality of clinical care and services as a whole (i.e. how long they had to wait to be seen) as being more valuable (Ferguson and Lim 2001). It is therefore important to remember this distinction when critically examining the quality of care and provision of a service and to encompass the perspectives of all stakeholders.

Common quality principles

Although it is acknowledged that the settings for delivering palliative care are different, and have characteristics unique to that setting, there are many common issues and, within quality terms, common principles: 'Regardless of the setting, for an organisation to be effective and therefore survive and prosper, management must have an understanding of the external environment in which the organisation operates and must anticipate and respond to change' (Ginter *et al.* 1992: 254).

One of the biggest challenges currently facing health care has been the speed of change and the emphasis on quality. Government has sought through its White Papers to seek improvements in the quality of care. Specifically, clinical governance requires that a comprehensive programme of quality improvement is in place in health care organizations. This is linked to the fact that societal changes have resulted in people being more consumer-orientated, less deferential and expecting greater accountability from professionals (Campbell *et al.* 2002). Technological advances, the drive to improve safety and quality of care and the need for accountability are challenging traditional and management system approaches and attitudes to care (Moss and Garside 2001).

The organizational context for quality improvement initiatives is a crucial determinant of their effectiveness (Walshe and Freeman 2002). Successful implementation requires cultural change and three fundamental steps:

- creating the necessary public awareness and consensus;
- ensuring health care professionals have the necessary knowledge, skills and tools for implementation; and
- ensuring organizational and other systems are created to sustain or extend change.

This final step puts the processes in place to ensure that high-quality care becomes part of the basic fabric of our society (Teno *et al.* 2001). Measurement provides the foundation for these and audit the evidence of opportunity for improvement.

What this means in practice is that standard-setting, audit, evaluation and all the components of a quality programme cannot be viewed in isolation from the organization and how it functions. Leadership is key, with strategic thinking, vision, knowledge-building, collaboration, persistence and management commitment important components to successful implementation.

The reality is no longer shall we use a system of quality improvement (to not do so would be an abrogation of professional and organizational responsibility; Walshe and Freeman 2002), but which one to use and how to use it. The following are examples: the Trent Hospice Audit Group (1998), Quality by Peer Review (Barker 2001), Support Team Assessment Schedule (Higginson and McCarthy 1989) and the Palliative Care Outcome Scale (Hearn and Higginson 1999).

What does this mean for practice?

Working within this current climate of change is challenging for any health care provider, not least providers of specialist palliative care. How can an individual provider of specialist palliative care demonstrate that it is providing high-quality care and a high-quality service?

Holistic multi-professional care underpins the philosophy of specialist palliative care; therefore, any attempts to measure that care should reflect the holistic nature of that care and the multi-professional delivery. Quality must encompass the whole organization, with the creation of a positive culture to enable quality to become part of everyone's business all of the time. Clinical governance provides a framework to enable the disparate activities of quality improvement to be brought together coherently.

In 2001, the NCHSPCS undertook a survey of all independent hospices in England and Wales to establish how many hospices had implemented clinical governance, the results of which are shown in Figure 37.3.

With the advent of clinical governance and the National Care Standards Commission, a number of providers have adopted external systems of review such as Quality by Peer Review and Health Quality Service. These systems propose to enable organizations to demonstrate compliance with national standards. Providers have adopted a number of more general approaches, such as Investors in People – whose focus is staff development – and adaptations of industrial quality systems, such as ISO 9000.[2] The European Foundation for Quality Management[3] has a non-prescriptive model, which assesses an organization's progress towards excellence. Some have adopted standards, such as the Trent Hospice Audit Group (1998), or specific mini audits, such as the Palliative Care Outcome Scale (Hearn and Higginson 1999) and the Support Team Assessment Schedule (Higginson and McCarthy 1989). For primary care, the Gold Standards Framework (Thomas 2001) and the Liverpool Integrated Care Pathway (Ellershaw *et al.* 2001) provide frameworks.

Providers of specialist palliative care services need to decide whether to adopt existing schemes or develop a quality approach themselves. If the former, then a number of questions should be posed in the selection process (Walsh and Walshe 1998):

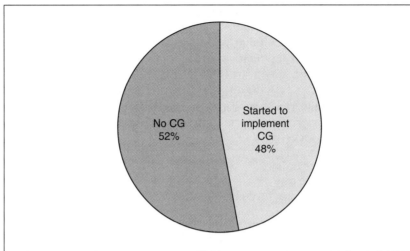

Figure 37.3 Clinical governance (CG) in voluntary hospices (after NCHSPCS 2002a).

1 What is the primary purpose of the scheme?

2 Is participation voluntary? How many organizations have participated?

3 At what level are the standards set, how were they developed, what do they cover and how are they measured?

4 Assessment method: Which data are needed? Who are the external assessors? How were they selected and trained?

5 Presentation of results: How is feedback delivered? Is it confidential to the organization?

6 Impact and follow-up: What is known of the effects on other organizations that have gone through the process and how will the process be followed up?

7 Costs: What are the fees charged? What are the opportunity costs in terms of time and preparation?

Using an existing external accreditation/review system can have benefits beyond those associated with just the assessment process, in terms of sharing good practice, collaborative working and benchmarking (Barker 2001). For those who choose to go it alone, some of the quality theories are discussed later.

Different settings for the provision of palliative care services

Palliative care is provided in a variety of settings by generalists and specialists: home, hospice, nursing home and hospital, with the latter remaining the most common setting in which people die. Each of these will face different challenges when looking at audit, evaluation and clinical governance. However, similar principles apply (Garside 1999). A large part of in-patient specialist palliative care services are provided within the voluntary sector, as can be seen from Table 37.1.

Table 37.1 UK hospice and specialist palliative care services

Services	n
Hospice units	208
Home care	334
Hospice at home	78
Day care	243
Hospital support teams	221
Hospital support nurses	100

Hospices and in-patient specialist palliative care services

The concept of hospice care grew out of the failure of the State to provide a cradle-to-grave service of the right quality (Clark 1993). As of 2002, there were 208 hospice units, of which 56 were NHS units and 152 were voluntary hospice units.[4]

Specialist teams

The evaluation of specialist teams will depend on whether they are based in a hospice, hospital or community as part of a primary care trust. Important issues for specialist palliative care teams in hospital and community relate to their role as an advisory team. How do you evaluate the advice given and how do you know whether that advice was actually followed in the first place? It is difficult separating the effect of a team from the effects of the input of specialists (Hearn and Higginson 1998). Donabedian (1988) also recognized this as a problem, noting that changes to a patient's health status (outcome) reflect all contributions to his or her care, including that of the patient; however, the direct effect of therapy interventions can be difficult to isolate. When looking at clinical incidents, the errors or omissions may be those of others outside the specialist team. How do you audit/ evaluate other people's practice? How do you raise the expectations of what basic quality palliative care is? 'For there to be a general improvement in the care of the dying, there must be consistent changes in the practice of a variety of clinicians who are not specialists in palliative medicine' (Butler *et al.* 1996: 33–4).

General palliative care

General palliative care is integral to good clinical practice and is provided by doctors, nurses and other health care professionals in hospitals, the community and care homes. In her Gold Standards Framework, Thomas (2001) proposes three 'acid tests' for evaluating care:

- Can we improve outcomes for hard measurable areas such as home death rate (or place of choice) and fewer crisis hospital admissions?
- What is the patient's and carer's experience of care?
- If a member of our family had cancer, what kind of care would we want for them?

Integrated care pathways

Integrated care pathways provide a method for implementing and monitoring best practice, and incorporating accepted guidelines and protocols into health care settings (Kitchener *et al.* 1996). Ellershaw *et al.* (2001) have developed the Liverpool Integrated Care Pathway for the Dying, which looks at the last 48 hours of a patient's life, enabling evaluation of the quality of care provided. This has been adopted as an evaluative and educational tool within a number of secondary and primary care settings.

Theorists and models of quality

As mentioned earlier, for those who wish 'to go it alone' there are a number of models that may be of assistance. Throughout the years, different theorists and models have been proposed as being appropriate for audit and evaluation, some of which are described below.

Donabedian (1980) provided a framework for quality assurance and standards development that consist of three interrelated components: structure, process and outcome. Structure is used to describe the physical, organizational and other characteristics of the system that provides the care. Process refers to the actions and behaviours and activities required of staff in giving the care as well as the care itself. Donabedian's structure, process and outcome has been used as a basis for developing standards.

Maxwell (1992) saw health care quality as more multi-dimensional than Donabedian and introduced six dimensions of quality equity, access, fairness, relevance, effectiveness and efficiency. These six dimensions of quality equate closely to the national service frameworks.

The components of Donabedian's structure, process and outcome and Maxwell's six dimensions of quality can be combined and used as a Don/Max grid (see Table 37.2) to identify what aspects of performance in a particular service are not covered adequately.

The PDSA cycle

Another virtuous circle as a tool, the PDSA cycle (Deming 1986), seeks to achieve continuing sustainable quality improvement. There are three key

Table 37.2　Don/Max grid (after Hurst 2002)

| | Donabedian | | |
Maxwell	*Structure*	*Process*	*Outcome*
Effectiveness			
Acceptability			
Efficiency			
Access			
Relevance			

questions to answer in the 'Plan–Do–Study–Act' (PDSA) cycle, which can be addressed in any order:

- What are we trying to accomplish?
- How will we know that a change is an improvement?
- What changes can we make that will result in improvement?

Standard setting

Clinical governance and the quality assurance cycle require standards to be set, which provide a baseline against which performance can be measured. 'They express values which are derived from changing knowledge, increasing sensibility, shifts in power and new perceptions of interest' (Williamson 1992: 121). Establishing clear, appropriate and acceptable standards is a fundamental problem in quality assurance work (Ellis and Whittington 1993). Any standards written should meet the RUMBA criteria (Wilson, cited in Higginbottom and Hurst 2001): relevant, understandable, measurable, behaviourable and achievable. Standard setting is, however, only a part of the quality cycle. It is better to write fewer standards and complete the audit cycle than to concentrate on writing many standards, which have no associated audit programme with them.

Audit cycle

Audit can begin at any point in the cycle. Standards or goals are set, which are compared with reality by observing practice, and the results are fed back to improve practice and new standards are set. The audit cycle is then repeated. Completing and repeating the audit cycle creates a quality spiral (Department of Health 1997).

Patient satisfaction

Patient satisfaction is at the heart of quality assessment (Department of Health 1998) and has been cited as the ultimate validator of quality of care (Donabedian 1966). Many tools have been designed to measure patient

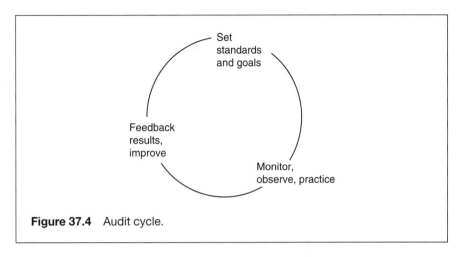

Figure 37.4   Audit cycle.

satisfaction, although there is little specifically in relation to palliative care services (Fakhoury 1998). Fakhoury addresses some of the methodological, theoretical and technological issues related to using satisfaction as a measure of the quality of palliative care.

> Multi-dimensional models of satisfaction with palliative care that would evaluate the care delivered taking into account the carers' and the patient's views and experiences are highly needed if we are to have an accurate assessment of carers' and patients' satisfaction with palliative care services.
>
> (Fakhoury 1998: 174)

Peer review

Multidisciplinary teamwork is the hallmark of palliative care audit, and peer review as part of the quality improvement programme must be multi-professional in its approach to reflect this philosophy. Multidisciplinary involvement in the process of peer review both for the reviewer and the reviewed means that individuals gain a much greater understanding of the organization as a whole and the value of teamwork. The National Council for Hospice and Specialist Palliative Care Services describes peer review as a valuable aspect of collaborative audit, having similar benefits to external assessment, but less threatening, ensuring assessors have local knowledge and the most relevant expertise (NCHSPCS 1997).

For peer review to succeed, there has to be a climate of mutual support and trust that encourages an innovative dynamic approach to problem solving (Morrison 1992). The most common reason why peer review fails is lack of support in the form of leadership and top management commitment.

Peer review can be external, as in systems such as Health Quality Service (1999) and Quality by Peer Review (2001) or internal within an organization.

Conclusions

Quality and its measurement is vitally important in the current climate of health care; however, the measurement of the quality of a service or the effectiveness of an intervention cannot be viewed in isolation. Quality and the culture of an organization are two sides of the same coin.

Patients' and professionals' views of quality differ and we must accommodate this in our measurement. We must also remember to close the loop, where areas for improvement have been identified, a plan of action must be agreed and implemented, then the service re-evaluated.

> We live in the roaring climate of change, a current so powerful today that it overturns institutions, shifts our values and shrivels our roots. Change is the process by which the future invades our lives, and it is important to look at it, not merely from the grand perspectives of history, but also from the vantage point of the living, breathing individuals who experience it.
>
> (Toffler, in Wright 1992: 3)

Notes

1   Cabinet Office (2000) *Care Standards Act*, Chapter c. 14 (http://www.hmso.gov.uk/acts/acts2000/20000014.htm).
2   ISO 9000 (2000) available at http://www.iso.org.uk/index.htm.
3   European Foundation for Quality Management (2002) available at http://www.excellenceteam.com/excel_model.htm.
4   Hospice Information (2002) *Directory 2002: Help the Hospices* (http://www.hospiceinformation.info).

References

Barker, E. (2001) Presentation to the *Conference on Interpreting the Challenges for Specialist Palliative Care Services*, October, Harrogate.

Buetow, S. and Roland, M.O. (1999) Clinical governance: bridging the gap between managerial and clinical approaches to quality of care. *Quality in Health Care*, 8: 184–90.

Butler, R.N., Burt, R., Foley, K.M. and Morrison, R.S. (1996) Palliative medicine: providing care when cure is not possible. A round-table discussion: Part I. *Geriatrics*, 51: 33–4.

Cambridge International Dictionary of English (2002) Cambridge: Cambridge University Press.

Campbell, S.M., Sheaff, R., Sibbald, B. *et al.* (2002) Implementing clinical governance in English primary care groups/trusts: reconciling quality improvement and quality assurance. *Quality and Safety in Health Care*, 11: 9–14.

Clark, D. (ed.) (1993) *The Future of Palliative Care: Issues of Policy and Practice.* Buckingham: Open University Press.

Deming, W.E. (1986) *Out of the Crisis.* Cambridge, MA: MIT Center for Advanced Engineering Study.

Department of Health (1989) *Working for Patients.* Working Paper 6, Medical Audit. London: HMSO.

Department of Health (1997) *The New NHS: Modern, Dependable.* London: HMSO.

Department of Health (1998) *A First Class Service: Quality in the New NHS.* London: HMSO.

Department of Health (2000a) *The Care Standards Act 2000.* London: HMSO.

Department of Health (2000b) *An Organisation with Memory.* Report of an Expert Group on Learning from Adverse Events in the NHS, chaired by the Chief Medical Officer. London: HMSO.

Department of Health (2000c) *The NHS Cancer Plan: A Plan for Investment, A Plan for Reform.* m01/25436. London: HMSO.

Department of Health (2000d) *The NHS Plan. A Plan for Investment: A Plan for Reform.* CM 4818-I. July 2000. London: HMSO.

Department of Health (2001a) *Manual of Cancer Services Standards.* London: HMSO.

Department of Health (2001b) *Shifting the Balance of Power Within the NHS: Securing Delivery.* London: HMSO.

Department of Health (2002a) *Shifting the Balance of Power within the NHS: The Next Steps.* London: The Stationery Office.

Department of Health (2002b). *Delivering the NHS Plan: Next Steps on Investment, Next Steps on Reform.* Cm 5503. London: The Stationery Office.

Donabedian, A. (1966) Evaluating the quality of medical care. *Milbank Memorial Fund*, Q44: 166–206.

Donabedian, A. (1980) *The Definition of Quality and Approaches to its Assessment.* Ann Arbor, MI: Health Administration Press.

Donabedian, A. (1988) The quality of care, how can it be assessed? *Journal of the American Medical Association*, 260(12): 1745.

Ellershaw, J., Smith, C., Overill, S., Walker, S.E. and Aldridge, J. (2001) Care of the dying: setting standards for symptom control in the last 48 hours of life. *Journal of Pain and Symptom Management*, 21(1): 12–17.

Ellis, R. and Whittington, D. (1993) *Quality Assurance in Health Care.* London: Edward Arnold.

Fakhoury, W.K.H. (1998) Satisfaction with palliative care: what should we be aware of? *International Journal of Nursing Studies*, 35: 171–6.

Ferguson, B. and Lim, J.N.W. (2001) Incentives and clinical governance, money following quality. *Journal of Management in Medicine*, 15(6): 463–87.

Garside, P. (1998) Organizational context for quality: lessons from the fields of organizational development and change management. *Quality in Health Care*, 7(suppl.): S8–S15.

Garside, P. (1999) The learning organization: a necessary setting for improving care? *Quality in Health Care*, 8: 211.

Ginter, P.M., Duncan, W.J. and Capper, S.A. (1992) Keeping strategic thinking in strategic planning: macro-environmental analysis in a state department of public health. *Public Health*, 106: 253–69.

Halligan, A. and Donaldson, L. (2001) Implementing clinical governance: turning vision into reality. *British Medical Journal*, 322: 1413–17.

Health Quality Service (1999) *The Health Quality Service Accreditation Programme*. London: HQS.

Hearn, J. and Higginson, I.J. (1997) Outcome measures in palliative care for advanced cancer patients: a review. *Journal of Public Health Medicine*, 19(2): 193–9.

Hearn, J. and Higginson, I.J. (1998) Do specialist palliative care teams improve outcomes for cancer patients? A systematic literature review. *Palliative Medicine*, 12: 317–32.

Hearn, J. and Higginson, I.J. (1999) Development and validation of a core outcome measure for palliative care: the palliative care outcome scale. *Quality in Healthcare*, 8: 219–27.

Higginbottom, M.J. and Hurst, K. (2001) Quality assuring a therapy service. *International Journal of Health Care Quality Assurance*, 14(4): 149–56.

Higginson, I.J. and McCarthy, M. (1989) Measuring symptoms in terminal cancer: are pain and dyspnoea controlled? *Journal of the Royal Society of Medicine*, 82: 264–7.

Hurst, K. (2002) *Managing Quality*. London: South Bank.

Kitchener, D., Davidson, C. and Bundred, P. (1996) Integrated care pathways: effective tools for continuous evaluation of clinical practice. *Journal of Evaluation in Clinical Practice*, 2: 65–9.

Klein, R. (1998) Can policy drive quality. *Quality in Health Care*, 7(suppl.): S51–S53.

Maxwell, R.J. (1992) Dimensions of quality revisited: from thought to action. *Quality in Health Care*, 1: 171–7.

Morrison, M.J. (1992) Promoting the motivation to change: the role of facilitative leadership in quality assurance. *Professional Nurse*, August, pp. 715–18.

Moss, F. and Garside, P. (2001) Leadership and learning: building the environment for better, safer healthcare (editorial). *Quality in Health Care*, (suppl. II): ii1–ii2.

National Council for Hospice and Specialist Palliative Care Services (1995) *Outcome Measures in Palliative Care*. Report of a Working Party on Clinical Guidelines in Palliative Care. London: NCHSPCS.

National Council for Hospice and Specialist Palliative Care Services (1997) *Making Palliative Care Better: Quality Improvement, Multiprofessional Audit and Standards*. London: NCHSPCS.

National Council for Hospice and Specialist Palliative Care Services (1999) *The Definition and Measurement of Quality in Palliative Care*. Briefing Paper No. 3, December. London: NCHSPCS.

National Council for Hospice and Specialist Palliative Care Services (2000) *Raising the Standard: Clinical Governance for Voluntary Hospices*. Occasional Paper No. 18, July. London: NCHSPCS.

National Council for Hospice and Specialist Palliative Care Services (2001) *Draft National Standards for Specialist Palliative Care for Carncer Services*. For information only. London: NCHSPCS.

National Council for Hospice and Specialist Palliative Care Services (2002a) *Turning Theory into Practice: Practical Clinical Governance for Voluntary Hospices*. Occasional Paper, June. London: NCHSPCS.

National Council for Hospice and Specialist Palliative Care Services (2002b) *Definitions of Supportive and Palliative Care*. Briefing Paper No. 11, September. London: NCHSPCS.

National Institute for Clinical Excellence (2002) *Service Configuration Guidance on Supportive and Palliative Care for Patients with Cancer*. First draft for stakeholders, July. London: NICE.

Normand, C. (1996) Economics and evaluation in palliative care. *Palliative Medicine*, 10: 3–4.

Ovretveit, J. (1992) *Health Service Quality: An Introduction to Quality Methods for Health Services*. Oxford: Blackwell.

Quality by Peer Review (2001) Presentation to the *Conference on Interpreting the Challenges for Specialist Palliative Care*, October, Harrogate.

Rycroft-Malone, J., Kitson, A., Harvey, G. *et al.* (2002) Ingredients for change: revisiting a conceptual framework. *Quality and Safety in Health Care*, 11: 174–80.

Shaw, C.D. (1980) Aspects of audit: the background. *British Medical Journal*, i: 1256–8.

Teno, J.M., Field, M.J. and Byock, I. (2001) The road taken to be traveled in improving end of life care. *Journal of Pain and Symptom Management*, 22(3): 714.

Thiagarajan, T. and Zairi, M. (1997) A review of total quality management in practice: understanding the fundamentals through examples of best practice application, Part 1. *The Total Quality Management Magazine*, 9(4): 270–478X.

Thomas, K. (2001) *Primary Care Handbook of Community Palliative Care: Practical Measures to Enable Best Supportive Care at Home for Dying Patients*. Calderdale and Kirklees Health Authority/Macmillan Cancer Relief. London.

Trent Hospice Audit Group (1998) *Palliative Care Core Standards: A Multidisciplinary Approach*. Sheffield: Trent Hospice Audit Group, University of Sheffield.

Walsh, N. and Walshe, K. (1998) *Accreditation in Primary Care*. Birmingham: Health Service Management Centre, University of Birmingham.

Walshe, K. and Freeman, T. (2002) Effectiveness of quality improvement: learning from evaluations. *Quality and Safety in Health Care*, 11: 85–7.

Williamson, C. (1992). *Whose Standards? Consumer and Professional Standards in Health Care*. Buckingham: Open University Press.

Wright, S. (1992) *Health for Nurses Series: Change Strategies*. Geneva: World Health Organization.

38

Leading and managing nurses in a changing environment

Matthew Hopkins

The leadership and management of nurses across the hospice and specialist palliative care world is undergoing a transformation. Complex drivers are underpinning this change, including:

- The changing needs and expectations of patients, carers and other service users, including demands for quicker access to services/in-patient beds and better information about treatment options.

- Health care commissioners are demanding improvements in access to services, quality of care and value for money.

- Voluntary sector organizations are facing increasing difficulties in securing adequate levels of charitable income to meet the cost pressures of increased patient throughput and dependency.

- Changes to the organization of palliative care delivery due to the introduction of clinical governance and the move towards a more flexible workforce.

These drivers are impacting against a backdrop of an inadequate supply of motivated and well-trained nurses, which are so fundamental to the care and management of dying patients and their families. Thus, the demands on nurse managers and leaders to seek new ways of working to optimize their current resources become greater and more challenging.

In this chapter, I aim to provide palliative care nurses with a framework for leading and managing nursing teams, within the constraints of a changing environment, to deliver the highest quality of nursing care possible to their patients. Some of the key environmental changes that have impacted on palliative care nursing are briefly discussed and a new model of nursing management is introduced. This new model, which comprises five components, aims to address the complexities of managing nurses within the palliative care workplace. It should be stressed that these components are as important to senior nurses as they are to clinical nurse specialists or to nurses just embarking on a leadership role for the first time.

Many of the points made in this chapter, while originating from mainstream nursing settings and health care organizations, I consider to be transferable to the palliative care setting. The key message here is that to achieve the right outcomes – in other words, doing the right things right – nurse leaders and managers must take account of the changing context in which they conduct their roles and deliver their services. They must, above all else, be consistent in their behaviour and actions with their teams and professional colleagues to be truly effective in their role.

The changing landscape

Over the past decade, there have been significant changes to the environment in which nurses practise. In the UK, these changes were driven by the implementation of a range of government-led initiatives, including:

- a shift towards a more customer-focused service with core standards of care that patients and their carers could expect to receive (Department of Health 1991);

- changes to professional regulation, brought about by the introduction of self-regulation, with the aim of developing and improving nursing professionalism (UKCC 1994).

Specialist palliative care services responded positively to these initiatives and developed their services to meet the needs of patients and improve the professional development of their nursing staff. However, these radical changes are essentially behind us and there are now perhaps more significant landscape changes taking place. The following issues, which I consider to be having a significant impact on specialist palliative care services in the UK and elsewhere, will be briefly discussed:

- Clinical governance – a driving force for change?
- Structural change and the drive for efficiency.
- The flexible workforce – shortages, pay, job evaluation.

Clinical governance, structural change and the flexible workforce

Clinical governance – a driving force for change?

As stated in Chapter 37, clinical governance was established as a central theme in the UK Government White Paper *A First Class Service: Quality in the New NHS* (Department of Health 1998). One of the aims outlined in this policy document was to strengthen clinical accountability. This was seen as the key to strategic control of the National Health Service (NHS), since it established a framework for providing evidence-based and rigorously audited practices, as well as professional accountability for those practices.[1] It was also intended as a systematic approach to quality assurance and improvement at local service level. The definition of clinical governance given in the original document was: 'a framework through which NHS organisations are accountable for continuously improving the quality of their services and safeguarding high standards of care, by creating an environment in which excellence in clinical care will flourish' (Department of Health 1998). In all areas of health care delivery, clinical governance has become a driving force of modernization. It has forced a sea change in the thinking of nursing leaders and has challenged traditional nursing strategy. One of the overarching principles of this new approach is to make health care work 'at the level of people' rather than solely on a theoretical level.

Palliative care services have been proud of their reputation for high-quality care and many services had already made significant progress with quality improvement strategies (Naysmith 2000). However, it has been noted that 'Clinical Governance offers a more systematic and reliable way of achieving continuous quality improvement than the methods employed by most hospices hitherto' (NCHSPCS 2000).

One example of this more structured approach is the requirement to involve patients and the public in service design, and to establish forums for patient representatives to feed back their experiences as users of the service. While some palliative care services have conducted satisfaction surveys (e.g. Addington-Hall *et al.* 1991; Clumpus and Hill 1999), few have in the past established systems for involvement of patients in service development. One reason given for this is that the bias inherent in these types of surveys, due to the sensitivities around interviewing dying patients and bereaved relatives of patients, adversely influences the survey results (Seymour and Ingleton 1999: 65). However, within a clinical governance framework, this rationale is no longer acceptable and palliative care services are now expected to involve patients and other service users more openly and proactively.

Another example is the move to integrate clinical effectiveness programmes into standard clinical practice. Specialist palliative care professionals have traditionally been at the forefront of the experimental use of pharmaceuticals and complementary therapies to manage distressing symptoms of advanced disease (Hadfield 2001). However, the new emphasis on evidence-based medicine challenges the historical practices of these palliative care professionals and forces neighbouring organizations to work together, sometimes for the first time, in designing collaborative research studies and in sharing resources for education and training (Naysmith 2000). The development of multi-centre evidence-based care pathways and clinical guidelines (e.g. in cancer pain management: Finlay *et al.* 2000) is another example of the positive way that clinical governance is impacting on palliative care practices.

These examples help to demonstrate the significant cultural shift required within palliative care services to improve the quality of services to patients. The challenges to traditional palliative care nursing practices that have no robust evidence base is leading to a review of the way that nurses organize themselves and care for their patients. Table 38.1 outlines some of the complex demands placed on nursing teams by the clinical governance agenda.

One of the key future challenges for palliative care nurse leaders is how to embrace the concepts of clinical governance and successfully integrate them into standard practice. As the list of activities in Table 38.1 demonstrates, the agenda is long and complex. Therefore, to meet this challenging agenda, the skills and abilities of nurses need to be optimized and continually updated, and the traditional practices reviewed, validated and, where necessary, new ways of working established.

Structural change and the drive for efficiency

The drive for improving efficiency in health care delivery across the Western world has stimulated a massive amount of restructuring in health care organizations, particularly in the UK. This restructuring has been instigated by the incumbent government, through the publication of a number of policy documents, as outlined in Table 38.2. The key structural changes that transpired from these documents, and their impact on specialist palliative care services in the UK, are outlined in Table 38.3. Within the hospice and palliative care sector in the UK, these structural changes have impacted on working relationships and partnerships within local communities and clinical networks. For example, as outlined in Table 38.3, neighbouring hospices are now required to work together across a geographical region or network to ensure that there is parity of service provision. However, faced with escalating costs, many UK hospices have struggled to attract adequate charity revenues to meet increasing expenditure[2] (NCHSPCS 1997). Therefore, the combination of structural change, greater demands for efficiency and lower revenues has led to some organizations undergoing major restructuring to create a more streamlined, integrated structure that emphasizes the seamless connection between institutional and community-based palliative care services.

This drive for greater efficiency has forced specialist palliative care services to demonstrate that they deliver evidence-based practice, including the use of evaluative research and outcome measures, in order to justify increasing costs. The new landscape is also leading to shifts in organizational cultures within the hospice sector. Traditional leadership styles are being replaced by business and commercial sector ideologies, for example organizations are now led by 'chief executives' rather than 'medical directors'. Meanwhile, frontline staff often struggle to maintain the traditional atmosphere and ethos of the organization. An example of this struggle is the conflict created when bed occupancy levels are used as a measure of organizational efficiency. For example, there may be instances where there is

Table 38.1   Demands on nursing teams related to the clinical governance agenda

Components	Examples of activities
1. Patient/service user and public involvement	Strategy and implementation plans for patient/service user and public involvement work 'Customer' care practice to ensure patient's/service user's privacy, dignity and confidentiality about themselves and their treatment (e.g. codes of conduct, attitudes and behaviours of staff)
2. Clinical audit	Integration of clinical audit with quality improvement programmes; for example, to audit compliance with evidence-based practice protocols, guidelines and care pathways (e.g. pressure area care, last 48 hours) Dissemination of lessons learned and quality improvements as a result of clinical audits
3. Risk management	Integration of all risk management activities (clinical, non-clinical, health and safety) Prevention and control of specific risks; for example, drug incidents, use of medical devices, lone workers, infections, pressure sores, violence/self-harm
4. Education, training and continuing personal and professional development	Links between training and continuous professional development (CPD) programmes and wider quality improvement programmes, and with individuals' personal development plans Time, financial and other support for staff undergoing formal education and for individuals' CPD activities
5. Clinical effectiveness programmes	Implementation and application of effective clinical practice (e.g. evidence-based guidelines for wound care, syringe driver use) Training for staff (e.g. in critical appraisal skills, literature, database and internet search skills)
6. Staffing and staff management	Performance appraisal, clinical supervision and mentoring schemes Deployment of appropriate staffing and skills; for example, minimum 'safe' numbers and mix, schemes of delegation and supervision, protocols for staff working in extended roles (e.g. nurse prescribing)
7. Use of information to support clinical governance and health care delivery	Health care records systems, including electronic patient/service user records (including communication of patient information with staff from other organizations) Processes to ensure confidentiality of information about patient/service users; for example, application of Data Protection Act (UK legislation on the control of information)

Source: Adapted from the 'Seven Components of Clinical Governance' framework devised by the Commission for Health Improvement (2002).

Table 38.2 Main policy documents that led to structural changes in health care organizations

Title	Key themes
The NHS Plan: A Plan for Investment, a Plan for Reform (Department of Health 2000b)	Sets out a long-term plan for reform and performance improvement within the NHS to ensure that it provides fast and responsive services at a consistent level of quality across the country. Also sets out strategies for cutting waiting time for treatment and improving health and reducing inequality
The NHS Cancer Plan: A Plan for Investment, a Plan for Reform (Department of Health 2000c)	Provides a detailed account of the government's comprehensive national programme for investment in and reform of cancer services in England, which aims to reduce death rates and improve prospects of survival and quality of life for cancer sufferers by improving prevention, promoting early detection and effective screening practice, and guaranteeing high-quality treatment and care throughout the country
Modernizing the NHS: Shifting the Balance of Power in London (Department of Health 2001)	Set out changes to the way NHS organizations were structured to shift the balance of power to patients, the public and the frontline clinical teams involved in their care and lead to improvements in efficiency and effectiveness of health care delivery

pressure on ward-based nursing staff to have a fast turnover of patients, sometimes facilitating early discharges or moving deceased patients off the ward soon after they have died, in order to accommodate a new admission. For some staff, this managerial pressure compromises the traditional nursing practices that are so much part of the hospice ethos and philosophy.

Inevitably, the need to adapt to an environment of greater scrutiny and performance review has driven palliative care providers to have more robust and responsive strategies for effectively managing their people. For example, the introduction of organization-wide professional development programmes to give staff better access to training and development, and the development of systems of open communication to engage and involve staff in change management.

But what does this mean for nurses? In real terms, it means busier wards and heavier caseloads. It also produces a requirement to work more flexibly and effectively, both individually and in teams. However, on the upside, it should also mean more effective individual performance management and development processes, including the realization of individual potential and of innovative new ways of working.

Table 38.3   The impact of structural changes on specialist palliative care services

New structure	Impact on specialist palliative care services
Primary care trust (PCT) Organizations established to assess need, plan and secure all health services for their care community. They provide most community services and commission health care delivery, working in partnership with secondary care providers and voluntary sector organizations (e.g. hospices)	Commissioning arrangements now managed and prioritized by local primary care delivery unit. This could threaten funding for specialist palliative care in some localities and lead to duplication of service provision
Clinical network Organizations established to bring together service providers to coordinate the provision of secondary and specialist services	Palliative care providers are now forced to work together across geographical boundaries to achieve parity in service provision. This could threaten the structure and practices of some providers
Strategic health authority (StHA) Established to replace health authorities and be responsible for the strategic development of the local health service and the performance management of PCTs and NHS Trusts	The relationship with the StHA is vital to ensure that local service development does not serve to increase the fragmentation of palliative care provision within geographical regions

The flexible workforce – shortages, pay, job evaluation

Within most service sector organizations, the most important resource is the people and much of the future success of health care services depends on the performance of those people. To complement the clinical governance-inspired service quality improvements and the structural change required to improve efficiency of service delivery, the UK government recognized that, to close the gap between present and desired level of service quality, workforce issues would need to be addressed, including:

- enhancing the skills of existing staff through training or professional development;
- developing a *new* group of staff with a set of skills and competencies to fit the new circumstances (Department of Health 1999).

The invisible workforce

The predictions that the nursing shortage of the early twenty-first century will be more severe and have a longer duration than has been previously experienced means that traditional strategies for recruiting and retaining staff will have limited success. The ageing nursing workforce, low unemployment and the global nature of this shortage compound the usual factors (earnings, multi-care delivery sites, the need for experienced nurses with specialized skills) that contribute to nursing shortages (Nevidjon and Erickson 2001).

Like other health care providers, hospices and specialist palliative care providers must be innovative in their recruitment of nursing staff at all levels and settings within the organization. They must differentiate themselves from other employers, be committed to adopting and implementing flexible working and family-friendly policies, be competitive on pay and conditions and aim to establish a reputation as a 'good' employer.

Flexible working

The key to ensuring effective service delivery under competitive workforce market conditions is to re-orientate and integrate workforce planning capacity across professional groups and disciplines to identify the skills and roles needed to meet evolving service needs. Flexible working schemes that match day-to-day nurse staffing with fluctuating workload demands are vital.[3] These working patterns must be efficient and also support nurses in maintaining a balance between their work and personal life (Buchan 2002).

One of the drivers for this change in approach in the UK was the White Paper *Agenda for Change* (Department of Health 2000a) implemented across the NHS to support the modernization agenda, helping to re-design jobs around the patient. As a response, some UK hospices are also adopting wide-ranging reforms to their pay and conditions, implementing flexible working schemes to enhance the efficiency of their staffing resource management, enabling the right people to be in the right place at the right time.

As part of the implementation of *Agenda for Change*, job descriptions for clinical and non-clinical roles (excluding doctors and senior managers) were evaluated against five categories – responsibility, freedom to act, knowledge, training and experience, skills and effort and environment – and each was given a weighting according to their relative importance and on an equal value basis. There is little doubt that job evaluation will have an important impact on nursing management in the voluntary hospice sector. The contrast between levels of responsibility and skills required in acute NHS units and voluntary sector hospices may be problematic. This process may also create barriers to the transfer of staff from the NHS, the major source of recruitment, to voluntary sector organizations that have not kept pace with these changes or are not paying comparable rates of pay. Therefore, nurse leaders and managers in the hospice sector must monitor this process closely and develop action plans for securing the necessary trained nursing staff to deliver care to patients across the various palliative care settings.

Summary

In summary, these are just three of the complex changes happening to the landscape of specialist palliative care delivery in both the mainstream health care and the voluntary sectors. Nurse managers and leaders must take stock of the impact of these changes on their staff, their organization and their profession. They need to adopt a new and innovative approach to their roles, planning for the impact of these changes and developing contingency plans and strategies for retaining, developing and growing their nursing teams. They must view the service they deliver from a different angle, first from the viewpoint of patients and their families and, second, using an objective measure of performance – in other words, looking from the outside in. They should ask themselves: is my nursing team delivering the best care possible by the right people and can I demonstrate evidence that the clinical team is constantly improving and learning?

The model described below will assist nurse leaders and managers in answering these questions and in building an effective and efficient nursing workforce to meet the future challenges.

A new model of nursing management

Introduction

This new model has been developed for palliative care nurse leaders and managers to apply when addressing the complexities of their work environment and the diversity of their teams. It provides a framework to help them achieve the highest quality of care, in collaboration and partnership with their staff, and improve retention rates.

The model is derived from a review of nursing and human resource management literature, and from a primary research study undertaken by myself in a UK voluntary sector specialist palliative care unit (Hopkins 2000). The study methodology included the collection of qualitative data through tape-recorded semi-structured interviews with a sample of five managers and 15 members of staff. As a comparator, two nurse managers from other organizations were also interviewed. A combined approach to the analysis of the data was adopted using both qualitative and quantitative methods. The qualitative data were coded and categorized from the transcripts using basic grounded theory and the themes that were developed, linked to the literature, provide the framework for the model.[4]

The themes were aggregated and summarized into five components of nursing leadership and management, producing the acronym SPEAR:

- Supervising and coaching
- Performance management

- **E**ducation, training and continuous professional development (CPD)
- **A**ctions and behaviours
- **R**eflective practice

As depicted in Figure 38.1, these components radiate out from the centre of the model, which contains the key aim of nursing: the delivery of *high-quality patient-focused care.*

The application of these five components will be discussed in detail, with supporting evidence from the literature. In addition to the five components,

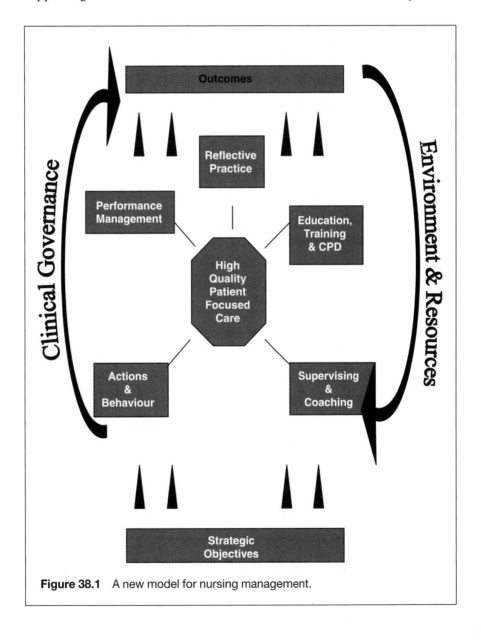

Figure 38.1   A new model for nursing management.

there is a key principle that underpins the model. As depicted in Figure 38.1, it is the *strategic objectives* of the organization, such as the continuous improvement in the quality of patient care, that act as the main drivers (hence the arrows) for all service delivery and for prioritizing service *outcomes*. In other words, whatever activity the nurse, doctor or other member of the multidisciplinary team is involved in, it should clearly contribute to the successful delivery of the strategic objectives and service outcomes of the organization. An example of a service outcome is the coordination of a safe and timely discharge package for a patient wishing to die at home.

However, it is important to acknowledge that these service outcomes and strategic objectives cannot be achieved without a suitable organizational culture,[5] adequate *resources* and a suitable *environment*. For example, the organizational approach to hierarchy, learning and development all reflect the organization's culture (Handy 1993), while, as noted earlier, the available resources and environment influence the development of the organization's strategic objectives (hence the direction of the arrow in the diagram).

Therefore, resources and environment are depicted in Figure 38.1 as parameters within which the nurse manager carries out their activities. The other parameter, as discussed in some detail earlier in the chapter, is *clinical governance*. As described, clinical governance provides a framework for the delivery of patient outcomes (hence the direction of the arrow in the diagram) by driving the modernization and continuous quality improvement of nursing care. Therefore, nurse managers need to take cognizance of their nursing team's practices in relation to examples of clinical governance activities outlined in Table 38.1.

In summary, the model focuses on the five components (SPEAR) of nursing management as the key activities in improving the quality of nursing care delivered by their nursing teams, within the context of strategic objectives and within the parameters of resources, environment and clinical governance. The first component to be discussed is *supervising and coaching*.

Supervising and coaching

> an intensive interpersonally focused, one-to-one relationship in which one person is designated to facilitate the development of competence in the other person.
>
> (Loganbill *et al.* 1982, cited in Timpson 1998)

Fulfilling the role of supervisor and coach is perhaps the most important component of leading, managing and developing nurses. To realize the potential of their teams, palliative care nurse managers should adopt these roles, using effective communication skills and developing trusting relationships, to identify the learning opportunities within the workplace and match them with the needs of individual nurses and teams. Table 38.4 lists the process and elements of coaching and supervising.

The role of the supervisor in the caring professions has a long history,

Table 38.4 Processes and elements of coaching and supervising

Coaching (Allison 1991)	*Supervising (Ash 1997: 21)*
• Dealing essentially with the development of skill through practice	• Recognizing and taking account of the effect on their supervisees of a stressful environment and workload
• Analysing the components of particular skills, techniques and the environment to assist learners	• Offering insights into working within a particular system, and information about the legislative and procedural framework
• Setting increasingly challenging exercises	• Being reliable and accessible
• Seeking to identify problems or weaknesses to be remedied	• Providing support in relation to senior management and a communication link
• Spotting potential, building on strengths and taking advantage of talent and opportunity	• Being alert to emergencies

and has been established in counselling, psychotherapy and social work practices for many years. In these settings, managers and professionals perform the role on a one-to-one basis with junior colleagues or in groups. Within the nursing profession, clinical supervision will be a term familiar to many nurses across the globe.

Clinical supervision – benefit or burden?

In the UK, clinical supervision has been endorsed by the government (Department of Health 1999) and has been discussed by many writers in the nursing literature (Faugier and Butterworth 1993; Kohner 1994; Johns 1995). However, there remains uncertainty about the tangible and measurable benefits of clinical supervision in achieving the strategic objectives of the organization or in achieving positive outcomes for patients. There is also considerable debate and disagreement within the health care literature about who should fulfil the role of a supervisor, and there is no single definition (Todd and Freshwater 1999). There are any number of models, some structured and based around competency, others closely linked to reflective practice and personal growth and development (Proctor 1986; Hawkins and Shohet 2000).

There is an emerging consensus that many clinical supervision models and processes neglect organizational objectives. There are few studies that provide empirical evidence of the benefits of clinical supervision to patient care and demonstrate a cost-efficient return on the considerable investment by organizations in establishing clinical supervision frameworks (Gray 2001).

Can managers supervise?

In some human resource management texts, the role of a supervisor is compared to that of a line manager, coach or mentor. While it is acknowledged that many managers do not supervise their staff well, despite training in feedback and coaching skills, there should be an emphasis on the purpose of supervision being to develop staff in a way that helps the achievement of the organization's goals (Mayo 1998; Lucas 2000).

However, there is fervent debate in the nursing literature about whether supervision is a role that managers can and should fulfil. Bond and Holland (1998) endorse the view that any manager performing clinical supervision is inappropriate, although they provide no conclusive evidence that such relationships are always detrimental. Timpson (1998) reflected that within nursing the notion of supervision is confused with control. Timpson (1998) argues this results from a patriarchal medical and management system.

Faugier (1992) notes that this sensitivity to seniority reduces the scope for recognition of personal limitations and the ability to listen to others. Reliability and consistency, in word and action, are important in helping the supervisee to feel safe and an atmosphere should be promoted in which deficits in knowledge, attitudes or skills may be explored without being interpreted as a negative comment on the employee personally.

While some authors suggest that clinical supervision prioritizes the needs of the individual over other outcomes such as organizational goals (Todd and Freshwater 1999), there is agreement that both managers and supervisors have a responsibility for service quality, maintenance of standards, retention of staff, identifying learning and development needs, and providing opportunities to meet these needs (Cowling *et al.* 1988). Therefore, the nurse manager has a considerable part to play in the supervision, training and development of their nurses.

Effective supervising and coaching

Supervising and coaching are activities that nurse managers should be involved in, not just for performance and quality monitoring purposes, but also to ensure that the team members are developing and continuously improving. It is accepted that managers supervising staff may regularly face conflicts between professional and managerial priorities, but this does not preclude the need for effective communication with staff to prevent or defuse such conflicts. The elements and processes of coaching and supervising overlap and it is vital that nurse managers acquire the necessary skills of both: effective communication skills, a consultative, supportive style and a challenging, motivating approach.

Performance management

> a continuous and holistic process, set firmly in the context of the business strategy and enhancing the performance of all the people in the organisation.
>
> (Industrial Society 1998: 3)

Performance management, for all health care professionals, is about optimizing the potential of individuals and teams to achieve the strategic objectives and service outcomes for patients and their families. Effective systems used by nurse managers include strategies for performance improvement and processes for development that are shared between managers and individuals and provide a valuable self-improving system (Pocock 1991; Armstrong 1994). For example, systems should include the following elements (Harrison 1997: 224):

- appraising and improving performance;
- ensuring continuous learning and development;
- setting objectives and establishing desired performance levels;
- giving recognition and rewards.

Performance management is well established in the health care setting, and can serve values such as professional autonomy and development (Edis 1995). However, he also argues that performance management approaches can lead to an emphasis on short-term gains in productivity where long-term people development is not considered a priority, and where little account is taken of the considerable diversity among the staff group within health care organizations.

In addition, in relation to personal development, Harrison (1997) notes that the balance between performance management and long-term development is rarely satisfactory and formal performance management systems frequently fail.

Development-based performance management, with its emphasis on self-assessment and reliance on the intrinsic elements of motivation and reward, is consistent with managing nurses working in specialist palliative care – although the motivations of nurses in these settings may differ from other groups. For nurses, the motivators are often 'needs-based', where job satisfaction and being able to fulfil the role effectively are more important than motivators such as money (Dartington 1994).

In this setting, the relationship with the line manager is very important in ensuring that performance management activities are beneficial to the individual, team and organization. For example, to achieve agreed outcomes, appraisal sessions should be genuinely developmental and motivating experiences and lead to three outcomes:

- feedback on performance;
- work planning; and
- diagnosis of training and development needs and action related to them.

In the current world of escalating demands for greater organizational efficiency and performance monitoring, specialist palliative care services can ill afford not to manage the performance of their staff more effectively than in the past. Good performance management strategies can motivate the high and low achievers within nursing teams, help with job satisfaction and retention, and help to provide clear direction for nurses' personal and professional development.

Education, learning and continuous professional development

> Learning is a relatively permanent change in behaviour that occurs as a result of practice or experience.
>
> (Bass and Vaughan 1967, cited in Harrison 1997)

The nurse manager can play a key role in promoting the three main concepts of continuous professional development: self-development, understanding the process of learning and the integration of learning at work. Nurse managers are central to identifying and evaluating the learning opportunities within the workplace and matching them with the needs of individuals, teams and the wider organization.

In my own experience, learning was often initiated by managers who identified skills deficits in their teams, perhaps after complaints or adverse incidents, and arranged external training courses as remedial action. Alternatively, the highly motivated members of the team would apply for a host of courses to fill gaps in their CVs or to make them more employable, sometimes with no relevance or tangible benefit to their patients, colleagues or to the organization. These approaches can produce difficulties within teams where nurses are not encouraged to develop a questioning approach to their work or to view the broader picture.

However, there is now a shift away from viewing educational institutions as the principal places where valid learning takes place towards recognition of the importance of the workplace as a site of learning (Dalziel 1995; Vaill 1996; Solomon 1999). Nurse managers should work to integrate learning and development activities into daily clinical practice and their staff should be encouraged to adopt an 'opportunistic' approach to skills development (Mumford 1991; Handy 1993; Barnett 1999). For example, the admission of a patient with a rare cancer diagnosis provides an opportunity for learning, as does the use of a new anti-cancer drug regime. The scope of palliative care, across many disease groups, produces continuous opportunities for learning and developing new nursing skills.

Managers need to foster the kind of individual and collective learning that not only produces changed behaviour in their staff, but also adds to the store of knowledge that the team or organization possesses. In addition to formal appraisal schemes, managers can enable their teams to identify areas for skills development and to initiate strategies to meet those gaps. A positive learning environment and access to 'someone who knows' are crucial to the successful of development of nurses (Galloway and Winfield 2000).

In summary, learning activities and opportunities should be formally structured but also permeate daily operations in the workplace so that a process of continuous development and improvement can take place. This demands time, good interpersonal skills, openness and shared leadership on the part of nurse managers.

Actions and behaviours

> If there is a burning issue and you don't feel that you can take it to your manager, then you have a huge problem on your hands.
>
> (nurse manager, quoted in Hopkins 2000)

As already discussed, the management and supervision of nurses is about maintaining quality of care through education and development, using coaching actions and supportive behaviours. In terms of the supervisory role of managers, the key attributes of this relationship, and the subsequent successful development of staff through supervision, actually relate to the ability of the supervisor, through effective use of interpersonal and communication skills, to engender an honest and open managerial style that earns respect and trust (Sloan 1999).

The results of my research study (Hopkins 2000) supported this view and found that critical success factors existed, in the form of actions and behaviours, in the relationship between managers and their teams. These can be summarized as: openness, trust, honesty, respect, credibility and consistency and reliability. These results also correlated with the work of Kohner (1994), who identified a range of actions and behaviours that were critical to the success of the manager–employee relationship (see Table 38.5).

Table 38.5 Comparison of my research with that of Kohner (1994)

Hopkins (2000)	Kohner (1994)
Openness	Compassion
Trust	Kindness
Honesty	Honesty
Respect	Wisdom
Credibility	Knowledge
Consistency and reliability	Availability

The study highlighted that palliative care nursing staff have concerns about the safety of exposing their 'weaknesses' in front of their manager. However, this perception may speak louder about the organizational culture than of the skills and integrity of the manager. Under workplace conditions where staff are empowered to take responsibility for their development, or to address issues of conflict with their managers, these concerns may be less profound. However, there is an equal responsibility on the part of nurses to overcome their fear of exposure and on managers to effect behavioural changes that lead to changes in organizational culture.

The study also identified that the experience and perception of the level of consistency of managerial approach appeared to be a prominent theme in promoting or hindering development. Therefore, it can be concluded that the key issue for nurse managers is to be consistent in their action and behaviour with their nursing teams.

This type of managerial style does not preclude the use of autocratic behaviour, as in some situations, such as with patient handling where there is risk of injury from not following agreed guidelines, a clear directive from a manager is warranted. Consistency is the key. However, it is not proposed that the manager should be everything to everyone and be 'best friends' with all staff. Instead, the recommendation is that managers develop relationships with their staff that are founded on achieving the organizational strategic objectives and good outcomes for the patients and their families. Table 38.6 outlines some actions related to each of the success factors that will assist managers in achieving such effective relationships.

These actions and behaviours will underpin the way that nurse managers perform and facilitate the other components of the model identified in this chapter. Of the factors, consistency in word and deed is perhaps the most important attribute that managers should strive for to be truly effective in their role.

Reflective practice

> On an individual level, reflection within the workplace is an essential component of life-long learning and continuous professional development.
>
> (Pringle 1999: 104)

Reflection is something that most nurses do subconsciously – it occurs at the end of most nursing interventions, during communication about patient progress and during handover between shifts or caseloads. While it is recognized that reflection is inherent in daily practice, the opportunities for facilitated reflection are rarely taken. There is some emerging evidence that it is extremely effective in improving performance and job satisfaction. For example, results from evaluative research conducted with home carers in Sweden showed that, as a result of facilitated problem-solving and reflection sessions, nurses' knowledge, understanding and practice improved (Olsson *et al.* 1998).

Table 38.6   Actions and behaviours that will assist in achieving effective relationships

Success factors	Examples of actions and behaviours
Openness	Being available, visible and willing to listen to staff and respond quickly to individual and team needs Being alert to individuals' changing development and personal needs
Trust	Maintaining confidentiality of personal information while being clear about the boundaries of information sharing within the organization (e.g. when information must be shared with others for safety and risk management purposes)
Honesty	Being able to say: 'I don't know – but let's find out together' Giving clear and constructive feedback on good and not-so-good performance
Respect	Leading by example and with integrity (e.g. behaving in a professional manner at all times) Treating staff as autonomous individuals within a team approach to delivering the service outcomes Always being clear and focused on the objectives and goal
Credibility	Being a knowledgeable practitioner (i.e. understanding the roles and limitations of the staff you manage) Delivering on agreed actions within agreed time-scales
Consistency and reliability	Communicating in a clear and consistent manner Treating individuals in a fair manner Consistently delivering on agreed actions

The benefits of reflection have been well documented in the nursing literature, particularly when linked to clinical supervision (Docherty 2000). However, reflective practice is a process in its own right. An example of this type of exercise is when multidisciplinary teams meet to debrief after a challenging or disturbing care episode. This is primarily used as a peer support session, but the learning from the discussion and sharing of views across hierarchical and professional boundaries should not be discounted.

Structured critical reflection, involving reviewing an important episode of care or patient case using a structured framework, allows practitioners to reflect on their personal work experiences and, ideally, those of the teams in which they practise, in order to learn and become more effective. Development opportunities exist in exposing, understanding and learning from and through the contradictions between desirable practice and actual practice (Johns 1994, 2001).

There are a number of models that can be useful by posing open questions about a critical incident or a challenging care pathway, to facilitate recognition of learning needs and the potential for improved performance next time round. This process can also help nurses to analyse their attitudes and behaviours and enable the development of self-determination, a process that can help individuals to grow both personally and professionally (Palmer *et al.* 1994; McDonald 2000; Gilbert 2001). For example, a structured reflection session after a critical incident, where a nurse was profoundly disturbed by the death of a patient, may elicit important information and enable the nurse to identify specific factors that made the experience so difficult. This, in turn, may enable the nurse to better understand the impact of caring for dying people on their personality, attitudes and behaviour.

Through facilitating reflective practice sessions, in the form of one-to-one or group meetings, managers can provide palliative care nurses, from health care assistants through to consultant nurses, with opportunities to learn from experience. This relationship between the nurses and line manager, where trust and respect can be created, is also fundamental to achieving the clinical governance agenda – safeguarding standards, developing professional expertise and delivering a quality service (Howell 1999).

Conclusions

In this chapter, I have tried to capture some of the contextual changes affecting the environment in which nurses lead and manage. The discussion has not intended to be exhaustive, but instead to raise key issues and encourage readers to reflect on their own environments and to analyse the impact of local change on themselves, their teams and organizations.

The discussion of the new model introduced in this chapter provides a detailed review of five components of managerial activity that will assist in addressing the complexities of the work environment and the diversity of the nursing and multidisciplinary teams. The ultimate aim is to achieve the highest quality of care possible, with and through the right people. It should be stressed again that these behaviours and activities are as important to senior nurses as they are to clinical nurse specialists or to nurses just embarking on a leadership role for the first time.

The model also clearly establishes the organization's strategic objectives, such as continuous improvement in patient care delivery, as the main driver for all service delivery, and there is no question that the outcomes and strategic objectives cannot be achieved without a suitable organizational culture and environment. It will be the changes in behaviour and application of different managerial activities that will help to change the culture of organizations. According to Timpson (1998), managers should develop a highly attuned sense of people perception, better understand the nature of their contribution, and their feelings, needs and expectations of their staff.

Notes

1 It is worth noting that these principles had previously been adopted within palliative care settings following work by Higginson and McCarthy (1989).

2 The charitable sector is more competitive with many new entrants competing for a diminishing amount of resources and the economic health of society is a key variable factor in charitable revenue growth. Furthermore, changes in charity legislation and the rate at which income tax if levied also impact on the achievement of revenue targets.

3 Flexible working schemes must also include a review of skill mix requirements and better utilization of other health professionals and support workers, together with more effective deployment of clinical nurse specialists and nurse practitioners in advanced roles.

4 The methodology provided a rich data set, which created a reliable and transferable set of results, although the scope of the study was limited by the relatively small sample.

5 Organizational culture will not be discussed here in great detail, but there is reference to the appropriate culture and environment required to support the successful application of the five components throughout the discussion.

References

Addington-Hall, J., Macdonald, L., Anderson, H. and Freeling, P. (1991) Dying from cancer, the view of bereaved family and friends. *Palliative Medicine*, 5: 207–14.

Allison, T. (1991) Counselling and coaching, in F. Neale (ed.) *The Handbook of Performance Management*. London: Institute of Personnel Management.

Armstrong, M. (1994) *Performance Management*. London: Kogan Page.

Ash, E. (1997) Taking account of feelings, in J. Pritchard (ed.) *Good Practice in Supervision*. London: Jessica Kingsley.

Barnett, R. (1999) Learning to work and working to learn, in D. Boud and J. Garrick (eds) *Understanding Learning at Work*. London: Routledge.

Bond, M. and Holland, S. (1998) *Skills of Clinical Supervision for Nurses*. Buckingham: Open University Press.

Buchan, J. (2002) Global nursing shortages (editorial). *British Medical Journal*, 324(7340): 751–2.

Clumpus, L. and Hill, A. (1999) Exploring the views of carers of cancer patients in an inner city locality. *International Journal of Palliative Nursing*, 5(3): 116.

Commission for Health Improvement (2002) *Organisational Review Handbook*. London: HMSO.

Cowling, A., Stanworth, M., Bennett, R., Curran, J. and Lyons, P. (1988) *Behavioural Sciences for Managers*, 2nd edn. London: Edward Arnold.

Dalziel, S. (1995) Learning and development, in M. Walters (ed.) *The Performance Management Handbook*. London: Institute of Personnel Management.

Dartington, A. (1994) Where angels fear to tread, in A. Obholzer and V. Zagier Roberts (eds) *The Unconscious at Work*. London: Routledge.

Department of Health (1989) *Working for Patients: Caring for the 1990s*. London: HMSO.

Department of Health (1991) *The Patient's Charter*. London: HMSO.

Department of Health (1997) *The New NHS: Modern, Dependable*. London: HMSO.

Department of Health (1998) *A First Class Service: Quality in the New NHS*. London: HMSO.

Department of Health (1999) *Making a Difference: Strengthening the Nursing, Midwifery and Health Visiting Contribution to Health and Healthcare*. London: HMSO.

Department of Health (2000a) *Agenda for Change: Modernising the NHS Pay System*. London: HMSO.

Department of Health (2000b) *The NHS Plan: A Plan for Investment, a Plan for Reform*. London: HMSO.

Department of Health (2000c) *The NHS Cancer Plan: A Plan for Investment, a Plan for Reform*. London: HMSO.

Department of Health (2001) *Modernising the NHS: Shifting the Balance of Power in London*. London: HMSO.

Docherty, B. (2000) Negotiating management and staff needs. *Nursing Times*, 96(14): 45–8.

Edis, M. (1995) *Performance Management and Appraisal in Health Services*. London: Kogan Page.

Faugier, J. (1992) The supervisory relationship, in T. Butterworth and J. Faugier (eds) *Clinical Supervision and Mentorship in Nursing*. London: Chapman & Hall.

Faugier, J. and Butterworth, T. (1993) *Clinical Supervision: A Position Paper*. Manchester: University of Manchester.

Finlay, I.G., Bowdler, J.M. and Tebbit, P. (2000) *Are Cancer Pain Guidelines Good Enough? Benchmarking Review of Locally Derived Guidelines on Control of Cancer Pain*. London: National Council for Hospice and Specialist Palliative Care Services.

Galloway, S. and Winfield, G. (2000) Using diaries to identify CPD need. *Nursing Standard*, 14(35): 31–2.

Gilbert, T. (2001) Reflective practice and clinical supervision: meticulous rituals of the confessional. *Journal of Advanced Nursing*, 36(2): 199–205.

Gray, W. (2001) Clinical governance: combining clinical and management supervision. *Nursing Management*, 8(6): 14–22.

Hadfield, N. (2001) The role of aromatherapy massage in reducing anxiety in patients with malignant brain tumours. *International Journal of Palliative Nursing*, 7(6): 279.

Handy, C. (1993) *Understanding Organisations*. London: Penguin.

Harrison, R. (1997) *Employee Development*. London: Institute of Personnel and Development.

Hawkins, P. and Shohet, R. (2000) *Supervision in the Helping Professions*. Buckingham: Open University Press.

Higginson, I. and McCarthy, M. (1989) Measuring symptoms in terminal cancer. *Journal of the Royal Society of Medicine*, 82: 1716.

Hopkins, M. (2000) Wise guides – the roles of supervisors in individual development. Unpublished MBA dissertation, Kingston Business School, Kingston University.

Howell, D. (1999) Reflective practice: advancing quality in palliative nursing care. *International Journal of Palliative Nursing*, 15(5): 212.

Industrial Society (1998) Managing best practice. *Performance Management*, 52: 1–2.

Johns, C. (1994) Clinical notes: nuances on reflection. *Journal of Clinical Nursing*, 3(2): 74.

Johns, C. (1995) Framing learning through reflection within Carper's fundamental ways of knowing in nursing. *Journal of Advanced Nursing*, 22: 226–34.

Johns, C. (2001) Reflective practice: revealing the (he)art of caring. *International Journal of Nursing Practice*, 7(4): 237.

Kohner, N. (1994) *Clinical Supervision in Practice*. London: King's Fund Centre.

Lucas, E. (2000) Coaching and the comfort zone. *Professional Manager*, 9(6): 10–12.

Mayo, A. (1998) *Creating a Training and Development Strategy*. London: Institute of Personnel and Development.

McDonald, J. (2000) Reflection in supervision. *Nursing Times*, 96(9): 49–52.

Mumford, A. (1991) Performance-related skills training, in F. Neale (ed.) *The Handbook of Performance Management*. London: Institute of Personnel Management.

National Council for Hospice and Specialist Palliative Care Services (1997) *Dilemmas and Directions: The Future of Specialist Palliative Care*. London: NCHSPCS.

National Council for Hospice and Specialist Palliative Care Services (2000) *Cost Analysis of Voluntary Hospice and Specialist Palliative Care Services: A User's Manual for the Year 2000/01*. London: NCHSPCS.

Naysmith, A. (2000) Clinical governance (editorial). *Palliative Medicine*, 14(3): 182.

Nevidjon, B. and Erickson, J.I. (2001) The nursing shortage: solutions for the short and long term. *Online Journal of Issues in Nursing*, 6(1): 4.

Olsson, A., Bjorkhem, K. and Hallberg, I. (1998) Systematic clinical supervision of home carers working in the care of demented people who are at home. *Journal of Nursing Management*, 6: 242.

Palmer, A., Burns, S. and Bulman, C. (1994) *Reflective Practice in Nursing: The Growth of the Professional Practitioner*. Oxford: Blackwell Scientific.

Pocock, P. (1991) Introduction, in F. Neale (ed.) *The Handbook of Performance Management*. London: Institute of Personnel Management.

Pringle, M. (1999) The inter-relationship between continuing professional development, clinical governance and revalidation for individual general practitioners. *Journal of Clinical Governance*, 7: 104.

Proctor, B. (1986) Supervision: a co-operative exercise in accountability, in M. Marken and M. Payne (eds) *Enabling and ensuring*. Leicester: National Youth Bureau and Council for Education and Training in Youth and Community Work.

Seymour, J. and Ingleton, C. (1999) Ethical issues in qualitative research at the end of life. *International Journal of Palliative Nursing*, 5(2): 65–6.

Sloan, G. (1999) Understanding clinical supervision from a nursing perspective. *British Journal of Nursing*, 8(8): 524–9.

Solomon, N. (1999) Culture and difference in workplace learning, in D. Boud and J. Garrick (eds) *Understanding Learning at Work*. London: Routledge.

Timpson, J. (1998) The NHS as a learning organisation: aspirations beyond the rainbow? *Journal of Nursing Management*, 6: 261–74.

Todd, G. and Freshwater, D. (1999) Reflective practice and guided discovery: clinical supervision. *British Journal of Nursing*, 8(20): 1383.

United Kingdom Central Council for Nursing and Midwifery (1994) *The Future of Professional Practice*. The Council's Statement for Education and Practice following Registration. London: UKCC.

Vaill, P.B. (1996) *Learning as a Way of Being*. San Francisco, CA: Jossey-Bass.

Conclusion

Sheila Payne, Jane Seymour and Christine Ingleton

In this book, we have explored 'palliative care' from many different perspectives, with a view to providing those who work in the field with a broad and critical understanding of the issues surrounding the care of people facing life-limiting illness and their companions. We now face the task of having to draw some conclusions: a daunting task given the complexity of the material that precedes these final words. We propose to proceed by asking some questions and trying to identify the factors that must be taken into account in moving towards the formulation of the answers to them.

Of course, the first question must be, 'do we know what palliative care is?' In asking this, we have moved full circle, since we set out in the Introduction to define palliative care. We do not intend to repeat that discussion, especially since it is revisited at various points in the book (see Chapters 2 and 3), but rather to tease out some of the tensions and common themes that have emerged. Of these, the most obvious tension is that between 'specialist' and 'general' palliative care. This tension is played out clearly in nursing, where debates seem set to continue about the remit, roles and boundaries of specialist nurses in palliative care, their different levels of specialism and exactly what is the 'added value' of specialist nursing care (see, for example, Corner 2003). As Corner notes, nurses in palliative care prioritize emotional and supportive care in their work and, as we have seen in this book (see Chapter 14), these aspects of care are likely to be highly valued by patients and their companions. However, there is no room for complacency: in spite of arguably widespread awareness of the core goals of palliative care and knowledge about how to reach them, too many nurses find it difficult to balance competing priorities and conflicting demands on their time, and work in poorly resourced organizations where these essential aspects of caring continue to be devalued and poorly articulated. Nor should we be deceived into thinking that 'specialists' in palliative care somehow have a monopoly on the skills and attributes that are required to provide good care to people with palliative care needs. Humility and a willingness to collaborate and learn from others, many of whom are experts and specialists in their own fields, can only enhance the quality of palliative and end-of-life care. O'Brien (2003) cites Kearney, who argued some years ago that, in meeting the broad spectrum of need in palliative care, attitudinal change is as important as attention to resource allocation:

> Patients with incurable illness must no longer be viewed as medical failures for whom nothing more can be done. They need palliative care, which does not mean a handholding second rate option, but treatment that most people will need at some point in their lives, and many from

the time of their diagnosis, demanding as much skill and commitment as is normally brought into preventing, investigating and curing illness.

(Kearney 1991: 170)

The issue of teamwork emerges as a further theme within the book (see Chapter 31). Mount (2003) draws our attention to the two goals of caring in clinical practice: (1) *hippocratic*, in which the controlling of disease from an objective standpoint is paramount; and (2) *askelepian*, in which the caregiver tries to enter the experience of suffering for the patient and his family, and focuses on preparing a space of safety and security for them (Kearney 2000; Mount 2003). With advances in medical technology, the boundaries between palliation and curative treatment are increasingly blurred, and both of these goals may remain intertwined in the care and treatment of patients at the most advanced stages of disease. Without a highly developed sense of teamwork, and in which the patient and his or her family is included as part of the team, the inevitable tensions between these two goals of caring cannot be resolved. Indeed, as Mount (2003) has observed so acutely and with characteristic humour: 'Whole person care requires a caregiver who is whole: until one comes along, use a team!' (p. 42). Teamwork is thus essential to high-quality palliative care. However, as we have seen in this book, a lack of attention to team dynamics means that nurses, doctors and other members of the 'multidisciplinary team' will tend to work in parallel and from their own somewhat insular and well-defended disciplinary perspectives, rather than jointly and from a position of shared understanding about the objectives of care (Corner 2003).

In discussing the problem of teamwork, Corner (2003) develops a taxonomy of cross-disciplinary working in which 'transdisciplinary working' is the ultimate goal. This model of teamwork involves developing a shared conceptual framework and working out together how to address common problems of patient care. In many health care settings, this may seem almost unattainable. Huntington's (1981, 1986) work with social workers and general practitioners demonstrated that difficulties lay within the social structures of the organizations rather than being attributable to individual professionals. So while current rhetoric emphasizes multidisciplinary teamworking, professional groups might seek to sustain power by developing and maintaining occupational cultures that emphasize differences and each profession's 'uniqueness' (Loxley 1997). Problems that need to be addressed to achieve efficient teamworking are: inadequate organizational support; lack of training in teamwork; lack of inter-professional trust; lack of clear goals; lack of continuity among team members; the dominance of particular discourses; and the exclusion of others (Opie and Bernhofen 1997). In addition, interdisciplinary educational initiatives may lessen these divisions and foster greater understanding.

One approach to understanding these common difficulties may be by analysing the complex dynamics of institutional cultures, professional enculturation and territoriality. For example, specialist palliative care providers may have to work across statutory and charitable organizations, across primary, secondary and tertiary health care services, and across health and social care services. Using a specific example from the UK, a community-based clinical nurse specialist providing care to a specific patient and family may have to work with NHS-funded general practitioners, a charitably funded hospice, a cardiologist or oncologist at a local general hospital, a radiologist at a distant regional cancer centre, a local authority-funded occupational therapist (to get adaptation to the home and obtain specialist equipment) and a social work team. The task of coordinating and managing the delivery of appropriate and timely care is formidable. It requires skills in liaison, management, planning and an understanding of how each of these very different organizations and professional groups operate. Analysis of these fundamental aspects of organizational work undertaken by nurses would benefit from further research.

Unlike some texts, in this book we have deliberately set out to highlight palliative care as a key issue for all health and social care professionals and, indeed, for all societies.

In the 2 years or so that it has taken to bring this book to completion, there has been a significant shift in understanding about what palliative care means, with palliative care now conceptualized as a public health issue, as well as a concern of clinical practice. In discussing this trend, Foley (2003) argues that, 'Since dying has a universal incidence, the incidence, *de facto*, makes it a public health concern. Dying is also associated with significant suffering, much of which is preventable' (p. 5). Foley draws attention to significant publications that develop the argument that palliative care should be seen as a public health issue (Bycock 2001; Rao *et al.* 2002; Singer and Bowman 2002). While seeing palliative and end-of-life care in this way is most common in North America, there is evidence of a concern to map out the huge variety of service provision, resources and models of care throughout the developed and developing countries of the world, and to facilitate dialogue about how best to mobilize scare resources in pursuit of better end-of-life care across the globe (Clark and Wright 2003; International Observatory on End of Life Care 2003, www.eolc/observatory.net). Such activity challenges us to look critically at the transferability of the Western model of palliative care and to think about some taken-for-granted assumptions we hold. Most obviously, the possibilities for palliative care must be understood in relation to the demography, epidemiology, politics, social and health care policies, economics and cultures of particular societies. One size certainly does not fit all. Changing patterns of disease and dying are likely to present new challenges not only to the technical aspects of medical and nursing care, but to the organizational aspects of provision.

Thinking of palliative care as a public health issue brings us to a further question that has emerged from the book: 'how is the issue of place of care associated with palliative care?' As well as marked differences between different societies and countries, we have seen throughout the book a concern to identify how 'places' impinge on palliative care and the whole experience of giving and receiving care. The technical and environmental qualities of particular places limit possibilities surrounding 'quality' care and the degree of comfort that may be achieved for a dying person; and different types of place may engender particular types of care practice and interpersonal relationships that influence fundamentally the experience of mortal illness, death and bereavement (Volicer *et al.* 2003). In palliative care, 'home' is often accepted as the ideal place in which to give care to a dying person and for death to occur. However, this assumption is beginning to come under critical review in recognition that this is a culturally contingent preference not necessarily shared by all. For example, in a study of older persons' views about home as a place of care at the end of life, Gott *et al.* (2002) report that older people do not always have access to the material or care resources that make care at home either possible or rewarding and that they worry about the possibility of dying alone, invasion of their privacy by visiting staff, and being a burden to their adult children, spouses and other family members and friends. Of course, places of care do not remain static: ill people move from place to place, often having to travel long distances between these to access the treatment they need. Payne *et al.* (2000) have shown that travel distance, and the difficulty of the journey (for example, whether it means negotiating rush hour traffic or narrow rural roads), causes inconvenience and hardship for many patients and their families.

Persons who give and receive care

In North America and some other Western cultures, personal choice and autonomy are held in high esteem. The cultural value placed on these aspects of personhood fundamentally influence the relationship of individuals to each other, and also their relationship with society as a whole. For example, they underpin different ethical positions in respect of end-of-life choices, the notion of a 'right to die' and euthanasia (see Chapters 19 and 20). Health technologies make possible the re-engineering of death and dying, such as in the use of organ transplantation, implantable defibrillation devices and heart pacemakers. Technological devices such as syringe driver pumps, Percutaneous Endoscopic Gastronomy (PEG) tubes and intravenous infusions make possible the delivery of medication, nutrition and fluids in ways that may sustain life and arguably prolong the dying process. However, to make choices effectively, information needs to be delivered at an appropriate pace and style for each individual (Fallowfield 2001). Who makes choices about how death is managed is also called into question. Perhaps new models of support are required to enable people to make choices for themselves. Finlay (2001) has argued for the use of 'death plans', which are analogous to birth plans in which pregnant women express their preferences about care during childbirth. In North America and elsewhere, advance directives or 'living wills' are starting to become popular. In these documents, people express their preferences for the types of life-sustaining interventions they would wish employed on their behalf, if they were unable to express their views at the time they are needed. While these initiatives are compatible with notions of choice and autonomy, they are based on assumptions that everyone can access and afford a range of high-quality health care and they also assume that choices remain stable – in other words, that people do not change their mind as they adapt to disability. Enshrined in these documents is the right that individuals have to reject or refuse to be cared for. It is this notion that many family members and health professionals find difficult to contemplate.

In this book, we have emphasized the important role played by patients' families, friends, neighbours and other companions (see Chapter 15). We have also argued that the collective term 'carers' may be understood in rather different ways by those supporting a dying person and health and social care workers. Much of the research evidence suggests that their role is largely unrecognized and insufficiently valued by many societies. A greater integration between health and social care than is currently the case in England, for instance, is likely to be required in the future. In the past, carers were predominantly women, either spouses or children of the dying person. Demographic trends with increased longevity, increased marital breakdown, geographical mobility and more dependence upon female income generation are all likely to impact on the availability of women to offer continuing (unpaid) care to family members. We know little about how people without immediate family members manage to make choices about provision of care and place of dying. It is possible that in future palliative care systems need to be seen as a wider approach to building services within communities as part of ensuring greater social cohesion and thereby accessing alternative forms of support rather than merely relying on kinship networks. For example, new communities for older people may be able to offer greater peer support and care. These may become self-help groups for older people, but they are based on the assumption that older people are willing and able to devote time to care-giving activities, which may not be the case.

'So, who will provide care?' This book has predominantly been focused on the activities of nurses, but palliative care services in many countries are heavily reliant on unpaid labour – volunteer workers – who may or may not have professional qualifications. Like carers, the contribution of this group of workers largely goes unresearched and unacknowledged. What evidence there is suggests that the employment of volunteers may be mutually beneficial for organizations and the individuals concerned (Field and Johnson 1993; Field *et al.* 1997; Payne 2002). Volunteer workers have tended to be drawn from middle-aged, middle-class women who have the time, motivation and sufficient economic resources to donate their labour to hospices and specialist palliative care services. Economic pressures to earn more and changing patterns of female employment may mean that new categories of people will need to be recruited or that services will need to employ more paid workers.

In the past, professional health and social care workers were predominantly young people. Large numbers of young (mostly female) school leavers became nurses. These women often had quite limited career options. In many developed countries, educational and employment opportunities have improved considerably for women, which means that nursing has become a less desirable career pathway. This has combined with more limited numbers of young people as a proportion of the total population. The profile of candidates entering nursing in the UK has changed over the past 5–10 years. Several factors are relevant here:

- The drive to raise the academic participation index (API; that percentage of 18- to 21-year-olds who access higher education).

- The introduction of accreditation of prior experiential learning (APEL).

- The drive to recruit more men, mature entrants and members of under-represented groups (for reasons of social justice).

The UK Central Council and, subsequently, the Nursing and Midwifery Council, have widened the entry gate to nursing courses. This has led to the recruitment of more students without 'traditional' educational qualifications. These changes present particular challenges in research-led universities and nurse academics remain concerned about nursing's lack of equal status within the academy (Carlisle *et al.* 1996). Sellers and Deans (1999) report similar concerns about status among nurse academics in Australia. The perceived risk of 'Cinderella' status for nursing in higher education institutions warrants careful deliberation. Nursing is seeking increased status through assimilation into educational institutions, including universities, that have conventionally gained their reputation through valuing and fostering theoretical knowledge rather than practical and interpersonal skills (Miers 2002). Furthermore, successful assimilation will also depend on the widespread acceptance of the importance of the 'better educated nurse'. However, in a study of 34 educational purchasers, Burke and Harrison (2000) report that in the UK there is continued scepticism about an all graduate nursing workforce and reservations that many nursing activities do not require graduate level skills. A more optimistic viewpoint is that a new model of nurse education can emerge and that nurses can take advantage of the cultural changes that are currently occurring within higher education (Miers 2002). Leaders in higher education are grappling with a number of challenges, which are relatively new to some disciplines, including: the development of lifelong, work-based and problem-based learning; the increasing emphasis placed on learning outcomes and transferable skills; the importance of graduate capabilities in terms of employability and core skills; the emphasis on teamwork as a part of these transferable skills; and the value of critical reflection as a means of acquiring these skills. These are not new concepts to many nurses. As we have seen in Part Four, nurses have played a prominent role in the development and application of many of these educational innovations. Arguably, nursing is now well placed to take a lead role in shaping these changes and take a lead on professional development within higher education.

Equity in palliative and end-of-life care

In many ways, palliative care can be regarded as a success story. As Chapter 2 illustrates, the ideas underpinning palliative care have spread around the world in a relatively short time. In our view, one of the major challenges for the future is to improve equity of access to good quality care during the end-of-life period. It is likely that advances in medicine and health technologies will mean that greater numbers of people will survive for longer with complex health and social care needs. Formerly acute diseases may become chronic diseases. This is likely to be combined with people experiencing greater numbers of co-morbidities, especially older people. The science of palliative medicine and palliative care nursing is going to be challenged by the management of highly complex symptomatology of multiple diseases. This may mean a different type of workforce is required in specialist palliative care. For example, one scenario might be that specialist professionals become advisers and consultants (on pain and symptom control) to generalists who actually deliver care in their usual health care environments. Greater prominence might be given to other team members such as counsellors, therapists, spiritual experts, nutritionists and psychologists, as their skills become better recognized and are more often demanded by patients and their families who wish to have a 'total package' of end-of-life care. From a public health perspective, it is no longer acceptable that people dying of diseases other than cancer are discriminated against. This may mean a breakdown in existing specialisms. As specialist palliative care is so closely identified with cancer care, it may threaten its existence as a separate specialty.

We believe that consumerism and the blurring of knowledge boundaries between professionals and the public who now have greater access to information, such as the internet (see Chapter 34), may influence issues of access and demands for improvement in end-of-life care. However, this is likely in our view to differentially advantage those with the knowledge, education and power to demand access to specialist palliative care. There are concerns that this will create greater divergence between those who have the skills to use health and social care systems and those who remain socially excluded. There is a danger that disease category, culture, ethnicity, social class and geographical location will remain the key drivers determining access rather than burden of illness. Nurses could have an important role in ensuring greater equity of access to end-of-life care, but they will have to be prepared to become more politically and socially assertive than they have generally been in the past. Whatever the configuration of services or the diversity of diseases, people will die and nurses are likely to have a central role in caring for them. As nurses, we are privileged to witness part of our common humanity – death. Palliative care belongs to everyone and, arguably, is a basic right for all those in need according to what it is possible to provide within societal constraints.

References

Burke, L.M. and Harrison, D. (2000) Education purchasers' views of nursing as an all graduate profession. *Nurse Education Today*, 20(8): 620–8.

Bycock, I.R. (2001) End of life care: a public health crisis and an opportunity for managed care. *American Journal of Managed Care*, 7: 1123–32.

Carlisle, C., Kirk, S. and Luker, K. (1996) The changes in the role of the nurse teacher following the formation of links with higher education. *Journal of Advanced Nursing*, 24(4): 762–70.

Clark, D. and Wright, M. (2003) *Transition in End of Life Care: Hospice and Related Developments in Eastern Europe and Central Asia*. Buckingham: Open University Press.

Corner, J. (2003) Nursing management in palliative care. *European Journal of Oncology Nursing*, 7(2): 83–90.

Fallowfield, L. (2001) Participation of patients in decisions about treatment for cancer (editorial). *British Medical Journal*, 323: 1144.

Field, D. and Johnson, I. (1993) Satisfaction and change: a survey of volunteers in a hospice organisation. *Social Science and Medicine*, 36(12): 1625–33.

Field, D., Ingleton, C. and Clark, D. (1997) The costs of unpaid labour: the use of voluntary staff in the King's Mill Hospice. *Health and Social Care in the Community*, 5(3): 198–208.

Finlay, I. (2001) Death plans (editorial). *Palliative Medicine*, 15: 179–80.

Foley, K.M. (2003) How much palliative care do we need? *European Journal of Palliative Care*, 10(2): 5–7.

Gott, M., Seymour, J.E., Bellamy, G., Clark, D. and Ahmedzai, S.H. (2002) Older people's reflections on home as a place of care during dying. *European Journal of Palliative Care*.

Huntington, J. (1981) *Social Work and General Medical Practice*. London: George Allen & Unwin.

Huntington, J. (1986) The proper contributions of social workers in health practice. *Social Science and Medicine*, 22: 1151–60.

Kearney, M. (1991) Palliative care in Ireland. *Irish College of Physicians and Surgeons*, 20(3): 170.

Kearney, M. (2000) *A Place of Healing: Working with Suffering in Living and Dying*. Oxford: Oxford University Press.

Loxley, A. (1997) *Collaboration in Health and Welfare*. London: Jessica Kingsley.

Miers, M. (2002) Nurse education in higher education: understanding cultural barriers to progress. *Nurse Education Today*, 22: 212–19.

Mount, B.M. (2003) Existential suffering and the determinants of healing. *European Journal of Palliative Care*, 10(suppl.): 40–2.

O'Brien, T. (2003) Response to Kathy Foley. *European Journal of Palliative Care*, 10(suppl.): 7–8.

Opie, A. and Bernhofen, D.M. (1997) Thinking teams and thinking clients: issues of discourse and representation in the work of health care teams. *Sociology of Health and Illness*, 19(3): 259–80.

Payne, S. (2002) Dilemmas in the use of volunteers to provide hospice bereavement support: evidence from New Zealand. *Mortality*, 7(2): 139–54.

Payne, S., Jarrett, N. and Jeffs, D. (2000) The impact of travel on cancer patients' experiences of treatment: a literature review. *European Journal of Cancer Care*, 9: 197–203.

Rao, J.K., Anderson, L.A. and Smith, S.M. (2002) End of life is a public health issue. *American Journal of Preventive Medicine*, 23(3): 215–20.

Sellers, E.T. and Deans, C. (1999) Nurse education in Australian universities in a period of change: expectations of nurse academics for the year 2005. *Nurse Education Today*, 19(1): 53–61.

Singer, P.A. and Bowman, K. (2002) Quality end of life care: a global perspective. *BMC Palliative Care*, 1(1): 4.

Volicer, L., Hurley, A.C. and Blasi, Z.V. (2003) Characteristics of dementia end of life care across care settings. *American Journal of Hospice and Palliative Care*, 20(3): 191–200.

Name index

Page numbers in *italics* refer to figures, tables and boxes.

Subject index

Page numbers in *italics* refer to figures, tables and boxes. Those in **bold** indicate main discussion.

THINKING NURSING

Tom Mason and Elizabeth Whitehead

- Important new nursing theory textbook

This major new text seeks to provide nursing students with an accessible overview of the theory which informs the application of nursing activity. The key disciplines that contribute to the nursing curriculum – such as sociology, psychology, public health, economic science and politics – are comprehensively discussed, with each chapter offering both a theoretical discussion and a section showing how the topic in question applies to nursing practice. Particular attention has been paid to pedagogy with brief boxed case studies, chapter summaries, glossaries of key words and further reading lists enabling easy use by students.

Contents:

Introduction – Thinking Sociology – Thinking Psychology – Thinking Anthropology – Thinking Public Health – Thinking Philosophy – Thinking Economics – Thinking Politics – Thinking Science – Thinking Writing – Conclusions – References – Index.

432pp   0 335 21040 6 (Paperback)   0 335 21041 4 (Hardback)

COUNSELLING SKILLS FOR NURSES, MIDWIVES AND HEALTH VISITORS

Dawn Freshwater

Counselling is a diverse activity and there are an increasing number of people who find themselves using counselling skills, not least those in the caring professions. There is a great deal of scope in using counselling skills to promote health in the everyday encounters that nurses have with their patients. The emphasis on care in the community and empowerment of patients through consumer involvement means that nurses are engaged in providing support and help to people to change behaviours.

Community nurses often find themselves in situations that require in-depth listening and responding skills: for example, in helping people come to terms with chronic illness, disability and bereavement. Midwives are usually the first port of call for those parents who have experienced miscarriages, bereavements, or are coping with decisions involving the potential for genetic abnormalities. Similarly, health visitors are in a valuable position to provide counselling regarding the immunization and health of the young infant. These practitioners have to cope not only with new and diverse illnesses, for example HIV and AIDS, but also with such policy initiatives as the National Service Framework for Mental Health and their implications.

This book examines contemporary developments in nursing and health care in relation to the fundamental philosophy of counselling, the practicalities of counselling and relevant theoretical underpinnings. Whilst the text is predominantly aimed at nurses, midwives and health visitors, it will also be of interest to those professionals allied to medicine, for example physiotherapists, occupational therapists and dieticians.

Contents
Introduction – The process of counselling – Beginning a relationship – Sustaining the relationship – Facilitating change – Professional considerations – Caring for the carer – Appendix: Useful information – References – Index.

128pp   0 335 20781 2 (Paperback)   0 335 20782 0 (Hardback)

COMMUNITY MENTAL HEALTH NURSING AND DEMENTIA CARE
PRACTICE PERSPECTIVES

John Keady, Charlotte L. Clarke and Trevor Adams (eds)

A rounded account of Community Mental Health Nurses' practice in dementia care has been long overdue. This is the first book to focus on the role of Community Mental Health Nurses in their highly valued work with both people with dementia and their families.

This book:

- Explores the complexity and diversity of Community Mental Health Nurse work
- Captures perspectives from along the trajectory of dementia
- Identifies assessment and intervention approaches
- Discusses an emerging evidence base for implications in practice

Contributions to this collection of essays and articles are drawn from Community Mental Health Nurse practitioners and researchers at the forefront of their fields.

It is key reading for practitioners, researchers, students, managers and policy makers in the field of community mental health nursing and/or dementia care.

Contents
Contributors – Acknowledgements – Editorial note – Foreword by Professor Mike Nolan – Introduction – Part One: Setting the scene: the landscape of contemporary community mental health nursing practice in dementia care – Voices from the past: the historical alignment of dementia care to nursing – Integrating practice and knowledge in a clinical context – Multidisciplinary teamworking – "We put our heads together" – Risk and dementia – Part Two: Dementia care nursing in the community: assessment and practice approaches – Assessment and therapeutic approaches for community mental health nursing dementia care practice – Cognitive-behavioural interventions in dementia – Turning rhetoric into reality – From screening to intervention – The community mental health nurse role in sharing a diagnosis of dementia – Group therapy – Psychosocial interventions with family carers of people with dementia – Admiral nurses – Normalization as a philosophy of dementia care – Assessing and responding to challenging behaviour in dementia – Part Three: Leading and developing community mental health nursing in dementia – Clinical supervision and dementia care – Multi-agency and inter-agency working – Higher level practice – Index.

Contributors
Trevor Adams, Peter Ashton, Gill Boardman, Angela Carradice, Chris Clark, Charlotte L. Clarke, Jan Dewing, Sue Hahn, Mark Holman, John Keady, Kath Lowery, Jill Manthorpe, Anne Mason, Cathy Mawhinney, Paul McCloskey, Anne McKinley, Linda Miller, Gordon Mitchell, Elinor Moore, Michelle Murray, Mike Nolan, Peter Nolan, Tracy Packer, Sean Page, Marilla Pugh, Helen Pusey, Assumpta Ryan, Alison Soliman, Vicki Traynor, Dot Weaks, Heather Wilkinson

306pp   0 335 21142 9 (Paperback)   0 335 21143 7 (Hardback)

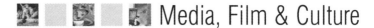
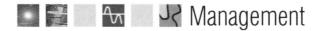

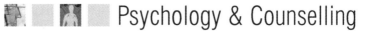
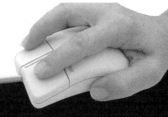